PEDIATRICS

A PRIMARY CARE

APPROACH

SAUNDERS TEXT AND REVIEW SERIES

PEDIATRICS

A PRIMARY CARE

APPROACH

CAROL D. BERKOWITZ, M.D.

Professor of Clinical Pediatrics
University of California Los Angeles School of Medicine
Los Angeles, California

Associate Chair and Program Director
Department of Pediatrics
Harbor-UCLA Medical Center
Torrance, California

W.B. SAUNDERS COMPANY
A Division of Harcourt Brace & Company
Philadelphia London Toronto Montreal Sydney Tokyo

W.B. SAUNDERS COMPANY
A Division of Harcourt Brace & Company

The Curtis Center
Independence Square West
Philadelphia, Pennsylvania 19106

Library of Congress Cataloging-in-Publication Data

Berkowitz, Carol D.
    Pediatrics: a primary care approach / Carol D. Berkowitz.—1st
ed.

        p.   cm.

    ISBN 0-7216-5623-4

    1. Pediatrics.   I. Title.
    [DNLM: 1. Pediatrics.   2. Primary Health Care.   WS 100 B513p
1996]
    RJ45.B43   1996   618.92—dc20
    DNLM/DLC   95-23414

Pediatrics: A Primary Care Approach   ISBN 0-7216-5623-4

Printed in the United States of America.

Last digit is the print number: 9   8   7   6   5   4   3   2   1

PREFACE

This book provides the reader with a logical and practical approach to the longitudinal care of children, discussing many of the common problems, both medical and psychosocial, that occur from infancy through adolescence. Emphasizing health maintenance and anticipatory guidance, the authors go beyond the traditional disease approach, which often frustrates clinicians who treat children according to symptoms and not diagnoses.

The authors wish to acknowledge the support, patience, and humor of their spouses and families. Likewise, the authors wish to thank their patients and their families for the knowledge and experience they provided. This book could not have been accomplished without the coordination and secretarial services of Sally Montoya. The authors are also most appreciative of the assistance of the staff at W.B. Saunders, in particular, William Schmitt and Anne-Marie Shaw, and of Martha Cushman.

CAROL D. BERKOWITZ

CONTRIBUTORS

SUDHIR K. ANAND, M.D.
Professor of Pediatrics, Charles R. Drew University of Sciences and Medicine, Los Angeles, California; Professor of Clinical Pediatrics, University of California Los Angeles School of Medicine, Los Angeles, California; Head of Pediatric Nephrology, King/Drew Medical Center, Los Angeles, California and Harbor–UCLA Medical Center, Los Angeles, California
Acute Renal Failure; Hypertension; Urinary Tract Infection

JILL M. BAREN, M.D.
Assistant Professor of Surgery and Pediatrics, Section of Emergency Medicine, Yale University School of Medicine, New Haven, Connecticut; Attending Physician, Emergency Department, Yale New Haven Hospital, New Haven, Connecticut
Approach to the Traumatized Child; Abdominal Trauma; Head Trauma

CAROL D. BERKOWITZ, M.D.
Professor of Clinical Pediatrics, University of California Los Angeles School of Medicine, Los Angeles, California; Associate Chair and Program Director, Harbor–UCLA Medical Center, Torrance, California
Caring for Twins; Circumcision; Sibling Rivalry; Toilet Training; Discipline; Fears and Phobias; Thumb Sucking and Other Habits; Enuresis; Encopresis; SIDS and Apnea; Craniofacial Anomalies; Vomiting; Diarrhea; Constipation; Abdominal Pain; Jaundice; Papulosquamous Eruptions; Maculopapular Rashes; Physical Abuse; Child Sexual Abuse; Failure to Thrive; Infants of Substance-Abusing Mothers; Divorce; Violence; Pediatric HIV

IRIS WAGMAN BOROWSKY, M.D., Ph.D.
Assistant Professor of Pediatrics, Division of General Pediatrics and Adolescent Health, University of Minnesota, Minneapolis, Minnesota; General Practitioner, University of Minnesota Hospital, Minneapolis, Minnesota
Telephone Management; Gifted Children; Injury Prevention; Attention Deficit/Hyperactivity Disorder

PAMELA S. COHEN, M.D.
Adjunct Member, Picower Institute, Manhasset, New York; Assistant Professor of Pediatrics, Division of Pediatric Hematology-Oncology, North Shore University Hospital, Manhasset, New York
Anemia; Bleeding Disorders; Lymphadenopathy; Cancer in Children

CARLO DI LORENZO, M.D.
Associate Professor of Pediatrics, University of Pittsburgh, Pittsburgh, Pennsylvania; Attending Staff, Children's Hospital of Pittsburgh, Pittsburgh, Pennsylvania
Gastroesophageal Reflux; Gastrointestinal Bleeding

ROBIN WINKLER DOROSHOW, M.D.
Professor of Pediatrics, University of California Los Angeles School of Medicine, Los Angeles, California; Associate Director, Pediatric Cardiology, Harbor–UCLA Medical Center, Torrance, California
Heart Murmurs; Cyanosis in the Newborn; Congestive Heart Failure

HELEN DUPLESSIS, M.D., M.P.H.
Assistant Professor, Department of Pediatrics, University of California Los Angeles School of Medicine, Los Angeles, California, and Harbor–UCLA Medical Center, Torrance, California; Director, Community Pediatrics, Harbor–UCLA Medical Center, Torrance, California
Diabetes Mellitus; Chronic Lung Disease; Osteomyelitis; Juvenile Rheumatoid Arthritis

GEETA GROVER, M.D.
Medical Education Coordinator, Ambulatory Care Services, Children's Hospital of Orange County, Orange, California
Talking to Parents; Talking to Children; Nutritional Needs; Sleep: Normal Patterns and Common Disorders; Dental Care; Normal Development and Developmental Assessment; Language Development: Speech and Hearing Assessment; Immunizations; Crying and Colic; Temper Tantrums; Breath-Holding Spells; Fever and Bacteremia; Common Oral Lesions; Strabismus; Infections of the Eye; Excessive Tearing; Developmental Hip Dysplasia; Rotational Problems of the Lower Extremity: In-Toeing and Out-Toeing; Angular Deformities of the Lower Extremity: Bow Legs and Knock Knees; Orthopedic Injuries and Growing Pains; Evaluation of Limp; Disorders of the Spine; Disorders of the Hair and Scalp; Diaper Dermatitis

KENNETH R. HUFF, M.D.
Assistant Professor of Pediatrics and Neurology, University of California, Los Angeles, Los Angeles, California; Chief, Division of Neurology, Department of Pediatrics, Harbor–UCLA Medical Center, Torrance, California
Febrile Seizures; Increased Intracranial Pressure; Hypotonia; Headaches; Tics; Seizures and Epilepsy

STANLEY H. INKELIS, M.D.
Professor of Pediatrics, University of California Los Angeles School of Medicine, Los Angeles, California; Director, Pediatric Emergency Medicine, Harbor–UCLA Medical Center, Torrance, California
Sore Throat; Nosebleeds; Neck Masses

ELAINE KAMIL, M.D.
Associate Professor of Pediatrics, University of California Los Angeles School of Medicine, Los Angeles, California; Associate Director, Pediatric Nephrology and Transplant Immunology, Cedars-Sinai Medical Center, Los Angeles, California
Hematuria; Proteinuria; Nephrotic Syndrome

JULIE E. NOBLE, M.D.
Associate Clinical Professor of Pediatrics, Harbor–UCLA Medical Center, Torrance, California
Primary Care: Introduction; Allergic Disease; Cough

ISIDRO B. SALUSKY, M.D.
Professor of Pediatrics, University of California Los Angeles School of Medicine, Division of Pediatric Nephrology, Los Angeles, California; Director, Pediatric Dialysis Program, Director, General Clinical Research Center, University of California Los Angeles School of Medicine, Los Angeles, California
Chronic Renal Failure

CHERYL P. SANCHEZ, M.D.
Clinical Instructor of Pediatrics, Division of Pediatric Nephrology, University of California Los Angeles School of Medicine, Los Angeles, California
Chronic Renal Failure

JAMES S. SEIDEL, M.D., Ph.D.
Professor of Pediatrics, University of California Los Angeles School of Medicine, Los Angeles, California; Chief, Division of General and Emergency Pediatrics, Harbor–UCLA Medical Center, Torrance, California
Respiratory Distress; Stridor and Croup; Wheezing and Asthma

MONICA SIFUENTES, M.D.
Assistant Clinical Professor of Pediatrics, University of California Los Angeles School of Medicine, Los Angeles, California; Assistant Program Director, Harbor–UCLA Medical Center, Torrance, California
Talking to Adolescents; Screening in Newborns; Screening in Older Children and Adolescents; Neonatal Examination and Nursery Visit; Well Child Care for Children with Trisomy 21; Well Child Care for Preterm Infants; Needs of Children with Physical and Sensory Handicaps; Reproductive Health; Fostering Self-Esteem; Vesicular Exanthems; Substance Abuse; Eating Disorders; Adolescent Depression and Suicide; Otitis Media; Hearing Impairments; Ambiguous Genitalia; Vaginitis; Sexually Transmitted Diseases; Menstrual Disorders; Orthopedic Complaints; Hepatitis; Acne

ERIC VASILIQUSKAS, M.D.
Clinical Instructor, Department of Pediatrics, University of California Los Angeles School of Medicine, Los Angeles, California; Clinical Research Fellow, Inflammatory Bowel Disease Center, Cedars-Sinai Medical Center, Los Angeles, California
Gastrointestinal Bleeding

CONTENTS

CHAPTER FIFTEEN

CHAPTER SIXTEEN

CHAPTER SEVENTEEN

CHAPTER EIGHTEEN

CHAPTER NINETEEN

CHAPTER TWENTY

CHAPTER TWENTY-ONE

CHAPTER TWENTY-TWO

CHAPTER TWENTY-THREE

CHAPTER TWENTY-FOUR

CHAPTER TWENTY-FIVE

CHAPTER TWENTY-SIX

CHAPTER TWENTY-SEVEN

CHAPTER TWENTY-EIGHT

CHAPTER TWENTY-NINE

CHAPTER THIRTY

CHAPTER THIRTY-ONE

CHAPTER THIRTY-TWO

CHAPTER THIRTY-THREE

SECTION III

ACUTE AND EMERGENT PROBLEMS

CHAPTER FIFTY-TWO

CHAPTER FIFTY-THREE

CHAPTER FIFTY-FOUR

CHAPTER FIFTY-FIVE

CHAPTER FIFTY-SIX

SECTION V

HEMATOLOGIC DISORDERS

CHAPTER FIFTY-SEVEN

CHAPTER FIFTY-EIGHT

CHAPTER FIFTY-NINE

SECTION VIII

ORTHOPEDIC DISORDERS

CHAPTER EIGHTY-FIVE

SECTION X

NEUROLOGIC DISORDERS

CHAPTER EIGHTY-SIX

CHAPTER EIGHTY-SEVEN

CHAPTER EIGHTY-EIGHT

SECTION XI

DERMATOLOGIC DISORDERS

CHAPTER EIGHTY-NINE

CHAPTER NINETY

CHAPTER NINETY-ONE

SECTION XII

THE NEW MORBIDITY

CHAPTER ONE HUNDRED

CHAPTER ONE HUNDRED ONE

CHAPTER ONE HUNDRED TWO

CHAPTER ONE HUNDRED THREE

CHAPTER ONE HUNDRED FOUR

SECTION XIII

Chronic Diseases Of Childhood And Adolescence

CHAPTER ONE HUNDRED FIVE

CHAPTER ONE HUNDRED SIX

CHAPTER ONE HUNDRED SEVEN

CHAPTER ONE HUNDRED EIGHT

CHAPTER ONE HUNDRED NINE

CHAPTER ONE HUNDRED TEN

CHAPTER ONE HUNDRED ELEVEN

CHAPTER ONE HUNDRED TWELVE

CHAPTER ONE HUNDRED THIRTEEN

SECTION I

PRIMARY CARE: SKILLS AND CONCEPTS

CHAPTER 1

PRIMARY CARE: INTRODUCTION

Julie E. Noble, M.D.

Primary care is defined as the comprehensive health care that patients receive from the same health care provider over a longitudinal period of time. The term was first used in the 1960s in response to the abundance of subspecialists and lack of generalists among practicing physicians. It is generally accepted that primary care physicians include pediatricians, family physicians, and internists. In 1966 the Millis Committee Report to the AMA on graduate medical education recognized the importance of primary care and recommended a national commitment to educating primary care physicians. Primary care was further defined in 1974 by Charney and Alpert, who separated it into component parts: first contact, longitudinal care, family orientation, and integration of comprehensive care. In order to understand the depth of primary care, the component parts should be explored.

First contact occurs when a patient arrives for medical care at the office of a primary care physician. The visit includes an intake history, complete physical examination, and an assessment of problems with treatment (if indicated). Of great importance is the establishment of the physician-patient relationship. Physicians become the primary medical resource and counselors to these patients and their families and the first contacts when successive medical problems arise.

Longitudinal care, the second component of primary care, implies continuity of care over a period of time. Physicians assume responsibility for issues concerning both health and illness. In pediatrics, such care involves monitoring growth and development, following school progress, screening for commonly found disorders, making psychosocial assessments, promoting health, and preventing illness with immunization and safety counseling programs.

Family orientation is the third component of primary care. Patients must be viewed in the context of their

environment and family. Otherwise, practitioners cannot adequately care for patients. In pediatrics, a child's problems become the family's, and the family's problems become the child's. This has become increasingly apparent with the emergence of problems of poverty, drug use, HIV exposure, teenage pregnancy, and gang involvement that have overtaken the pediatric population. The psychosocial forces in a particular child's life are intricately interwoven, and their assessment is an essential component of the primary care of that child.

As pediatric medical problems become more complex, many health and educational resources may be utilized to supplement care. Primary care physicians integrate and coordinate these services in the best interest of patients, thus providing **integration of comprehensive care,** the fourth component of primary care. Working with social service agencies, home care providers, educational agencies, and government agencies, physicians can use multiple resources for the benefit of patients. Understanding the resources of the community is an important part of a primary physician's education.

When patients select a primary care provider, they have identified a medical "home." That home incorporates the physical, psychological, and social aspects of individual patients into comprehensive health care services, thus meeting the needs of the whole person. To make that home work for patients, geographic and financial accessibility are key elements. The most important aspect of a home is that it is a place where patients feel "cared for."

SUBSPECIALIST CARE

Medical knowledge and technology have made amazing advancements in the past several decades. Total

1

knowledge of all fields is impossible for individual physicians. As a result, the role of the subspecialist physician has developed as an adjunct to that of the primary care physician. Primary care physicians seek subspecialist consultation when the suspected or known disease process is unusual or complicated, when it demands specialized technology, or when they have little experience with the disease. Generally, subspecialists evaluate patients and concentrate on the organ system or disease process in their area of expertise.

Primary care physicians can use a subspecialist for either a consultation or referral. When initiating a consultation, primary physicians send patients for advice. Consulting physicians assess the patients with a history and physical examination, focusing on their specialty. They then recommend possible additional laboratory tests, offer a diagnosis and treatment plan, and send the patients back to their primary care physicians for coordination of further care.

Use of the subspecialist is termed **secondary care.** For example, an eight-year-old girl with weight loss and persistent abdominal pain has an upper GI x-ray series that reveals a duodenal ulcer. She is sent by her primary care physician to a pediatric gastroenterologist for **consultation,** with a request for an endoscopy to allow definitive diagnosis and up-to-date management guidelines. The girl then returns to the primary care physician with recommendations for treatment and further care.

Primary care physicians can also generate a referral to a subspecialist, which differs from a consultation. A **referral** requests that the subspecialist assume complete care of the patient. This transfer of a patient to a tertiary care site establishes a subspecialist as the coordinator of further health care for the patient. For example, a four-year-old boy with recurrent fevers, hepatosplenomegaly, and blasts on peripheral blood smear is referred to a pediatric oncologist for diagnosis, the latest treatment, and ongoing medical care.

When requesting advice from subspecialists, whether on a consultative or referral basis, primary care physicians should outline specific questions with a probable diagnosis to be addressed by the subspecialist. For example, a consultation requesting evaluation of a child with hematuria is inappropriate. The primary care physician should perform a basic diagnostic evaluation and should make the most likely diagnosis. The child can then be referred appropriately. A child diagnosed with nephritis should be sent to a pediatric nephrologist, whereas a child diagnosed with Wilms' tumor should be sent to a pediatric oncologist.

When primary care physicians and subspecialists function cooperatively and offer the three levels of care (primary, referral, and consultative), patients receive the highest quality medical care. However, the number of generalist physicians has declined over the last several decades as the number of subspecialist physicians has risen excessively. This imbalance of physician supply has resulted in a decreased accessibility to primary medical care by underserved populations and an overuse of subspecialists by patients. In general, care provided by subspecialists is characterized as being more expensive and procedure-driven. Labora-

tory studies are ordered with increased frequency by subspecialists, further inflating the cost of medical care. If patients have no longitudinal health care and see multiple providers, repeat laboratory studies are often ordered. Primary care is believed to deliver more cost-effective, improved medical care. With the spiraling cost of medical care, there is currently a nationwide movement to produce more primary care physicians.

LABORATORY TESTS

For most conditions, studies have shown that the diagnosis is revealed by the history and physical examination in over 95% of cases. Thus good communication skills are a basic tenet of primary care. Patients' complaints often concern unnecessary laboratory tests, which increase the cost of medical care and the prescription of unnecessary medications. To lessen these problems, the primary care physician should use laboraratory tests and medications discriminately, recognizing their value as well as their potential iatrogenic effects.

In primary care, laboratory tests should be used to help confirm a condition suspected on the basis of the history or physical examination or diagnose a condition that may not be apparent after a thorough history and physical assessment. In pediatrics, especially, the value of each test result should be weighed against the inconvenience, discomfort, and possible side effects in children. Tests can be used as screening tools to prevent disease or to identify a disease early so that treatment can begin and symptoms can be minimized. Laboratory studies can provide a variety of other information, including data to establish a diagnosis, knowledge necessary to select therapy or to monitor a disease, and information about the risk of future disease. Organ function, metabolic activity, and nutritional status can also be assessed, and evidence of neoplastic or infectious disease can be provided. In addition, laboratory studies can be used to identify infectious and therapeutic agents or poisons.

Screening laboratory tests are used when the incidence of an unsuspected condition is high enough in a general population to justify the expense of the test. (See Chapter 6, Screening in Newborns.) Subclinical conditions such as anemia, lead poisoning, and hypercholesterolemia are part of some health maintenance assessments.

Physicians must remember that there is variability in test results and that laboratory error can occur. Laboratory results should always be viewed in the context of the patient. The sensitivity of a test, the ability of the test to detect low levels, and the specificity of a test for the substance being measured must also be considered by the physician when evaluating a test result.

COST CONTAINMENT

In recent years, cost containment for medical care has become a primary economic concern in the United States. Health care costs are increasing at rates well above inflation. Currently there is a national movement to decrease the financial burden of the cost of medical care. Traditional medicine has operated on a fee-for-service basis; that is, if a physician saw a patient, the physician would be reimbursed for services provided. Some have suggested that this plan has given physicians a financial incentive to generate more services and see patients more than is necessary.

Many alternative ways to run the business of medicine are being explored. One of the more popular alternatives is **managed care,** which replaces traditional insurance programs with a system that integrates financing with appropriate case-managed health care for its enrollees. It relies on a monthly capitation fee for each enrollee in the plan, which contracts with selected physicians and hospitals to furnish comprehensive health services. Cost containment depends on control of services provided. That control is provided through physician selection, financial incentives for physicians, and monitoring and utilization review of services provided. Preventive health issues and patient education are important services that keep the enrolled population healthy. Each member of the managed care organization is supplied with a primary care physician to ensure comprehensive longitudinal care. This physician serves as a gatekeeper for initial contact, restricting subspecialist referrals to only appropriate cases. Each member also has a case manager, who may be the physician or a nurse, to coordinate services and provide individual patients with a health care plan.

Managed care organizations vary in structure. The managed care organizations may be **health maintenance organizations (HMOs),** groups that offer coverage of health services for a fixed premium either from a group, network, or staff model, or **individual practice associations (IPAs),** which contract with physicians who provide health care from their offices. Managed care plans may also be **preferred provider organizations (PPOs),** where the program contracts with providers for services, usually on a discounted fee-for-service basis. These organizations will prosper if they manage to restrict services to their members. It is hoped that the patients' best interests will be the cornerstone for decisions regarding patient care.

Utilization review, the review of the appropriateness of health care services, and the development of management outlines for physicians to decrease variability and cost in disease treatment are essential elements of managed health care. These elements impose greater control over physicians as they decide medical management of individual cases.

Goals of managed care include not only cost containment but the reduction of fragmented and duplicative care for patients. Currently many patients see several different providers for the same illness and inappropriately utilize the emergency room for minor illnesses. A designated primary care physician should eliminate these problems. In the past decade enrollment in HMOs in the United States has more than tripled. No data clearly indicate whether managed care is resulting in medical cost savings, however, and it remains to be seen whether managed care is the answer for the health care crisis in the United States.

The issue of cost containment has also spawned additional movements toward shorter hospital stays and outpatient management of diseases that used to be treated in the hospital. Improved technology now allows many surgical conditions that a few years ago required hospital stays of several days to be performed on an outpatient basis, with the patient discharged hours after the procedure. Gallbadder surgery is an example of this new management. Other conditions, such as sepsis and treatment of osteomyelitis, have also moved to the outpatient arena as treatments have advanced. The development of oral rehydration therapy now allows patients with dehydration to be treated as outpatients, without intravenous therapy, eliminating the possible complications associated with intravenous access. Even respirator care in chronically ill patients can be done in the home setting. Medical advances are increasing the value of outpatient care and the importance of primary care physicians in supplying and coordinating care.

This book is designed to be a practical guide to help most primary care physicians treat and manage common pediatric problems, both medical and biosocial. It is not a comprehensive treatise on all pediatric conditions. In large part the book has been divided into chapters by symptom or complaint rather than by disease because most patients in primary care usually present with a symptom. The authors hope that this book makes caring for children easier.

Selected Readings

American Association of Medical Colleges. Policy on the generalist physician. Academic Medicine 68:1–6, 1993.

Alpert, J. J. Primary care: the future for pediatric education. Pediatrics 86:653–659, 1990.

Blin, R. D., and N. M. Matlin. Health care systems: a pediatric perspective. Pediatr. Rev. 9:5–10, 1987.

Iglehart, J. K. The American health care system: managed care. N. Engl. J. Med. 327:742–747, 1992.

Noe, D. A., and R. C. Rock. Laboratory Medicine: The Selection and Interpretation of Clinical Laboratory Studies. Baltimore, Williams & Wilkins, 1994.

Sia, C. C. J. The medical home: pediatric practice and child advocacy in the 1990s. Pediatrics 90:419–423, 1992.

Starfield, B. Primary Care. Concept, Evaluation, and Policy. New York, Oxford University Press, 1992.

CHAPTER 2

TALKING TO PARENTS

Geeta Grover, M.D.

H$_x$ An eight-month-old boy with a one-week history of cough and runny nose and a two-day history of vomiting, diarrhea, and fever, with temperature of 101° F (38.3° C), is evaluated in the emergency department. The mother is very concerned because her son's appetite has decreased and he has been waking up several times at night for the last two days.

A nurse interrupts and says that paramedics are bringing a five-year-old trauma victim to the emergency department. The appearance of the eight-month-old child is quickly assessed; he seems active and alert. Bilateral otitis media is diagnosed. Before leaving the examination room the physician says to the mother: "Your son has a viral syndrome and infection in his ears. I am going to prescribe an antibiotic that you can begin giving him today. Give him Tylenol as needed for the fever. Don't worry about his vomiting and diarrhea; just make sure that he drinks plenty of liquids and don't give him milk or milk products for a few days. Bring him back here or to his regular doctor if his fever persists, he doesn't eat, he has too much vomiting or diarrhea, he looks lethargic, or if he isn't better in two days."

Questions

1. Did this mother receive more information than she can be reasonably expected to remember?
2. Did the physician address the mother's concerns sufficiently?
3. Was the mother given a chance to acknowledge that she had understood the diagnosis and treatment plan?
4. What are some barriers to effective doctor-patient communication?
5. How does the setting itself influence communication?

Effective communication in the pediatric setting involves the exchange of information between physicians, parents, and children. In addition, observing the interaction between parents and children gives physicians an opportunity to assess parenting skills and the dynamics of the parent-child relationship. The communication needs of both parents and children are quite different; this makes the exchange of information challenging. Parental concerns should be addressed in a sensitive, empathetic, and nonjudgmental manner. A nonthreatening, pleasant demeanor and age-appropriate language help facilitate communication with children (see Chapter 3, Talking to Children).

Pediatrics encompasses not only the traditional medical model of diagnosis and treatment of disease but also maintenance of the health and well-being of children through longitudinal care and the establishment of ongoing relationships between physicians and families. Personal relationships between physicians and families create an atmosphere in which information can be exchanged openly. The pediatrician's role in such relationships is to not only diagnose and treat, but also to listen, advise, guide, and teach.

The doctor-patient relationship is truly a privilege. Mutual respect is essential for the development of a healthy relationship between physicians, parents, and children. Through practice and continued awareness of interpersonal abilities, physicians can develop good communication skills. All physicians eventually develop their own personal interviewing and examination style. What seems awkward and difficult at first soon becomes routine and even enjoyable as physicians become more comfortable with patients.

PARENTAL CONCERNS

Parents' preconceived ideas and concerns regarding their children's illnesses can greatly influence the exchange of information between physicians and patients. At health maintenance or well child care visits, parents have questions and concerns regarding their children's development, nutrition, and growth. Often these questions stem from discussions with other parents or information received through the media. Although such concerns may seem trivial to pediatricians, they may be extremely important to parents. When evaluating children brought in for illness, it is important to ask parents what concerns them the most. Parental fears may be much different than medical concerns. Failure to give parents the opportunity to ask questions or to address these concerns in a sensitive manner may lead to dissatisfaction and poor communication.

THE PEDIATRIC INTERVIEW

Pediatric interviews are conducted in a variety of settings for many different reasons. The first interaction between the physician and parents may be during the prenatal interview before the birth of the child, in the hospital following the delivery, or in the doctor's office during the well baby visit. Later, the physician may see children in the office for regular health maintenance visits or in the office, emergency department, or hospital for an acute illness.

The specific clinical situation dictates the information

that needs to be gathered and the appropriate interviewing techniques. During the prenatal visit, physicians should discuss common concerns and anxieties about the new baby with prospective parents. In addition, parents have an opportunity to interview physicians and evaluate their offices and staffs.

In the emergency setting, physicians must elicit pertinent information needed to make decisions regarding management within a short period of time. Absence of long-term relationships can make communication in the emergency department particularly challenging. Focused, closed-ended questions should be used primarily. The periodic health maintenance visit is at the opposite end of this spectrum. Here the use of broad, open-ended questions is more appropriate; closed-ended questions should be used as needed for clarification.

COMMUNICATION GUIDELINES

Overall principles, applicable regardless of the setting, include interacting with the child and family in a professional yet sensitive and nonjudgmental manner. Common courtesies, such as knocking before entering the room, dressing and behaving in a professional manner, introducing oneself, and addressing parents and children by their preferred names, are always appreciated and welcomed. Taking a few moments to socialize with families develops a more personal relationship that may allow more open conversation about sensitive and emotional issues.

The medical visit may be divided into three parts: the interview, the physical examination, and the concluding remarks. Examples of doctor-parent and doctor-child communications for each of these components are given in Table 2–1.

The Interview

The goal of the interview is to ascertain the chief complaint and determine the appropriate medical history. The interview usually begins with open-ended questions to give parents and children an opportunity to discuss their concerns and outline their agenda for the visit. Closed-ended questions can then be used to clarify and further define the information presented. It often becomes necessary to guide the interview, especially when parents have several broad issues on their agenda for that visit and time does not permit their discussion.

Physicians should gently acknowledge parental concerns and define time limitations. These actions allow physicians to focus on the most salient issues of that visit. Physicians should limit their use of medical jargon (scientific terms) and be aware of nonverbal communication. Practitioners should empathize with parents; this makes them feel that their situation is truly understood even if physicians can do very little to help them. Pauses and silent periods should be used, especially when discussing emotionally difficult issues, to convey to parents and children that their physician

TABLE 2–1. Communication Guidelines and Techniques

Technique	Example
The Interview	
Open-ended questions	"How is Susie?"
Closed-ended questions	"Does she have a cough?"
Repetition of important phrases	"She has had a high fever for four days now?"
Clarification	"What do you mean by 'Susie was acting funny'?"
Pauses and silent periods	
Limit medical jargon	"Susie has an ear infection" vs. "Susie has otitis media"
Guide the interview	"Right now I am most interested in hearing about the symptoms of this illness"
Be aware of nonverbal communication	Use eye contact and phrases such as "I see"
Acknowledge parental concerns	"Worrying about hearing loss is understandable"
Empathize	"A fever of 104° F can be very frightening"
Remember common courtesies	Knock before entering
Recognize personal limitations	"I am not an expert in this area. I would like to consult with a colleague"
Summarize	"So she has had fever for four days but the rash and cough began one week ago?"
The Physical Examination	
Show consideration for the child	"It's OK to be afraid"
Inform	"That took me some time, but her heart sounds normal"
Explain procedures	"You may feel a little uncomfortable during the rectal examination"
Avoid exclamations	"Wow! I have never seen anything like this"
Concluding Remarks	
Provide closure	"Our time is over today. May we discuss this at the next visit?"
Minimize discharge instructions	
Be specific	"I am going to treat her with amoxicillin" vs. "I'll prescribe an antibiotic"
Compliment	"You're doing a great job"
Confirm parental understanding	"Please repeat for me Susie's diagnosis and treatment instructions"

cares enough to listen. Physicians should not underrate their own knowledge, but at the same time they should recognize their limitations and use consultants appropriately. Finally, physicians' understanding of the chief complaint and history should be summarized so parents have an opportunity to clarify points of disagreement.

The Physical Examination

Parents keenly observe physicians' interactions with children during the examination. It is an important time for physicians to build a therapeutic relationship with children (for further discussion see Chapter 3, Talking to Children). The transition between the history and physical examination can be made by briefly telling children and parents what to expect during the examination. Practitioners should show consideration for children's fears. Clinicians often find it helpful to speak to families at periodic intervals during the examination regarding their observations. Prolonged periods of silence as the doctor listens or palpates may be anxiety-provoking for families. Physicians should be sure to explain any procedures that either they or their staff are going to perform at a level that is appropriate for both parents and children. In addition, physicians should try to avoid exclamations or comments to themselves during the examination (e.g., "Wow, that's some murmur!"), which may be alarming to families.

Concluding Remarks

This portion of the visit, which is all too easy to rush through, is extremely important. Closure can be provided by either summarizing the diagnosis or outlining plans for the following visit. Parents should be asked to participate by acknowledging closure and helping to develop a management plan. It is important to assess parental readiness for knowledge (especially in emotionally difficult situations) and keep family resources and limitations in mind. Discharge instructions should be minimized; physicians should be specific and the number of diagnoses, medications, and "PRN" instructions (indications for seeking medical advice such as "return PRN for high fever") should be limited. When complicated discharge instructions are given, additional physician time may be required to ensure parental understanding. Complimenting parents on their care of their children can boost their self-esteem and confidence and may minimize calls and questions. Parental understanding should be confirmed; parents should be asked to repeat the diagnosis and treatment plan. Simply asking parents if they have understood is not enough, because parents often say "yes" out of respect for the physician's time or embarrassment that they have not understood what has been said. For example, the physician could say, "I want to be sure that I've spoken clearly enough. Please repeat for me [child's name] diagnosis and treatment instructions."

BARRIERS TO EFFECTIVE COMMUNICATION

Barriers to effective communication may be divided into systems barriers and interpersonal barriers (Table 2–2). The primary systems barriers are the setting itself and lack of continuity of care. Because of access problems within the health care system (i.e., lack of health insurance coverage) today, many children receive only episodic care from different physicians in acute care clinics or emergency departments. Without the benefit of long-term relationships, doctor-patient communication may suffer.

Interpersonal barriers include physician time constraints, frequent interruptions, and cultural insensitivity. Frequent interruptions or apparent impatience on the part of physicians conveys to parents and children that either they do not care or they are too busy for them. Language differences may pose a significant barrier depending on the region in which physicians practice. Ideally, physicians themselves should be able to speak to parents and children. If translators must be used, children should not play this role, if possible, because this places them in an awkward situation. Parents of other patients should not be used because this violates patients' privacy. Physicians should be sensitive to cultural differences (e.g., gender issues, views on illness, folk remedies, and beliefs). Suggesting treatments that are not culturally acceptable or are contrary to folk wisdom simply decreases compliance with prescribed treatment plans. For example, many Eastern cultures believe in the concept of "hot" and "cold" foods and illnesses. Suggesting to a mother that she feed primarily "hot" foods to a child she believes to have an illness that is also "hot" may not be acceptable to her. Such information is rarely volunteered and must be elicited through sensitive patient interviewing.

Case Resolution

The doctor-patient interaction presented in the case history illustrates several of the points discussed here. The physician did not acknowledge parental concerns or make sure that the mother had understood the diagnosis and treatment plan. The mother was presented with more information than she could have reasonably been asked to remember. This interaction could have been improved (1) if the physician conveyed to the mother that her concerns were appreciated and (2) then reassured her that her child was going to be all right. Furthermore, the physician could have told the mother the name and dosage schedule of the antibiotic to be prescribed and limited the number of PRN instructions.

Selected Readings

American Academy of Pediatrics. Guidelines for Health Supervision II. Elk Grove Village, IL, American Academy of Pediatrics, 1988.

Grover, G., C. D. Berkowitz, and R. J. Lewis. Parental recall after a visit to the emergency department. Clin. Pediatr. 33:194–201, 1994.

Korsch, B. M., B. F. Freemon, and V. F. Negrete. Practical implications of doctor-patient interaction analysis for pediatric practice. Am. J. Dis. Child. 12:110–114, 1971.

Stein, M. T. Interviewing in a pediatric setting. In Dixon, S. D., and M. T. Stein. Encounters with Children. Chicago, Year Book Medical Publishers, 1987.

Wissow, L. S., D. L. Roter, and M. E. H. Wilson. Pediatrician interview style and mother's disclosure of psychosocial issues. Pediatrics 93:289–295, 1994.

TABLE 2–2. Barriers to Effective Communication

Systems Barrier	Example
Lack of continuity of care	Episodic care that is primarily illness driven
The setting itself	Emergency departments and acute care clinics
Interpersonal Barriers	
Physician time constraints	Appearing impatient or preoccupied
Frequent interruptions	
Cultural insensitivity	Suggesting treatments that are not acceptable within the family's belief systems

CHAPTER 3

TALKING TO CHILDREN

Geeta Grover, M.D.

H$_x$ The moment you walk into the examination room, the two-year-old girl begins to cry and scream uncontrollably. She clings to her mother and turns her face away. The mother appears embarrassed and states that her daughter reacts to all physicians this way. After reassuring the mother that you have received such welcomes before, you sit down at a comfortable distance from the girl and her mother. You smile at the girl and compliment her on her dress, but she does not seem to be interested in interacting with you at this point. You begin your interview with the mother and try not to look at the girl. Out of the corner of your eye, you see that her crying is easing a bit and that she is looking at you very carefully. Without moving from your chair, you hand her your stethoscope with a clip-on toy teddy bear attached to it. She accepts it hesitantly and begins to examine it as you and the mother continue talking.

Questions

1. How does children's age influence their understanding of health and illness?
2. Should physicians speak directly with children about their illnesses?
3. At what age can children begin to communicate with physicians about their illnesses?
4. How can positioning and placement of children in the examination room affect the overall tone and quality of the visit?

Effective doctor-patient communication, which is difficult enough when patients are adults, becomes even more challenging when patients are children. In pediatrics, interviewing involves balancing the needs of both parents and children. Whereas parents may be more focused on issues pertaining to disease, treatment, or aspects of parenting, children look to physicians with different needs and concerns, depending on their age. To have a meaningful and satisfying exchange with children, pediatricians must take into account children's developmental maturity and how this affects their concepts of health and illness. As children grow and develop, their understanding of health and illness increases.

DEVELOPMENTAL APPROACH TO COMMUNICATING WITH CHILDREN

An appreciation of the cognitive stages of development helps pediatricians develop a healthy relationship with their patients by allowing them to communicate with the children in an age-appropriate manner. Piaget defined four stages of cognitive development, which occur in the same sequence but not at the same rate in all children (Table 3–1). Children in the sensorimotor stage (birth–2 years of age) experience the world and act through sensations and motor acts. They are developing the concepts of object permanence, causality, and spatial relationships. Children in the preoperational stage (2–6 years) understand reality only from their own viewpoint. As egocentric thinkers, they are unable to separate internal from external reality, and fantasy play is important. School-age children (6–11 years) are capable of concrete operational thinking. These children can reason through problems that relate to real objects. Older children (> 11 years) have the capacity for abstract thought, which defines the stage of formal operations.

An appreciation of how children's cognitive development affects their understanding of illness and pain aids physicians in developing therapeutic relationships. Bibace and colleagues have outlined a developmental approach to children's understanding of illness: Children's explanations of illness are classified into six categories consistent with Piaget's cognitive developmental stages. Children two to six years of age view illness as caused by external factors near the body (phenomenism and contagion). Young children engage

TABLE 3–1. Piaget's Stages of Cognitive Development

Age*	Stage	Characteristics
Birth–2 yr	Sensorimotor	Experiences world through sensations and motor acts
2–6 yr	Preoperational	Egocentric thinking; imitation and fantasy play
6–11 yr	Concrete operational	Mental processes only as they relate to real objects
> 11 yr	Formal operations	Capacity for abstract thought

*Approximate ages.

TABLE 3–2. Children's Concepts of Illness

Age	Concept of Illness	Example
	Preoperational	How do people get colds?
2–6 yr	Phenomenism	"From the sun"
	Contagion	"When someone else gets near them"
	Concrete Operational	How do people get colds?
7–10 yr	Contamination	"You're outside without a hat and you start sneezing. Your head would get cold—the cold would touch it—and then it would go all over your body"
	Internalization	"In winter, people breathe in too much air into their nose and it blocks up the nose"
	Formal Operations	How do people get colds?
>11 yr	Physiologic	"They come from viruses, I guess"
	Psychophysiologic	How do people get a heart attack?
		"It can come from being all nerve-racked. You worry too much, and the tension can affect your heart"

Modified and reproduced, with permission, from Bibace, R., and M.E. Walsh. Development of children's concepts of illness. Pediatrics 66:912–917, 1980.

in so-called magical thinking; proximity alone provides the link between cause and illness. Children 7 to 10 years of age should be able to differentiate between self and nonself. At this stage they begin to understand that although illness may be caused by some factor outside the body, illness itself is located inside the body (contamination and internalization). Children over 11 years of age understand physiologic and psychophysiologic explanations for illness (Table 3–2).

A similar developmental sequence applies to children's understanding of pain. Gaffney and Dunne have outlined a developmental approach to this understanding. Younger children may attribute pain to punishment for some transgression or wrongdoing on their part. They may not understand the relationship between pain and illness (e.g., "pain is something in my tummy"). Children with concrete operational thought can appreciate that pain and illness are related, but they may have no clear understanding of the causation of pain (e.g., "pain is a feeling you get when you are sick"). Older children and adolescents begin to understand the complex physical and psychological components of pain. For example, they realize that although the bone in the arm is broken, pain is ultimately felt in the head (e.g., "pain goes up some nerves from the broken bone in my arm to my head").

GUIDELINES FOR DOCTOR-CHILD COMMUNICATION

Successful communication with children depends not only on spoken words but also nonverbal cues and the environment itself. A pleasant, child-friendly environment with bright colors, wall decorations, and toys helps make children feel more comfortable. Health care practitioners should be sincere, because children are extremely sensitive to nonverbal cues. Pediatricians

should take a few minutes to enjoy children; this not only gives children a chance to evaluate their physicians, but also allows clinicians to begin assessing areas of development. A general principle of the pediatric examination is to begin with the least invasive portions of the examination (e.g., heart, lungs, abdomen) and save the most invasive for last (e.g., oropharynx, ears). Pediatricians should maintain their self-control in difficult situations. If they approach their limit, they should step outside for a few minutes or ask someone for assistance. Overall guidelines for communicating with children are provided in Table 3–3. Age-specific guidelines are outlined below.

Birth to Six Months

Examination of children of this age is usually pleasant. Although verbal interaction is limited, it is important to play with children, hold them, and talk to them. By watching physicians interact with their children, new parents have an opportunity to learn how to behave with their infants. Infants have not yet developed a fear of strangers and can usually be easily examined either in parents' arms or on the examination table.

Seven Months to Three Years

This is perhaps the most challenging age group with regard to developing rapport and performing examinations. After entering the examination room, pediatricians should take a few moments to converse or play with children. Such actions help put children at ease and allow them to get to know their doctors. Children who are one to two years of age will probably busy themselves, exploring the room during the history taking. By acknowledging them periodically, physicians build rapport that will help later during the examination. Two- to three-year-old children are usually very apprehensive of the examination. Physicians should get down to children's eye level when speaking to them. Reassurances such as, "You're not going to get any shots today," can help alleviate their fears. Because stranger anxiety has developed, physicians should try to do as much of the examination as possible with children in parents' laps. Distractions such as stethoscope toys, flashing penlights, or keys may be helpful.

TABLE 3–3. Physician-Child Communication

Do's	Don'ts
Provide a pleasant environment	Limit the child's participation
Pay attention to nonverbal cues	Threaten the child
Be sincere and honest	Compare the child to others
Enjoy the child	Get into power struggles
Speak age appropriately	
Get down to the child's eye level	
Examine from least to most invasive	
Respect the child's privacy	
Maintain self-control	
Have a sense of humor	

Three to Six Years

Children's expressive capabilities are growing at tremendous rates during this period. Children can usually be engaged in conversation. They should be given repeated opportunities for participation, but they should not feel pressured to take part. Children may doubt physicians' true intentions and will probably only speak once their comfort level has been achieved. Children should be involved; they can be asked simple questions regarding their illness (e.g., "where does it hurt?"). In addition, children should be given some control during the examination (e.g., "should I look in your mouth next or your ears?"), and they should be allowed to handle physicians' equipment. Knowing what to expect next and having some control over the examination can help to decrease fear and increase cooperation.

Seven to Eleven Years

Examination of children in this age group can be rewarding. Physicians should make a point to speak directly with children and not just to parents concerning the chief complaint and history. Children can usually provide a good history regarding their illness, although their concept of time may be misleading. For example, a "long, long time" may mean hours, days, or months, and parents need to clarify this. Children should be asked about school, friends, and favorite activities. Answers to such questions give physicians an idea of children's social and emotional well-being, which may be affecting their physical health. Physicians sometimes overlook children's need for privacy at this age. Drapes should be used appropriately during the examination, and physicians should be sensitive to the presence of other children or adults in the room.

Physicians should begin to involve older children in the management of their illness. Children's understanding of their illness and its management should be assessed (e.g., children with asthma could be asked "What is this inhaler for? When are you going to use it? Show me how."). Children should be given an opportunity to express their fears and anxieties, and these concerns should be discussed (e.g., "Asthma can be scary, especially when you can't catch your breath. Have you ever felt like that? Tell me about it."). Children should be involved in the management of their illness, which allows them to develop a sense of responsibility for their own health and medical care.

Over Twelve Years

Communication with adolescents is discussed in detail in Chapter 4, Talking to Adolescents.

BARRIERS TO EFFECTIVE COMMUNICATION WITH CHILDREN

The manner in which adults speak to children is influenced by what they think children can understand.

Clinicians tend to overestimate the understanding capabilities of younger children and underestimate those of older children. Lack of appreciation for the cognitive sophistication of children may lead to frustration for all involved. Younger children are presented with information they may not be able to comprehend, and older children may feel frustrated because they are being spoken to in a childlike manner.

Another potential barrier in communicating with children is limiting their participation. Physicians tend to elicit information from children but exclude them from diagnostic and management information. Older children want to know about their illness and are capable of learning about management.

All physicians have been frustrated or pushed to the limit at one time or another when working with children. In such situations, practitioners should remember that children are probably not trying to irritate physicians on purpose. Crying or lack of cooperation generally stems from fear or a sense of lack of control over the situation. Pediatricians should avoid taking part in a battle over power or control with children. Threatening remarks (e.g., "If you're not good, I'll have to give you a shot") or comparisons between children (e.g., "Your brother is younger than you, and he didn't cry") not only are ineffective but may make the situation worse. A clear perspective, empathy, and a sense of humor are much more useful.

Case Resolution

In the case presented in the opening scenario, you learn from the mother that her daughter has been in good health. The mother has brought in the child for a routine health maintenance visit. You assess that her development is normal and that her immunizations are up-to-date. As you and the mother talk, the child appears more relaxed and less frightened. She begins to respond to your questions and cooperate with the examination, but she chooses to remain on her mother's lap.

Selected Readings

Bibace R., and M. E. Walsh. Development of children's concepts of illness. Pediatrics 66:912–917, 1980.

Gaffney, A., and E. A. Dunne. Developmental aspects of children's definitions of pain. Pain 26:105–117, 1986.

Ginsburg, H., and S. Opper. Piaget's Theory of Intellectual Development, 3rd ed. Englewood Cliffs, NJ, Prentice-Hall, 1988.

Greenspan, S. I. The Clinical Interview of the Child, 2nd ed. Washington, DC, American Psychiatric Press, 1991.

Lewis, C. C., R. H. Pantell, and L. Sharp. Increasing patient knowledge, satisfaction, and involvement: randomized trial of a communication intervention. Pediatrics 88:351–358, 1991.

McGrath, P. J., and K. D. Craig. Developmental and psychological factors in children's pain. Pediatr. Clin. North Am. 36:823–836, 1989.

Perrin, E. C., and P. S. Gerrity. There's a demon in your belly: children's understanding of illness. Pediatrics 67:841–849, 1981.

Perrin, E. C., and J. M. Perrin. Clinicians' assessments of children's understanding of illness. Am. J. Dis. Child. 137:874–878, 1983.

TALKING TO ADOLESCENTS

Monica Sifuentes, M.D.

H$_x$ This is a first-time visit for a quiet, shy, adolescent girl who is accompanied by her mother. The mother is concerned because her daughter's grades have been dropping, and she has been fatigued and irritable. The mother reports no new activities or recent changes in the family's schedule and no new stressors at home. Both parents are employed, the girl has the same friends she has always had, and her siblings are currently doing well academically. The girl is healthy and has never been hospitalized.

After the mother leaves the room, the girl is interviewed alone.

Questions

1. When interviewing adolescents, what is the significance of identifying their stage of development?
2. What are important areas to cover in the adolescent interview?
3. What issues of confidentiality and competence need to be discussed with adolescents before conducting the interview?

Adolescence is a time of unique change. Unlike other periods in life when individuals have at least some knowledge or experience to guide them, adolescence is stereotypically characterized by feelings of physical awkwardness, emotional turmoil, and social isolation. Unfortunately, the teenage years are dreaded by most parents, who often feel ill equipped to handle the wide range of children's responses. So instead of "taking the bull by the horns," parents choose the route of quiet observation. They fully intend to "be there" for their children but wait to be approached. Hence many adolescents do not have the guidance or advice of parents during the teenage years and spend the time alone or in the company of friends or acquaintances. Most adolescents pass through this period uneventfully. In fact, many individuals go through this period gladly, finally being permitted to drive a car or go out on a date.

Physicians must use a different approach when interviewing adolescents. Information must come directly from patients rather than parents, unlike with other pediatric patients. The interview should focus on several psychosocial issues that may be uncomfortable to discuss. The goal of the interview is the discovery of any problems that might interfere with a relatively smooth passage through adolescence.

STAGES OF ADOLESCENCE

Adolescents are stereotypically labeled as difficult, complex, time-consuming patients with problems or complaints that lead to uninteresting diagnoses. In addition, they are often accompanied by overbearing, demanding parents, or sometimes no parents at all.

The quality and quantity of information obtained during the medical and psychosocial interview can be greatly enhanced by taking developmental milestones into consideration. Adolescence can be divided into three developmental stages: early, middle, and late (Table 4–1). For example, interest in discussing long-term educational goals varies depending on the age of the adolescent. Most 18-year-olds are prepared to discuss college plans, specific vocational interests, and employment opportunities. In contrast, 12-year-olds are still anchored in the concreteness of early adolescence and often are ill prepared to discuss higher education. School experiences are much more important to this age group and should therefore be the focus of discussion. Peer pressure is most prominent during middle adolescence; 14-year-olds with friends who smoke cigarettes and drink beer probably use the same recreational materials.

Knowledge of these differences allows interviewers to better explain instructions and diagnoses to teenagers. For example, 19-year-olds can better understand the effects of untreated or recurrent chlamydia cervicitis on long-term fertility than 13-year-olds. This is not to say that physicians should not tell sexually active 13-year-olds with chlamydia about these possible effects, but they should use more concrete wording and repeat the information at future visits. Age guidelines are not rigid, however, and each interview should be individually tailored to the particular adolescent and the circumstances surrounding the visit.

TABLE 4–1. Developmental Milestones During Adolescence

	Early Adolescence (11–13 years)	Middle Adolescence (14–16 years)	Late Adolescence (17–21 years)
Thought processes	Concrete	± Abstract	Abstract
Parental supervision	+	±	−
Risk-taking behavior	+	±	−
Peer pressure	±	++	+

Modified from March, C.A., and M.S. Jay. Adolescents in the emergency department: an overview. Adolesc. Med. State Art Rev. 4:2, 1993.

ISSUES OF CONFIDENTIALITY AND COMPETENCE

The discussion of **confidentiality** can be approached in two ways. Each method has distinct advantages as well as disadvantages. Interviewers should use the approach that they find most comfortable; this allows conversation to flow more naturally.

The first approach involves informing adolescents at the beginning of the interview that most issues discussed are held in confidence and not repeated to anyone. Exceptions are suicidal or homicidal behavior and sexual or physical abuse. In any of these instances, other professionals are told of the disclosed information, and parents may ultimately find out. The advantages to this approach are that discussion of these "logistics" at the beginning of the interview is less awkward, and the ground rules are clear at the beginning. This contributes to an atmosphere of trust and honesty. The disadvantage is possible inhibition of adolescents who are unsure about disclosing particular incidents (e.g., those concerning sexual abuse); some teenagers are now almost certain not to share this information for fear of involving other professionals or family members. Interviewers should be nonjudgmental, reassuring, and patient in order to reduce the possibility of such an occurrence.

The second, less popular approach to the discussion of confidentiality involves informing adolescents at the end of the interview or when and if one of the exceptions to maintaining confidentiality arises. Proponents of this approach argue that adolescents tend to respond more honestly to questions when they do not believe physicians will inform others, including their parents or legal guardians. Physicians have a legal responsibility, however, to report sexual and physical abuse; in cases of suicidal or homicidal behavior, it is in the patient's best interest to inform other professionals of this disclosure. The disadvantages to this method are that these issues often arise at very emotional times during the interview, and it is difficult to interrupt the patient to discuss mandated reporting. If physicians wait until the end of the interview to inform adolescents about mandated reporting, however, patients may leave the office feeling deceived and probably will not return for future visits. Most health care providers prefer to inform adolescents at the onset of the interview about confidentiality with the hope that it contributes to the development of a trusting relationship.

Assessments of adolescents' ability to make health-related decisions is another important aspect of the interview. **Competence** is the ability to understand the significance of information and assess the alternatives and consequences sufficiently to then identify a preference. Various factors besides age must be considered such as level of maturity, intelligence, degree of independence, and presence of any chronic illness. This last factor is included because adolescents with chronic conditions have presumably already participated in decisions regarding their health care. Regardless, it may be difficult to assess competence from just one visit. It may not even be necessary to make that assessment emergently, except in certain cases such as pregnancy.

Although it is imperative to interview adolescents alone, every attempt should be made to involve parents in all health-related decisions. Although specific state laws allow physicians to treat minors in emergent situations and in cases of suspected venereal disease without parents' consent, physicians should urge adolescents to inform their parents of any problems disclosed during the interview. The ultimate decision rests with adolescents. Physicians can offer to help adolescents discuss delicate issues with parents by role-playing or by sitting in on the adolescent-parent conversation.

PSYCHOSOCIAL REVIEW OF SYSTEMS

A large part of the adolescent interview involves taking an adequate psychosocial history. The approach known by the acronym **HEADSSS** (**h**ome environment, **e**mployment and education, **a**ctivities, **d**rugs, **s**exual activity/sexuality, **s**uicide and depression, **s**afety) allows interviewers to evaluate the critical areas in adolescents' lives that may contribute to a less than optimal environment for normal growth and development (see Questions Box). Questions about sexuality must be asked in a nondirected, nonjudgmental fashion, giving adolescents time to respond. This information is useful to assess risks for conditions such as HIV. An inquiry about both sexual and physical abuse is indicated during this part of the interview.

ISSUES THAT NEED IMMEDIATE ATTENTION

Many issues discussed during the psychosocial interview can be a source of anxiety for adolescents. Some problems must be taken more seriously than others, and some demand immediate attention. Suicidal ideation with or without a previous attempt definitely requires a more in-depth analysis of the gravity of the problem. Physicians should make sure that adolescents feel they can make a verbal contract to call someone if they feel like hurting themselves. Mental health professionals should assess these situations. Other issues that require immediate attention include possible danger to others, possible or confirmed pregnancy, and sexual or physical abuse.

CONCLUDING THE INTERVIEW

The adolescent interview should be conducted at a time when adolescents are relatively healthy and the interviewer has set aside time for a thorough discussion. All topics need not be addressed at one visit. Issues that arise at one visit can be readdressed at the next visit. The number of appointments needed to solve a particular problem is unlimited.

At the end of each visit, the interview should be summarized; any difficult topics should be mentioned, and the issue of confidentiality should be reviewed. Adolescents should then be asked to identify a person whom they can trust or confide in should any problems arise before the next visit. In some instances, this issue may already have been addressed. Adoles-

Questions: Talking to Adolescents: HEADSSS*

H: Home environment
- With whom does the adolescent live?
- Have there been any recent changes in the living situation?
- How are things between parents at home?
- Are the parents employed?

E: Employment and **education**
- Is the adolescent currently in school?
- What are his or her favorite subjects?
- How is the adolescent performing academically?
- Has the adolescent ever been truant or expelled from school?
- Are the adolescent's friends attending school?
- What are the adolescent's future education/employment goals?

A: Activities
- What does the adolescent do in his or her spare time?
- What does the adolescent do for fun? Is the adolescent ever bored?
- Who does the adolescent spend time with?

D: Drugs
- Has the adolescent ever used any illicit drugs? Has the adolescent ever used tobacco? What about steroids? Alcohol?
- Is the adolescent still using these drugs? Are friends using or selling any drugs?

S: Sexual activity/sexuality
- What is the adolescent's sexual orientation?
- Is the adolescent sexually active?
  - If so, what was the age of the adolescent's sexual debut?
  - How many sexual partners does the adolescent have?
  - Does the adolescent (or the partner) use condoms?
  - Does the adolescent (or the partner) use contraception?
- Does the adolescent have a history of sexual or physical abuse?

S: Suicide/depression
- Is the adolescent ever sad or tearful? Tired and unmotivated?
- Has the adolescent ever felt that life is not worth living or ever thought of or tried to hurt himself or herself? More importantly, does the adolescent have a suicide plan?

S: Safety
- Does the adolescent use a seat belt and bicycle helmet?
- Does the adolescent enter into high-risk situations?
- Is there a firearm in the adolescent's home? If so, does the adolescent know about firearm safety?

---

*For more detailed information, see the references by Goldenring and Cohen.

cents should also be given the opportunity to express any other concerns not covered in the interview and ask questions that may have arisen during the interview.

Physicians should frankly inform adolescents about any significant risk factors or risk-taking behaviors that have been identified. In addition, physicians should give adolescents positive feedback for strengths and accomplishments and acknowledge that things are going well. They should tell adolescents about available resources such as teen hotlines and offer follow-up visits or opportunities to talk.

Case Resolution

The adolescent in the case history should first be informed about confidentiality and the specific exceptions to maintaining it. Nonthreatening topics such as home life, school, and outside activities should first be explored, followed by questions regarding sexuality, sexual activity, and illicit drug use. Suicidal behavior or depression and safety issues should also be reviewed.

Selected Readings

Alderman, E. M., and A. R. Fleischman. Should adolescents make their own health-care choices? Contemp. Pediatr. 10:65–82, 1993.

Anderson, M. M. Principles of care for the ill adolescent. Adolesc. Med. State Art Rev. 2:441–458, 1991.

Cheng, T. L., et al. Confidentiality in health care: a survey of knowledge, perceptions and attitudes among high school students. J.A.M.A. 269:1404–1407, 1993.

Council on Scientific Affairs, American Medical Association. Confidential health services for adolescents. J.A.M.A. 268:1420–1424, 1993.

English, A. Treating adolescents: legal and ethical considerations. Med. Clin. North Am. 74:1097, 1990.

Goldenring, J. M., and E. Cohen. Getting into adolescent heads. Contemp. Pediatr. 5:75–90, 1988.

King, N. M. P., and A. W. Cross. Children as decision makers: guidelines for pediatricians. J. Pediatr. 115:10–16, 1989.

TELEPHONE MANAGEMENT

Iris Wagman Borowsky, M.D., Ph.D.

H$_x$ The mother of an otherwise healthy 10-month-old girl calls and tells you that her daughter has a fever. The girl's rectal temperature has been 103–104° F (39.4–40.0 °C) for the past two days. Although she is cranky with the fever, she plays normally after receiving acetaminophen. The girl is eating well and has no runny nose, cough, vomiting, diarrhea, or rash.

Questions

1. How do telephone and face-to-face encounters between physicians and patients differ?
2. What are some general guidelines for effective doctor-patient communication over the telephone?
3. What historical information is necessary for appropriate telephone management?
4. What points are important to cover in home treatment advice?

Parents frequently call their pediatricians seeking medical advice about their children. It is estimated that pediatricians spend over 25% of their total practice time engaged in "telephone medicine." Telephone medicine serves two purposes: (1) it provides a service and (2) it controls costs and overcrowding by reducing unnecessary visits to the office and emergency department. Most calls concern upper respiratory symptoms, fever, rash, trauma, or GI complaints—the same problems most commonly seen in the office.

Telephone management of illnesses differs in that it requires pediatricians to give advice based on history alone and precludes the opportunity to see the child, much less do a careful physical examination. For example, a practitioner in the emergency department who does not know the patient or family may choose to see the child if questions about the child's general health or the feasibility of continued contact with the family arise. On the other hand, a primary care physician who knows the patient and family and can follow the child's progress by telephone may advise home management for a child with a similar history. Pediatric practice settings, whether in an emergency department or primary care office, should have an organized approach to telephone care. In addition to physicians, nurse practitioners, and physician's assistants, telephone care systems may include trained and supervised nurses and nonmedical office staff using protocols.

TELEPHONE COMMUNICATION SKILLS

Parents commonly call their pediatricians because they are worried about their child. The friendly voice of a health care worker who is ready to lend an ear goes a long way toward reassuring an anxious parent. Calls should begin with a "verbal handshake." Staff should identify themselves and the place where the call is received and offer to help. They should learn the caller's name, his or her relationship to the child, and the child's name and gender; these names, as well as the child's gender, should be used in the conversation, thus creating a more personal atmosphere.

Telephone calls for medical advice are often received in busy environments such as emergency departments or clinics where patients are waiting to be seen. It is easy to be abrupt under these circumstances and not give complete attention to callers. If calls are not emergencies, practitioners can always take the caller's telephone number and return the call as soon as possible. If callers do not feel that their concerns have been fully acknowledged, they are likely to feel dissatisfied, even if they are given sound advice. Furthermore, research on doctor-patient relationships suggests that lack of friendliness or warmth in the doctor-patient relationship and patient dissatisfaction are associated with noncompliance with medical advice. Interestingly, studies have shown that the length of a patient visit does not correlate with patient satisfaction. Telephone encounters do not necessarily have to be lengthy; the average length of a call is reported to be three to five minutes, depending on the setting. Calls must be pleasant, however, and they must address callers' concerns. Open-ended questions such as "Tell me about your child's illness" or "Are there any other symptoms?" are useful at the beginning of a call because they give callers an opportunity to explain the situation without interruptions.

Establishing rapport over the telephone is more difficult than it is in person because the practitioner is limited to verbal communication. In face-to-face encounters, physicians can use words as well as means of nonverbal communication such as facial expressions, eye contact, gesturing, and touch to convey warmth and empathy. Practitioners should use various aspects of **verbal communication** to convey sincere interest in callers' concerns, and they should pay attention to these verbal cues in callers. Many components of verbal communication, in addition to words themselves, including vocal expression, pace, articulation, tone, volume, and pauses, affect telephone interactions. Health care professionals should speak clearly and use vocabulary that callers understand; **medical jargon should be avoided.** A friendly yet respectful tone and a calm, professional manner should be maintained.

Careful listening is crucial to obtaining the information necessary to make medical decisions over the telephone. One of the major goals of health care professionals is to recognize and respond to callers' main concerns and expectations. This can be difficult, because most callers do not specifically tell their major concerns to their physicians. Researchers have found the following questions useful in the identification of parents' chief concerns: "What worries you the most about your child's (use child's name) illness?" and "Why does that worry you?"

For callers who ramble, health care professionals may need to focus the conversation. Asking the question "What can I do to help?" should clarify the reason for the call. If information needs to be verified, practitioners can summarize what they have heard and ask if they have understood correctly.

Angry callers may strike a nerve, resulting in defensive or confrontational behavior by health care professionals. Responding to anger with arguments, however, is time-consuming, stressful, and pointless. Practitioners should be warm and understanding so that callers who want to discuss their feelings feel comfortable. Acknowledging anger may encourage open discussion and problem-solving (e.g., "You sound upset. Is there anything I can do to help?"). Empathizing with callers (e.g., "I don't blame you for being upset," "That must have been very frustrating") may also help.

Practitioners can build confidence in callers by complimenting them on the way they have handled things so far (e.g., "You did the right thing by giving [child's name] Tylenol and a lukewarm sponge bath for the fever. That is exactly what I would have done" or "I'm glad that you called about this"). They may even be able to offer reassurance to parents who are not managing their child's illness correctly by commenting that many parents try the same treatment. A different treatment approach can then be suggested.

Before the end of the conversation, callers can be given an opportunity to ask questions and encouraged to call again if additional problems occur.

TELEPHONE HISTORY TAKING

How much history should be obtained over the telephone? Enough information should be gathered to make an appropriate decision. Questions should be directed at **determining whether an emergency exists** and **making a diagnosis.** For example, if the mother of a 20-day-old girl reports that her daughter has a temperature of 102° F (38.9° C), the infant must be seen immediately. If diarrhea is the chief complaint, some additional information would be helpful before giving advice (e.g., "How many bowel movements did the girl have in the last 24 hours? Is there any blood in the diarrhea? Does she have a fever? Is she drinking less

than usual? Is there any decrease in urine output?"). An older child with the same chief complaint of fever may be safely managed at home, depending on the answers to other questions about additional symptoms.

Pediatricians typically follow an organized approach to history taking for acute care visits that includes the chief complaint, history of present illness, pertinent review of systems, medical history, and family and social history. A similarly **organized framework** should be used to obtain a history over the telephone (see Questions Box). Specific questions should then be asked to clarify the child's condition and obtain all the information necessary to make a good decision. A child's medical history may affect a practitioner's management of the current problem. For example, knowing that a child who has been exposed to chickenpox has asthma and is receiving steroids or has leukemia is crucial in providing the appropriate telephone advice.

Practitioners can refer to several texts on pediatric telephone decision making (see Selected Readings). These books outline protocols for common chief complaints to serve as guides for history taking and management over the telephone. The most efficient way to provide such medical advice is to obtain critical information that affects decisions about diagnosis and management instead of asking all possible questions. For example, with a child who is vomiting or has diarrhea, the state of hydration is critical; with a cough, the occurrence of breathing difficulty; and with head trauma, loss of consciousness. Methods of teaching telephone management skills include role playing, listening to mock calls by "simulated" mothers, and reviewing tapes of actual calls.

Because most childhood illnesses are mild and self-limited, evaluation of the safety of medical advice obtained over the telephone requires large samples to detect poor outcomes associated with mismanagement. Research has described a "wellness bias" in which practitioners, who primarily see patients with mild, self-limited illnesses, may downplay the severity of reported symptoms and choose the most benign diagnostic possibility. This bias may be more pronounced in a telephone encounter, where the physician cannot see the child. One study reported telephone encounters in which physicians seemed to make a decision early in the conversation and then "shut out" additional information that should have led to the consideration of more

---

Questions: Telephone Management (all callers)

- How old is the child?
- What is the child's chief problem? What are the child's symptoms?
- How long has the child had these symptoms?
- How is the child acting?
- Does the child have any chronic illnesses?
- Is the child taking any medications?
- What is the caller most worried about?

serious diagnoses. The safest approach is to always have a high index of suspicion for a serious condition. Questions can then be asked to confirm or dispel those suspicions.

TELEPHONE ADVICE

Pediatricians should formulate an **assessment and management plan** based on the child's history. If the situation is an emergency, this should be explained to the caller, and appropriate follow-up plans should be made (i.e., sending an ambulance for life-threatening conditions such as respiratory depression or uncontrollable bleeding, advising the caller to bring the child by car to the emergency department or physician's office within a specified amount of time for potentially dangerous complaints, such as right lower quadrant pain or possible fracture). If the call is not an emergency, then health care professionals must decide if and when the child should be seen by a physician and the appropriate home treatment.

Research shows that parents need and expect to receive an explanation of their child's illness. Practitioners should clearly state what the child's illness seems to be, what probably caused it, and what the parents can expect (e.g., length of time that the child is likely to be sick, additional symptoms that may appear).

Before giving any treatment advice, health care professionals should ask callers the following questions: "What have you done so far?," "Have you given the child any medications?," and "How is this treatment working?" If the therapy appears appropriate, callers should be complimented and encouraged to continue the treatment. The regimen should be modified as indicated. Instructions for home treatment should be clear and as easy to implement as possible. If the instructions are complicated or lengthy, callers may want to write them down. When prescribing medication, ask if the child has any known drug allergies, and give the dose, frequency of administration, and information about possible side effects. Practitioners should verify that the caller can follow the telephone advice (e.g., a parent has a thermometer and knows how to use it). If pediatricians plan to check up on children by telephone, they should confirm that callers (or relatives or neighbors) have a telephone and record the number.

Practitioners should confirm that callers understand the information and instructions and agree with the plan. Asking questions such as "What questions do you have?" encourages callers to raise uncertainties and ask for needed clarification. Most importantly, if the decision is to manage at home, callers should always receive specific instructions about when to call back (e.g., child has fever for more than two days, irritability, decreased urination). Parents who seem unduly anxious or uncomfortable with home treatment should be given the opportunity to have their child seen by a physician.

DOCUMENTATION

All calls for medical advice should be documented in a telephone log book or the child's medical record, for both medical reasons (e.g., better follow-up, improved continuity of care) and legal purposes. The form used for documentation should include the date and time of the call; the name, identity, and telephone number of the caller; the name and age of the child; the chief complaint; other symptoms; possible diagnoses; advice given; and the name of the person who took the call.

Case Resolution

In the case history at the beginning of this chapter, the pediatrician learns several facts that lead to the recommendation that the child be seen that day (the next day if the call is made at night). These facts include the child's age, the height and duration of the fever, and lack of any symptoms of localized infection.

Selected Readings

Brown, J. L. Pediatric Telephone Medicine: Principles, Triage and Advice, 2nd ed. Philadelphia, J.B. Lippincott, 1994.

Francis, V., B. M. Korsch, and M. J. Morris. Gaps in doctor-patient communication: patient's response to medical advice. N. Engl. J. Med. 280:535–540, 1969.

Isaacman, D. J., et al. Pediatric telephone advice in the emergency department: results of mock scenario. Pediatrics 89:35–39, 1992.

Katz, H. P. Telephone Medicine: Triage and Training—A Handbook for Primary Health Care Professionals. Philadelphia, F. A. Davis, 1990.

Kosower, E., S. H. Inkelis, and J. S. Seidel. Telephone T.A.L.K.: a telephone communication program. Pediatr. Emerg. Care 7:76–79, 1991.

Schmitt, B. D. Pediatric Telephone Advice. Boston, Little, Brown, 1980.

Wood, P. R., J. H. Littlefield, and D. M. Foulds. Telephone management curriculum for pediatric interns: a controlled trial. Pediatrics 83:925–930, 1989.

Yanovski, S. Z., et al. Telephone triage by primary care physicians. Pediatrics 89:701–706, 1992.

SCREENING IN NEWBORNS

Monica Sifuentes, M.D.

H$_x$ A six-day-old infant is brought to the office by the parents because of an abnormal neonatal screening test for galactosemia. The family recently moved to the area. The parents report that their daughter has been doing well. Initially she seemed a bit sleepy, but she is now taking short naps during the day and waking every two to three hours at night for feedings. The infant is breast-fed, with occasional formula supplementation. She wets seven to eight diapers per day and has had normal, soft, seedy stools since birth.

The infant, the product of a 39-week gestation, was born via normal spontaneous vaginal delivery to a 28-year-old gravida II para II woman in good health. The mother received appropriate prenatal care beginning at 14 weeks' gestation and had no problems during the pregnancy. She reportedly used no alcohol, drugs, or medications, and the results of all prenatal laboratory tests were normal. At birth the infant weighed 6 lb, 13 oz (3100 g) and was 19 inches (48.25 cm) long. She was discharged 18 hours later at the parents' insistence.

The family history is unremarkable. The four-year-old sibling is healthy and developmentally normal.

The infant's current weight is 6 lb, 6 oz (2900 g). The physical examination is entirely within normal limits.

Questions

1. What are the proposed benefits of newborn screening?
2. What newborn screening tests are most commonly performed?
3. How are results of newborn screening tests reported to physicians?
4. What measures should be taken when results of newborn screening tests are abnormal?
5. What are the most common causes of false-positive and false-negative tests?

Newborn screening programs were initially developed over 30 years ago. The goal was early identification of specific metabolic disorders in newborn infants; the hope was prevention, or at least amelioration, of known catastrophic outcomes associated with the delayed treatment of these conditions. Neonatal screening for multiple metabolic disorders is now routine. All 50 states in the United States require newborn screening for phenylketonuria and congenital hypothyroidism. In addition, screening tests for over 50 other disorders are now available.

Each state requires newborn screening for different conditions. The incidence of a specific disorder, the availability of effective treatment for the condition, and the financial advantages of providing early diagnosis and treatment all influence state requirements. For example, in a state where the African-American population is large, screening for hemoglobinopathies such as sickle cell anemia is particularly recommended.

Primary care physicians must participate in the standard screening program of the state in which they practice. Because all neonates must be screened and certain conditions may be life-threatening in the newborn period, it behooves pediatricians and other health care practitioners to become familiar with all aspects of the state-mandated program that affects them. Table 6–1 lists the conditions for which most states require neonatal screening.

Some newborn tests may not be state-mandated. Anonymous samples may be collected and analyzed for purely epidemiologic reasons or in conjunction with a research protocol. These results are never reported to the families or physicians. For example, random newborn screening tests may be used to determine the prevalence of HIV within a given community.

NEWBORN SCREENING PRACTICES

Parental Education and Informed Consent

The AAP recommends that all infants have a blood specimen taken for newborn screening before discharge from the nursery. All parents should therefore be informed of the state screening program either at the prenatal visit or during the initial newborn examination. Written materials that explain the screening program may be useful. Health care providers are responsible for educating parents regarding the method for obtaining the blood specimen, the risks and benefits of the screening tests, the conditions to be screened, and the implications of positive results. It is important to tell parents that positive results do not necessarily mean that their infant has a particular disorder; the results must be repeated and confirmed by more sensitive methods. In addition, parents should know that disorders in some children are missed either because of sampling errors, faulty testing, or inadequate accumulation of the abnormal metabolite at the time of testing.

TABLE 6–1. Neonatal Screening Tests Mandated by Most States in the United States

Disorders and Incidence*	No. of States	Symptoms Without Treatment	Special Considerations
Congenital hypothyroidism 1:3600–5000	50	Mental retardation, poor growth, constipation, poor appetite	Late onset of disorder in 10% of cases
Phenylketonuria (PKU) 1:10,000–25,000	50	Mental retardation, seizures, eczema	Neonatal symptoms usually absent
Galactosemia 1:60,000–80,000	45	Lethargy, feeding intolerance, vomiting, jaundice, hepatomegaly, sepsis, seizures, cataracts	Approximately 25% of unrecognized infants develop sepsis (usually *Escherichia coli*) by week 1–2 of life
Hemoglobinopathies (sickle cell disease; 1:400 African-Americans)	42	Anemia, sepsis, vaso-occlusive crisis, osteomyelitis	Clinical diagnosis is rarely made before 1 year of age if disorder not identified by newborn screening
Maple syrup urine disease 1:250,000–300,000	23	Feeding intolerance, vomiting, lethargy, severe ketoacidosis, coma, death	Death within first 2 weeks of life is not uncommon; characteristic urine odor of maple syrup or curry

*Other disorders screened for by some states: Homocystinuria (1:50,000–200,000), 21 states; biotinidase deficiency (1:40,000–70,000), 16; congenital adrenal hyperplasia (21-OH deficiency) (1:12,000), 13; tyrosinemia (<1:400,000), 7; cystic fibrosis (1:2000) (whites), 3; toxoplasmosis (1:500), 3.

Modified from Clayton, E.W. Newborn screening: legal requirements and beyond. Contemp. Pediatr. 10:35, 1993, and Buist, N.R.M., and J.M. Tuerck. The practitioner's role in newborn screening. Pediatr. Clin. North Am. 39:202–203, 1992.

Legal requirements for obtaining signed informed consent differ from state to state. Theoretically, all parents have given informed consent if practitioners have discussed the state-mandated program with them and they have agreed to participate. Although consenting parents are not required to sign any forms, parental refusal is important to document on newborns' charts regardless of state laws. Primary care practitioners must be particularly alert for signs and symptoms of undiagnosed metabolic disorders in children who have not been screened for these conditions.

Specimen Collection and Handling

Proper specimen collection and handling are essential components of a successful screening program because they may influence the results. The Committee on Genetics of the AAP has published specific guidelines regarding timing of the test, type of blood specimens that are acceptable, indications for rescreening, and influence of treatments such as transfusions and dialysis.

Recommendations concerning **timing of the test** stipulate that all newborns be screened before discharge from the nursery as close to the time of discharge as possible, and before day seven of life. If the test is performed before infants are 24 hours old (as in the case of early discharges), the test should be repeated at one to two weeks of age.

An adequate **blood specimen** can often be obtained from a heel stick. Cord blood is unacceptable for routine newborn screening because specific metabolites measured in certain tests such as phenylalanine (used to test for phenylketonuria) do not accumulate until after birth when infants have been on a normal protein diet. One drop of blood may be sufficient. Only 3μL are needed for each disk on the filter paper, but the sample must saturate the paper evenly. The use of needles and glass capillary tubes for blood collection is discouraged because they may cause hemolysis or microtears in the filter paper. The specimens must be individually air dried in a horizontal position, thus avoiding contamination and excessive exposure to heat. They should be mailed to the laboratory within 24 hours of collection.

Rescreening is currently mandated only for newborns who are less than 24 hours old (early discharges). Retesting should occur between one and two weeks of age. Infants who appear symptomatic for a metabolic disorder should be retested as well, even if initial screening results are normal. Reports indicate that initial screening tests for congenital hypothyroidism are normal in 6 to 12% of patients who have the disease.

If possible, blood samples should be obtained prior to any transfusions or dialysis. Otherwise, screening tests should still be performed as outlined above, and arrangements should be made to have them repeated at an appropriate time (i.e., at 2–3 months of age).

Other specific circumstances must also be taken into consideration when performing newborn screening tests, including prematurity, illness, hyperalimentation therapy, and antibiotic administration. Premature infants may have a low T_4 level consistent with their gestational age. Studies have reported that ill infants exposed to topical iodinated antiseptic agents can have transient hypothyroidism as well. Hyperalimentation may influence the measurement of certain amino acids. Parenteral antibiotics may inhibit the growth of bacteria used in some assays. As with transfusions and dialysis, initial specimens should still be obtained. Results should be interpreted cautiously, however, and often tests must be repeated.

Inadequate specimen collection and handling can lead to test inaccuracies, delays in reporting results to physicians, and unnecessary repetition of screening tests. Therefore, all individuals who are involved in the newborn screening process should adhere strictly to the procedures discussed above.

Reporting of Results

In most states, all results of neonatal screening tests, whether normal or abnormal, are reported to the physician of record. Normal results are mailed to the physician for placement in the patient's medical record.

Abnormal results are usually reported by telephone or letter, depending on the significance of the abnormality. Results are also sent to the hospital where the infants were born for inclusion in the medical record. The physician of record is responsible for contacting the parents regarding the need for confirmatory testing. If a newborn is no longer under the care of this physician or if the family cannot be located, state and local public health departments can be called on to assist in the search for the infant and family.

Diagnostic and Therapeutic Considerations

All abnormal results, whether borderline or clearly significant, should be evaluated by primary care physicians. In addition, a complete physical examination should be performed. Depending on the nature of the suspected disorder, initiation of treatment before repeat laboratory results are known may be appropriate. For example, prophylactic antibiotics should be administered if sickle cell anemia is suspected. After confirmatory results have been received, the treatment can be modified or halted. The ultimate decision for the initiation of early treatment, however, lies with practitioners.

Potentially life-threatening conditions in the newborn period such as galactosemia, maple syrup urine disease, and congenital adrenal hyperplasia are particularly important to evaluate and treat emergently. Depending on the clinical picture, the suspected disorder, and the experience of the practitioner, telephone consultation with a specialist or immediate referral to a regional medical center may be necessary.

If the confirmed disorder is inherited, such as cystic fibrosis or sickle cell disease, the siblings of affected infants should be carefully evaluated. Laboratory tests may be required in some instances. Families should be offered reproductive counseling for future pregnancies in addition to written information about the newly diagnosed condition.

THE FUTURE OF NEWBORN SCREENING PROGRAMS

Future screening programs will probably become more sophisticated as the inherited pattern or defect associated with particular conditions is better defined using DNA technology. The polymerase chain reaction, which amplifies a specific area of DNA, has already been applied to studies concerning the early detection of several important viral infections such as HIV and herpes simplex. This method has also proved to be particularly helpful in screening certain families who are known to have a specific mutation. At present,

the cost and labor intensiveness of this technology preclude its use for general newborn screening purposes.

No single program for screening, identification, and treatment of metabolic disorders is ideal. The decision to add metabolic disorders to existing state-mandated newborn screening programs is a complicated issue. Three questions must be asked. What is the expected effect of early intervention on the patient's outcome? Could identification of this disorder lead to increased availability of medical and educational resources for affected infants and their families? What are the broader public health consequences of undiagnosed, untreated infectious conditions (e.g., unrecognized maternal HIV infection)? Pediatricians should be involved in decisions concerning the addition of new disorders to existing newborn screening programs because they are key players in the implementation of these programs.

Case Resolution

The infant should be examined carefully for any stigmata of a metabolic condition such as hepatomegaly, lethargy, irritability, or poor weight gain. She should be placed on a soy formula until the repeat results are returned. The mother can pump her breasts to maintain her supply of milk pending the results of the repeat test. With early diagnosis and treatment, the infant's outcome is excellent.

Selected Readings

American Academy of Pediatrics, Committee on Genetics. Issues in newborn screening. Pediatrics 89:345–349, 1992.

American Academy of Pediatrics, Committee on Genetics. Newborn screening fact sheets. Pediatrics 83:449–464, 1989.

American Academy of Pediatrics, Section on Endocrinology and Committee on Genetics, American Thyroid Association Committee on Public Health. Newborn screening for congenital hypothyroidism. Pediatrics 91:1203–1209, 1993.

Buist, N. R. M., and J. M. Tuerck. The practitioner's role in newborn screening. Pediatr. Clin. North Am. 39:199–211, 1992.

Clayton, E. W. Issues in state newborn screening programs. Pediatrics 90:641–646, 1992.

Clayton, E. W. Newborn screening: legal requirements and beyond. Contemp. Pediatr. 10:34–46, 1993.

Irons, M. Screening for metabolic disorders. Pediatr. Clin. North Am. 40:1073–1085, 1993.

Kling, S. Newborn screening: an overview of newborn screening programs in the United States and Canada, 1990. Springfield, IL, Illinois Department of Health, 1993.

Listernick, R., L. Frisone, and B. L. Silverman. Delayed diagnosis of infants with abnormal neonatal screens. J.A.M.A. 267:1095–1099, 1992.

Newborn screening for sickle cell and other hemoglobinopathies. Pediatrics 83(suppl):813–914, 1989.

SCREENING IN OLDER CHILDREN AND ADOLESCENTS

Monica Sifuentes, M.D.

Hx

Before a 13-year-old girl enters a new school, she is required to have a physical examination. She has not seen a physician in five years and has been healthy. Currently she has no medical complaints. Her examination is completely normal.

Questions

1. What are the important components of the history and physical examination in apparently healthy older children and adolescents?
2. What laboratory tests should be performed at health maintenance visits? Why?
3. What are the results of screening tests likely to show?

Older children and adolescents are relatively healthy individuals who infrequently visit physicians. Visits are often for acute complaints such as pharyngitis or bronchitis and are therefore very problem-oriented. Statistics regarding health maintenance visits in this age group are not readily available, because patients go to several different sites for health care and often do not receive comprehensive care at any of these places. Older children and adolescents seek treatment for both acute and chronic conditions in private offices, public health clinics, public hospitals, and emergency rooms. It is estimated that less than 15% of adolescents go to pediatricians for health care in general, and the same percentage probably applies to older children.

This all too common practice contributes to missed opportunities for adequate health screening for preventable conditions. Screening tests can also be used to identify treatable conditions such as hypertension, anemia, and tuberculosis. Ideally, older children and adolescents should receive recommended booster immunizations; counseling concerning sexual activity, contraception, and STDs, including HIV; guidelines for adequate nutrition; education about tobacco, drugs, and alcohol; and information about physical fitness and exercise.

Guidelines for preventive child and adolescent health care have been published by the Committee on Practice and Ambulatory Medicine of the AAP, the federal Child Health and Disability Prevention Program (CHDP), the section on adolescent health of the AAP, and the AMA (Table 7–1).

TABLE 7–1. Preventive Health Services by Age and Procedure

Procedure	Early				Middle			Late			
	11	12	13	14	15	16	17	18	19	20	21
Health Guidance											
Parenting*		•				•					
Development	•	•	•	•	•	•	•	•	•	•	•
Diet and fitness	•	•	•	•	•	•	•	•	•	•	•
Lifestyle†	•	•	•	•	•	•	•	•	•	•	•
Injury prevention	•	•	•	•	•	•	•	•	•	•	•
Screening											
History											
Eating disorders	•	•	•	•	•	•	•	•	•	•	•
Sexual activity‡	•	•	•	•	•	•	•	•	•	•	•
Alcohol and other drug use	•	•	•	•	•	•	•	•	•	•	•
Tobacco use	•	•	•	•	•	•	•	•	•	•	•
Abuse	•	•	•	•	•	•	•	•	•	•	•
School performance	•	•	•	•	•	•	•	•	•	•	•
Depression	•	•	•	•	•	•	•	•	•	•	•
Risk for suicide	•	•	•	•	•	•	•	•	•	•	•
Physical Assessment											
Blood pressure	•	•	•	•	•	•	•	•	•	•	•
Body Mass Index	•	•	•	•	•	•	•	•	•	•	•
Comprehensive exam		•				•				•	
Tests§											
Cholesterol			1			1				1	
TB			2			2				2	
GC, chlamydia, and HPV			3			3				3	
HIV and syphilis			4			4				4	
Pap smear			5			5				5	
Immunizations											
MMR		•									
Td						•					
HBV			6			6				6	

*A parent health-guidance visit is recommended during early and middle adolescence.
†Includes counseling regarding sexual behavior and avoidance of tobacco, alcohol, and other drugs.
‡Includes history of unintended pregnancy and STDs.
Reproduced, with permission, from Elster, A. (ed.). American Medical Association Guidelines for Adolescent Preventive Services (GAPS): Recommendations and Rationale. Baltimore, Williams & Wilkins, 1994, p. 179.
§1: Perform screening test once if family history is positive for early cardiovascular disease or hyperlipidemia. 2: Screen if positive for exposure to active tuberculosis or patient lives or works in high-risk situation (e.g., homeless shelter, jail, health care facility). 3: Screen at least annually if sexually active. 4: Screen if high-risk for infection. 5: Screen annually if sexually active. 6: Vaccinate if high-risk for hepatitis B infection.

THE HEALTH MAINTENANCE VISIT

Questions asked during a health maintenance visit should initially be simple and focus on how children feel in general. More specific questions can then be formulated from the initial responses. In healthy patients, the medical history can be obtained using a questionnaire that parents and children complete in the waiting room. If this method is used, a separate form should be given to adolescents if they are accompanied by one or both parents. The information is then reviewed at the start of the interview. Chronic medical conditions also should be addressed at this time.

Medical History

Older children and adolescents should always be questioned directly about their medical history (see Questions Box: Screening in Older Children and Adolescents). Parents should be encouraged to participate only after their children have responded to questions or if invited by children or adolescents themselves. The degree of parental participation is also influenced by the current cognitive as well as developmental stage of patients.

Psychosocial History

The psychosocial component of the interview should be conducted with older children or adolescents alone as well as together with parents (see Questions Box). General questions about school, outside activities or hobbies, and family are often less threatening than inquiries about friends and tobacco or drug use. More sensitive topics relating to sexuality and sexual activity should be addressed after parents have left the room. Subjects initially discussed with parents should also be reviewed in their absence.

A useful tool for conducting the psychosocial interview has been developed and refined by physicians who specialize in pediatrics and adolescent medicine. Known by the acronym **HEADSSS**, it reviews the essential components of the psychosocial history: **h**ome, **e**ducation or **e**mployment, **a**ctivities, **d**rugs, **s**exual activity, **s**uicide or depression, and **s**afety (see Chapter 4, Talking to Adolescents).

Family History

Significant illnesses such as hypertension, hyperlipidemia, obesity, and diabetes in first- and second-degree family members should be reviewed. Family use of alcohol, tobacco, and illegal substances should also be determined. Age and cause of death in immediate family members should also be recorded.

Medications and Allergies

Prescription as well as nonprescription medications should be reviewed along with the indications and frequency of usage.

Physical Examination

The height and weight of patients should be plotted on a growth curve, with particular attention paid to the velocity of growth. The blood pressure should also be noted.

Aspects of the physical examination that are influenced by puberty should be emphasized. The skin should be carefully inspected for acne, and clinicians should offer treatment whether or not patients state that they have skin problems. The oropharynx should be examined for any evidence of gingivitis or other signs of poor hygiene or malocclusion. The neck should be palpated for adenopathy and the thyroid gland for hypertrophy or nodules, especially in adolescent females. The back should be examined for any evidence of scoliosis, which is important to diagnose during this time of rapid growth.

Assessment of the pubertal development of the breasts and pubic hair in preadolescent or adolescent females and the genitalia and pubic hair in adolescent males is essential. The Tanner stage can then be correlated with other signs of puberty, such as the appearance of acne and body odor. For example, the adolescent female with Tanner stage 4 breasts and immature pubic hair distribution may have a problem such as testicular feminization syndrome.

The abdomen should be palpated for organomegaly, the testicles for masses, and the external female

---

Questions: Screening in Older Children and Adolescents

Questions for both the patient and parent:
- How has the child or adolescent been lately? Does he or she have any complaints or concerns?
- How does the child or adolescent like school?
- What activities does the child or adolescent currently participate in? Does he or she have any hobbies?
- With whom does the child or adolescent live?
- Are there any significant illnesses in the immediate or extended family, such as hypertension, diabetes, or cancer?
- Does the child or adolescent take any medications (prescribed or over-the-counter) regularly?

Questions for the child or adolescent alone:
- Do you have any questions or concerns?
- How are things at home? Are there any problems with parents or siblings?
- Are you attending school?
  - Do you like school?
  - Have you ever been truant?
- Do you have friends?
- What do you do for fun?
- Do you or your friends use tobacco, drugs, or alcohol?
- Are you or your friends sexually active?
- Do you or any of your friends use contraception?
- Are you ever really sad?
  - Have you ever thought of, or tried to commit, suicide?
  - Do you have access to a gun?

genitalia for lesions. A speculum examination should be performed in sexually active females or in adolescents with a vaginal discharge or unexplained bleeding. (See Chapter 21, Reproductive Health, for additional indications for a pelvic examination.) A rectal examination is reserved for patients with chronic abdominal pain or a history of sexual activity.

Immunizations

Practitioners should verify that patients received the primary immunization series, and they should administer MMR boosters (if not given at five years of age) as well as dT boosters. A Mantoux skin test for tuberculosis also should be given. Sexually active adolescents in particular should receive the first in the series of the hepatitis B vaccine if it has not previously been administered. Other immunizations, such as influenza, pneumococcal, and meningococcal vaccines, should be considered on an individual basis.

Laboratory Tests

A hemoglobin level must be determined to check for anemia and a urinalysis must be performed, especially in sexually active adolescents, to assess for protein, blood, and pyuria. Other suggested screening tests include hearing and vision tests and a cholesterol and lipid profile. Cholesterol screening remains controversial, but it is important to consider in patients who are morbidly obese or have a positive family history for hyperlipidemia or premature atherosclerotic heart disease.

In addition to the above laboratory tests, sexually active adolescents should be screened for STDs. A cervical culture for gonorrhea, a fluorescent antibody test for chlamydia, and a Pap smear should be performed on adolescent females. Males should be screened if they are symptomatic or have a history of multiple partners and unprotected intercourse. In addition, an RPR test for syphilis should be obtained, especially if another venereal disease is evident or suspected. HIV testing is not usually emergently indicated and should be offered in the clinically appropriate setting after patients have received pretest counseling.

Patient Education

At the conclusion of the health maintenance visit, positive as well as negative findings should be reviewed with patients and their parents. Depending on the nature of these findings and the age of patients, practitioners may initially choose to address these findings with patients alone. All recommended screening laboratory studies and immunizations should also be reviewed before administration, including the need for further follow-up with tests such as the Mantoux test. Subsequent vaccine doses must be outlined for patients or parents. The timing of the next visit and reasons for this visit should be discussed.

The remainder of the visit should then be spent addressing any specific concerns of patients and parents, highlighting health care problems (e.g., obesity, high blood pressure), and identifying any factors that may be related to high-risk behavior such as drug or alcohol use. Older children or adolescents who are not participating in any deleterious activities should be praised for their positive behavior as well as provided with information regarding injury prevention.

PREPARTICIPATION PHYSICAL EXAMINATION FOR SCHOOL-AGE AND ADOLESCENT ATHLETES

The preparticipation physical examination (PPE) is essentially the "sports physical" that many schools require for participation in organized athletic programs. The primary objective of the PPE is to evaluate young athletes for musculoskeletal abnormalities that may lead to further injuries. Pediatricians can use this required visit as an opportunity to perform an annual comprehensive health maintenance examination on older children and adolescents.

Controversy exists about the appropriate location for performance of the PPE. Community physicians are often asked to perform limited en masse examinations at schools, or a group of clinicians is asked to perform the examinations in the gymnasium using "stations." Either way, the patient does not truly receive a complete physical examination or assessment, and neither approach lends itself to privacy. In addition, parents have a false sense of security and believe that their children have received adequate medical care. Ideally, primary care physicians should perform the PPE in their office during a scheduled visit at least four to six weeks before the beginning of the athletic season. At this time they should perform the general health maintenance examination, including the various screening tests.

History

The medical history for the PPE should primarily focus on previous athletic participation and any injuries that may have occurred (see Questions Box: Prepar-

---

Questions: Preparticipation Physical Examination

- What sport(s) does the child or adolescent wish to participate in?
- Has the child or adolescent ever experienced a sports injury? If so, how much time did the athlete miss doing sports activities as a result of this injury?
- Does the child or adolescent have any medical conditions?
- Is the child or adolescent taking any medications?
- Does the child or adolescent have any allergies?
- Has the child or adolescent ever had syncope, palpitations, or angina during exercise?
- Does the child or adolescent have a family history of sudden, early, nontraumatic deaths?

ticipation Physical Examination). A standard questionnaire developed by the AAP for this purpose may be used in the office setting. In addition, many practitioners record the results of the physical examination as well as their recommendations regarding the degree of athletic participation on this standard form (Table 7–2).

Physical Examination

A complete physical examination should be performed as previously described, and specific attention should be paid to the musculoskeletal system. The "two-minute orthopedic examination" consists of a head-to-toe assessment of all muscle groups and joints; any

---

TABLE 7–2. Sports Participation Health Record

This evaluation is only to determine readiness for sports participation. It should not be used as a substitute for regular health maintenance examinations.

NAME _____ AGE _____ (YRS) GRADE _____ DATE _____

ADDRESS _____ PHONE _____

SPORTS _____

The Health History (Part A) and Physical Examination (Part C) sections must both be completed, at least every 24 months, before sports participation. The Interim Health History section (Part B) needs to be completed at least annually.

PART A — HEALTH HISTORY:
To be completed by athlete and parent

YES NO

1. Have you ever had an illness that:
   a. required you to stay in the hospital?
   b. lasted longer than a week?
   c. caused you to miss 3 days of practice or a competition?
   d. is related to allergies (ie, hay fever, hives, asthma, insect stings)?
   e. required an operation?
   f. is chronic (ie, asthma, diabetes, etc)?
2. Have you ever had an injury that:
   a. required you to go to an emergency room or see a doctor?
   b. required you to stay in the hospital?
   c. required x-rays?
   d. caused you to miss 3 days of practice or a competition?
   e. required an operation?
3. Do you take any medication or pills?
4. Have any members of your family under age 50 had a heart attack, heart problem, or died unexpectedly?
5. Have you ever:
   a. been dizzy or passed out during or after exercise?
   b. been unconscious or had a concussion?
6. Are you unable to run 1/2 mile (2 times around the track) without stopping??
7. Do you:
   a. wear glasses or contacts?
   b. wear dental bridges, plates, or braces?
8. Have you ever had a heart murmur, high blood pressure, or a heart abnormality?
9. Do you have any allergies to any medicine?
10. Are you missing a kidney?
11. When was your last tetanus booster? _____
12. For Women
   a. At what age did you experience your first menstrual period? _____
   b. In the last year, what is the longest time you have gone between periods?

EXPLAIN ANY "YES" ANSWERS _____

I hereby state that, to the best of my knowledge, my answers to the above questions are correct.

Date _____

Signature of athlete _____

Signature of parent _____

PART B — INTERIM HEALTH HISTORY:
This form should be used during the interval between preparticipation evaluations. Positive responses should prompt a medical evaluation.

1. Over the next 12 months, I wish to participate in the following sports:
   a. _____
   b. _____
   c. _____
   d. _____
2. Have you missed more than 3 consecutive days of participation in usual activities because of an injury this past year?
   Yes _____ No _____
   If yes, please indicate:
   a. Site of injury _____
   b. Type of injury _____
3. Have you missed more than 5 consecutive days of participation in usual activities because of an illness, or have you had a medical illness diagnosed that has not been resolved in this past year?
   Yes _____ No _____
   If yes, please indicate:
   a. Type of illness _____
4. Have you had a seizure, concussion or been unconscious for any reason in the last year?
   Yes _____ No _____
5. Have you had surgery or been hospitalized in this past year?
   Yes _____ No _____
   If yes, please indicate:
   a. Reason for hospitalization _____
   b. Type of surgery _____
6. List all medications you are presently taking and what condition the medication is for.
   a. _____
   b. _____
   c. _____
7. Are you worried about any problem or condition at this time?
   Yes _____ No _____
   If yes, please explain: _____

I heareby state that, to the best of my knowledge, my answers to the above questions are correct.

Date _____

Signature of athlete _____

Signature of parent _____

TABLE 7–2. Sports Participation Health Record *Continued*

PART C: PHYSICAL EXAMINATION RECORD

NAME _____ DATE _____ AGE _____ BIRTHDATE _____

Height _____ Vision: R _____/_____, corrected _____, uncorrected _____

Weight _____ L _____/_____, corrected _____, uncorrected _____

Pulse _____ Blood Pressure _____ Percent Body Fat (optional) _____

	Normal	Abnormal Findings	Initials
1. Eyes			
2. Ears, Nose, Throat			
3. Mouth & Teeth			
4. Neck			
5. Cardiovascular			
6. Chest and Lungs			
7. Abdomen			
8. Skin			
9. Genitalia—Hernia (male)			
10. Musculoskeletal: ROM, strength, etc.			
a. neck			
b. spine			
c. shoulders			
d. arms/hands			
e. hips			
f. thighs			
g. knees			
h. ankles			
i. feet			
11. Neuromuscular			
12. Physical Maturity (Tanner Stage)		1. 2. 3. 4. 5.	

Comments re: Abnormal Findings: _____

_____

_____

PARTICIPATION RECOMMENDATIONS:

1. No participation in: _____

_____

2. Limited participation in: _____

3. Requires: _____

_____

4. Full participation in: _____

Physician Signature _____

Telephone Number _____ Address _____

Reproduced, with permission, from Sports Medicine: Health Care for Young Athletes, 2nd ed. Elk Grove Village, IL, American Academy of Pediatrics, 1991.

TABLE 7–3. The Two-Minute Orthopedic Examination

Instructions	Points of Observation
Stand facing examiner	Acromioclavicular joints, general habitus
Look at ceiling, floor, over both shoulders; touch ears to shoulders	Cervical spinal motion
Shrug shoulders (examiner resists)	Trapezius strength
Abduct shoulders 90 degrees	Deltoid strength
Full external rotation of arms	Shoulder motion
Flex and extend elbows	Elbow motion
Arms at sides, elbows 90 degrees flexed; pronate and supinate wrists	Elbow and wrist motion
Spread fingers; make fist	Hand or finger motion and deformities
Tighten (contract) quadriceps; relax quadriceps	Symmetry and knee effusion; ankle effusion
"Duck walk" four steps (away from examiner with buttocks on heels)	Hip, knee, and ankle motion
Back to examiner	Shoulder symmetry, scoliosis
Knees straight, touch toes	Scoliosis, hip motion, hamstring tightness
Raise up on toes, raise heels	Calf symmetry, leg strength

Reproduced, with permission, from Sports Medicine: Health Care for Young Athletes, 2nd ed. Elk Grove Village, IL, American Academy of Pediatrics, 1991, p. 54.

deformities, anomalies, or evidence of previous injuries are noted (Table 7–3).

Laboratory Tests

Routine laboratory screening tests, except for those performed during the general health maintenance visit, are not recommended for the PPE. Screening young athletes for anemia or proteinuria has not been found to be particularly helpful. Such screening may be useful with highly competitive professional athletes, however.

Exclusion Criteria

Medical exclusion criteria for athletic participation are based on information obtained in the medical as well as family history. Findings such as stature consistent with Marfan's syndrome, cardiac arrhythmia, or the midsystolic click of mitral valve prolapse may be discovered during the physical examination. Specific conditions, such as the athlete with one eye or one kidney, should be evaluated on an individual basis by a physician qualified to assess the safety of the particular sport for the athlete (contact/collision versus limited contact).

Significant historical clues include a family history of sudden, nontraumatic death; premature coronary artery disease in a first- or second-degree relative; a history of palpitations, angina, or syncope during exercise; and recent, documented infection with EBV. Controversy exists regarding when athletes can return to collision sports after infectious mononucleosis. The most common causes of unexpected death during athletics include cardiomyopathies, anomalous coronary arteries, heart valve defects, primary cardiac rhythm disorders, and pulmonary hypertension.

Special circumstances to consider during the PPE are menstrual disorders and the female athlete; exercise-induced bronchospasm; anabolic steroid use; and eating disorders that may be associated with certain activities such as gymnastics, ballet, and wrestling.

Case Resolution

The young adolescent described in the case history should first be interviewed with the parent and then alone. Her medical and psychosocial history should be reviewed. A complete physical examination should be performed as well as a pelvic examination if she is sexually active. General laboratory screening tests should be performed and the results reviewed with the patient. The remainder of the visit should be spent discussing issues such as nutrition, exercise, illicit substance abuse, sexuality and sexual activity, and safety. Results of the physical examination and screening tests should then be discussed with the parent who accompanied her to the office. If necessary, a follow-up visit should be scheduled. Otherwise, the adolescent should be seen annually.

Selected Readings

American Academy of Pediatrics, Committee on Sports Medicine and Fitness. Medical conditions affecting sports participation. Pediatrics 94:757–760, 1994.

Cromer, B. A., C. S. McLean, and F. P. Heald. A critical review of comprehensive health screening in adolescents. J. Adolesc. Health 13:1S–65S, 1992.

Elster, A. (ed.). American Medical Association Guidelines for Adolescent Preventive Services (GAPS): Recommendations and Rationale. Baltimore, Williams & Wilkins, 1994.

Igra, V., and S. G. Millstein. Current status and approaches to improving preventive services for adolescents. J.A.M.A. 269:1408–1412, 1993.

National Cholesterol Education Program (NCEP). Highlights of the report of the expert panel on blood cholesterol levels in children and adolescents. Pediatrics 89:495–501, 1992.

Rowlett, J. D., D. E. Greydanus, and D. R. Patel. The Adolescent Health Maintenance Examination. In Section on Adolescent Health Newsletter, American Academy of Pediatrics 12:73–95, 1991.

Sports Medicine: Health Care for Young Athletes, 2nd ed. American Academy of Pediatrics, 1991.

Steiner, N. J., L. S. Neinstein, and J. Pennbridge. Hypercholesterolemia in adolescents: effectiveness of screening strategies based on selected risk factors. Pediatrics 88:269–275, 1991.

U.S. Preventive Services Task Force. Screening for adolescent idiopathic scoliosis: policy statement. J.A.M.A. 269:2664–2672, 1992.

HEALTH MAINTENANCE AND ANTICIPATORY GUIDANCE

CHAPTER 8

NEONATAL EXAMINATION AND NURSERY VISIT

Monica Sifuentes, M.D.

Hx You are performing a discharge examination on a one-day-old infant, who was born at 39 weeks' gestation to a 28-year-old healthy primigravida via normal vaginal delivery. There were no complications. The infant weighed 7 lb, 1 oz (3200 g) and was 19.7 inches (50 cm) long at birth. The mother received prenatal care beginning at 10 weeks' gestation; had no prenatal problems, including infections; and used no drugs, alcohol, or tobacco during the pregnancy. Her blood type is O positive, and she is negative for the hepatitis B surface antigen and nonreactive for syphilis. The father is also healthy.

On physical examination, the infant is average size-for-gestational-age with a length and head circumference in the 50th percentile. Aside from small bilateral subconjunctival hemorrhages, the rest of the physical examination is entirely normal.

Questions

1. What parts of the maternal history are important to review before performing the infant's physical examination?
2. What aspects of the physical examination of newborns are essential to explain to parents?
3. What physical findings mandate a more extensive work-up prior to discharge?
4. What are important points to cover with parents at the discharge examination of a normal term newborn?
5. What laboratory studies, if any, should be performed prior to discharge?

The purpose of the newborn nursery visit is to answer the question foremost in a parent's mind: "Is the baby normal?" By performing a physical examination in the parents' presence during the infant's first 24 hours of life, pediatricians can play a major role in allaying parental anxiety. In addition, medical problems that the newborn may experience in this important transitional period to extrauterine life may be detected. Treatment can be initiated, if necessary, before discharge from the nursery.

PEDIATRIC PRENATAL VISIT

Ideally, the pediatrician has spoken with the parents at a prenatal visit before meeting them in the hospital. This meeting provides a time when the parents are able to interview the physician as well as the rest of the office staff regarding general policies and procedures for well child appointments, sick visits, and contacting the physician after hours. It also is a time to discuss what will take place at the hospital and explain the role of allied health professionals (e.g., lactation specialists) in the overall care of the mother and newborn. For pediatricians and other health care practitioners, the prenatal visit is a time to gather vital medical information regarding the current pregnancy, inquire about any problems with previous deliveries, and review any pertinent family history. In addition, it is important that physicians be sensitive to cultural rituals or ceremonies surrounding the birth of an infant and inquire about any specific familial preferences before delivery. Whether the infant is born at a birthing center or in the more traditional hospital setting, arrangements should be made to accommodate the wishes of the family. The prenatal visit also allows physicians to assess any psychosocial issues that may negatively influence initial maternal-infant bonding, such as maternal drug use, paternal uninvolvement, or the absence of a supportive social network. Other issues such as breast-feeding, circumcision, and child passenger safety can also be introduced.

NEONATAL NURSERY VISIT

The timing of the newborn visit and its length depend on several factors, including the type of delivery (vaginal delivery or cesarean section), the history of prenatal care, and the occurrence of any perinatal complications, such as severe, prolonged bradycardia or meconium aspiration. These complications may warrant early neonatal examination in the nursery. Other reasons for a more lengthy initial visit include suspected congenital anomalies (e.g., congenital heart disease, hydronephrosis) as noted on prenatal fetal ultrasound, a history of prematurity, the presence of maternal fever or sepsis, ABO or Rh incompatibility, and any evidence of infant drug withdrawal.

EVALUATION

Perinatal History

The prenatal history and results of maternal laboratory tests, such as blood type, RPR status, and chlamydial and gonococcal cultures, should be noted (see Questions Box). Perinatal events should then be reviewed before performing the physical examination of the neonate. This review helps the physician focus the examination on findings consistent with the maternal history. The occurrence of any unusual circumstances surrounding the delivery must also be explained to the parents at this time. They may be very puzzled by a sudden change in plans such as the need for an emergent cesarean section. It is also important to be prepared to discuss the medical implications of such events and to address any concerns the parents may have concerning the newborn infant.

Physical Examination

Every attempt should be made to perform the neonatal physical examination at the bedside. This gives the physician an opportunity to meet with parents and gives parents a chance to have all their initial questions answered immediately. In certain circumstances, such as when the infant is premature or when the mother is particularly exhausted during postpartum, a bedside examination may be impossible to perform. In any event, physicians or other health care providers should speak to parents about the results once the examination has been completed.

The neonatal examination should be performed with the infant completely unclothed and the infant's body temperature maintained. A search for congenital anomalies is the priority. The infant's birth weight, length, and head circumference should be plotted; physicians should keep in mind that these measurements are often made in the delivery room and may be subject to error. Temperature, respiratory rate, and heart rate should be reviewed via the nursery record.

The infant's overall appearance should be noted, particularly for the presence of any dysmorphic features. Physicians should determine whether the infant looks normal or has any abnormal facial features such as low set ears and widely spaced eyes. The presence and location of any rashes or birthmarks should also be carefully noted; the location aids in the diagnosis of the lesion.

Head

Head size and shape, including the size of the fontanelle and the position of the sutures, should be evaluated. A cephalohematoma, which is a subperiosteal bleed that does not cross the suture line, appears as a unilateral lump on the side of the head and can be quite disfiguring. This should be differentiated from a caput succedaneum, which occurs at the crown of the head crossing the midline, and can be indented by pressure. Both conditions occur commonly and are often a source of concern to parents.

Eyes

The eyes should be evaluated for subconjunctival hemorrhages, extraocular movements, and the presence of red reflexes. Any difficulty in obtaining a red reflex should be taken seriously, because conditions such as congenital cataracts are important to diagnose early in life.

Ears

The placement, size, and shape of the pinnae should be noted as well, along with any preauricular pits or appendages. The presence of a significant auricular abnormality suggests an associated renal anomaly.

Nose

The nose should be checked carefully. Choanal atresia is an important condition to rule out, because infants are obligate nose breathers until three months of age.

Questions: Neonatal Examination

- Did the mother receive prenatal care? If so, since what month of gestation?
- Were all prenatal studies normal?
- Does either parent have a history of STDs, such as syphilis, gonorrhea, or herpes?
- Does either parent have a history of alcohol, tobacco, or illicit drug use?
- Did the mother take any prescribed or over-the-counter medications routinely during pregnancy?
- Did the mother have any complications, such as bleeding or decreased fetal movement, during the pregnancy?
- Does the neonate have any siblings? If so, what are their ages?
- Is anyone available to help with the new baby or siblings?

Mouth

The oropharynx should be examined closely for any defects in the hard palate. A bifid uvula may indicate a submucosal defect of the soft palate that may be difficult to appreciate without palpation (see Chapter 44, Craniofacial Anomalies). Common normal findings in the oropharynx, including Epstein's pearls located at the midline on the hard palate and epithelial cysts along the gum line, should also be noted. Loose natal teeth should be removed to prevent the possibility of aspiration.

Chest

The neck should be palpated for sternocleidomastoid hematomas and the clavicles for fractures, especially in infants who are large-for-gestational-age. Chest wall deformities such as a pectus excavatum should be noted. The presence of breast buds and supernumerary nipples are of no clinical consequence, although widely spaced nipples suggest Turner's syndrome.

Heart

Cardiac murmurs should be appreciated and documented. The presence of a murmur does not always indicate complex congenital heart disease, however. Each case should be evaluated on an individual basis, and advice from specialists in pediatric cardiology should be sought as necessary. Equal and symmetric pulses should also be palpated in all extremities.

Abdomen

The abdomen should be palpated for any masses or organomegaly (e.g., polycystic kidneys, hepatosplenomegaly) that warrant further investigation.

Genitalia

In female neonates, the labia majora are often swollen, making an examination of the hymen difficult, but clitoral size should be noted. Parents should be told that the physiologic vaginal discharge and the presence later of a bloody discharge are a normal neonatal response to maternal estrogen withdrawal. In uncircumcised male infants, it is imperative that the foreskin be retracted sufficiently to reveal the location of the urethra. A testicular examination can rule out hydroceles, inguinal hernias, and cryptorchidism.

Skeleton

The Ortolani test is performed to evaluate the newborn for congenital hip dislocations. The "clunk" felt when performing the examination is the relocation of the femoral head of the affected hip in the joint capsule. In contrast, a "click" may indicate normal perinatal ligament laxity. The spine should be palpated completely to the sacrum. Sacral defects, deep sacral pits, or sacral tufts of hair warrant an investigation for such conditions as spina bifida occulta. Fingers and toes should be counted.

TABLE 8–1. Normal Physical Findings in Newborns

Skin
Milia, erythema toxicum, salmon patch, nevus flammeus, hemangiomas, Mongolian spots, lanugo (body hair)
Head
Cephalohematoma, caput succedaneum
Face
Swollen overall appearance
Eyes
Swollen eyelids, subconjunctival hemorrhages
Ears
Preauricular appendages/pits, folded pinnas
Nose
Flattened nose, milia over bridge
Mouth and Throat
Epstein's pearls, epithelial pearls, natal teeth, shortened frenulum
Chest
Supernumerary nipples, breast buds, galactorrhea, pectus excavatum or carinatum
Genitalia
Females: swollen labia, hymenal tags, vaginal discharge
Males: hydrocele, undescended testicle (palpated in inguinal canal)
Hips
Click
Extremities
Feet turned up, in, or out, but malleable
Neurologic Examination
Primitive reflexes: Moro, grasp, rooting, stepping

Neurologic Examination

Primitive reflexes such as the Moro, rooting, grasp, and stepping reflexes are a primary component of the neonatal neurologic examination. In addition, tone, sensation, and deep tendon reflexes should be evaluated. Tone can be assessed by holding the infant upright below the shoulder girdle or by observing the crying infant; all extremities should be in the flexed position.

Normal findings of the nursery physical examination are summarized in Table 8–1. Emergent findings that must be addressed immediately when noted at the initial nursery examination include evidence of hydrocephalus, a ductal dependent cardiac lesion, a diaphragmatic hernia, an abdominal mass, or a possible chromosomal abnormality such as trisomy 13 or trisomy 18. The physical conditions associated with trisomy 21 are rarely life-threatening, although its suspicion does warrant a careful examination and evaluation for cardiac and abdominal anomalies (see Chapter 18, Well Child Care for Children With Trisomy 21).

Laboratory Tests

The only laboratory test required of all newborns prior to discharge from the nursery is the newborn screening heel stick for inheritable conditions such as phenylketonuria and hypothyroidism. Mandated neonatal screening varies by state and depends on the prevalence of a particular disease in a given region (see Chapter 6, Screening in Newborns).

Other laboratory tests that are often performed include a serum glucose, especially in lethargic, polycythemic, or jittery infants, and a hematocrit in jaundiced or ruddy-appearing newborns. In cases of ABO or Rh incompatibility, a serum bilirubin and a Coombs' test are often necessary to obtain after confirming the maternal and infant blood types.

Imaging Studies

Routine x-rays are not indicated in neonates whose newborn examination is normal or who have minor abnormalities such as pectus excavatum. Vertebral x-rays are appropriate in the neonate with a deep sacral pit or sacral tuft of hair for the diagnosis of spina bifida occulta. Clavicular x-rays are indicated if swelling or pain is located in the clavicular area or if an asymmetric Moro reflex is elicited. A chest x-ray and ECG are warranted for a significant murmur. A renal ultrasound is appropriate in the infant with significant ear deformities. More extensive studies are necessary if an emergent physical finding is discovered.

MANAGEMENT

The administration of intramuscular vitamin K and the application of ophthalmic ointment or silver nitrate in the newborn's eyes is universal. Because of the possibility of maternal infection with HIV, many institutions are reevaluating the timing of the vitamin K administration. They are waiting until all maternal blood is washed from the infant before giving the injection. The infant is then kept in the transitional nursery in an isolette for the initial few hours following delivery to ensure the maintenance of an adequate body temperature and stable vital signs. Serum glucose is often monitored as well.

If desired, the circumcision is usually performed on the day of discharge (see Chapter 10, Circumcision). Local anesthesia is now universally recommended for the procedure, but its use remains at the discretion of the physician and parents. Following the procedure, the parents are instructed to leave the gauze or Plastibell in place. It will fall off spontaneously. Petroleum ointment may also be placed on the corona of the penis to prevent its sticking to the diaper. The physician should be notified if excessive bleeding or oozing occurs (e.g., soaking of the diaper with blood) after discharge from the nursery.

DISCHARGE PLANNING/COUNSELING

Before the infant is discharged to home, physicians should discuss normal variants found on the physical examination with parents. Abnormal physical findings

and their relevance should also be explained. If any further studies were performed other than routine neonatal screening, parents should also be informed of the results.

Other topics that should be covered at the bedside include breast-feeding versus bottle feeding, sleeping and elimination patterns in the newborn, umbilical cord care, bathing the newborn, and safety issues such as car seats. In addition, the timing of the first dose of the hepatitis B vaccine should be discussed. It can be administered prior to hospital discharge or at the first follow-up visit. Guidelines regarding when to call the office or emergency department should also be addressed. These include a fever of 100.4° F (38.0° C), irritability, lethargy, and evidence of dehydration. Parents should be encouraged to call the physician's office about any concern they may have, especially if they are first-time parents, and to trust their own instincts. A follow-up visit should be arranged for one to three weeks after discharge.

Case Resolution

In the case presented at the beginning of the chapter, the parents should be told that the weight, length, and head circumference are all normal. The subconjunctival hemorrhages should be shown to the parents and their self-limited nature explained. Routine neonatal screening, feeding, sleeping, elimination, bathing, and safety should be reviewed. Prior to discharge, the infant should receive the hepatitis B vaccine. A follow-up appointment should be made for one to three weeks of age.

Selected Readings

American Academy of Pediatrics, Vitamin K Ad Hoc Task Force. Controversies concerning vitamin K and the newborn. Pediatrics 91:1001–1003, 1993.

American Academy of Pediatrics and the American College of Obstetrics and Gynecologists. Guidelines for Perinatal Care, 3rd ed. Elk Grove, IL, American Academy of Pediatrics, 1992.

Britton, J. R., H. L. Britton, and S. A. Beebe. Early discharge of the term newborn: a continued dilemma. Pediatrics 94:291–295, 1994.

Conrad, P. D., R. B. Wilkening, and A. A. Rosenberg. Safety of newborn discharge in less than 36 hours in an indigent population. Am. J. Dis. Child. 143:98–101, 1989.

Hurt, H. Early discharge for newborns—when is it safe? Contemp. Pediatr. 11:68–88, 1994.

Schmitt, B. D. Characteristics of newborn babies. *In* Your Child's Health, 2nd ed. New York, Bantam Books, 1991.

Schmitt, B. D. The first weeks at home with your new baby. *In* Your Child's Health, 2nd ed. New York, Bantam Books, 1991.

CHAPTER 9

CARING FOR TWINS

Carol D. Berkowitz, M.D.

H$_x$ An expectant mother visits you. She has been advised by her obstetrician that ultrasound shows she is pregnant with twins. She asks about care of twins and what special considerations she should keep in mind as she looks forward to the delivery. In particular, she is concerned about the feeding schedule and whether she will be able to breast-feed.

Questions

1. What is the incidence of multiple births?
2. What is the difference between fraternal and identical twins?
3. What major medical problems may affect twins?
4. What developmental and behavioral problems are associated with raising twins?

Counseling the mother of twins is a unique opportunity for pediatricians. In the past, twins were often not diagnosed before delivery. With the advent of ultrasound, the diagnosis is made prenatally in over 90% of cases. Many societies have been fascinated with twins, and many myths and superstitions surround their birth. Some people believe that a mother of twins must have been unfaithful to her husband because a father cannot sire two children. To prevent the recurrence of twins, the Khoikhain remove one of the father's testicles.

Part of the fascination with twins relates to the concern about being able to tell them apart. Mark Twain wrote, "My twin and I got mixed up in the bath when we were only two weeks old, and one was drowned, but we never knew which." Researchers have noted marked differences in temperament and responsiveness of twins. Twins are different, and maintaining the individuality of each twin is important both for the parents and for the health care provider.

Parents of twins often have many questions that concern their care, but they rarely pose them to health care providers. In one study in which 18 out of 29 mothers breast-fed their twins, only three received information about breast-feeding from their physicians. One mother had been told by her obstetrician that she could not breast-feed her twins. Physicians should become knowledgeable about caring for twins. They can help the parents of twins with problems related to feeding, sleeping, and behavior.

EPIDEMIOLOGY

The overall incidence of twin births is about 1 in 87. Twins account for just slightly more than 1% of all births, and 20% of infants born under 30 weeks' gestation are twins. The average incidence of monozygotic or identical twins, which is the same for all women regardless of race and age, is about 1 in 250 births. The incidence of dizygotic or fraternal twins varies among different groups. In the United States it is 0.6 per 100 in Caucasians and 0.9 per 100 in African Americans. The occurrence of dizygotic twins may be inherited recessively in some families. The likelihood of dizygotic twins is believed to be higher in low socioeconomic classes and in mothers between the ages of 35 and 40. In older mothers the incidence is 10-fold that of teenage mothers. Births of twins increase after the fifth pregnancy, the use of oral contraceptives, and the use of fertility drugs. After the use of such drugs twin births reportedly occur in up to 50% of cases.

PATHOPHYSIOLOGY

Monozygotic twins result from the splitting of a single egg. They may share a placenta (monochorionic and monoamniotic) (Fig. 9–1A and 1B). When splitting occurs early (after several cell divisions of the zygote), each fetus develops its own chorion and amnion, leading to dichorionic and diamniotic placentas. Dizygotic twins result from two eggs, and each egg is fertilized by a different sperm. Dizygotic twins have two placentas (Fig. 9–1C). Although these placentas may fuse together like two pancakes, they are always dichorionic and diamniotic (Fig. 9–1D).

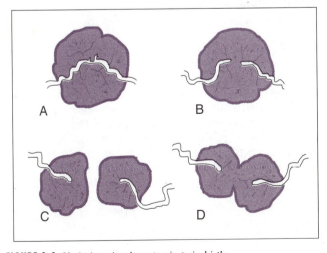

FIGURE 9–1. *Variations in placentas in twin births.*
A. *Monochorionic, monoamniotic placenta, cords close together.*
B. *Monochorionic, monoamniotic placenta, cords further apart.*
C. *Dichorionic, diamniotic placentas, separate.*
D. *Dichorionic, diamniotic placentas, fused.*

Following the birth, it is important to determine whether twins are monozygotic or dizygotic. About 50% of families specifically request this information. If transplantation becomes a concern, this knowledge is also significant. Monozygotic twins have a higher incidence of malformations. Different sex twins are almost always dizygotic, although monozygotic twins of different sexes have been reported in the literature. This occurs when one twin loses a Y chromosome and becomes a phenotypic female with Turner's Syndrome (XO). Occasionally the male twin may be XXY and have Klinefelter's syndrome.

To determine whether twins are monozygotic or dizygotic, a number of procedures can be undertaken. Visual or pathologic examination of the placenta is helpful. About two-thirds of monozygotic twins have a common chorion and share one placenta. Finding a single chorion usually means the twins are monozygotic, unless the placentas of dizygotic twins have fused together (see above). Examination of hair whorls, iris patterns, ear configuration, eye color, dental morphology, and fingerprint patterns may give a clue to the type of twinning. Laboratory evaluation to determine the nature of twinning begins with human leukocyte antigen (HLA) testing. The HLA genes are on chromosome 6. Dizygotic twins have a 20% chance of having the same HLA type. If the HLA types are the same, the next step involves testing blood group types. If the blood group types are the same, enzyme and protein analysis should be undertaken. Enzymes, such as phosphoglucomutase, and proteins, such as haptoglobin and transferrin, should be evaluated. Agreement in all these areas suggests that the twins are monozygotic.

DIFFERENTIAL DIAGNOSIS

Diagnosing twins is not difficult, but physicians should be aware that twins may have problems.

Perinatal Complications

The perinatal mortality of monozygotic twins is eight times that of singletons and four times that of dizygotic twins as a result of many factors, including small size and prematurity. Twins have a mean gestational age of 262 days, as opposed to 280 days for singletons. The mean gestational age for monozygotic twins is less than for dizygotic twins. In addition, hydramnios is 16 times more likely to occur in twin pregnancies. Other perinatal complications associated with twin births include pregnancy-induced hypertension, placenta previa, antepartum hemorrhage, prolapse of the cord, abnormal presentation, and uterine inertia. In 41% of twin pregnancies, both twins are delivered by vertex presentation. In 37% of births, one twin is breech, and in 8%, both twins are breech.

Congenital Malformations

Monozygotic twins have a higher incidence of congenital malformations. Anomalies that have been reported with increased incidence include anencephaly and spina bifida, holoprosencephaly, VATERL, and limb defects association (**v**ertebral defects, imperforate **a**nus, **t**racheoesophageal fistula, **r**enal dysplasia, and **l**imb defects), sirenomelia (mermaidlike extremity), and extrophy of the cloaca. In addition to malformations, twins may suffer from deformations secondary to crowding. Growth in twins tends to be normal until 30 to 34 weeks, when the combined weight of twins reaches 8 lb, 13 oz (4 kg).

Postnatal Complications

Smaller twins have an increased incidence of hypoglycemia. Twin-to-twin transfusions, which may account for persistent growth differences, are seen in 10 to 15% of monochorional pregnancies. Artery-to-vein shunts result in one twin transfusing the other, and this may be diagnosed prenatally by ultrasound of the placenta, which shows one sac with oligohydramnios and the other sac with polyhydramnios. Artery-to-artery shunts and vein-to-vein shunts can also be anticipated by ultrasound and result in twin-to-twin transfusions.

EVALUATION

History

A general medical history should be obtained, including a history of the pregnancy. Any specific medical complaints should also be addressed (see Questions Box).

Physical Examination

The initial evaluation of newly born twins involves assessment of gestational age and determination of the presence of any medical problems or anomalies (see Chapter 8, Neonatal Examination). Older twins should undergo health maintenance visits where routine as well as specific complaints are addressed.

Laboratory Tests

The twins should be assessed in the newborn period for the presence of anemia or polycythemia with a hemoglobin determination. Hypoglycemia may occur in the newborn period and can be assessed with a rapid test, such as a Dextrostix or a serum glucose. If the twins are premature, they may have many of the problems seen in preterm infants, such as respiratory distress syndrome and necrotizing enterocolitis.

Older twins should receive an appropriate evalua-

Questions: Caring for Twins

- Did the mother have any problems during the pregnancy?
- How long did the pregnancy last?
- Did the mother take any medications, including fertility drugs?
- Did either twin have any problem after the delivery or in the newborn nursery?
- Which was twin A (first-born twin) and which was twin B (second-born twin)?

tion for age, with a specific focus on any behavioral concerns.

MANAGEMENT

The focus of the management of twins involves counseling the mother about issues related to routine care. Mothers often care for two or more children at the same time, but twins are two children who are developmentally and chronologically at the same point in time. *Twins Magazine* (800-821-5533), which is published bimonthly, contains pertinent articles and lists organizations to help parents of twins.

Feeding is a major issue. Breast-feeding is both physically and emotionally possible. Wet nurses have fed up to six infants at a time, and the difficulty appears more with timing and positioning of the infants rather than with the supply of milk. Some suggestions about breast-feeding twins follow.

1. Feed both infants at the same time, with one on each breast. The infants may be put in a number of positions. The mother can be sitting and cradling one infant while holding the other infant like a football. Alternatively, the mother may cradle both infants, so that they are lying over one another, or she may have both infants under her arms in a football position. Both infants may not be hungry at the same time, however, which may present a problem.

2. Feed the infants at different times. The mother breast-feeds one infant and then the other. The mother starts with the more vigorous feeder. This approach may pose a problem; both infants may be hungry at the same time.

3. Breast-feed one infant and bottle-feed the other, which gives the mother a free hand. Bottle-feeding presents certain difficulties too, primarily cost.

Research shows that mothers who bottle-feed their twins use powder rather than concentrated formula and wean their infants from formula earlier than is recommended. Breast-feeding mothers tend to breast-feed their infants longer for economic reasons. One problem with formula feeding concerns storage, that is, making up enough formula and having enough room to keep a supply of milk. It is suggested that a half-day supply be prepared to reduce the needed storage space. Another suggestion involves the use of plastic-bag nursers because they take up less room. Some physicians recommend sticking to a feeding schedule for twins. A mother can let the first infant feed on demand but wake up the second one when the first one is done. Eighty percent of parents of twins acknowledge that they prop the bottle instead of holding it, and they should be counseled about this.

Twin infants on solid foods should be given two meals a day instead of three. Putting strained baby food in the bottle to facilitate feeding is also an option. Most parents of twins use one dish and one spoon and feed both infants at the same time using this technique.

Sleeping is also a consideration. Many parents use one crib with a partition, but the twins may disturb one another. A play pen is bigger and provides more room. Twins on apnea monitors should not sleep next to each other, however, because their wires can become entangled. Twin strollers, which are available in different types, are useful. Some strollers have seats adjacent to each other, but sometimes these are too wide to fit through a doorway. Other strollers have the infants facing each other, which may be a problem because of fighting.

Children should have separate dressers, clothing areas, and toys. Diapers are also an issue. Disposable diapers are more convenient, but the cost is high. Diaper services are less expensive, and many parents choose to use cloth diapers and rinse them out themselves. Toilet training is reportedly easier with some twins because one twin learns from the other.

It is important to counsel parents about **car seats.** Parents who cannot afford the cost of two car seats may resort to placing one twin in the car seat and the other on the seat of the car, a dangerous practice that is illegal in all states in the United States. Parents should be advised about the need for car seats for both infants. Consideration can be given to renting car seats.

Bathing should be done separately in the interests of safety.

Having twins is a **financial hardship** for some families. Some mothers must leave work 2 to 3 months before delivery because of their large size. Prematurity necessitates prolonged hospitalization. Physicians should consider whether a discount should be given if twins are seen at the same time.

Maternal fatigue is another important issue. One mother said that her physician should be aware that she was like a zombie because she was not getting enough sleep. Physicians frequently recommend that mothers rest when infants rest. With twins, however, this is rarely possible because of the so-called "ping-pong" effect. While one infant sleeps, the other gets up, and as soon as the second one falls asleep, the first one is up again.

Help from fathers is variable in families with twins. Physicians should check with mothers about how much help they are receiving from husbands. If help is not forthcoming, they should schedule a family meeting at one month. It is also important to suggest that mothers of twins obtain outside aid, including help from high school students after school and even mothers-in-law.

Lastly, **maintenance of individuality** for twins may be challenging. Researchers suggest that mothers can bond to only one infant at a time, a concept called monotropy. For this reason, twins are often dressed alike and given similar names. This may facilitate the bonding process. To help with individual development, physicians are encouraged to examine each child individually. Twins should not be referred to as "the twins" but by their respective names. As twins get older, issues related to classrooms and birthday parties frequently arise, and they should be consulted concerning their preferences. It is often recommended that twins be in different classrooms and that they be allowed to have individual birthday parties.

PROGNOSIS

Although twins have a higher incidence of perinatal problems, appropriate anticipatory guidance and routine health maintenance result in normal growth and development.

Case Resolution

The mother in the case scenario is advised that breast-feeding is not only possible but recommended. She is told about the options for timing and positioning of the infants. The issues of family history and child passenger safety are also discussed.

Selected Readings

Baldwin, V. J. Pathology of Multiple Pregnancy. New York, Springer-Verlag, 1994.

Becker, P. G. Counseling families with twins: birth to 3 years of age. Pediatr. Rev. 8:81–86, 1986.

Blickstein, I., and M. Lancet. The growth discordant twin. Obstet. Gynecol. Surv. 43:509–515, 1988.

Dungy, C. I., L. Cooper, and D. Wacker. Behavioral problems and twins. J. Dev. Behav. Pediatr. 14:336–339, 1993.

Grether, J. K., B. K. Nelson and S. K. Cummings. Twinning and cerebral palsy: experience in four northern California counties, births 1983 through 1985. Pediatrics 92:854–858, 1993.

Taffel, S. M. Health and demographic characteristics of twin births: United States, 1988. National Center for Health Statistics. Vital Health Statistics 21(50), 1992.

CHAPTER 10

CIRCUMCISION

Carol D. Berkowitz, M.D.

H$_x$ An expectant mother visits you prenatally. She talks about circumcision in addition to issues relating to breast-feeding and car passenger safety. Her husband is circumcised. She understands that the medical indications for circumcision are few and asks your opinion about circumcision in the newborn period.

Questions

1. What are the benefits of circumcision in neonates?
2. What are the indications for circumcision in older children?
3. What are the techniques used to perform circumcision?
4. What are the complications of circumcision?

Male circumcision, a procedure in which the foreskin of the penis is removed, has been performed for over 4000 years. It is routinely performed in certain groups, most notably among Jewish and Muslim people. In many other cultures (e.g., Abyssinian, Australian [aborigine], Polynesian), circumcision is presumably performed to facilitate intercourse. Circumcision can be viewed as a ritual procedure, but its role as a medical one is open to greater controversy.

The benefits of male circumcision have been debated for years. Disadvantages of routine circumcision in infants concern cost effectiveness and the risk of complications. The procedure is sometimes viewed as an archaic and maiming ritual. Female circumcision, which may involve clitorectomy or resection and closure of the labia minor or majora, is infrequently practiced in Western culture and is not discussed here. There are no medical benefits attributable to female circumcision.

Circumcision in newborns has been performed in a routine and preventive manner, much the same way immunizations are administered. Primary care physicians should be aware of the risks and benefits of the procedure to be able to counsel parents and make referrals to consultants when certain medical conditions arise.

EPIDEMIOLOGY

The prevalence of circumcision, a procedure that became increasingly popular in the United States in the 1950s and 1960s, once ranged from 69 to 97% depending on cultural mores. Changing cultural patterns have resulted in a lower frequency of circumcision. In recent years the prevalence has decreased to about 59%. The prevalence of circumcision in Australia is reported to be 70%; in Canada, 48%; and in the United Kingdom, 24%. Circumcision is the second most common surgical procedure after vasectomy in males.

A reported 10% of uncircumcised males ultimately require circumcision as adults because of complications of phimosis and balanitis. Uncircumcised males with diabetes are particularly prone to these complications.

PATHOPHYSIOLOGY

In uncircumcised males, the foreskin adheres to the glans until about the age of 6 years. This adhesiveness, or crusting, may be controlled by androgens. A gradual, normal lysing of the adhesive bands connecting the foreskin to the underportion of the glans then occurs. Nonphysiologic phimosis occurs as a result of scarring of the preputial wing. Lysing of adhesions in an effort to treat the phimosis usually leads to further adhesions. If the foreskin is retracted and remains in that position, paraphimosis develops.

BENEFITS

It has been stated that circumcision facilitates penile hygiene by removing the foreskin, which may serve as a repository for bacteria, smegma, and dirt. Retractability of the foreskin increases with age (Table 10–1), and thus penile hygiene is easier to achieve in older children. The term **phimosis** refers to inability to retract the foreskin. In male infants beyond the newborn period, phimosis is the major indication for circumcision. Phimosis is normal in children up to about 6 years of age but is nonphysiologic if urination results in ballooning of the foreskin, regardless of age. When the retracted foreskin acts as a tourniquet in the midshaft of the penis, **paraphimosis** occurs, preventing the return of lymphatic flow. Paraphimosis is believed to be iatrogenic or matratrogenic, that is, related to the mother's retracting the foreskin. In the past, mothers were advised to retract the foreskin in an effort to lyse adhesions. This is no longer routinely recommended because adhesions are thought to be normal.

Balanitis, or inflammation of the glans, is not uncommon in young infants. It is frequently associated with *Candida* infection, and the glans is swollen and erythematous. Posthitis, or inflammation of the foreskin, is also often secondary to *Candida* infection. Other organisms, including gram-negative microbes, may be associated with balanitis. The presence of recurrent balanitis is an indication for circumcision. In older males, indications for circumcision include phimosis, paraphimosis, balanitis, posthitis, and balanoposthitis.

Bacterial colonization of the skin also leads to possible balanitis and posthitis. Group B streptococci, which bind to the foreskin of adults, causing balanitis, may be transmitted sexually. The incidence of STDs, particularly herpes and condyloma acuminatum, is increased in uncircumcised men.

Penile cancer, which is reported in 0.7 to 0.9 per 100,000 men in the United States, is also thought to be

TABLE 10–2. Complications Associated With Circumcision

Bleeding
Infection
Repeat circumcision
Phimosis
Skin bridges
Urinary retention
Meatitis
Inclusion cysts
Penile lymphedema
Urethrocutaneous fistulae
Penile cyanosis
Penile necrosis
Wound dehiscence

related to lack of circumcision of the penis. Only a few isolated cases of cancer of the penis occur in circumcised men. The reported mortality of penile cancer is 25%. This type of cancer appears to be associated with infection with human papillomavirus types 16 and 18. Whether lack of circumcision, poor hygiene, or the presence of STDs is responsible for the increased incidence of penile carcinoma is unclear.

Cervical carcinoma among the partners of uncircumcised men has been reported with increased incidence. Human papillomavirus types 16 and 18 are believed to play a role here. Herpes simplex virus type II has also been linked with cervical cancer. The link between uncircumcised males and cervical carcinoma is inconclusive.

UTIs reportedly occur ten times more often in uncircumcised male infants than in circumcised infants. In young uncircumcised boys, UTIs are directly related to colonization of the foreskin with urotoxic organisms. Pyronephritogenic, fimbriated *Escherichia coli* bind to the inner lining of the foreskin within the first few days of life. Other bacteria preferentially bind to this mucosal surface, including fimbriated strains of *Proteus mirabilis* and nonfimbriated *Pseudomonas, Klebsiella,* and *Serratia* species. The incidence of UTIs has increased as the rate of circumcision has decreased. In addition, complications associated with UTIs, particularly bacteremia, meningitis, and subsequent death, have occurred.

RISKS

The risks related to circumcision are related to complications from the procedure. These are listed in Table 10–2 and discussed in Management.

PARENT COUNSELING

Parents of Newborns

In the newborn period, proper counseling of the parents, including a discussion of the risks and benefits of circumcision, is important. Parents should be informed about the benefits of circumcision, including a reduction in occurrence of UTIs, STDs, and cancer of the penis and cervix. Problems related to the foreskin itself, such as phimosis, paraphimosis, posthitis, and balanitis, should also be discussed.

TABLE 10–1. Retractability of the Foreskin in Boys by Age

Age	Percentage With Retractable Foreskin
Birth	4%
6 months	15%
1 year	50%
3 years	80%
6 years	90%

It is appropriate to tell parents that boys who are not circumcised in the neonatal period may need to be circumcised later in life. In addition, parents should be told that approximately 10% of circumcised neonates require a second circumcision. Parents should be informed about the risks associated with circumcision in newborns, which are discussed in greater detail in the following text. In older individuals, risks include hemorrhage, infection, and injuries to the penis and urethra.

Research has shown that parents are more influenced by friends than by physicians regarding their ultimate decision about circumcision. Counseling during the second trimester of pregnancy results in no change in parents' decision about circumcision. The last reported survey of physician attitudes, conducted in 1979, showed that 41% recommended routine circumcision, 15% did not, and 38% had no recommendations (no answers: 5%). Pediatricians usually advised against circumcision, and younger physicians were more often opposed to the practice.

Parents of Older Infants

The need for circumcision in young male infants who present with UTIs is problematic. The evaluation usually tries to determine the existence of other predisposing conditions that could lead to the UTI. Investigators disagree on the need for circumcision following the initial UTI in uncircumcised boys. No clear-cut evidence indicates that circumcision at this time decreases the incidence of future UTIs, so the decision is parental rather than medical. In older children who present with phimosis, paraphimosis, balanitis, or balanoposthitis, circumcision is usually recommended to prevent recurrences of these problems. A history including the duration of symptoms and whether the child has had similar episodes in the past helps formulate the appropriate management.

MANAGEMENT

The medical attitude toward circumcision has changed over the last 40 years, with an initial inclination toward circumcision, followed by a move away from circumcision. The present position on circumcision as described by the Task Force on Circumcision of the AAP suggests that newborn circumcision has potential medical benefits and advantages as well as disadvantages and risks. When circumcision is considered, the benefits and risks should be explained to the parents, and informed consent should be obtained. Parents should be advised that the frequency with which third-party payers reimburse for circumcisions, particularly for routine circumcisions in the newborn period, has decreased.

Contraindications

Circumcisions should only be performed in completely healthy neonates. Contraindications to circumcision are well defined. Any abnormalities of the penis, such as hypospadias, absence of any portion of the foreskin, or chordee, preclude circumcision. Prematurity is a contraindication. Circumcision should be delayed in premature infants until they are ready for discharge. A family history of bleeding diatheses is also a contraindication to circumcision. Infants from such families should be assessed for evidence of coagulation problems. If these are present, circumcision should not be carried out. Infants with meningomyelocele should also not be circumcised because it is easier to fit such boys with an external collecting device if they are uncircumcised.

Circumcision Procedure

Numerous techniques are used to perform circumcisions. These procedures may involve clamp techniques with Gomco, Mogen, or Plastibell clamps. Any of these techniques is believed to give comparable results in the hands of trained, experienced operators. Formal surgical excision may also be carried out, usually in older children and adults. Three guidelines should be followed to decrease the incidence of complications: (1) marking of the coronal sulcus in ink, (2) dilation of the prepucial wing, and (3) retraction of the foreskin so that the urethral meatus is visualized. This prevents cutting the meatus. Electrocautery should never be used in conjunction with metal clamps because of the danger of extensive injury.

Appropriate anesthesia in newborns has been recently emphasized. The pain and stress of circumcision is evidenced by changes in infant state and behavior. Local anesthesia may be carried out with a dorsal penile nerve block using 1% lidocaine without epinephrine in a dose of 3–4 mg per kg. However, it is unclear whether local anesthesia makes any difference in overall symptomatology of the infant.

Complications

A number of complications are associated with circumcision in newborns (see Table 10–2). The most common complication is **bleeding,** which may occur in 0.1 to 35% of cases. This wide variation may reflect differences in method, technique, and skill. Bleeding can usually be controlled using local pressure or with 1:1000 adrenaline-soaked gauze. The second most frequently seen complication is **infection,** reported in up to 8% of circumcised infants. Neonatal sepsis may occur secondary to infections following circumcision. Plastibell clamps, which are associated with a higher incidence of infection than Gomco clamps, generally require intravenous antibiotics. Gomco-related infections usually respond to local treatment with hydrogen peroxide and 3% hexachlorophene.

In addition, true **phimosis** may occur if removal of the foreskin is insufficient. If the foreskin is inadequately freed up from the inner prepucial epithelium, a concealed penis, with the shaft retracted backwards into the abdominal wall, may develop. **Skin bridges** may form between the glans and the shaft, leading to accumulation of smegma or the tethering of the erect penis.

In the immediate postsurgical period, urinary retention may occur secondary to tight surgical bandages. Meatitis and meatal ulcers, believed to be caused by irritation from ammonia, are also reported in 8 to 31% of circumcised males. Inclusion cysts that represent implantation of smegma are also seen. Additional injuries following circumcision may include penile lymphedema, urethrocutaneous fistulae secondary to misplaced sutures, penile cyanosis secondary to tight Plastibell clamps, and penile necrosis. Wound dehiscence, which involves separation of the penile skin from the mucous membrane, and denudation of the penile shaft may occur more frequently with Gomco than Plastibell clamps.

Case Resolution

In the case history at the beginning of this chapter, the risks and benefits of circumcision should be discussed with the mother. The father should be encouraged to participate in the decision-making process.

Selected Readings

Anderson, G. Circumcision. Pediatr. Ann. 18:205–213, 1989.

Herzog, L. W. Urinary tract infections and circumcision: a case-control study. Am. J. Dis. Child. 143:348–350, 1989.

Larsen, G. L., and S. D. Williams. Postneonatal circumcision: population profile. Pediatrics 85:808–812, 1990.

Poland, P. L. The questions of routine neonatal circumcision. N. Engl. J. Med. 322:1312–1315, 1990.

Report of the Task Force on Circumcision, American Academy of Pediatrics. Pediatrics 84:388–391, 1989.

Schoen, E. J. Circumcision updated—indicated? (Commentary.) Pediatrics 92:860–861, 1993.

Schoen, E. J. The status of circumcision of newborns. N. Engl. J. Med. 322:1308–1312, 1990.

Wellington, N., and M. J. Rieder. Attitudes and practices regarding analgesia for newborn circumcision. Pediatrics 92:541–543, 1993.

Wiswell, T. E., and D. Geschke. Risks from circumcision during the first month of life compared with those for uncircumcised boys. Pediatrics 83:1011–1015, 1989.

Wiswell, T. E., and H. L. Tencer. Circumcision in children beyond the neonatal period. Pediatrics 92:791–793, 1993.

CHAPTER   11

NUTRITIONAL NEEDS

Geeta Grover, M.D.

H$_x$ At a routine health maintenance visit, a mother asks if she may begin giving her 4-month-old daughter solid foods. The infant is taking about 4 to 5 ounces of formula every 3 to 4 hours during the day (about 32 oz per day) and sleeps from 12 PM to 5 AM without awakening for a feeding. Her birth weight was 7 pounds, and her present weight and height (13 pounds and 25 inches, respectively) are at the 50th percentile for age. The physical examination, including developmental assessment, is within normal limits.

Questions

1. What are some of the parameters that may be used to decide when infants are ready to begin taking solid foods?
2. Up to what age are breast milk or infant formulas alone considered to be adequate intake for infants?
3. At what age do infants double their birth weight? At what age do they triple their birth weight?
4. What problems are associated with the early introduction of solid foods?

Good nutrition is essential for normal growth and development. The physician plays an important role not only in assessing the growth of children from infancy through adolescence but also in providing counseling for parents regarding the nutritional needs of maturing children. The primary care physician should be knowledgeable about key nutritional concepts in children, including growth patterns and nutritional requirements of normal children and how they vary with age; feeding patterns of infants and children; assessment of nutritional status; and common feeding and nutritional disorders.

GROWTH PATTERNS AND NUTRITIONAL REQUIREMENTS OF NORMAL CHILDREN

Monitoring the growth and nutritional status of infants and children is an integral component of well child care. The average normal expected increases in weight, height, and head circumference for the first several years of life are listed in Table 11–1.

The energy and nutritional requirements of children vary with age. Postnatal growth is most rapid during the first 6 to 12 months of life. Hence caloric and protein needs are very high at this time. The average daily energy and protein needs of children from birth to 18 years of age are presented in Table 11–2.

TABLE 11–1. Normal Expected Increase in Weight, Height, and Head Circumference of Infants and Children

Normal Weight Gain in Children	
Age	Expected Weight Increase
0–3 mo	25–35 g/day
3–6 mo	12–21 g/day
6–12 mo	10–13 g/day
1–6 yr	5–8 g/day
7–10 yr	5–11 g/day
Normal Height Increase in Children	
Age	Expected Height Increase
0–12 mo	10 in/yr (25 cm/yr)
13–24 mo	5 in/yr (12.5 cm/yr)
2 yr–puberty	2.5 in/yr (6.25 cm/yr)
Normal Increase in Head Circumference	
Age	Expected Increase in Head Circumference
0–3 mo	2 cm/mo
4–6 mo	1 cm/mo
7–12 mo	½ cm/mo
Total increase:	12 cm in the first year

On average, newborns weigh 7.7 lb (3.5 kg), are about 20 inches (50 cm) long, and have a head circumference of 14 inches (35 cm). They lose about 5 to 10% of their birth weight during the first several days of life and usually regain this weight by the age of 10 to 14 days. During the first several months of life, weight gain serves as an important indicator of children's general well-being. Failure to gain weight during this time may be a clue to a wide variety of problems, ranging from underfeeding to malabsorption. Newborns gain about 30 g/day (roughly 1% of their birth weight per day) for the first three months of life, and about 10 to 20 g/day for the rest of the first year. Infants double their birth weight by 6 months of age and triple their birth weight by 12 months of age. On average, children weigh about 10 kg at one year of age, 20 kg at 5 years of age, and 30 kg at 10 years of age. A rough rule of thumb that can be used to estimate the expected weight of a child based on age is:

$$2 \times (\text{age in years}) + 10 = \text{weight (kg)}$$

FEEDING PATTERNS OF INFANTS AND CHILDREN

Liquid Foods

Breast milk or one of the several iron-fortified infant formulas provides complete nutrition for infants during the first 4 to 6 months of life. During the first month or 2 of life, infants take about 2 to 3 ounces of formula (approximately 10 minutes on each breast) every two to three hours.

Because breast milk is more easily digested than formula, it passes out of the stomach in 1½ hours. Formula may take up to 4 hours. Therefore, during the first 4 to 6 weeks of life, breast-fed infants want to feed more frequently (8–12 times in 24 hours) than formula-fed infants (6–8 times in 24 hours), with an increased number of nighttime feedings as well. By about 3 to 5 months of age, breast-fed and bottle-fed infants do not differ in the number of nighttime feedings, although some breast-fed infants continue to awaken out of habit.

Most infants 6 months of age or less consume about 4 to 5 ounces per feeding every 4 to 5 hours. Under rou-

tine circumstances, breast milk is preferred to infant formulas because it has emotional, nutritional, and immunologic advantages. Breast-feeding allows infants and mothers to develop a unique relationship that can be emotionally satisfying.

The composition of breast milk varies over time. Colostrum, the first milk produced after delivery, is high in protein, immunoglobulins, and secretory IgA. Colostrum gradually changes to mature milk 7 to 10 days after delivery. The nutrient content of human milk of mothers who deliver preterm compared to those who deliver at term may vary considerably. Individual assessment may be necessary to determine the appropriateness of breast milk for preterm infants.

Nutritionally, breast milk is uniquely tailored to meet the specific needs of human infants. Human milk provides approximately 20 kcal/oz, the same as routine infant formulas. Table 11–3 compares the composition of human milk and several infant formulas. Human milk has relatively low amounts of protein when compared to cow's milk (1% vs. 3%), yet the levels are sufficient to provide for satisfactory growth of infants.

Qualitative differences also make human milk more desirable. The casein-to-whey ratio in human milk is about 40:60, making it easier to digest than most infant formulas, which have a casein-to-whey ratio of 80:20 (equivalent to cow's milk). Fat is the primary source of calories in human milk. The fat in cow's milk, which contains primarily saturated fatty acids, is not as well digested by infants as human milk fat, which is predominately composed of polyunsaturated fats. Lactose is the major carbohydrate of both human and cow's milk, but it is present in higher concentrations in human milk.

Human milk from well-nourished women should provide adequate amounts of all vitamins and other micronutrients. However, vitamin K, vitamin D, iron, and fluoride are not present in sufficient quantities to satisfy all nutritional needs over a prolonged period, and supplementation should be considered. The AAP recommends that all newborns receive a prophylactic dose of 0.5 to 1 mg of parenteral vitamin K in the immediate newborn period to help prevent bleeding disorders. The vitamin D content of human milk is low compared to cow's milk. Exclusively breast-fed infants may require 400 IU per day of vitamin D supplementation, especially if exposure to sunlight is limited, to prevent rickets. Although human milk contains less iron than iron-fortified formulas (fortified to about 12 mg/L of iron), the bioavailability of the iron in human milk is greater. Breast-fed infants do not need iron supplementation until the sixth month of life. Exclusively breast-fed infants and infants who are fed ready-

TABLE 11–2. Energy and Protein Needs of Children

Age (years)	Calories (kcal/kg/day)	Protein (g/kg/day)
0–1	90–120	2.5–3.0
1–7	75–90	1.5–2.5
7–12	60–75	1.5–2.5
12–18	30–60	1.0–1.5

TABLE 11–3. Composition of Breast Milk and Select Infant Formulas (calories: 20 kcal/oz)

Formula	Protein	Carbohydrate	Fat
Human milk (mature)	40% casein and 60% whey	Lactose	Human milk fat
Cow's milk	80% casein and 20% whey	Lactose	Butterfat
Enfamil 20	Nonfat cow's milk and whey (60% whey, 40% casein)	Lactose	Coconut, soy, palm olein, and sunflower oils
Isomil	Soy protein	Corn syrup and maltose	Soy and coconut oils
Nutramigen	Casein hydrolysate	Corn syrup solids and cornstarch	Corn oil
Pregestimil	Casein hydrolysate	Corn syrup solids, dextrose, and cornstarch	MCT, corn and safflower oils
ProSobee	Soy protein	Corn syrup solids	Coconut, palm olein, and sunflower oils
Similac 20	Nonfat cow's milk (80% casein, 20% whey)	Lactose	Coconut and soy oils

Abbreviation: MCT, medium-chain triglycerides.

to-eat formulas or formulas prepared with bottled water should all receive supplementation with 0.25 mg of fluoride per day (see Chapter 13, Dental Care).

Human milk has several immunologic advantages, which are both allergy-protective and infection-protective, over standard cow milk-based formulas. Its allergy-protective characteristics are attributed, in part, to the decreased intestinal permeability associated with human milk compared to standard formulas. The host defense factors present in human milk include immunoglobulins, complement, and cellular components (e.g., macrophages, neutrophils, lymphocytes). Studies have shown that the incidences of both viral and bacterial illnesses are lower in exclusively breast-fed infants compared to their formula-fed peers.

Breast-feeding is the recommended method of infant feeding during the first 6 months of life, but it is not always possible and is occasionally contraindicated. Although maternal infection is usually not a contraindication to breast-feeding, maternal HIV infection is one exception to this recommendation in the United States. This is not necessarily true, however, in many developing countries, where the risk of death during the first year of life without breast-feeding is greater than the risk of HIV infection. Antibiotics are generally safe during breast-feeding, but certain other drugs are contraindicated (Table 11–4).

Solid Foods

Supplemental foods may be added to infants' diets between the age of 4 to 6 months. Solid foods should be introduced as soon as infants require the additional calories and are developmentally mature (e.g., infant can sit and support the head). Early introduction of solid foods has been associated with an increased incidence of food allergy and may contribute to overeating and obesity. Factors that indicate infants may be ready for solid foods include (1) current weight twice that of birth weight, or about 13 pounds; (2) consumption of more than 32 ounces of formula per day; (3) frequent feeding (regularly more than 8 to 10 times per day or more often than every three hours); and (4) persistent unsatisfaction due to hunger.

The quantity of formula should be limited to no more than 32 ounces to allow for the introduction of solid foods. An iron-fortified infant cereal, most commonly rice cereal, is usually the first solid food offered to infants. Other single-grained cereals, such as barley cereal

or oatmeal, are also appropriate early supplemental foods. Fruits and vegetables may be introduced within a few weeks. The order is not as important as the need to add only one new food at a time—no more than one to two new foods per week. Meats may be introduced after 6 months of age.

Commercially prepared infant juices are an important source of vitamin C for infants and may provide a smooth transition to solid foods. About 2 ounces of apple juice can be given at 4 to 6 months of age. This can be gradually increased to about 4 ounces per day. Once infants have accepted the juice, a small quantity of cereal can be added to it and offered to infants with a spoon. Solid foods should not be mixed in the bottle; caregivers should wait until the infant can accept spoon

TABLE 11–4. Drugs and Breast-feeding

Contraindicated	Avoid or Use With Great Caution	Probably Safe But Use With Caution
Antineoplastic agents	Anthroquinolones (laxatives)	Anesthetics
Amphetamine	Aspirin	Acetaminophen
Bromocriptine	Atropine	Aldomet
Clemastine	Birth control pills	Antibiotics (not tetracycline)
Cimetidine	Bromides	Antithyroids (not methimazole)
Chloramphenicol	Calciferol	Antiepileptics
Cocaine	Cascara	Antihistamines*
Cyclophosphamide	Danthron	Antihypertensives/ cardiovascular agents
Cyclosporine	Dihydrotachysterol	Bishydroxycoumarin
Diethylstilbestrol	Estrogens	Chlorpromazine*
Doxorubicin	Ethanol	Codeine*
Ergots	Metoclopramide	Digoxin
Gold salts	Metronidazole	Dilantin
Heroin	Narcotics	Diuretics
Immunosuppressants	Phenobarbital*	Furosemide
Iodides	Primidone	Haloperidol*
Lithium	Psychotropic drugs	Hydralazine
Meprobamate	Reserpine	Indomethacin
Methimazole	Salicylazosulfapyridine (sulfasalizine)	Methadone*
Methamphetamine		Muscle relaxants
Nicotine (smoking)		Prednisone
Phencyclidine (PCP)		Propranolol
Phenindone		Propylthiouracil
Radiopharmaceuticals		Sedatives
Tetracycline		Theophylline
Thiouracil		Vitamins
		Warfarin

*Watch for sedation.
Reproduced, with permission, from Behrman, R.E., (ed.). Nelson Textbook of Pediatrics, 14th ed. Philadelphia, W.B. Saunders, 1992, p. 428.

feedings. It is not unusual for infants to reject their first several spoonfuls of cereal, because the tastes and textures are new. If they refuse the feeding, it should be stopped. Solid foods should be reintroduced in one week.

Precooked infant cereals, such as rice cereal, can be mixed with a variety of liquids, including breast milk, formula, infant fruit juices, or water. Initially, the cereal should be mixed to a thinner consistency (e.g., about 1 tablespoon of cereal to 2 oz of liquid), and once infants have accepted the new taste and texture, the mixture should gradually be worked to a thicker consistency. By about 7 to 8 months of age, infants should be taking 4 to 6 tablespoons of cereal mixed with enough liquid to give the mixture the consistency of mustard. Mixed cereal grains may be introduced to older infants.

A wide variety of commercially prepared baby foods designed to be developmentally appropriate and labeled by stage (i.e., first-, second-, third-stage) are available. The jars of different stages contain the amount of food that an infant at a given age should be able to eat at one sitting. This is not always the case, however, and opened jars of baby food may safely be stored in the refrigerator for 2 to 3 days. Infants should not be fed directly from the jar, because saliva on the spoon mixes with the remaining food and digests it, causing it to liquify. Vegetables and meats may be offered at room temperature but should be warmed slightly for greater palatability. Fruits and desserts may be at room or refrigerator temperature.

First-stage foods, for infants 4 to 6 months of age, include strained infant juices, single-grain cereals, and puréed fruits and vegetables, such as bananas, carrots, and peas. These foods contain no egg, milk, wheat, or citrus, to which some infants may be sensitive. Second-stage foods, for infants from about 6 to 9 months of age, are smooth, mixed-ingredient foods, such as mixed vegetables, or meat dinners, such as chicken noodle. Third-stage foods, or junior foods, are for infants about 9 to 10 months of age who can sit well without support, have some teeth, and have begun self-feeding. These more coarsely textured foods contain a wider variety of nutrients, such as vegetable and meat dinner combinations. Finger foods, such as crackers, cheese wedges, or cookies, can also be introduced by 9 to 10 months of age, once infants have developed a pincer grasp. Most infants are eating the same meals as the rest of the family (table foods) by about one year of age. Foods that can easily be aspirated, such as raw carrots, nuts, and hard candies, should be avoided, however, until children are over 4 years of age.

Baby foods can be prepared at home as long as they are finely puréed or strained and contain enough liquid to make them easy for infants to swallow. One danger of preparing foods at home is that sugar, salt, or spices can be easily added to make foods palatable to adults. These ingredients are not necessary for infants. In addition, home-grown, home-prepared vegetables may be contaminated with high levels of nitrates (e.g., due to contaminated well water) and nitrites (e.g., in vegetables such as carrots, beets, and spinach). Nitrates and nitrites have been implicated in the development of methemoglobinemia in children.

Weaning from the breast or bottle to a cup usually occurs at 6 to 12 months of age but may be delayed up to 18 months of age in some children. Homogenized, vitamin D-fortified cow's milk may be given at 12 months of age. Skim milk or lowfat milk (2% milk fat) should not be given before two years of age.

DIET OF CHILDREN AND ADOLESCENTS

The caloric and protein needs of children decrease in the second year of life, paralleling the decrease in growth rate during this time. Milk intake also decreases, and may drop to 16 ounces per day by 24 to 36 months of age. Except for increased caloric requirements, the diet of school-age children and adolescents should be similar to that of normal adults. Evidence that foods eaten during childhood may have long-lasting effects on adult health is increasing, and it is important that children develop healthy eating habits early in life. Atherosclerosis, osteoporosis, and obesity are some of the diseases that may have their beginnings during childhood.

ASSESSMENT OF NUTRITIONAL STATUS IN INFANTS AND CHILDREN

History

Nutritional assessment begins with a complete dietary history. The dietary assessment should emphasize the quantity, quality, and variety of foods in the diet. Any special or restricted dietary habits should be noted (e.g., vegetarian diet). A 3-day food record listing the types and quantities of food eaten throughout the day can be very helpful in evaluating the dietary history.

In addition, the child's routine medical, family, and social history all may influence nutritional status. For example, the economic status of families may affect the variety and type of foods that they may be able to purchase, and the level of education of parents influences their ability to understand the concepts of a healthy diet. Poverty and ignorance regarding nutritional needs are among the most common reasons for malnutrition in children.

Physical Examination

Height, weight, and head circumference should be measured routinely and plotted on a longitudinal basis on appropriate growth curves. Changes in the rate of growth over time are more useful than a single measurement in time in the assessment of nutritional problems. Calculation of the height age (age for which the child's height is at the 50th percentile), weight age (age for which the child's weight is at the 50th percentile), and ideal weight for actual height may be useful when deviations from normal are noted.

In addition to the overall impression regarding nutritional status, certain findings on physical examination may be characteristic of particular nutritional disor-

TABLE 11–5. Physical Signs of Nutritional Deficiency Disorders

System	Sign	Deficiency
General appearance	Reduced weight for height	Calories
Skin/hair	Pallor	Anemias (iron, B_{12}, vitamin E, folate, and copper)
	Edema	Protein, thiamine
	Nasolabial seborrhea	Calories, protein, vitamin B_6
	Dermatitis	Riboflavin, essential fatty acids, biotin
	Photosensitivity dermatitis	Niacin
	Acrodermatitis	Zinc
	Follicular hyperkeratosis (sandpaper-like)	Vitamin A
	Depigmented skin	Calories, protein
	Purpura	Vitamins C, K
	Scrotal, vulval dermatitis	Riboflavin
	Alopecia	Zinc, biotin, protein
	Depigmented, dull hair	Protein, calories, copper
Subcutaneous tissue	Decreased	Calories
Eye (vision)	Poor adaptation to dark	Vitamins A, E, zinc
	Poor color discrimination	Vitamin A
	Bitot spots, xerophthalmia, keratomalacia	Vitamin A
	Conjunctival pallor	Nutritional anemias
	Fundal capillary microaneurysms	Vitamin C
Face, mouth, neck	Angular stomatitis	Riboflavin, iron
	Cheilosis	Vitamins B_6, niacin, riboflavin
	Bleeding gums	Vitamins C, K
	Atrophic papillae	Riboflavin, iron, niacin
	Smooth tongue	Iron
	Red tongue (glossitis)	Vitamins B_6, B_{12}, niacin, riboflavin, folate
	Parotid swelling	Protein
	Caries	Fluoride
	Anosmia	Vitamins A, B_{12}, zinc
	Hypogeusia	Vitamin A, zinc
	Goiter	Iodine
Cardiovascular	Heart failure	Thiamine, selenium, nutritional anemias
Genital	Hypogonadism	Zinc
Skeletal	Costochondral beading	Vitamins D, C
	Subperiosteal hemorrhage	Vitamin C, copper
	Cranial bossing	Vitamin D
	Wide fontanelle	Vitamin D
	Epiphyseal enlargement	Vitamin D
	Craniotabes	Vitamin D, calcium
	Tender bones	Vitamin C
	Tender calves	Thiamine, selenium
	Spoon-shaped nails (koilonychia)	Iron
	Transverse nail lines	Protein
Neurologic	Sensory, motor neuropathy	Thiamine, vitamins E, B_6, B_{12}
	Ataxia, areflexia	Vitamin E
	Ophthalmoplegia	Vitamin E, thiamine
	Tetany	Vitamin D, Ca^{++}, Mg^{++}
	Retardation	Iodine, niacin
	Dementia, delirium	Vitamin E, niacin, thiamine

Reproduced, with permission, from Behrman, R.E., and R.M. Kleigman (eds.). Nelson's Essentials of Pediatrics, 2nd ed. Philadelphia, W.B. Saunders, 1994.

ders. The evaluation of the hair, skin, eyes, lips and oral mucosa, dentition, and musculoskeletal system should be emphasized, because the examination of these areas is most likely to show the effects of malnutrition. Muscle wasting, hepatosplenomegaly, skeletal deformities, decayed teeth, rough dry skin, easily pluckable hair, and irritability may all be clues to inadequate nutrition (Table 11–5).

Laboratory Tests

Suspected malnutrition or nutrition-related disorders, based on history and physical examination, can be further investigated with laboratory studies. Tests that may be used in the evaluation of anemia, one of the most common nutrition-related disorders seen in children, include a CBC, reticulocyte count, serum iron, ferritin, and total iron-binding capacity. Investigation of suspected malnutrition begins with an assessment of protein status, with measures of indicators such as serum albumin, total protein, and prealbumin. Liver function tests and a lipid profile may also be useful in the evaluation of suspected malnutrition. Screening tests that may be used in the evaluation of failure to thrive (FTT) include thyroid function studies, urinalysis, and bone age. More specific tests, such as serum vitamin levels (e.g., folate or vitamin B_{12} levels in suspected malabsorption) or hormone assays (e.g., growth hormone levels in the evaluation of FTT), may be obtained in certain instances.

COMMON FEEDING AND NUTRITIONAL PROBLEMS OF CHILDHOOD

Several GI problems have been attributed to diet. A small amount of spitting up is seen in the majority of children, especially during the first 6 months of life. However, vomiting can be a sign of several disorders, ranging from viral GI tract infections to more severe illnesses such as pyloric stenosis, urinary tract infection, and GI obstruction (see Chapter 78, Vomiting). Constipation, which is seen more commonly in formula-fed than breast-fed infants, may be due to insufficient fluid intake (see Chapter 82, Constipation). The simple addition of 4 to 6 ounces of water to an infants' diet or temporary use of apple or prune juice may solve the problem. Enemas and suppositories should not be recommended routinely.

Underfeeding or a diet that is not nutritionally balanced may result in FTT (see Chapter 98, Failure to Thrive). The opposite problem, obesity, is one of the most common nutritional problems of children in the United States. The prevalence of this condition in children 6 to 11 years of age is estimated to be about 20 to 25%. Finally, the eating disorders, anorexia nervosa and bulimia, are estimated to affect about 1 in 100 adolescent females 16 to 18 years of age (see Chapter 101, Eating Disorders).

Nutritional disorders include malnutrition and deficiencies of vitamins and minerals. Table 11–5 lists the characteristics of various vitamin and mineral deficiencies. Anemia is one of the most common nutrition-related problems seen in children. Malnutrition is one of the leading causes of childhood morbidity and mortality worldwide. Although primary protein-calorie malnutrition (PCM) is rare in most parts of the United States, surveys conducted on pediatric wards have demonstrated that about one third of pediatric inpatients with chronic disease have evidence of some degree of PCM.

The most common deficits were weight for height below 90% of standard (i.e., evidence of acute malnutrition) and height for age less than 95% of standard (i.e., evidence of chronic malnutrition). The two forms of PCM are marasmus (severe caloric depletion) and kwashiorkor (inadequate protein intake). Untreated PCM can result in impaired growth, poor intellectual development, and impaired immune functioning.

Case Resolution

The infant described in the case history is probably ready to begin some solid foods because she is consuming 32 ounces of formula per day and continues to be hungry. In addition, she has reached a weight of 13 pounds and has almost doubled her birth weight. The mother is counseled to begin feeding her daughter a single-grain infant cereal mixed with either formula or juice. (The cereal should be fed by spoon, not given in a bottle.) Within a few weeks, once the infant is taking the cereal well, other first foods such as fruits and vegetables may be introduced.

Selected Readings

Barness, L. A. Nutrition update. Pediatr. Rev. 15:321–326, 1994.

Deen, D. Nutritional assessment for the primary care pediatrician. Pediatr. Ann. 19: 244–262, 1990.

Forbes, G. B. Nutrition. *In* Hoekelman, R. A. (ed.). Primary Pediatric Care, 2nd ed. St. Louis, Mosby-Year Book, 1992, pp. 168–196.

Greer, F. R. Formulas for the healthy term infant. Pediatr. Rev. 16:107–112, 1995.

Howard, C. R., and M. Weitzman. Breast or bottle: practical aspects of infant nutrition in the first 6 months. Pediatr. Ann. 21:619–631, 1992.

Klish, W. J. Special infant formulas. Pediatr. Rev. 12:55–62, 1990.

Lawrence, R. A. Breast-feeding: A Guide for the Medical Profession, 3rd ed. St. Louis, C.V. Mosby, 1989.

Lawrence, R. A. The pediatrician's role in infant feeding decision making. Pediatr. Rev. 14:265–272, 1993.

CHAPTER 12

SLEEP: NORMAL PATTERNS AND COMMON DISORDERS

Geeta Grover, M.D.

H$_x$ During a routine 6-month health maintenance visit, a mother states that although her 6-month-old son falls asleep very easily at about 10 PM every night while breast-feeding, he wakes every two to three hours and cries until she nurses him back to sleep. A review of the dietary history reveals that the infant is breast-fed about every three hours and was begun on rice cereal 2 weeks ago. His immunizations are current; he should receive his third dose of DPT/OPV/Hib today. The boy has no medical problems, and his physical examination is normal.

Questions

1. How old are most infants when they can begin to sleep through the night (at least five hours at a stretch) without a feeding?
2. What factors contribute to frequent nighttime wakings during infancy?
3. What advice can be given to parents to facilitate an infant's sleeping through the night?

Sleep disorders are common during infancy and childhood. Getting children to go to bed, fall asleep, stay asleep, and stay in bed can be no small challenge. Parents frequently ask pediatricians about sleep-related problems at routine health maintenance visits. Age-appropriate suggestions on how to help children sleep well are usually welcomed by parents.

EPIDEMIOLOGY

Bedtime struggles and frequent night wakings occur in 20 to 25% of children under 3 years of age. In preschool-age children, nighttime fears (e.g., fear of noises, fear of the dark) or separation anxiety often contribute to these problems. As children get older, nightmares and night terrors may contribute to difficulties with night wakings. About 5% of individuals experience nightmares, which usually begin before the age of 10 years and are seen more often in girls than in boys. Night terrors are a specific form of partial night waking from deep sleep that may begin during the preschool years. The incidence in children is reported to be 1 to 4%, with the greatest frequency between 5 and 7 years of age. Such terrors are more common in boys than in girls, and a familial tendency has been reported. Febrile illness and obstructive sleep apnea may be predisposing factors.

In most Western countries, children are expected to sleep in their own beds. However, in many cultures, it is not uncommon for infants and young children to sleep in their parents' bed (the "family bed"). **Cosleeping** is not a problem in and of itself, and the decision to cosleep, like the decision to breast- or bottle-feed, is an entirely personal one. Parents who are interested in cosleeping should be cautioned that bed-sharing is not a solution to sleep problems, however; in the long term it may even contribute to them. Parents who share a bed with their children commonly have to lie down with them for 20 to 30 minutes to get them to fall asleep. Several studies have shown that cosleeping infants are two to three times more likely to have night awakenings than those who sleep alone. Furthermore, infants who are both breast-feeding and bed-sharing sleep the shortest periods prior to awakening.

PATHOPHYSIOLOGY

To understand the problems associated with sleep, the physiology of normal sleep and the development of normal sleep behavior in children must be understood.

Sleep States

Normal sleep is divided into two distinct states, **rapid eye movement (REM)** and **nonrapid eye movement (NREM)** sleep. REM sleep develops at about 29 weeks' gestation and then persists throughout life. It is an active, lighter stage of sleep that occurs in association with rapid eye movements. Other features of REM sleep include suppression of muscle tone; rapid, irregular pulse and respiratory rate; and body twitches. Dreams occur during REM sleep. The EEG pattern of REM sleep is very similar to stage 1 NREM sleep.

NREM sleep begins at about 32 to 35 weeks' gestation. During NREM sleep, pulse and respiratory rates are slower and more regular, and body movements are minimal. Most of the restorative functions of sleep occur during this state. After the first several months of life, NREM sleep may be further divided into four stages ranging from drowsiness to very deep sleep. Each stage represents a progressively deeper state of sleep and has a characteristic EEG tracing: stage 1 has low-voltage, fast activity; stage 2 is notable for the presence of sleep spindles and K complexes against a low-voltage background; and stages 3 and 4 are identified by varying amounts of high-amplitude, slow waves known as delta waves (Fig. 12–1).

The Sleep Cycle

REM and NREM sleep together make up the sleep cycle. Typically, the deepest sleep takes place during the first several hours of the night, with lighter stages of NREM sleep and REM sleep occurring during most of the rest of the night. Although sleep stages are the same in both infants and adults, several differences concerning the onset and duration of REM and NREM sleep between infants and adults exist. First, the sleep cycle is shorter in infants (50–60 minutes) than in adults (90–100 minutes), which means that infants have more periods of active REM sleep as compared to adults. Second, the total amount of time spent in REM sleep decreases with increasing age. Term newborns spend about 50% of their total sleep time in REM sleep (up to 80% in premature infants); this decreases to about 30% by 3 years of age and to 20% by adulthood. Third, infants may have very little REM latency, entering their first REM cycle very shortly after falling asleep. Adults, in comparison, generally enter their first REM period about 90 minutes after the onset of sleep.

Sleep-Wake Patterns

Sleep patterns follow a normal developmental sequence in children; the amount of sleep children need changes with maturation (Fig. 12–2). Healthy term newborns sleep 16 to 17 hours per day. Because they are unable to sleep for more than a few hours at a time, sleeping and waking periods are fairly evenly distributed throughout the day and night. Many infants are able to sleep through the night (at least 5 hours uninterrupted) by the age of 3 months; most infants are capable of this by 4 months. Brief arousals are a normal

FIGURE 12–1. *Brain wave patterns in waking and sleep. (Reproduced from Ferber, R. Solve Your Child's Sleep Problems. New York, Simon & Schuster, 1985, p. 24. Copyright 1985 by Richard Ferber, M.D. Reprinted by permission of Simon & Schuster, Inc.)*

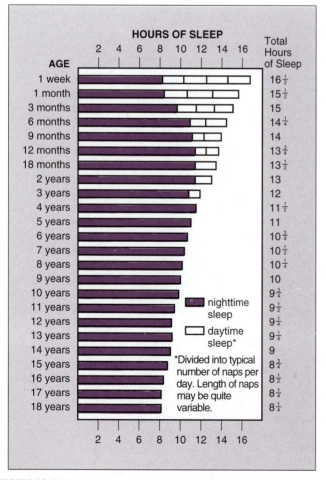

FIGURE 12–2. *Typical sleep requirements in childhood. (Reproduced from Ferber, R. Solve Your Child's Sleep Problems. New York, Simon & Schuster, 1985, p. 19. Copyright 1985 by Richard Ferber, M.D. Reprinted by permission of Simon & Schuster, Inc.)*

part of the sleep cycle at all ages, but children should be able to return to sleep on their own without requiring parents' attention. Children should definitely be able to fall asleep on their own by the age of 4 to 6 months. Otherwise, parental participation to fall asleep becomes a habit required at every awakening throughout the night.

By 12 months of age, infants sleep about 14 hours per day, divided into two naps during the day and a period of about 10 hours at night. During the second year of life, most children stop napping in the morning. By 2 years of age, they require about 13 hours of sleep per day (1 to 2 hours in an afternoon nap and 11 to 12 hours at night). Most children take an afternoon nap until 3 years of age, and some children continue this until 5 years of age. The amount of nighttime sleep children need gradually continues to decline, decreasing from about 12 hours during the preschool years to about 8 to 9 hours during adolescence.

Sleep Abnormalities

The etiology of sleep disorders can be complex, involving the interaction of children's temperamental characteristics, psychosocial stressors in the home, parental childrearing philosophies, and the developmental nature of normal sleep states and sleep cycles.

DIFFERENTIAL DIAGNOSIS

The differential diagnosis of sleep disorders may be divided into problems associated with falling asleep and frequent night wakings (Table 12–1). Falling asleep may present two types of difficulties: problems associated with settling children to sleep and bedtime refusal.

In infants, **inappropriate sleep-onset associations** are the most common reason for difficulty settling to sleep. These infants require parental participation (e.g., hold-

TABLE 12–1. Differential Diagnosis of Sleep Disorders

Difficulty Falling Asleep

Inappropriate sleep-onset associations
Poor and inconsistent limit setting
Sleep schedule disturbances
Separation anxiety
Nighttime fears (e.g., fears of the dark, monsters)
Family and social stresses
Overstimulation
Acute illness
Underlying medical problems
Medications (e.g., antihistamines, stimulants, codeine, anticonvulsants)

Nighttime Waking

Normal variation
Night waking for feeding beyond first several months
Learned behavior; lacks self-soothing or comforting behaviors
Poor and inconsistent limit setting
Nightmares
Night terrors, sleepwalking, and sleeptalking
Family and social stresses
Acute illness
Underlying medical problem
Medications (e.g., cold remedies)

---

ing, rocking, feeding) to fall asleep. They have not learned the critical skills of self-calming and initiating sleep on their own. Because these infants do not have the self-soothing behaviors necessary to fall back asleep after normal nighttime arousals, they may also have nighttime wakings. Brief arousals are a normal component of sleep. Nighttime wakings are different, because parents' participation is needed to resettle children. The difficulty that the children experience falling back to sleep on their own, not the waking itself, is the problem.

An example of an inappropriate sleep-onset association is the child who needs to be nursed or fed to fall asleep. The term **"trained night feeder"** has been coined to describe children who need to be fed before going back to sleep after normal nighttime awakenings. Although they are developmentally old enough to receive all nutrition during the day, they have become conditioned to require nighttime feedings. These children are often nursed or bottle-fed until they fall asleep and only then placed in the crib. They are conditioned to require feeding to initiate sleep, and when they experience normal nighttime arousals, they require the breast or bottle to go back to sleep.

The term **"trained night crier"** refers to children who, like "trained night feeders," lack the self-comforting and self-initiating skills necessary to fall asleep on their own. Trained night criers awaken, cry, and want to be held, comforted, or entertained before they can go back to sleep.

Acute illness may also be a cause of sleep disturbances. Children with otitis media may awaken at night because of pain. They may continue to experience awakenings even after the infection has resolved, however, and they require comforting or some sort of attention to fall asleep again.

In children between the ages of 9 and 18 months, **separation** and **separation anxiety** may also affect sleep patterns. Children may cry when parents leave the room

and have difficulty settling to sleep. Ability to climb out of the crib or bed can be associated with nighttime wakings in older toddlers. The transition from a crib to a bed is usually made between 2 and 3 years of age. Children who can climb out of their cribs or beds may come out of their rooms repeatedly for drinks of water, trips to the bathroom, or sleeping in the parents' bed. Such factors as nighttime fears of the dark influence sleep behaviors during the preschool years (3 to 5 years of age). Children's growing needs for autonomy and control over their environment may lead to bedtime refusals during both the toddler and preschool years.

Disorders of the sleep-wake cycle may contribute to sleep schedule irregularities. The circadian clock inherent in humans is about 24 hours and requires daily resetting or entrainment to function on a precise 24-hour schedule. Regular and consistent structure needs to be provided by parents, because development of children's sleep-wake rhythms depend on an interaction of the child's inherent biologic rhythms with the environment. Entrainment requires predictable occurrence of time cues such as light and dark, mealtime, and bedtime.

Irregular sleep-wake cycles may be seen in children living in chaotic environments with irregular mealtimes and sleep-wake schedules. A delayed sleep phase and regular but inappropriate sleep-wake schedule are the most common forms of sleep rhythm disturbance. Children with **delayed sleep phase** have a resetting of their circadian rhythm; they are not sleepy at bedtime and have excessive morning sleepiness. This is a common problem, because the inherent circadian clock has a cycle closer to 25, not 24, hours. This clock has not been entrained to a 24-hour schedule in these children.

Examples of **regular but inappropriate sleep-wake schedules** include children who nap at the "wrong" time (e.g., a child who regularly naps at 7 PM for one hour and then has trouble going to bed at 9 PM) and infants who seem to have day and night confused. These children sleep most of the day and stay up most of the night.

Night terrors (pavor nocturnus), **sleepwalking** (somnambulism), and **sleeptalking** (somniloquy) are all forms of partial awakenings that occur during deep or stage 4 NREM sleep, most often during the transition from stage 4 NREM sleep to the first REM sleep period. Sleepwalking and sleeptalking usually occur during the school-age years, whereas night terrors begin during the preschool years.

Both nightmares and night terrors may begin during the preschool years and may continue throughout childhood. Night terrors are different from nightmares and occur during a different stage of the sleep cycle. With night terrors, children usually sit up in bed and cry or scream inconsolably for up to 15 minutes. They may appear dazed and have signs of autonomic arousal such as tachycardia, tachypnea, and sweating. These children cannot be consoled. When they finally go back to sleep, they do not remember the event in the morning. Because parents are often frightened by the experience, they may think the child is having a seizure or is suffering from an emotional disturbance and may seek medical advice. Although attacks may be precipitated by stressful events or fatiguing daytime activities, night terrors do not indicate excessive stress or emotional disturbance in children's lives unless they recur.

Nightmares usually occur during the last third of the night during REM sleep, whereas night terrors more often take place during the early part of the night. Nightmares are scary dreams that may awaken children, who can often remember them. Children can usually be consoled by parents but are reluctant to go back to sleep because of their fears.

Excessive daytime sleepiness can be a symptom of medical problems such as depression, sleep apnea, or illness. Viral illness is perhaps the most common medical cause of such sleepiness in children. Inadequate sleep at night may also be a potential cause of sleepiness during the day. Narcolepsy, a disorder of excessive sleepiness, is characterized by an overwhelming desire to sleep during the daytime despite adequate sleep at night. Its symptoms include excessive daytime sleepiness, cataplexy, sleep paralysis, and hypnagogic hallucinations. Cataplexy is an abrupt loss of muscle tone that is usually precipitated by an emotional reaction such as laughter or anger. Sleep paralysis is an inability to move or speak that occurs as patients fall asleep or awaken. Hypnagogic hallucinations, which can be visual or auditory, occur while falling asleep.

Narcolepsy affects about 0.05 to 0.1% of the general population. The prevalence increases to 50% when the family history is positive. The exact genetic basis of inheritance is unknown. The age of onset is usually between 10 and 20 years. The diagnosis is often delayed or missed for months to years in some cases because not all symptoms may be present initially. Diagnosis is important because pharmacologic therapy with CNS stimulants may provide some symptomatic relief.

EVALUATION

History

Evaluation of children with sleep difficulties begins with a thorough, detailed sleep history taken from both parents and children, if old enough (see Questions Box).

Evaluation should also include an assessment of children's temperament and psychological well-being. Children's developmental status and level of function should also be evaluated.

Physical Examination

Physical examination is important to rule out organic causes of sleep difficulties. Acute illness (e.g., otitis media), obstructive sleep apnea resulting from adenoidal or tonsillar hypertrophy (most commonly), colic, gastroesophageal reflux, and any CNS disease or abnormality may all alter the sleep-wake cycle.

Laboratory Tests

Laboratory assessment is usually not necessary. An EEG may be useful if a central abnormality such as a seizure disorder is suspected. Polysomnography, the

---

Questions: Sleep

- Does the child have regular nap times and bedtimes, or do these depend on changing parental schedules?
- What activities does the child participate in during the evening before going to bed?
- Where does the child sleep?
- Does the child sleep in his or her own room or in the parents' room in his or her own bed or crib?
- Does anyone else sleep in the room?
- Is the child able to fall asleep on his or her own, or does he or she require the parent's participation?
- Does the child require feeding or fluids at night?
- What typically happens when the child wakes at night? Which parent attends to the child? What does the parent do?
- Is there a family history of sleep disturbances?
- Is there any stress within the home due to marital or financial difficulties that may affect the home environment and cause the child to be anxious or stressed?
- Is the child taking any medications that may affect sleep patterns?
- How long has the child been having sleep disturbances?
- Does the child experience problems every night or only intermittently?

---

simultaneous monitoring of EEG, ECG, chin muscle tone, eye movements, and respirations during a night of sleep in a sleep laboratory may be very useful in certain children when significant sleep disturbances such as apnea are suspected.

MANAGEMENT

The goal of management is to help children develop a healthy pattern of sleeping, not simply eliminate the immediate problem. Healthy sleep associations include providing a consistent schedule of naps and bedtime, along with a pleasant bedtime routine. It is important to put infants in their cribs while they are relaxed and drowsy but not already asleep. This gives them the opportunity to develop skills to put themselves to sleep. If they become accustomed to being fed or rocked until they fall asleep, they will seek the same means of falling asleep every time they normally wake up during the night. In addition, overstimulation in the evening may make settling to sleep difficult for toddlers or young children. Instead, a routine such as a bath followed by a story in the child's bedroom with a clearly defined end point when the parent leaves the child in the crib or bed sleepy but awake may help facilitate sleep. Children must learn to fall asleep on their own.

Trained night feeders and trained night criers are infants who have not learned to fall asleep on their own. The basic treatment for these children is to put them in their cribs when they are sleepy but awake and ignore the subsequent crying. Their last memory before falling asleep should not be of their mothers holding or feeding them. If the crying persists, the contact with the infants should be brief and boring. If they awaken for a feeding, parents should try to stretch the interval between waking and feeding so that children have an opportunity to practice self-calming techniques.

Specific sleep disorders can be addressed individually. Older toddlers and preschoolers who delay going to bed or refuse to stay in their room at night need clear, firm limits. It is important that these children have consistent bedtime routines and nighttime interventions for when they awaken. A gate may need to be installed in the bedroom doorway to prevent children who refuse to stay in their rooms at night from moving about the house and potentially hurting themselves or disturbing others. Parents of children who have night terrors may require reassurance that their children are not suffering from significant emotional problems or stressors. A night-light may help alleviate the anxieties of preschoolers who are unable to sleep at night because of their fears of darkness. Disturbances of the sleep-wake schedule can be corrected over time by gradually shifting children's schedules in the desired direction. For example, children with a delayed sleep phase who go to bed very late can have their morning wake-up time progressively advanced about 15 minutes per day; this is followed by a progressive advancement in their bedtime until the desired schedule is reached.

PROGNOSIS

Unfortunately, infants with sleep problems tend to grow into children with sleep problems. Researchers have found that about 40% of infants with sleep problems at the age of 8 months still had a problem at 3 years. It is to the parents' advantage to help their children develop healthy sleep habits rather than ignore the problems and hope that the children outgrow them.

Case Resolution

The 6-month-old infant described in the case history has disordered sleep associations. He has been conditioned to nighttime feedings, although he is old enough not to require them for nutrition. The physician suggests several things the mother can do to try to solve her son's sleep problem. She can begin by gradually lengthening the interval between daytime feedings to four to five hours. When he cries at night, she can wait progressively longer before feeding him and can then eventually eliminate the feedings altogether. He will learn to fall asleep on his own without requiring feeding.

Selected Readings

American Academy of Pediatrics: "Sleep Problems." *In* Guidelines for Health Supervision II. Elk Grove Village, IL, American Academy of Pediatrics, 1988, pp. 132–136.
Dement, W. C. Some Must Watch While Some Must Sleep. New York, W.W. Norton, 1976.
Ferber, R. Sleeplessness, night awakening and night crying in the infant and toddler. Pediatr. Rev. 9:1–14, 1987.
Ferber, R. Solve Your Child's Sleep Problems. New York, Simon & Schuster, 1985.
Schmitt, B. D. Sleep. *In* Your Child's Health, rev. ed. New York, Bantam Books, 1991.
Weissbluth, M. Sleep learning: the first four months. Pediatr. Ann. 20:228–238, 1991.

C H A P T E R   1 3

DENTAL CARE

Geeta Grover, M.D.

H$_x$ The parents of a 9-month-old girl bring her to the office because they are concerned because their daughter has no teeth yet. Growth and development have proceeded normally, and the physical examination is unremarkable.

Questions

1. What is the mean age and range for the eruption of the first tooth?
2. What is meant by the term "mixed dentition?"
3. At what age should fluoride supplementation begin?
4. When should oral hygiene using a toothbrush begin?

Pediatricians play an important role in the maintenance and evaluation of the oral health of children. Routine examination and screening of the oral cavity allow physicians to monitor normal development of teeth and screen for early signs of disease and abnormalities that involve the teeth or supporting structures. Parental counseling regarding preventive dental care and oral hygiene is also important.

NORMAL ANATOMY OF THE ORAL CAVITY

The oral cavity consists of teeth and supporting structures. Individual teeth have four major compo-

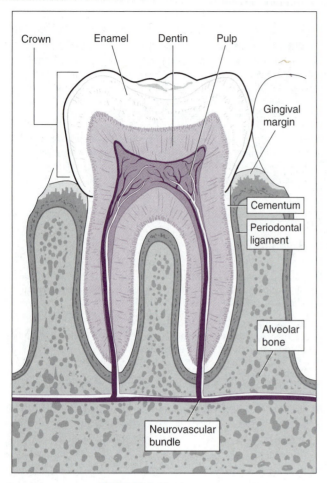

FIGURE 13–1. *Tooth anatomy.*

mately two thirds of root development is complete, and the tooth protrudes through the gingiva. **Exfoliation** of the primary teeth may be referred to as the final stage of tooth development. Table 13–1 summarizes the chronology of tooth development for both the primary and permanent teeth.

Normal Dentition

There is a relationship between the pattern of tooth eruption and skeletal maturation ("poor man's bone age"). Knowledge of the chronology of dental development can help physicians monitor normal growth and development and identify specific disease.

Primary Dentition

The period of primary dentition begins with the eruption of the first tooth, usually at about 6 months of age (normal range: about 4 to 12 months). In the vast majority of infants, the first tooth to appear is the mandibular central incisor. The **incisors** (central and lateral) erupt first; these are followed by the **first molars,** the **cuspids,** and the **second molars.** The pneumonic device used to recall this sequence is "forward-forward-back-forward-back" (incisor-incisor-molar-cuspid-molar). Maxillary teeth generally erupt 1 to 2 months after their mandibular counterparts. The 20 primary teeth should all be in place by the age of 24 to 36 months. In general, it is more important to know that one tooth should appear per month once eruption has

nents (Fig. 13–1): the outer layer, or **enamel;** the inner layer, or **dentin,** which constitutes the bulk of the tooth; the **pulp,** which contains the neurovascular structures; and the **root,** which secures the tooth into its socket in the maxilla or mandible. The **supporting structures** consist of the **bones of the face** (maxilla and mandible) and the **periodontal tissues** (gingiva, alveolar bone, periodontal ligament, and cementum). The visible portion of an erupted tooth is called the **crown.**

GROWTH AND DEVELOPMENT OF TEETH

Unlike the other calcified tissues of the body, which are mesodermal, the teeth originate from both ectoderm (enamel) and mesoderm (dentin and pulp). Tooth development occurs both pre- and postnatally in four stages, which may be summarized as growth, calcification, eruption, and exfoliation. **Growth** begins at about 6 weeks of gestation with the establishment of the organic matrix of the primary teeth. **Calcification,** or hard tissue formation, which involves the deposition of enamel, first occurs at about 3 to 4 months' gestation; the permanent teeth also begin to develop at this time. Although the major part of enamel deposition of the primary teeth has occurred by birth, this process may continue until the age of 12 to 16 years in one or more of the permanent teeth. **Eruption** occurs when approxi-

TABLE 13–1.   Chronology of Human Dentition

Primary or Deciduous Teeth

	Eruption		Shedding	
	Maxillary	*Mandibular*	*Maxillary*	*Mandibular*
Central incisors	6–8 mo	5–7 mo	7–8 yr	6–7 yr
Lateral incisors	8–11 mo	7–10 mo	8–9 yr	7–8 yr
Cuspids (canines)	16–20 mo	16–20 mo	11–12 yr	9–11 yr
First molars	10–16 mo	10–16 mo	10–11 yr	10–12 yr
Second molars	20–30 mo	20–30 mo	10–12 yr	11–13 yr

Secondary or Permanent Teeth

	Eruption	
	Maxillary	*Mandibular*
Central incisors	7–8 yr	6–7 yr
Lateral incisors	8–9 yr	7–8 yr
Cuspids (canines)	11–12 yr	9–11 yr
First premolars (bicuspids)	10–11 yr	10–12 yr
Second premolars (bicuspids)	10–12 yr	11–13 yr
First molars	6–7 yr	6–7 yr
Second molars	12–13 yr	12–13 yr
Third molars	17–22 yr	17–22 yr

Adapted, with permission, from Behrman, R.E. (ed.). Nelson Textbook of Pediatrics, 14th ed. Philadelphia, W.B. Saunders, 1992, p. 40.

FIGURE 13–2. *Primary dentition* (A) *and permanent dentition* (B). (From Zitelli, B. J., Davis, H. W. [eds.]. Atlas of Pediatric Physical Diagnosis, 2nd ed. Philadelphia, J. B. Lippincott, 1992, with permission.)

begun than it is to remember how many teeth should be present at a given age.

During the period of primary dentition, extra space between the teeth may be apparent. This space is actually normal and beneficial because it gives the larger permanent teeth more room. Crowding of the primary teeth may be an early indication of similar problems with the permanent teeth.

The time of eruption of primary teeth varies considerably. Late eruption is probably no cause for concern in children who are otherwise growing and developing normally. Significant delays in eruption, especially when associated with other developmental delays, however, may be associated with a variety of nutritional and systemic disturbances such as rickets, Down's syndrome (trisomy 21), hypopituitarism, and hypothyroidism.

Teething, the eruption of the primary teeth, is a normal part of development that usually occurs uneventfully. However, many symptoms have been attributed to teething by parents, grandparents, and physicians. Low-grade fever; drooling; local, temporary discomfort at the site of tooth eruption; and increased fussiness are some of the symptoms more commonly ascribed to teething. Otitis media, upper respiratory infection, and diarrhea are all common conditions during infancy whose appearance may coincide with the eruption of primary teeth. High fever, irritability, or signs of systemic illness should not be attributed to teething alone; further evaluation is necessary.

An eruption hematoma, a bluish swelling of the overlying gum, may precede the eruption of a tooth. It usually ruptures when the tooth appears and requires no further treatment. Symptoms of teething may be treated with acetaminophen, infant teething rings, and infant teething gels (if used correctly). Several other teeth remedies that have been suggested include hard or frozen bagels, ice, or firm rubbing of the gums. Caution is warranted when preparations containing topical anesthetics are used, because cases of seizures secondary to excessive absorption of the anesthetic have been reported.

Mixed Dentition

Mixed dentition occurs during the transition from primary to permanent dentition. It begins at about 6 years of age with the exfoliation of the primary teeth, usually the central incisors, followed by the eruption of the first permanent molars. The early appearance of primary teeth may herald the early eruption of permanent teeth. This stage continues until the last primary tooth has been shed, at about 12 years of age.

Two common, normal variations may give the children an awkward appearance temporarily. Either the maxillary permanent incisors may erupt in a widely spaced, outwardly inclined position ("ugly-duckling" stage) or the mandibular incisors may erupt behind the primary incisors ("double teeth"). These variations generally self-correct as dental development continues.

Permanent Dentition

Permanent dentition begins with the exfoliation of the last primary tooth, usually the cuspid or second molar, at 10 to 12 years of age. The permanent teeth number 32 (Fig. 13–2). Each of the four quadrants of the mouth contains two incisors, one cuspid, two premolars (bicuspids), and three molars (the third molar is the wisdom tooth).* The manner in which the teeth of the mandibular and maxillary arches fit together is referred to as **occlusion.** Normally, the maxillary incisors slightly

---

*The wisdom teeth generally erupt between the age of 17 and 22 years. The timing of their eruption is highly variable, however.

overlap their mandibular counterparts. Occlusion is fully established on completion of the permanent dentition, but it may be altered during the pubertal growth spurt secondary to jaw growth.

PREVENTIVE DENTAL CARE

Pediatricians can begin preventive oral health counseling during routine health maintenance visits. The role of nutrition, oral hygiene, daily fluoride intake, and nonnutritive sucking can be discussed with parents and children at this time. The American Academy of Pediatric Dentistry recommends that all children have their first visit to the dentist for examination and oral health counseling by 12 to 18 months of age.

Nutrition

Proper nutrition is essential to the development of healthy teeth. **Vitamins A, C, and D** as well as **calcium** and **fluoride** are particularly important in the formation of teeth. Maintenance of a diet low in sugar to help prevent caries is also important. It is particularly critical that pediatricians inform parents about nursing bottle caries, because these caries may harm both the primary teeth and any unerupted permanent teeth (see Chapter 45, Common Oral Lesions, for a more complete discussion).

Oral Hygiene

Counseling parents about oral hygiene should begin during their child's first year of life. During infancy, parents can **wipe children's teeth and gums** with a damp washcloth after feedings. A soft **toothbrush** moistened with **water** may be used after several teeth have appeared. **Toothpaste** may be introduced to children between the ages of two and three years. Parents should be warned that children of this age often swallow the toothpaste. A small, pea-sized amount should be used to minimize fluoride ingestion. **Flossing** should also be initiated when children are two to three years of age. It is usually not necessary before this age because tooth-to-tooth contact before this time is minimal.

Parents should continue to brush and floss their children's teeth at least once a day until the age of 6 years, when children should be encouraged to perform additional brushings themselves, with supervision. Although children usually begin to brush their teeth independently at age six, they still require assistance with flossing. Not until the age of 8 to 10 years do children have the fine motor coordination necessary to brush and floss effectively.

Fluoride

Fluoride is one of the most effective prophylactic agents in the prevention of dental caries. Dramatic reductions in the rate of dental caries have been demonstrated when systemic fluoride therapy is begun during infancy. Fluoride may be provided both systemi-cally and topically (e.g., fluoride-containing toothpaste and rinses or direct application in the dentist's office).

Systemic fluoride is incorporated into the enamel of the developing tooth, thus serving as an effective preeruptive cariostatic agent. Fluoride in the saliva provides a topical cariostatic effect by interfering with plaque-related microorganisms. For maximum protection against caries, **systemic fluoride** should be provided while teeth are developing; **topical fluoride** may be applied after teeth begin to erupt.

At present, it is recommended that systemic fluoride therapy begin at 6 months of age. Fluoridation of drinking water is the most effective way of providing systemic fluoride. The optimal concentration of fluoride in the local water supply varies in accordance with the climate (climate determines the amount of water children drink); it ranges between 0.7 and 1.2 ppm. Fluoride supplements may be prescribed in the form of drops or tablets based on children's age and the amount of fluoride in the drinking water (Table 13–2). Infants who are breast-fed or drink premixed formula require full fluoride supplementation until they begin drinking fluoridated water. Ideally, supplementation should be continued until all of the permanent teeth, excluding the third molars, have erupted, which is usually between 12 and 14 years of age (see Table 13–1). The American Association of Pediatrics recommends that supplementation continue until 16 years of age to ensure maximum benefit.

Although acute fluoride toxicity is rare, ingestion of large amounts can be potentially fatal (e.g., 500 mg of fluoride is a lethal dose for a 3-year-old child). To avoid accidental overdoses, no more than 120 mg of supplemental fluoride should be prescribed at one time. Chronic ingestion of excessive amounts of fluoride may result in enamel fluorosis. Fluorosis is the result of disruption in enamel formation; therefore, it can only be caused by the preeruptive ingestion of systemic fluoride. Small white specks on the enamel surfaces of teeth are the only signs of mild fluorosis, whereas pitting and brown discoloration of teeth surfaces are associated with severe fluorosis.

Nonnutritive Sucking

Nonnutritive sucking is a normal and essential activity for infants and young children. They may suck as a means of enjoyment, to cope with stress, or for comfort. Sucking is initially a reflex activity but later becomes an

Age	Water Fluoride Content (ppm)		
	< 0.3	0.3–0.6	> 0.6
Birth–6 mo	0	0	0
6 mo–3 yr	0.25	0	0
3–6 yr	0.50	0.25	0
6–16 yr	1.00	0.50	0

TABLE 13–2.   Fluoride Supplementation*

*Fluoride daily doses are given in milligrams.
Reproduced with permission from the Committee on Nutrition: Fluoride Supplementation for Children: Interim Policy Recommendations Pediatrics 95:777, 1995.

adaptive or learned behavior. The thumb, fingers, and pacifier are the most common objects used for sucking. An estimated 70% of children still practice some form of nonnutritive sucking at the age of 12 months. This decreases to 40% by the age of 24 months and to 1% by the age of 6 years. Most children discontinue the habit themselves by the age of 3. Generally, nonnutritive sucking has no long-term effects on permanent dentition if the habit ceases by the age of 4 or 5 years (see Chapter 31, Thumb-sucking and Other Habits). The most common dental problem associated with prolonged sucking is development of malocclusions.

Case Resolution

The parents of the infant in the case history should be reassured that the absence of teeth in their 9-month-old daughter is normal. Her first tooth may not appear until she is 12 months old. As long as she is growing and developing normally, there is no cause for concern.

Selected Readings

Griffen, A. L., and S. J. Goepferd. Preventive oral health care for the infant, child and adolescent. Pediatr. Clin. North Am. 38:1209–1226, 1991.

Jaber, L., I. J. Cohen, and A. Mor. Fever associated with teething. Arch. Dis. Child. 67:233–234, 1992.

Nazif, M. M., et al. Oral disorders. *In* Zitelli, B.J., and H.W. Davis. Atlas of Pediatric Physical Diagnosis, 2nd ed. Philadelphia, J.B. Lippincott, 1992.

Nowak, A. J. Promoting oral health in the school-age child. Contemp. Pediatr. 11:27–51, 1994.

Nowak, A. J. What pediatricians can do to promote oral health. Contemp. Pediatr. 10:90–106, 1993.

Schusterman, S. Pediatric dental update. Pediatr. Rev. 15:211–218, 1994.

CHAPTER 14

NORMAL DEVELOPMENT AND DEVELOPMENTAL ASSESSMENT

Geeta Grover, M.D.

Hₓ The parents of a 12-month-old child are concerned that she is not walking yet. They report that she sat independently at seven months and began crawling at eight months. She can pull herself up to stand while holding on but is not cruising. Her birth and medical history are both unremarkable. The physical examination is within normal limits.

Questions

1. What are the major areas in which development is assessed?
2. What are the gross motor, fine motor, and personal/social milestones for a 12-month-old child?
3. What tests are useful for assessing child development?
4. How is developmental delay in children defined?

Development is the acquisition of motor and cognitive skills during childhood. These skills may be divided into five major domains or areas: gross motor, fine motor/adaptive, personal/social, language, and cognitive. Monitoring the growth and development of children is an integral part of the assessment of pediatric patients. This chapter discusses the major areas of development and the principles that govern them.

Four principles apply to all aspects of development. First, development is a continuous process that proceeds in the cephalocaudal direction and parallels neuronal myelination; therefore, developmental milestones reflect the maturation of the nervous system. Second, the sequence of development is the same in all children, but the rate of development may vary from child to child (e.g., all children must walk before they run, but the age at which children walk or run varies from child to child). Third, the rate of attainment of milestones in one area may not parallel that in another. Fourth, certain primitive reflexes must be lost before corresponding voluntary movements can be attained (e.g., the asymmetric tonic neck reflex must disappear before children can roll over).

PATHOPHYSIOLOGY

Development is influenced by both biological and environmental factors. Biological factors such as prematurity, exposure to drugs in utero, or the presence of chronic disease may place children at increased risk for developmental problems and delays. Environmental factors influencing development include parental attitudes and actions, sociodemographic factors, and cultural and societal influences. The quality of parental stimulation may influence the rate of acquisition of certain skills, especially cognitive and language abilities in preschool-age children. Poverty and other social factors may make it difficult for parents to provide their child with an optimal environment for growth and development.

Development in Newborns and Infants

Normal, full-term newborns enter the world capable of responding to visual, auditory, olfactory, oral, and tactile stimuli. They can be quieted and can even soothe themselves. Newborns can signal needs (e.g., crying when hungry or wet), but they have a limited ability to respond to caregivers, primarily exhibiting disorganized and seemingly purposeless movements when stimulated. These patterns of movements may be primitive reflexes or postural reactions.

Primitive reflexes are mediated by the brainstem; they are involuntary motor responses that are elicited by appropriate peripheral stimuli. They are present at birth and disappear during the first six months of life. Normal motor development appears to be related to the suppression of these reflexes (Fig. 14–1). Persistence or reappearance of these reflexes may indicate the presence of brain damage. **Postural reactions, which are ultimately smoothly integrated into adult motor function** (see Fig. 14–1), appear between 2 and 9 months of age. These reactions help maintain the orientation of the body in space and the interrelationship of one body part to another.

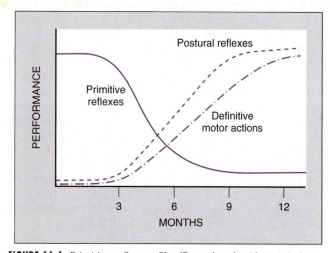

FIGURE 14–1. *Primitive reflex profile. (Reproduced, with permission, from Capute, A.J., et al. Primitive Relex Profile. Baltimore, University Park Press, 1978, p. 10.)*

TABLE 14–1. Selected Primitive Reflexes

Moro Reflex
Allowing the infant's head to drop back suddenly results in abduction and upward movement of the arms followed by adduction and flexion. This reflex disappears by 4 months.

Rooting Reflex
Touching the corner of the infant's mouth results in lowering of the lower lip on the same side and movement of the tongue toward the stimulus.

Sucking Reflex
Placing an object in an infant's mouth causes vigorous sucking.

Grasp Reflex
Placing a finger in an infant's palm causes the infant to grasp it; the infant reinforces the grip as the finger is drawn upward. A similar response is seen in the foot grasp. Both these reflexes disappear by 2–3 months.

Placing Reflex
Stroking the anterior aspect of the tibia against the edge of a table results in the lifting of the infant's leg to step onto the table.

Stepping Reflex
Holding the infant upright and slightly leaning forward produces alternating flexion and extension movements of the legs that simulate walking. This reflex disappears by 5–6 weeks.

Asymmetrical Tonic Neck Reflex
With the infant lying supine, turning the head to one side results in extension of the extremities on that side and flexion of the opposite extremities ("fencer position"). This reflex disappears by 3–4 months.

The profile generated by combining primitive reflexes and postural reactions can be used to monitor the course of normal development and identify cases of problematic development. Persistence of primitive reflexes or failure of development of postural reactions can signal developmental problems. Authorities estimate that there are over 70 primitive reflexes and postural reactions. Researchers do not agree on which of these reflexes or reactions are the most useful in the monitoring of development. The seven most commonly used primitive reflexes are described in Table 14–1, and selected postural reactions are presented in Table 14–2.

Normal Development

A developmental assessment should include an evaluation of milestones in each of the five major areas. **Gross motor skills** are overall movements of large muscles (e.g., sitting, walking, running). **Fine motor/adaptive skills** involve use of the small muscles of the hands, the ability to manipulate small objects, problem-solving skills, and eye-hand coordination. **Language skills** include hearing, understanding, and use of language. **Personal/social skills** involve socialization and ability to care for personal needs. **Cognitive skills** in-

TABLE 14–2. Selected Postural Reactions

Righting Reactions
These allow the body to maintain normal postural relationships of the head, trunk, and extremities during all activities. The different reactions appear at different ages, beginning shortly after birth and ranging up to 12 months of age.

Parachute Reactions
When held in ventral suspension and suddenly lowered (downward parachute), infants extend their arms as if to protect themselves from a fall; similar reactions are seen with lateral, forward, and backward stimulation. These reactions appear at 4–9 months.

TABLE 14–3.   Normal Pattern of Development

Gross Motor Skills		Personal/Social Skills	
Newborn	Reflex head turn; moves head side to side	Newborn	Regards face
1 mo	Lifts head when prone	6 wk	Spontaneous social smile
2 mo	Lifts shoulders up when prone	6 mo	Discriminates social smile
3 mo	Lifts up on elbows; head steady when upright	7 mo	Displays stranger anxiety; plays peek-a-boo (7–9 mo)
4 mo	Lifts up on hands; rolls from front to back; no head lag when pulled to sitting from supine position	12 mo	Drinks from a cup
5 mo	Rolls back to front	15–18 mo	Uses a spoon, spilling a little
6 mo	Sits alone 30 seconds or more	2 yr	Washes and dries hands
7–8 mo	Crawls/sits well	3 yr	Uses a spoon well; uses buttons
9–10 mo	Pulls to stand	4 yr	Washes and dries face; engages in cooperative play
10–11 mo	Cruises	5 yr	Dresses without assistance
12 mo	Walks	**Language Skills***	
15 mo	Walks backwards	Newborn	Alerts to bell
18 mo	Runs; kicks a ball	2 mo	Cooing; searches with eyes for sound
2 yr	Walks up and down stairs (taking one step at a time and holding on; stands on one foot [2.5 yr])	4 mo	Turns head to sound of voice or bell; laughs (3 mo)
3 yr	Walks up stairs alternating steps; rides a tricycle	6 mo	Babbles
4 yr	Walks down stairs alternating steps/hops on one foot	8 mo	Mama/dada nonspecific
5 yr	Skips	9 mo	Understands the word "no"
Fine Motor/Adaptive Skills		12 mo	Mama/dada specific; follows one-step command with gesture/3–5-word vocabulary
1 mo	Tracks horizontally to midline	14 mo	Follows one-step command without gesture
2 mo	Tracks past midline/tracks vertically	16 mo	Can point to several body parts
3 mo	Unfisted for >50% of the time; tracks 180 degrees; visual threat; discovers midline	2 yr	50-word vocaulary; two-word sentences; uses pronouns indiscriminately
4 mo	Reaches for bright object; brings object to mouth	2.5 yr	Gives first and last names; uses plurals
5 mo	"Rakes" at bright object	3 yr	250-word vocabulary; three-word sentences; speech intelligible to strangers 75% of time; uses pronouns discriminately
6 mo	Transfers object from one hand to the other	**Cognitive Skills**	
7 mo	Three-finger pincer grasp	Newborn–2 yr	Sensorimotor
9 mo	Neat pincer grasp bangs cubes in midline	2–6 yrs	Preoperational
14 mo	Tower of two cubes; scribbles spontaneously	6–11 yrs	Concrete operational
18 mo	Tower of four cubes	>11 yrs	Formal operations
2 yr	Copies vertical and horizontal line; tower of six cubes	**Miscellaneous Cognitive Milestones**	
3 yr	Copies circle	24 mo	Concept of today
4 yr	Copies "+" (3.5 yr)	30 mo	Concept of tomorrow
5 yr	Copies square; draws person with three parts (4.5 yr)	36 mo	Concept of yesterday
6 yr	Copies triangle; draws person with six parts	7 yr	Concept of right and left

*Detailed milestones are presented in Chapter 15, Table 15–1.

volve the ability to use higher mental processes including comprehension, memory, and logical reasoning.

Table 14–3 outlines the normal pattern of development with regard to each of these skills. Development is an orderly and sequential process, and children must proceed through several stages before any given milestone is attained. Therefore, the physician should document not only *what* children can do but *how* they do it. For example, to sit without support, children first achieve head control. Several stages later they are able to sit in a "tripod" position with arms extended in front for support, and finally sit with the head steady and back straight without support (Fig. 14–2).

Gross Motor Skills

The primary goal of gross motor development is walking. The first step toward this goal is head control. By six months of age children are able to sit without support for a few seconds. At 9 to 10 months children are able to pull themselves to a standing position, and by 12 to 14 months of age they are able to walk. Children then learn to run, negotiate stairs, hop on one foot, and skip—in that order.

Fine Motor Skills

Development of the two-finger pincer grasp is the major goal of fine motor development during the first year (Fig. 14–3). The hands primarily remain in a fisted position until 3 months of age. Infants also discover the midline at this age, and shortly thereafter they may play with the hands in the midline. 5-month-old children begin "raking" at desired objects; by 6 months of age they are able to transfer objects from one hand to the other. By 7 months they have a three-finger pincer grasp, and by 9 to 12 months they have developed the two-finger grasp, which allows them to manipulate small objects such as raisins and pencils. By 14 months they begin to scribble, and by 3 to 5 years they are able to copy geometric shapes. Early preference for the use of one hand over another should be assessed for the presence of paresis or other neuromuscular problems. Handedness may develop at 3 years but often is not firmly established until the age of 4 to 5 years.

Language Skills

The development of normal speech and language skills is discussed in Chapter 15, Language Development.

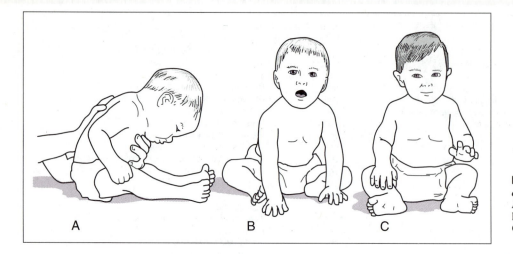

FIGURE 14–2. *Stages in the development of sitting.*
A. *Head control.*
B. *"Tripod sitting."*
C. *Head steady and back straight without support.*

Personal/Social Skills

These skills enable children to interact and respond to the surrounding world. The spontaneous social smile appears at 6 weeks of age followed by the discriminate social smile at 6 months. Stranger anxiety appears at 7 months, when games such as peek-a-boo become appealing.

Cognitive Skills

These abilities allow children to think, reason, problem-solve, and understand the surrounding environment. The concept of object permanence or object constancy, the realization that objects may exist even if they cannot be seen, develops at approximately 7 to 9 months of age. The understanding of time comes much later. Children develop the concept of "today" at 24 months of age, "tomorrow" at 30 months, and "yester-day" at 36 months. It is extremely important that health care providers realize that children's perception and understanding of pain, disease, and illness are guided by their stage of cognitive development. The psychologist Piaget generated complex generalizations by observing what children did and how they did it; his theories are the cornerstone of knowledge in this area. Piaget's four stages of cognitive development are presented in Table 14–4.

Developmental Delay

Children are said to be developmentally delayed if they fail to reach developmental milestones at the expected age. This age ranges widely because of the wide variation among normal children. Individual children may be delayed in one area or several areas of development.

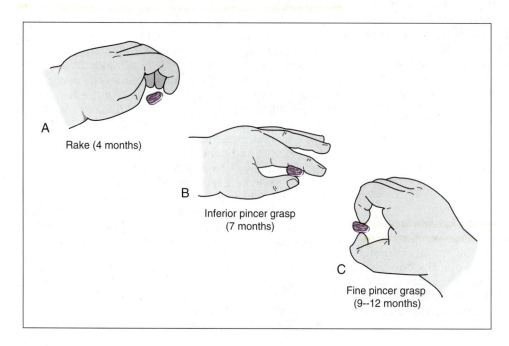

Rake (4 months)

Inferior pincer grasp (7 months)

Fine pincer grasp (9--12 months)

FIGURE 14–3. *Development of the pincer grasp.*
A. *Rake (4 months).*
B. *Inferior pincer grasp (7 months).*
C. *Fine pincer grasp (9–12 months).*

TABLE 14–4.   Stages of Development of Piaget

Sensorimotor (birth–2 years)
Children approach the world through sensations and motor actions. They develop a sense of object permanence, spatial relationships, and causality.
Preoperational (2–6 years)
Children's mental processes are linked to their own perception of reality. They do not separate internal and external reality.
Concrete Operational (6–11 years)
Children can perform mental operations in their heads if they relate to real objects. They develop concepts of conservation of mass, volume, and number.
Formal Operations (>11 years)
Children develop the capacity for abstract thought.

DIFFERENTIAL DIAGNOSIS

Three factors are involved in the differential diagnosis of children with developmental delays: (1) determination of the area or areas of development in which delay is apparent; (2) if motor delay is evident, determination of whether the condition is progressive or nonprogressive; and (3) assessment to see if developmental milestones previously achieved are lost or if age-appropriate milestones were achieved at all.

Children with an early history of normal development who subsequently experience a slowing of developmental progression, often associated with cognitive delays or seizures, may have a metabolic defect. Children who attain developmental milestones and subsequently lose them may have a neurodegenerative disease (e.g., multiple sclerosis, adrenoleukodystrophy) or a lesion of the spinal cord or brain. The presence of habitual rhythmic body movements (e.g., body rocking, head banging) may be a sign of a pervasive developmental disorder such as autism.

Cerebral palsy, the classic example of nonprogressive motor abnormality, is a form of static encephalopathy characterized by abnormal movement and posture. The type of cerebral palsy depends on which area of the brain is injured. Spastic cerebral palsy, seen most commonly, is secondary to upper motor neuron injury. The ataxic form of the disease is related to lesions of the cerebellum or its pathways. Dyskinetic cerebral palsy manifests as uncontrolled and purposeless movements that often result from a basal ganglia lesion (e.g., athetosis following bilirubin deposition in the basal ganglia [kernicterus]). The onset of symptoms is either in infancy or early childhood. The key factor in making the diagnosis is establishing that the motor deficits are static and nonprogressing.

EVALUATION

When evaluating children for possible delays in development, it is important to remember that there is a great deal of variation in the age of attainment of milestones. In addition, the rate of acquisition of milestones in one area of development may not parallel that in another. Routine and ongoing assessment of a child's level of development at all periodic health maintenance visits through observation, history, physical examination, and screening tests allows the physician to form a longitudinal view of the child. The physician is thus able to iden-

tify and differentiate true deficits and delays from temporary setbacks.

History

Evaluation of children for suspected delays in development includes a complete history (see Questions Box). Family history is important, because other family members may have relatively delayed attainment of milestones. Perinatal factors that place children at high risk for developmental difficulties include a history of maternal drug or alcohol use during pregnancy, prematurity in the infant, and congenital infections. Other historical risk factors for developmental delay include history of seizures, sepsis, or meningitis, exposure to lead or other toxins, and poor feeding or growth. Environmental factors such as stressful home conditions, history of abuse or neglect, and lack of stimulation may also contribute to delayed development.

Physical Examination

Both height and weight should be checked. Abnormal growth (i.e., height or weight less than the fifth percentile or head circumference either less than the fifth percentile or greater than the 90th percentile) may be a risk factor for developmental delay. The presence of congenital anomalies (e.g., cataracts, hypertelorism, spinal bifida) or neurocutaneous lesions (e.g., café au lait spots) may be suggestive of chromosomal anomalies or other genetic diseases. Neuromuscular examination should emphasize age-appropriate milestones. Abnormalities in muscle tone (e.g., hypotonia, hypertonia) or bulk or strength may be clues to the presence of neuromuscular disease (e.g., muscular dystrophy), cerebral palsy, or Down's syndrome.

Laboratory Tests

Age-appropriate assessment of the child's vision and hearing should be performed if signs of motor, cognitive, or language delays are apparent. Chromosomal studies may be conducted if dysmorphic features are noted on the physical examination. Evidence of cognitive or motor delays may warrant metabolic studies (e.g., organic and amino acids).

Imaging studies of the head such as MRI scans or EEGs may be necessary if the child has a history of seizures or an abnormal neurologic examination.

Questions: Normal Development

- Has anyone in the child's family had developmental problems or delays?
- Did the mother use any drugs or alcohol during pregnancy?
- Was the child premature?
- Does the child have a history of seizures?
- Has the child had meningitis or sepsis?
- Does the child have any history of not feeding well or poor growth?
- Is the child's home environment characterized by any stresses (e.g., divorce, limited financial resources)?

Developmental Testing

Developmental screening tests provide an assessment of children's performance on age-appropriate tasks in each area and allow for comparison with peers. Used regularly at routine well child care visits, these tests can help identify, in a timely manner, potential developmental problems and delays.

Many infant/child assessment scales are currently used. The Gesell Developmental Schedules, first developed by Arnold Gesell and colleagues in 1925, are primarily of historical significance today. They emphasize the importance of maturation of the central nervous system and deemphasize the influence of the environment. The Bayley Scales of Infant Development, first published in 1933 by Nancy Bayley, is one of the most commonly used scales today. It has three sections: mental, motor, and behavior. The final Bayley score is numerically equal to an IQ score for children 1 to 30 months of age. Both these assessments should be administered by trained examiners.

Unlike the above assessment scales, the Denver Developmental Screening Test or the Denver-II, the most recent version, is designed to be used by practitioners as a screening instrument for children from birth to 6 years of age. The test, divided into four areas (gross motor, fine motor/adaptive, personal/social, and language), consists of 125 tasks or items and takes 15 to 20 minutes to administer. It assesses the presence of developmental delays rather than simply giving each child an overall numerical score. Examiners should be trained in the administration of the Denver-II prior to using it. Studies examining the accuracy of the Denver-II in identifying children with developmental problems have shown that it has a high sensitivity but a limited specificity. Therefore, potentially normal children may be referred for additional evaluation.

MANAGEMENT

Children with identified developmental delays in one or more areas should be referred to the appropriate specialist, agency, or state program for further testing and assessment. Detailed neurologic examination may be necessary if gross motor delays are identified. Language delays may warrant formal hearing and speech assessment by an audiologist or speech pathologist. Cognitive impairment requires formal psychometric assessment, which in some cases can be performed through the child's school.

PROGNOSIS

The goal of early identification and intervention is to allow individual children to reach their maximum potential. Identification and treatment of underlying disease (e.g., hypothyroidism or infection) prevents further damage. Removal of children from adverse home environments or placement of children from impoverished home environments in early intervention programs can greatly stimulate their developmental potential. The prognosis for children with mild developmental delays can sometimes be improved greatly from participation in such infant stimulation programs.

Case Resolution

The parents of the child described in the case history may be reassured that their child is developing normally for her age. Although the majority of children begin walking at about 12 months of age, commencement of walking anywhere up to the age of 15 months is considered to be within normal limits.

Selected Readings

Capute, A. J., et al. Primitive Reflex Profile. Baltimore, University Park Press, 1978.

First, L. R., and J. S. Palfrey. The infant or young child with developmental delay. N. Engl. J. Med. 330:478–483, 1994.

Frankenburg, W. K., et al. Denver II Screening Test and Screening Manual, Denver, Denver Developmental Materials, Inc. 1990.

Illingworth, R. S. The Development of the Infant and Young Child, 9th ed. New York, Churchill Livingstone, 1987.

Illingworth, R. S. The Normal Child, 10th ed. New York, Churchill Livingstone, 1991.

Vaughan, V. C. Assessment of growth and development during infancy and early childhood. Pediatr. Rev. 13: 88–96, 1992.

CHAPTER 15

LANGUAGE DEVELOPMENT: SPEECH AND HEARING ASSESSMENT

Geeta Grover, M.D.

H$_x$ The parents of a 3-year-old girl bring her to see you. They are concerned because their daughter has only an 8- to 10-word vocabulary, and she does not put words together into phrases or sentences. They report that she seems to have no hearing problems; she responds to her name and follows directions well.

In general, she has been in good health. Her development, aside from delayed speech, is normal. During the physical examination, which is also normal, the girl does not speak.

Questions

1. What language skills should children have at 1, 2, and 3 years?
2. Approximately how many words should 3-year-olds have in their vocabulary?
3. By what age should children's speech be intelligible to strangers at least 75% of the time?
4. What factors may be associated with delayed speech development?
5. What tests are used to assess children's hearing, speech, and language development?

The ability to communicate through language is a uniquely human skill. Speech refers to the production of sounds, whereas language involves both comprehension and expression; it is the use of words, phrases, and gestures to convey intent. Normal hearing is essential for the development of speech and language.

The development of normal speech and language skills is an extremely important developmental milestone, that is eagerly awaited by parents. Normal patterns of language development should be as familiar to pediatricians as all other aspects of child development (see Chapter 14, Normal Development and Developmental Assessment). It is important that children with suspected language delays be referred to specialists as early as possible. Children with delayed speech or language development should be suspected of having a hearing deficit. Diminished hearing is an important cause of delayed language development.

EPIDEMIOLOGY

Handicapping sensorineural hearing loss is estimated to affect approximately 1/1000 live births in the United States. Many more infants are born with less severe hearing impairments, and still others develop hearing impairments during childhood. The prevalence of moderate to severe bilateral hearing loss is 1.5–2/1000 in children under 6 years of age. If less severe hearing losses and transient losses secondary to middle ear effusions are included, the prevalence increases significantly.

Language disorders may affect 5 to 10% of all children; they are one of the most common childhood disabilities. Although speech and hearing problems are common, they are often missed or minimized, and referral for evaluation and remediation is delayed significantly. Some researchers have estimated that the time from parents' first suspicion that their child may have a hearing loss to referral by the pediatrician to an audiologist for evaluation is as much as 12 months. On average, children with profound congenital hearing losses are not identified until they are approximately 2½ to 3 years of age, and children with less severe hearing losses may not be diagnosed until they are 4 years of age.

CLINICAL PRESENTATION

Lack of response to sound at any age, failure to achieve age-appropriate expressive language skills, and parental concern regarding a child's hearing are the most important signs of hearing or language impairment. Deaf infants coo normally and may even babble; therefore, an infant's vocalizing does not preclude a hearing loss.

PATHOPHYSIOLOGY

The left hemisphere of the brain is responsible for language skills in 94% of right-handed adults and approximately 75% of left-handed adults. Peripheral auditory stimuli are transmitted to the primary auditory areas in both temporal lobes. Sounds then undergo a series of analyses, primarily in three main areas in the left cerebral cortex: Wernicke's area (or auditory association area), which is responsible for the comprehension of language; Broca's area (or motor encoding area), which is responsible for the preliminary conversion of language into motor activity; and the primary motor cortex and supplementary motor cortex, which control the movements necessary for speech. This complex process is responsible for the comprehension and production of language.

Speech and language develop in a predictable, orderly

TABLE 15–1. Receptive and Expressive Language Milestones (birth to three years)*

	Receptive Milestones
Newborn:	Alerts to sound (e.g., startling, widening eyes, crying)
4 mo:	Orients to sound (i.e., looks to where sound came from); responds to own name
9 mo:	Understands "no"
12 mo:	Follows one-step commands accompanied by gesture (e.g., "bring me the bottle")
14 mo:	Follows one-step commands without gesture
17 mo:	Can point to several body parts
24 mo:	Follows two-step commands (e.g., "come here and sit down")
36 mo:	Listens to stories
	Expressive Milestones
2 mo:	Cooing (vowel sounds)
4 mo:	Laughs, "ah-gooing"
6 mo:	Babbling (consonants added to vowel sounds)
8 mo:	Indiscriminate use of "mama" and "dada"
12 mo:	Discriminate use of "mama" and "dada"; 3–5-word vocabulary; one-word utterances; immature "jargon-ing" (i.e., essentially gibberish with intonation and inflection)
16 mo:	Mature jargoning (i.e., gibberish with occasional intelligible word)
24 mo:	50-word vocabulary; two-word sentences; indiscriminate use of pronouns
36 mo:	250-word vocabulary; three-word sentences; discriminate use of pronouns; 75% of speech intelligible to strangers

*The language skills appropriate for each age should be viewed as general guidelines.

sequence. Language skills can be either receptive or expressive. Early receptive milestones refer to ability to hear and respond to sound, whereas later milestones reflect ability to understand spoken words. Early expressive milestones relate to speech production; later, children use language to convey their intent to others. In the first year of life, receptive skills are more advanced than expressive skills.

Knowledge of normal receptive and expressive language skills (Table 15–1) is essential to recognition and identification of developmental delays. Table 15–2 lists "danger signals" that indicate possible delays and serves as a guide for referral to specialists. It is most important to remember that by the age of three years, 75% of children's speech should be intelligible to strangers.

DIFFERENTIAL DIAGNOSIS

The various causes of delayed language development include hearing loss, disorders of CNS processing,

TABLE 15–2. Danger Signals in Language Development

Inconsistent or lack of response to auditory stimuli at any age
No babbling by 9 months
No intelligible speech by 18 months
Inability to respond to simple directions or commands (e.g., "sit down," "come here") by 24 months
Speech predominantly unintelligible at 36 months
Dysfluency (stuttering) of speech noticeable after five years
Hypernasality, inappropriate vocal quality, pitch, or intensity at any age

TABLE 15–3. Causes of Delayed Language Development

Hearing impairment
Perinatal risk factors leading to hearing impairment
Disorders of central nervous system processing
  Global developmental delay
  Mental retardation
  Autism
  Developmental language disorders
Disorders of language production (disorders of articulation)
Presence of anatomic abnormalities (e.g., cleft lip, cleft palate)
Environmental deprivation

anatomic abnormalities, and environmental deprivation (Table 15–3). Although birth order (e.g., the belief that younger children speak later than first-born children because older siblings speak for them), laziness (e.g., "Don't give him what he wants when he points. Make him ask for it"), and bilingualism are commonly believed to lead to speech and language delay, their contributory role has never been proved.

Hearing loss, which may lead to language delays, is either congenital or acquired. The majority of cases of congenital deafness are the result of genetic factors. The TORCH infections (**to**xoplasmosis, **r**ubella, **c**ytomegalovirus, **h**erpes simplex, **s**yphilis), especially CMV and rubella, are the most common nongenetic causes of hearing loss in the newborn period. Factors associated with high risk for infant hearing loss are outlined in Table 15–4.

The leading cause of acquired hearing loss in older infants and children is meningitis. On the basis of etiology, hearing loss can be divided into two categories: central (cortical hearing impairment) and peripheral. Peripheral causes are further subdivided into two broad groups: conductive (problems with transmission of sound through the external or middle ear) and sensorineural (inadequate transduction of sound waves into

TABLE 15–4. Factors Associated With High Risk for Infant Hearing Loss

Neonatal Period (birth to 28 days)
Family history of hereditary childhood hearing loss
In utero infection (e.g., TORCH infections [toxoplasmosis, rubella, cytomegalovirus, herpes simplex, syphilis])
Anatomical malformations of the head and neck region
Low birth weight (<1500 g)
Hyperbilirubinemia at a level requiring exchange transfusion
Exposure to ototoxic medications (e.g., aminoglycoside antibiotics)
Bacterial meningitis
Severe neonatal asphyxia or low Apgar score
Mechanical ventilation for 5 days or more
Stigmata of syndromes known to be associated with hearing loss
Infants and Children (28 days to 3 years of age)
Family history of hereditary hearing loss
Parental suspicion that the child does not hear
Bacterial meningitis or other infections associated with hearing loss
Severe head trauma (associated with loss of consciousness or skull fracture)
Stigmata of syndromes known to be associated with hearing loss
Exposure to ototoxic medications
Recurrent or persistent otitis media with effusion

Adapted, with permission, from the Joint Committee on Infant Hearing 1994 position statement. Pediatrics 95:152–156, 1995.

neural activity at the level of the inner ear or cranial nerve VIII).

Otitis media with effusion is the most common cause of conductive hearing loss in children (see Chapter 46, Otitis Media). Fluid in the middle ear can decrease sound conduction by an average of 25 decibels (dB). Other conditions that may result in conductive hearing loss include impaction of cerumen in the external ear canal, perforation of the tympanic membrane, atresia or stenosis of the ear canal, otosclerosis, abnormalities of the ossicles, and cholesteatoma. Injury to cranial nerve VIII or damage or maldevelopment of inner ear structures due to ototoxic agents, noise, cochlear agenesis, or perilymphatic fistula of the round or oval window membrane may lead to sensorineural hearing loss. Mixed hearing loss, a combination of conductive and sensorineural loss, may be seen in some children with developmental abnormalities.

Disorders of CNS processing include global developmental delay, mental retardation, autism, and developmental language problems. Developmental language disorders produce speech or language delays in children in the absence of hearing loss, anatomic abnormalities of the vocal tract, mental retardation, or global developmental delay. "Late talkers," or children who have normal comprehension but simply begin speaking late, have mild developmental language problems. Children who are completely nonverbal have more severe problems.

Anatomic abnormalities may also result in both speech and language delays. Cleft palate is the abnormality most commonly associated with difficulties in speech production. Children with cleft palate characteristically have hypernasal speech secondary to velopharyngeal incompetence (i.e., dysfunction of the soft palate). In addition, conductive hearing losses may result from chronic serous otitis media, which is common in these children. The presence of a submucous cleft palate, characterized by a bifid uvula, diastasis of the muscles in the midline of the soft palate with intact mucosa, and notching of the posterior border of the hard palate, should be considered in children without an overt cleft palate who have recurrent symptomatic serous otitis media and phonation difficulties.

Environmental deprivation is an uncommon cause of delayed language development. It requires historical or physical evidence of severe deprivation (e.g., profound FTT, physical or sexual abuse) or emotional trauma (e.g., domestic violence).

EVALUATION

History

At present, an estimated 70% of children with acquired hearing loss are initially identified by their parents. Therefore, parental suspicion that their children do not hear should be sufficient reason to initiate a formal hearing evaluation. When evaluating children less than 3 years of age, pediatricians must rely primarily on parental reports of children's language capabilities (see Questions Box). Children 3 years of age

and older can usually be engaged in conversation during the visit, but younger children are more likely to be uncooperative or remain silent when confronted by strangers or new situations.

Historical factors such as a family history of childhood deafness, exposure to ototoxic agents (e.g., aminoglycoside antibiotics) neonatal asphyxia, hyperbilirubinemia, maternal cocaine abuse, or low birth weight provide valuable information in the identification of high-risk infants (see Tables 15–2 and 15–4).

Questions: Language Development

- Is there any family history of childhood deafness?
- Has the child been exposed to any ototoxic agents (e.g., aminoglycoside antibiotics)?
- Is there a history of neonatal asphyxia, hyperbilirubinemia, or low birth weight?
- Has the child ever had bacterial meningitis?
- Did the mother have a TORCH infection during pregnancy?
- Are the child's language capabilities appropriate for age?
- Do the parents feel that their child has difficulty hearing?

Physical Examination

Examination should include a thorough assessment of the head and neck region. Microcephaly may indicate the presence of mental retardation or structural abnormalities. Abnormalities of the external ear (e.g., microtia) may be associated with sensorineural hearing loss. Otoscopic examination of the ear is essential. Presence of a middle ear effusion may be associated with a conductive hearing loss. The tympanic membrane should be examined for evidence of scarring or perforation, often secondary to recurrent otitis media. Tympanometry (impedance audiometry) performed in the office can provide information regarding the mobility of the tympanic membrane and the presence of middle ear effusions. Tympanometry is not a hearing test but rather an assessment of middle ear functioning.

Physical stigmata of any syndromes that may be associated with deafness (Table 15–5) should be noted.

Laboratory Tests

The advantages of early identification of hearing loss cannot be overemphasized. The 1994 position statement of the Joint Committee on Infant Hearing has endorsed universal hearing evaluation of all infants prior to discharge from the newborn nursery and no later than 3 months of age. The use of high risk criteria (see Table 15–4) to identify the population of infants to be screened is estimated to exclude approximately 50% of infants with hearing impairment. Until universal screening can be implemented, however, these factors should be used.

The evaluation of any child with delayed language development or suspected hearing loss begins with a hearing assessment. Various techniques are available, depending on the child's age and the degree of sophis-

TABLE 15–5. Syndromes Commonly Associated With Hearing Impairment

Autosomal Dominant Conditions

Brachio-otorenal syndrome
Goldenhar's syndrome (facioauriculovertebral dysplasia)
Stickler syndrome
Treacher Collins syndrome
Waardenburg's syndrome

Autosomal Recessive Conditions

Alport's syndrome
Jervell and Lange-Nielsen syndrome
Pendred's syndrome
Usher's syndrome

Chromosomal Disorders

Trisomy 13 s
Trisomy 18q s

Miscellaneous Disorders

CHARGE association (coloboma, congenital heart disease, choanal atresia, growth and mental retardation, genitourinary anomalies, ear anomalies and genital hypoplasia)
Congenital rubella syndrome

---

tication required. The brainstem auditory evoked response (BAER) may be used in children at any age, including newborns. This electrophysiologic measure, which does not require a child's cooperation, records brain waves as a function of sound stimuli (most commonly clicks). The BAER provides an objective assessment of the integrity of auditory pathways. Behavioral audiometry, which involves rewarding children visually for turning their heads toward sounds can be used in infants over 6 to 8 months of age. Conventional pure tone audiometry with headphones can be used in children over the age of 3 to 4 years and allows for the evaluation of each ear independently. Within the frequency range of normal hearing (500–2000 hertz), a hearing threshold of 0 to 15 dB defines the normal range. A hearing threshold of 15 to 25 dB indicates minimal hearing loss; 25 to 40 dB, mild; 40 to 65 dB, moderate; 65 to 95 dB, severe; and 95 dB or greater, profound.

Language assessment may be aided by the use of screening tests such as the Denver Developmental Screening Test or the Early Language Milestone Scale (Coplan, J.; Austin, TX, PRO-ED, 1987). These tests are used to supplement the clinical history of a child's language abilities.

MANAGEMENT

The first three years of life are extremely important to language development. Hearing impairment is one of the most common causes of delayed language development in young children. The history, physical examination, and initial screening can be used to suggest referral to various specialists (e.g., audiologists, speech pathologists, child psychologists, otolaryngologists) for further clarification of hearing, speech, or language deficits and treatment. Early identification of hearing impairment and its degree of severity allow for early intervention in the form of amplification of sound, special education for children, and counseling and support services for the families with affected children.

As soon as a diagnosis of significant hearing loss is made, **hearing aids** may be provided. **Cochlear implants** are experimental at present, but they may be useful in children with acquired hearing loss, such as toddlers with meningitis. With severe hearing loss, training in **sign language** and **lip reading,** which are most helpful for those children who already know a language, may be begun as early as possible. Special education is of prime importance in the management of children with language difficulties. The Education for All Handicapped Persons Act, federal legislation passed in 1975, requires that public schools provide an individualized and appropriate education for all children with disabilities. A knowledge of available community resources (e.g., special schools) can aid pediatricians in providing **support services** such as special community agencies and support groups for handicapped children and their parents.

Case Resolution

The child described in the case history has delayed development of expressive language skills. At the age of three years, she should have a 250-word vocabulary and speak in three-word sentences; in addition, her speech should be primarily intelligible to strangers. Because of the delay, she should be referred immediately for a hearing assessment and speech and language evaluation. Hearing loss is an important diagnosis to rule out. Simply because her parents report no hearing problems does not mean she does not have a deficit. She may have learned to respond to nonverbal cues, or she may hear only some things.

Selected Readings

Coplan, J. Evaluation of the child with delayed speech or language. Pediatr. Ann. 14:203–208, 1985.

Coplan, J. Normal speech and language development: an overview. Pediatr. Rev. 16:91–100, 1995.

Epstein, S., and J. S. Reilly. Sensorineural hearing loss. Pediatr. Clin. North Am. 36:1501–1520, 1989.

Joint Committee on Infant Hearing. Joint Committee on Infant Hearing 1994 position statement. Pediatrics 95:152–156, 1995.

Klein, S. K. Evaluation for suspected language disorders in preschool children. Pediatr. Clin. North Am. 38:1455–1467, 1991.

Montgomery, T. R. When "not talking" is the chief complaint. Contemp. Pediatr. 11:49–70, 1994.

Rapin, I. Hearing disorders. Pediatr. Rev. 14:43–49, 1993.

CHAPTER 16

GIFTED CHILDREN

Iris Wagman Borowsky, M.D., Ph.D.

H$_x$ A 3-year-old girl is brought to your office for well child care. Her parents believe that she may be gifted because she is much more advanced than her sister was when she was the same age. The parents report that their younger daughter walked at 11 months of age and was speaking in two-word sentences by 18 months. She is very "verbal," has a precocious vocabulary, and constantly asks difficult questions such as, "How do voices come over a radio?" The girl stays at home with her mother during the day but recently began going to a preschool program two mornings a week. She enjoys preschool and plays well with children her own age. She also likes to play with her sister's friends from school.

The girl is engaging and talkative. She asks questions about what you are doing during the examination and demonstrates impressive knowledge of anatomy. The physical examination is normal.

Questions

1. How are gifted children identified?
2. What characteristics are associated with giftedness?
3. What are the best approaches for dealing with the education of gifted children?
4. What is the role of the pediatrician in the management of gifted children?

Giftedness has been defined in several ways. The psychometric definition of giftedness is based on scores obtained on standardized intelligence tests. The two most frequently used cut-off points are two standard deviations above the mean (intelligence quotient [IQ] = 130–135) and three standard deviations above the mean (IQ = 145–150). Children with these scores are in the upper 2% and 0.1% of the IQ distribution, respectively. IQ, which is considered to be fairly stable after the age of 3 or 4 years, is the best single predictor of scholastic achievement at all levels, from elementary school to college.

A second definition of giftedness is based on real-life achievements or performance of exceptional skills rather than on test scores. Children with special talents (other than general intelligence) in areas such as music, mathematics, ice skating, chess, or drama fit this description. Other definitions of giftedness recognize motivation, commitment, perseverance, high self-esteem, and creativity as personality traits that allow children with above average ability to develop exceptional talents.

EPIDEMIOLOGY

The prevalence of giftedness depends on the somewhat arbitrary definitions of giftedness and the varied approaches for identification of gifted children. Traditional screening systems identify 3 to 5% of students for participation in gifted programs in schools. Some schools use an alternative system, where 10 to 15% of children are recognized as above average. In an effort to foster giftedness in these children, schools offer them enriched programs.

Intellectual giftedness in children has been associated with the social, economic, and educational background of their families. Factors that correlate with higher IQ scores in children are more years of parental education, higher IQ scores of mothers, increased family income, smaller family size, and longer intervals between siblings. Children from low-income and minority backgrounds are less likely to be identified as gifted than other children. African Americans, Hispanics, and Native Americans are underrepresented by 30 to 70% in gifted programs in the United States.

Larger head size at one year of age and greater height and weight at four years of age have also been reported in children with high IQs. Although researchers have found that academically gifted children, as a group, begin to walk, verbalize, and read earlier, such factors are not useful for predicting giftedness in individual children.

EVALUATION

One of the primary goals of child health promotion is **developmental monitoring.** The early identification of developmental delays, which allows for prompt intervention, is one of the primary purposes of such monitoring. Techniques for developmental assessment include **review of developmental milestones** with parents and discussion of parental concerns, **informal observation** of children in the office, and **formal screening with standardized tests** such as the Denver Developmental Screening Test.

Identification of Gifted Children

Although parents' first concern is usually to confirm that their child is developing normally, it is not uncommon for parents to ask if their child is gifted. Such questions are typically motivated by parents' desire to optimally encourage their child's development. Sharing

TABLE 16–1. Factors Used in the Identification of Giftedness in Children

Intelligence tests
Standardized achievement tests
Grades
Classroom observations
Parent and teacher rating scales
Evaluation of creative work in a specific field (e.g., poems, drawings, science projects)

---

information and observations with parents during developmental monitoring may facilitate parent-child interaction and child development. In a competitive society, the pediatric provider should look for signs that above average abilities are the result of undue pressures placed on children, such as incessant teaching or overscheduling of time.

Infancy and early childhood may not be the best time to determine whether a child is gifted. Age of attainment of developmental milestones and performance on standardized tests (e.g., Bayley Scales of Infant Development) during the first two years of life are both unreliable predictors of intellectual giftedness. Reasons for this lack of reliability may include weaknesses in the tests and variable rates of child development that result in transient precocity or delay. Tests that focus on visual memory tasks in infants may be better predictors of later academic intelligence; this possibility requires more research. In addition, many special talents that comprise giftedness, such as creativity or artistic or musical ability, may not manifest themselves until children are older.

The determination of giftedness in older children may involve several factors (Table 16–1). The early identification of giftedness allows for the development of an appropriate educational program that is optimally matched to a particular child's ability to learn. Without early identification and intervention, intellectually gifted children may become disillusioned with school, lose interest in learning, fail to develop study skills because they are never challenged to think and work hard, and develop a pattern of underachievement that may be difficult to reverse by the middle grades.

Special Groups of Gifted Children

Giftedness is harder to identify in some children. In **physically disabled children,** giftedness is often obscured by their obvious physical handicap, which demands attention. These children may participate in special programs where their physical needs are the major concern at the expense of their academic or artistic potential. In addition, poor self-esteem associated with the disability may prevent these children from realizing their potential. To identify giftedness in physically disabled children, parents and teachers must make a concerted effort to search for potential and encourage its development. Strengthening a child's capacities may involve training in the use of a wheelchair or computer or taking frequent breaks to prevent fatigue.

Giftedness also commonly goes unnoticed in **learning-disabled children.** It is quite possible for exceptional and poor abilities to coexist in a given child. In fact, an estimated 10% of gifted children have a reading problem, reading two or more years below grade level. Albert Einstein, Auguste Rodin, and John D. Rockefeller are famous examples of brilliant individuals who had reading and writing problems. An extreme example of the occurrence of both extraordinary and deficient abilities together in one individual is the "child savant." Affected children possess amazing abilities in one area (e.g., music, drawing, mathematics, memory), but they are retarded in other respects. In addition, they have behavioral problems that resemble autism, such as repetitive behavior, little use of language, and social withdrawal.

Learning disabilities may obscure children's talents, thus preventing awareness of their potential. Conversely, children's giftedness may mask their weaknesses, depriving them of needed help. Worst of all, gifted-learning disabled children may manage to barely "get by" in the regular classroom setting and fail to receive recognition for strengths or weaknesses. Large differences on intelligence and achievement tests between scores in different areas, such as language and spatial abilities, may indicate both giftedness and a learning disability. Attention should be given to both weaknesses and strengths. Research suggests that programs that focus on strengths, not deficits, however, enhance self-esteem in gifted learning, disabled children and can be extremely beneficial in their academic development.

The identification of giftedness is also difficult in **underachieving children.** Parents may approach the pediatrician with the following frustrating problem: their child is doing poorly at school, although they believe that the child is bright because of the child's abilities and participation in advanced activities at home. Underachievement may result from a learning disability; poor self-esteem; lack of motivation; or the absence of rewards, either at home or at school, for succeeding in academics.

As previously stated, giftedness is less likely to be recognized in children from low-income or ethnically diverse families. Many of the tests used to identify giftedness have been "normed" on white, English-speaking, middle-class children. In the absence of tests that are sensitive to socioeconomic differences, other means for identifying giftedness, such as assessment of creative work and teacher and student nominations, should be stressed. Schools with students from low-income or minority backgrounds tend to use their limited resources to help students who are doing poorly in school, not those students who are gifted. Research has shown that programs for gifted children from such backgrounds benefit all students by creating positive role models and promoting the school as a place for the cultivation of excellence.

MANAGEMENT

At Home

Loving, responsive, stimulating parenting should be encouraged for all children, including gifted children. Parents of gifted children may feel inadequate, fearing that their child is smarter than they are. The pediatrician can provide **parental reassurance** by telling parents, "You must have been doing something right for your child to have been identified as gifted." Children's librarians, periodicals written for parents and teachers of gifted children (e.g., *The Gifted Child Today*), and the local chapter of the National Association for Gifted Children are good resources for parents.

Parents are often overwhelmed with complex questions from their precocious preschool children about issues ranging from homelessness and world hunger to theology and the creation of the universe. The pediatrician should tell parents that they (1) should not be afraid to admit that they do not know all the answers and (2) should work together with their child to find the answers.

The pediatrician may need to warn parents about putting too much pressure on their gifted children. For example, enrolling children in multiple classes often leaves little free time for unstructured play. Play affords many opportunities for self-learning, interaction with peers, and development of creativity and initiative. Parents of infants, toddlers, and preschoolers should be encouraged to take cues from their children. If children have a rich environment with plenty of objects and books to explore, diverse experiences, and stimulating interactions, they will develop their own interests. Other educational materials and special instruction can then be provided in a particular area of interest.

Gifted children are often mistakenly considered to fit the stereotype of troubled, socially awkward "nerds." With the exception of children at the genius extreme (IQ >180), gifted children are generally more sociable, well-liked, trustworthy, and emotionally stable than their peers, with lower rates of mental illness and delinquency. Nevertheless, they have the same emotional needs as do other children. Gifted children may prefer to play with older children whose interests and abilities are closer to their own. This should be allowed as long as these relationships are healthy.

Parents should be encouraged to treat gifted children the same way they do their other children. Siblings of gifted children may become resentful if attention is centered on their brother or sister. They may feel inferior, particularly if gifted children surpass them in school. Tensions may be magnified if gifted children become friends with their older sibling's friends. All tensions should be openly discussed within the family. To preserve a sense of self-worth and competence in siblings, the pediatrician should recommend to parents that they set aside special time to spend with each of their children. Parents should encourage other talents (e.g., musical or athletic abilities) in siblings. Older siblings should receive the special privileges and responsibilities that come with age, such as staying up later or doing different chores. Any tensions within the family should be openly addressed.

At School

Parents often seek advice from their pediatrician about educational planning for gifted children. A learning environment with the optimal degree of challenge—hard enough to require new learning and stave off boredom, but not so hard as to be discouraging—is the goal for all children. Parents of young children should look for preschools with flexible programs and capable teachers to accommodate children with precocious skills. Parents of school-age children must decide whether **acceleration** (starting school earlier or skipping grades) or **enrichment** (staying in the same grade but supplementing the regular curriculum) is more appropriate (Table 16–2). The choice depends on the particular child.

Parents and teachers of gifted children are usually concerned that children in accelerated programs may have problems with social adjustment if their classmates are older. Existing evidence suggests gifted children benefit socially from acceleration, however. Gifted children in accelerated programs participate in school activities (except contact sports) more often than gifted children placed with classmates of the same age. Even when gifted children are placed with children their own age, they tend to make friends with older children with whom they share more interests. Gifted children also make up any curricular content missed by grade-skipping. Because the process may be difficult to reverse, it may not be the best option when the decision is a borderline one.

Enrichment involves keeping gifted children with same-age classmates but supplementing the regular curriculum. Regular class placement with a teacher who is willing to offer extra work (e.g., special projects) in addition to grade-level assignments, part-time programs to supplement regular classwork (e.g., field trips, foreign language classes), "honors" classes that group bright children together for their basic curriculum, and independent study by the family at home are all examples of enrichment programs. These programs may work well for some gifted children, depending in

TABLE 16–2.   Acceleration Versus Enrichment in Gifted Education

	Advantages	Disadvantages
Acceleration	May provide suitable academic challenge	Difficult to reverse
	May have social benefits	May have to skip more than one grade to be properly challenged
	Can be offered by all schools	
	Inexpensive	
Enrichment	Classmates are same age	May be expensive
	May expose children to subjects they would not otherwise learn	Inadequate for highly gifted children
	Appropriate for mildly gifted children	May isolate gifted from nongifted children and encourage "elite" label
		May lead to excessive homework if children have to make up work of regular class

large part on the resources and funding available and the experience, creativity, and enthusiasm of the teachers involved.

Some enrichment programs may isolate gifted from nongifted children, however, and encourage labeling of the gifted students as "elite." If children are required to make up the regular class work that they miss when they are involved in the enrichment program, they may find themselves overloaded with homework.

Often a **combination of acceleration and enrichment** programs is the best option. Either acceleration or enrichment alone may not be enough for the brightest children. Acceleration may not be sufficient for markedly advanced children who would have to skip two or three grades to be appropriately challenged. The pediatrician should recommend that parents work closely with teachers to achieve the best learning environment for their children. Some factors that should be considered are age, physical size, motor coordination, emotional maturity, personality, and particular areas and degrees of giftedness of the child. Acceleration may be a better option for a large, outgoing child than for a small one. Gifted children should be asked what they would like to do.

When evaluating the suitability of an educational situation for their gifted child, parents should watch for some warning signs. Excessive homework should neither be expected nor tolerated, as it cuts into the child's time to play and develop socially. The emphasis in gifted education should be on broadening perspectives, not increasing busy work. If gifted children are developing a sense of elitism or peer animosity, the nature and

philosophy of the program should be questioned. Boredom with schoolwork, the lack of a need to study, signs of depression, or symptoms suggestive of school phobia such as recurrent abdominal pain or headaches on school mornings should prompt investigation of the suitability of the child's program.

Case Resolution

In the case presented, the physician should reaffirm the parents' observations that their child is gifted. The parents should be encouraged to explore programs in which their daughter's talents may be fostered, but at the same time, they should understand that even gifted children need time for play and unstructured activities.

Selected Readings

Ciba Foundation Symposium. The origins and development of high ability. 178:1–258, 1993. (Entire issue on giftedness.)

Feiring, C., and L. T. Taft. The gifted learning disabled child: not a paradox. Pediatr. Ann. 14:729–732, 1985.

Fisch, R. O., et al. Children with superior intelligence at seven years of age: a prospective study of the influence of perinatal, medical and socioeconomic factors. Am. J. Dis. Child. 130:481–487, 1976.

Mills, C. J. Academically talented children: the case for early identification and nurturance. Pediatrics 89:156–157, 1992.

Pediatr. Ann. 14:691–768, 1985. (Entire issue on the gifted child.)

Shapiro, B. K., et al. Giftedness: can it be predicted in infancy? Clin. Pediatr. 28:205–209, 1989.

Schecter, N. L., and S. M. Reis. The gifted child. In: Levine, M.D., W. B. Carey, and A. C. Crocker (eds.). Developmental-Behavioral Pediatrics. Philadelphia, W. B. Saunders, 1992, pp. 589–596.

CHAPTER 17

IMMUNIZATIONS

Geeta Grover, M.D.

H_x An 8-month-old infant is evaluated in the emergency department for a history of fever for 2 days. The mother reports that her daughter has been pulling at her ears and is not sleeping well at night. The girl's past medical history is unremarkable. She is taking no medications except for acetaminophen for fever, and no family members are ill at home. Review of her immunization history reveals that she has received immunizations only at 2 and 4 months.

On examination, the girl's temperature is 101° F (38.3° C), but she is alert and appears nontoxic. Except for bilateral otitis media, the rest of the examination is within normal limits. Discharge orders for appropriate immunizations to be given today in addition to antibiotics and antipyretic medications are written. The nurse questions the orders to give immunizations to an ill infant.

Questions

1. According to the recommended schedule of immunizations, what immunizations should infants have received by the age of 8 months?
2. Can febrile infants with conditions such as otitis media be immunized?
3. What are the contraindications to immunizations?
4. What are some of the barriers that prevent children from being immunized?

Immunizations are one of the simplest and most cost-effective preventive health care measures available today. They are an essential component of comprehensive well child care, and immunization coverage levels of infants and children are a measure of quality of preventive health services. The immediate goal of immunizations is to prevent disease in susceptible individuals, but the ultimate goal is to eradicate disease in populations. The global eradication of smallpox in 1980 is an example of disease eradication through immunizations and effective public health control measures. The incidence of vaccine-preventable diseases has declined tremendously in the United States as a result of immunizations. The reported number of cases of diphtheria, measles, mumps, pertussis, poliomyelitis, rubella, and tetanus have declined by 97% or more during this century.

Over 95% of school-age children in the United States are fully immunized by the time they are 5 or 6 years of age because of the enforcement of laws requiring adequate immunizations prior to school entry. However, according to a recent study by the CDC, only 11 to 58% (median: 44%) of children are adequately immunized by their second birthday, with 20% or fewer age-appropriately immunized (each dose of vaccine given no later than 30 days after the recommended age for its administration). This disparity between immunization levels at 5 years of age versus 2 years of age is the **immunization dichotomy,** which states that although children are adequately immunized by the time of school entry, they are inadequately protected during the first few years of life. This is the period when they are most susceptible to the morbidity and mortality associated with vaccine-preventable diseases. The previously high immunization rates in the United States are now slowly declining.

An example of the high cost of inadequate immunization is an increase in the occurrence of vaccine-preventable disease. This is currently best represented by the recent measles epidemic. In 1983, the United States had 1500 cases of measles, an all-time low. This number rose to about 25,000 at the peak of the epidemic in 1990, with case fatality rates as high as four deaths per 1000 cases in some areas.

TYPES OF IMMUNIZATION

Active immunity is the development of specific immunity within the host in response to contact with infectious organisms (e.g., bacteria, viruses). Natural active immunity is spontaneously obtained through community-acquired contact with the organism and protects the host against subsequent exposures to that organism (e.g., as in chickenpox). When the morbidity and mortality associated with infections is significant (e.g., with measles or diphtheria), electively induced immunity, or immunoprophylaxis, is considered. Immunoprophylaxis may be accomplished by means of active immunization.

Vaccines may either contain live and attenuated or killed (inactivated) infectious agents. Although live vaccines are more likely to induce long-lasting or permanent immunity than killed vaccines, they carry the risk of causing vaccine-induced disease in recipients or spreading the vaccine strain to secondary hosts. Killed vaccines are noninfectious, but they can only induce immunity for relatively short periods. They therefore require booster injections to maintain immunity.

In **active immunization,** a vaccine that contains all or part of a microorganism or a modified product of that microorganism (e.g., toxoid, purified antigen, genetically engineered antigen) is administered to evoke an immunologic response without producing significant clinical illness. This immunologic response protects recipients from future exposures to the involved microorganism.

Passive immunization, in contrast to active immunization, involves providing preformed human or animal antibodies to individuals who have no active immunity against a particular infectious agent but have already been exposed or are at high risk for exposure. Indications for the use of passive immunizations include high risk of developing significant complications from certain disease exposure (e.g., immunocompromised children exposed to varicella or measles); insufficient time for adequate protection by active immunization alone (e.g., postexposure rabies); certain immunodeficiency states that result in deficient antibody synthesis; and preexposure prophylaxis with immune globulin against hepatitis A (e.g., for persons traveling to high-risk areas). Passive immunization provides immediate, relatively brief protection. In contrast, active immunization requires time to develop but provides prolonged or lifelong immunity.

CURRENT RECOMMENDED IMMUNIZATION SCHEDULE

Whether to immunize for a particular disease in a given region depends on the severity of the disease and the probability of exposure as compared to the cost and effectiveness of the vaccine. The earliest a vaccine may be administered is the youngest age at which children can mount a protective immunologic response to it. For example, measles, mumps, and rubella (MMR) vaccine is usually given at 12 to 15 months of age because transplacentally acquired maternal measles antibodies may persist up to 12 months of age.

TABLE 17–1. Routine Childhood Vaccinations in the United States

Vaccine	Type	Route
DTP	Toxoids and inactivated bacteria	IM
DTaP	Toxoids and bacterial components	IM
HBV	Inactivated viral antigen: yeast-derived recombinant or plasma-derived	IM
Hib	Polysaccharide-protein conjugate	IM
MMR	Live viruses	SC
Poliovirus		
OPV	Live virus (trivalent)	Oral
IPV	Inactivated virus (trivalent)	SC

Modified, with permission, from Committee on Infectious Diseases, American Academy of Pediatrics. Active and passive immunization. In 1994 Red Book: Report of the Committee on Infectious Diseases, 23rd edition. Elk Grove Village, IL, American Academy of Pediatrics, 1994, p. 11.

Abbreviations: DTP, diphtheria and tetanus toxoids and pertussis vaccine; DTaP, diphtheria and tetanus toxoids and acellular pertussis vaccine; HBV, hepatitis B virus vaccine; Hib, *Haemophilus influenzae* type b conjugate vaccine; MMR, measles-mumps-rubella vaccine; OPV, oral poliovirus vaccine; IPV, inactivated poliovirus vaccine; IM, intramuscular; SC, subcutaneous.

TABLE 17–2.   Recommended Childhood Immunization Schedule

Recommended Age	Immunization(s)
Birth	HBV
2 months	DTP, OPV, Hib, HBV
4 months	DTP, OPV, Hib
6 months	DTP, OPV,* Hib,† HBV*
12–15 months	Hib, MMR
12–18 months	DTP or DTaP if older than 15 months
4–6 years	DTP or DTaP, OPV, MMR‡
14–16 years	dT (repeat every 10 years throughout life)

*The third dose of OPV and HBV may be given at any time between 6 and 18 months of age.

†Currently three Hib conjugate vaccines are available for use in infants: HbOC (HibTITER), PRP-T (ActHIB), (OmniHIB), and PRP-OMP (PedvaxHIB). The fourth, PRP-D (ProHIBit) is recommended only for children 12 months of age and older. Children who receive the PRP-OMP at 2 and 4 months of age do not require a dose at 6 months.

‡The second dose of MMR may be administered at either 4 to 6 or 11 to 12 years of age.

Adapted, with permission, from Committee on Infectious Diseases, American Academy of Pediatrics. 1994 Red Book: Report of the Committee on Infectious Diseases, 23rd edition. Elk Grove Village, IL, American Academy of Pediatrics, 1994. (The reader is referred to this source for a more detailed discussion of immunization recommendations.)

Abbreviations: DTP, diphtheria and tetatnus toxoids and pertussis vaccine; DTaP, diphtheria and tetanus toxoids and acellular pertussis vaccine; dT, diphtheria and tetanus toxoids; HBV, hepatitis B virus vaccine; Hib, *Haemophilus influenzae* type b conjugate vaccine; MMR, measles-mumps-rubella vaccine; OPV, oral poliovirus vaccine.

In the United States, recommendations for childhood immunizations are made by two organizations, the Committee on Infectious Diseases of the AAP and the United States Public Health Service Immunization Practice Advisory Committee (ACIP). In developing countries, the Expanded Program on Immunization (EPI) of the World Health Organization (WHO) prepares guidelines for immunization practices.

Children are currently required to receive immunizations against nine different diseases from birth until the time of school entry in the United States. Although many of these vaccines are provided in combination form, all require more than one dose. The current recommended schedule of immunizations for normal children includes the following vaccinations: hepatitis B virus (HBV); diphtheria, tetanus, and pertussis (DTP); oral poliovirus (OPV); *Haemophilus influenzae* type b (Hib); and MMR. The composition and route of administration of each vaccine is provided in Table 17–1, and the recommended schedule of administration according to the AAP is summarized in Table 17–2. Six visits are required prior to school entry to immunize children fully.

HBV

About 300 million people worldwide are infected with HBV. Although an effective vaccine to combat hepatitis B infection has been available for use in high-risk individuals since 1982, the incidence of the infection continued to increase through 1989. The recommendation for universal immunization of all children against hepatitis B came because of this failure of selective immunization to control the disease. Two types of vaccines have been licensed in the United States, a recombinant vaccine containing particles of hepatitis B surface antigen (HBsAg) and one that contains HBsAg purified from the plasma of chronic carriers of HBsAg.

Only the recombinant vaccine is currently available in the United States, however. The recommended three doses may be administered at birth, 2, and 6 to 18 months of age, or at 2, 4, and 6 to 18 months of age.

DTP

Diphtheria, tetanus, and pertussis can each produce very serious illness with high mortality rates, especially in young infants. DTP vaccine contains diphtheria and tetanus toxoids and whole-cell, killed *Bordetella pertussis*. The toxoids are obtained by formalin inactivation of the respective bacterial toxins. DTP is administered at 2, 4, and 6 months of age; booster doses are given at 15 to 18 months and 4 to 6 years.

Unlike the whole-cell vaccine, acellular pertussis vaccines are prepared from one or more purified components of *B. pertussis* and then combined with diphtheria and tetanus toxoids (DTaP). The DTaP vaccine has the advantage of lower rates of common systemic reactions, including vaccine-associated seizures, fever, and local reactions, than the whole-cell preparation. DTaP is presently licensed and recommended for use in children 15 months of age and older. The dT vaccine contains about one-tenth the dose of diphtheria toxoid compared to the pediatric preparation of diphtheria and tetanus toxoids (DT); dT is administered to individuals over the age of 7 years. At present, pertussis immunization of persons 7 years of age or older is not routinely indicated. Adults at high risk may receive acellular pertussis vaccine.

OPV

Poliomyelitis is an acute viral infection that affects the spinal motor neurons. Poliovirus, an enterovirus, has a propensity for CNS invasion. Transient or permanent paresis of one or more of the extremities may result. Trivalent poliovirus vaccine that immunizes against polio is available either as a live-attenuated vaccine that is administered orally (OPV) or as an inactivated vaccine that is given parenterally (IPV). OPV is the vaccine of choice for primary immunization of infants and children. Administration should occur at 2 and 4 months of age, with booster doses at 6 to 18 months and 4 to 6 years. IPV should be given to adults who need the polio vaccine, immunocompromised children, and to children living with immunocompromised individuals such as persons with cancer or HIV infection. The live virus is excreted in the stool, and it may infect exposed individuals and cause paralysis.

Hib

Before the availability of the Hib vaccine, Hib was a major cause of such serious illnesses in young children as epiglottitis, meningitis, and septic arthritis. Between 1985, when the first Hib vaccine was licensed, and 1991, the incidence of Hib disease in the United States decreased 80 to 90%. Four Hib conjugate vaccines are currently available in the United States. The Hib polysaccharide, polyribose ribosyl phosphate, is linked to various protein antigens such as diphtheria or tetanus toxoids to augment the immune response, particularly in young infants. Hib vaccine is administered either at 2, 4, and 6 months of age, with a booster dose at 12 to 15 months, or at 2, 4, and 12 months, depending on the particular vaccine conjugate used.

MMR

Measles can be a severe illness with significant mortality due to complications such as pneumonia, especially in young children. Orchitis, seen more commonly in adolescents and adults, is the most serious complication of mumps infection. Although rubella is a mild disease in childhood, infection of susceptible women during the first trimester of pregnancy can result in congenital rubella infection, a serious multisystem infection in neonates. To prevent development of measles, mumps, and rubella, MMR, a trivalent vaccine containing live attenuated viruses, was developed. This vaccine is administered at 12 to 15 months of age and again at either 4 to 6 years (ACIP recommendation) or 11 to 12 years (AAP recommendation).

SIDE EFFECTS AND CONTRAINDICATIONS

Common side effects following vaccination include local reactions such as erythema, swelling or tenderness at the site of the injection, and low-grade fever (temperature: 100.4° F [38° C]) especially following DTP immunization. Side effects are common, whereas adverse reactions, such as an anaphylactic reaction to a vaccine, are quite uncommon.

A guide to contraindications and precautions to vaccine administration is presented in Table 17–3. Low-grade fever, minor acute illness (e.g., otitis media), mild diarrheal illness in children who otherwise appear well, and current antimicrobial therapy are not contraindications to vaccine administration. Other common misconceptions about contraindications to vaccine ad-

TABLE 17–3. General Contraindications and Precautions for Vaccines (DTP/DTaP, OPV, IPV, Hib, HBV, and MMR)

True Contraindications and Precautions

Anaphylactic reaction to a vaccine (this contraindicates further doses of that vaccine)

Anaphylactic reaction to a vaccine constituent (this contraindicates the use of vaccines containing that substance)

Moderate or severe illness with or without a fever

Not True Contraindications (vaccines may be given)

Mild to moderate local reaction (e.g., soreness, redness, swelling) following a dose of an injectable antigen

Mild, acute illness with or without a low-grade fever

Current antimicrobial therapy

Convalescent phase of illness

Prematurity

Recent exposure to an infectious disease

History of penicillin or other nonspecific allergies or relatives with such allergies

Adapted from Committee on Infectious Diseases, American Academy of Pediatrics. 1994 Red Book: Report of the Committee on Infectious Diseases, 23rd edition. Elk Grove Village, IL, American Academy of Pediatrics, 1994. (The reader is referred to this source for a more detailed discussion of immunization recommendations.)

ministration include prematurity and a personal or family history of seizures. Generally, premature infants should be immunized at the same chronologic age as other infants; full, not reduced, vaccine doses should be used. A history of seizures usually is not a contraindication to pertussis immunization unless the seizure followed a previous immunization for pertussis. The role of pertussis vaccine in causing epilepsy or permanent neurologic damage, if any, remains as yet unconfirmed. Children who have had seizures do have an increased risk of vaccine-associated seizures, which are usually febrile convulsions with no permanent sequelae.

True contraindications to vaccine administration are anaphylactic reactions to a vaccine; immunocompromise (live-virus vaccines); pregnancy (live-virus vaccines); moderate or severe febrile illness (e.g., pneumonia, meningitis, suspected bacteremia); and severe prior reaction to a particular vaccine. Specific contraindications include fever greater than 105.0° F (40.5° C) within 48 hours after administration of a previous dose of DTP and administration of OPV to immunologically normal children living in a home with an immunocompromised child. (MMR may be administered to such normal siblings because transmission of these viruses does not occur.) Children with chronic illness, acquired or congenital immunodeficiency, malignancy, and those on chronic corticosteroid therapy should be individually evaluated regarding appropriate vaccinations.

Although live-virus vaccines usually are not given to immunocompromised children, exceptions to this guideline do exist. For example, it is recommended that children infected with HIV should receive MMR because of the severity of measles as compared to the potential risks of the vaccine. OPV is contraindicated because possible vaccine-associated poliomyelitis in these children may occur. These children can receive IPV instead.

OTHER CONSIDERATIONS

Informed Consent

Although the risk of serious adverse reactions following immunizations is small, informed consent has become an important issue in the last several years. The National Childhood Vaccine Injury Act of 1986 requires notification of patients or parents about vaccine risks and benefits. Distribution of standardized vaccine information pamphlets prior to vaccine administration and written informed consent is required for administration of all vaccines.

Simultaneous Administration of Multiple Vaccines

In general, immune responses to one vaccine do not interfere with those of other vaccines.* Simultaneous administration of routine immunizations is not contraindicated. Live virus vaccines not administered on the same day should be given at least 30 days apart because

---

*Simultaneous administration of the yellow fever and cholera vaccines limits their effectiveness.

the immune responses to the live virus vaccines may interfere with each other. In addition, live vaccines (e.g., MMR) may have decreased efficacy when administered shortly before or within several months after the administration of immune globulin (IG). The duration of this effect depends on the dose of IG. Exceptions include OPV administration and simultaneous administration of hepatitis B IG, tetanus IG, and rabies IG given in conjunction with the corresponding inactivated vaccine or toxoid in postexposure situations.

Immunization of Children Not Immunized During Infancy

Children not immunized during the first year of life should be vaccinated according to the appropriate schedule (Table 17–4). Pertussis vaccination is not routinely recommended for children 7 years of age or older, and Hib vaccination is also unnecessary after 5 years of age.

Interruptions in the Immunization Schedule

An interruption does not require restarting the entire immunization schedule. Immunizations should resume from the point of interruption, regardless of the time since the last dose.

Unknown or Undocumented Immunization Status

Children with unknown or undocumented immunization status should receive all appropriate vaccinations. No evidence indicates that immunization of already immune individuals with MMR, Hib, HBV, OPV, or DTP (dT for those age 7 years or more) is harmful.

SPECIAL VACCINES AND NEW VACCINES

Aside from the primary series of childhood immunizations that all children are required to receive, several other vaccines are available for use in specific circumstances. Influenza vaccine is recommended for children who are immunocompromised or those who have chronic cardiovascular or pulmonary disease or any other underlying condition that may make them more susceptible to complications after influenza infection. Pneumococcal vaccine is recommended for children with sickle cell disease, anatomic or functional asplenia, nephrotic syndrome, and immunocompromise, but can only be given to children over 2 years of age. Several vaccinations, including vaccines for cholera, yellow fever, and tuberculosis, are available for persons traveling abroad. The requirements for different countries may be obtained from the Centers for Disease Control. Vaccine technology is increasing every day. Some combination vaccines are already available (e.g., Hib conjugate and DTP combination [DTP-HbOC]), and in the future it is likely that even more vaccines already in routine use will be combined. Varicella vaccine has recently been licensed for use in all healthy children over the age of 1 year who have not had varicella. Vaccines against hepatitis A, rotavirus, HIV, herpes

TABLE 17–4. Recommended Immunization Schedule of Children Not Immunized in the First Year of Life

Recommended Time/Age	Immunization(s)
Younger Than 7 Years	
First visit	DTP, OPV, Hib,* HBV, MMR
Interval after first visit	
1 month	DTP, HBV
2 months	DTP, OPV, Hib†
≥8 months	DTP or DTaP,‡ OPV, HBV
4–6 years	DTP or DTaP,§ OPV,§ MMR
14–16 years	dT (repeat every 10 years throughout life)
7 Years and Older	
First visit	dT, OPV,‖ MMR, HBV
Interval after first visit	
2 months	dT, OPV, HBV
8–14 months	dT, OPV, HBV
11–12 years	MMR#
10 years after last dT	dT (repeat every 10 years throughout life)

*If the child is 5 years of age or older, Hib is not indicated.
†The second dose of Hib is indicated only in children whose first dose was received when younger than 15 months of age.
‡DTaP may be given to children older than 15 months. DTaP is not recommended for primary immunization (e.g., first three doses) at any age.
§DTP or DTaP and OPV are not required if the fourth dose was given after the fourth birthday.
‖Routine poliovirus immunization is not indicated in the United States for persons 18 years or older.
#Minimal interval between doses of MMR is one month.
Adapted, with permission, from the Committee on Infectious Diseases, American Academy of Pediatrics. 1994 Red Book: Report of the Committee on Infectious Diseases, 23rd edition. Elk Grove Village, IL, American Academy of Pediatrics, 1994.
Abbreviations: DTP, diphtheria and tetanus toxoids and pertussis vaccine; DTaP, diphtheria and tetanus toxoids and acellular pertussis vaccine; dT, diphtheria and tetanus toxoids; HBV, hepatitis B virus vaccine; Hib, *Haemophilus influenzae* type b conjugate vaccine; MMR, measles-mumps-rubella vaccine; OPV, oral poliovirus vaccine.

simplex, RSV, group B streptococcus, and CMV are all investigational at the present time.

PUBLIC HEALTH PERSPECTIVE ON IMMUNIZATIONS

Worldwide Immunization Programs

Dramatic declines in the rates of vaccine-preventable diseases have occurred worldwide; these are largely a result of the efforts of the WHO through the EPI and the United Nations Children's Fund (UNICEF). At the time of the inception of the EPI in 1974, fewer than 5% of children in the developing world were immunized. The objectives of the EPI are to reduce the morbidity and mortality from diphtheria, pertussis, tetanus, measles, poliomyelitis, and tuberculosis by making immunizations against these diseases available to all the world's children. Today, 75 to 85% of the children in the developing world are protected by immunizations, and the rate continues to rise. The goal is the immunization of at least 85% of all 1-year-old children by the year 2000.

National Immunization Coverage Rates and Year 2000 Goals

Although the United States spends more money on health care than any other nation, it lags behind many other countries with regard to most aspects of child health, including immunizations. In 1992, the United States ranked 88th worldwide with regard to the percentage of 1-year-olds fully immunized against polio, and the ranking for DTP was 115. Studies consistently show that nonwhite children and children from economically disadvantaged populations are far less likely to be adequately immunized than their peers.

In response to the current low levels of vaccine coverage of infants and young children in the United States, the U.S. Public Health Service has made immunization coverage of children one of its national year 2000 health goals. By the year 2000, 90% of 2-year-old children and 95% of school-age children should be appropriately immunized with the recommended immunizations.

Barriers to Immunization

Immunization coverage is a good example of the difference between the capacity to provide a service compared to availability, affordability, and ultimate utilization. Reasons for failure to immunize all children fully by 2 years of age may be classified into three main groups (Table 17–5): parental barriers, provider barriers, and systems barriers.

Perhaps the two most significant barriers involve economic factors (not just parental) and those known collectively as the "missed opportunities to vaccinate." One economic factor is cost. In 1980 the cost to completely immunize one child in the public sector was $6.69; in 1990, this value had risen to $91.20 (not taking into account the Hib or HBV immunizations), and this figure continues to increase today. A second economic factor is lack of health insurance coverage. In 1990, about 15% of children under the age of 18 had

no health insurance coverage, which makes access to health care difficult. One of the easiest "missed opportunities" to remedy is the failure of health care providers to review immunization status at all health care visits. Misinformation regarding contraindications to vaccination also means that many children are not immunized on schedule.

Possible solutions include such creative ideas as providing immunizations at federally funded programs such as Women, Infants, and Children (WIC) or on-site in child care settings. Such ideas acknowledge the busy and complex schedules of young families today and make access to preventive services easier. Decreasing administrative barriers, especially for economically disadvantaged families; improved, centralized tracking and monitoring systems; and continuing education for health care providers regarding appropriate contraindications are a few of the other solutions currently available. Universal access to health care, a system that eliminates all financial barriers to health care, will also help make health care more accessible and ensure children's immunization status.

Case Resolution

The infant described in the case history should be immunized today. She should receive DTP, OPV, Hib, and HBV. Minor illness, including low-grade fever and otitis media, is not a contraindication to immunization.

TABLE 17–5. Barriers to Immunization

Parental Barriers
Financial (15% of children uninsured in the United States)
Lack of knowledge regarding value of immunizations
Concerns about adverse reactions
Provider Barriers: "Missed Opportunities to Vaccinate"
Using inappropriate contraindications (e.g., minor illness)
Failure to review the immunization record during all visits to the health care provider, including visits to emergency departments
Failure to administer all required immunizations at one visit
Systems Barriers
Economic
Limited clinic hours and locations
Administrative
Requiring appointments in advance for immunizations

Selected Readings

Barker, W. H., R. A. Strikase, and P. D. Brugliera (eds.). Immunization in medical education. Am. J. Prev. Med. (Suppl.) 10:1–94, 1994.

Bellanti, J. A. Basic immunologic principles underlying vaccination procedures. Pediatr. Clin. North Am. 37:513–530, 1990.

Committee on Infectious Diseases, American Academy of Pediatrics. Active and passive immunization. In 1994 Red Book: Report of the Committee on Infectious Diseases, 23rd edition. Elk Grove Village, IL, American Academy of Pediatrics, 1994, pp. 7–71, 602–617.

General Recommendations on Immunization. Recommendations of the Advisory Committee on Immunization Practices (ACIP). M.M.W.R. 43:1–38, 1994.

Hoekelman, R. A. New immunization practices and prophecies. Pediatr. Ann. 22:707–710, 1993.

Peter, G. Childhood immunizations. N. Engl. J. Med. 327:1794–1800, 1992.

Zell, E. R., et al. Low vaccination levels of U.S. preschool and school-age children. J.A.M.A. 271:833–839, 1994.

CHAPTER 18

WELL CHILD CARE FOR CHILDREN WITH TRISOMY 21

Monica Sifuentes, M.D.

H$_x$ A 9-month-old girl with trisomy 21 whom you have known since birth is brought to your office for well child care. She and her parents have been doing well and report no intercurrent problems or illnesses since her last visit. Her past medical history is significant for a small ventricular septal defect, which has since closed spontaneously, and one episode of otitis media at 7 months of age. Her weight gain has been good—along the 25th percentile on the trisomy 21 growth chart. She now sleeps through the night and has a bowel movement once a day. She has received all of the recommended immunizations for her age without any problems. Except for an oral fluoride supplement, she takes no medications.

The infant can now roll from a supine to prone position but is still unable to sit unassisted. She grasps objects in both hands, however, and babbles appropriately with her siblings. Since she was 1 month old she has been enrolled in an early intervention program. An occupational therapist visits her at home twice a month.

On physical examination, she has typical facial features consistent with trisomy 21, a single palmar crease on each hand, and diffuse hypotonia.

Questions

1. What is the prevalence of trisomy 21 (Down syndrome) in the general population? What is the association of maternal age with trisomy 21?
2. What are the clinical manifestations of this syndrome?
3. What medical conditions are associated with trisomy 21 in the newborn period, during childhood, and in adolescence? When should screening tests for these conditions be performed?
4. What is the role of early intervention services for these patients and their families?
5. What specific psychosocial issues should be included in your anticipatory guidance and health education?
6. What is the prognosis for children with trisomy 21?

Trisomy 21, or Down syndrome, is one of the most common genetic disorders causing developmental delay. Infants and children with trisomy 21, like children with other developmental disabilities and chronic illnesses, need to be evaluated and monitored for associated conditions concurrently with their well child visits. The primary care provider is thus in the unique position to offer affected children routine health care maintenance and follow-up for intercurrent illnesses or chronic problems, as well as anticipatory guidance for families. In addition, the general pediatrician has the opportunity to develop rapport with children and families given the frequency of well child visits. Such relationships are particularly important when considering the complex medical and social implications of raising children with trisomy 21. An important goal of the well child visit is to provide children with trisomy 21 and their families with counseling about educational, social, and financial resources and support to ensure a healthy and productive transition into adulthood.

EPIDEMIOLOGY

The prevalence of trisomy 21 is approximately 1 in 800 to 1000 live births. Although the degree of mental retardation is variable, some authors claim it is responsible for up to one-third of all cases of moderate to severe mental retardation. Trisomy 21 occurs more commonly in males than in females, with a male-female ratio of 1.3:1.0.

The vast majority of cases of Down syndrome are caused by trisomy 21. This chromosomal nondisjunction occurs in the egg 95% of the time and in the sperm 5%, and it is strongly influenced by maternal age. For a 35–39-year-old woman, the risk of having a child with trisomy 21 is 6.5 times greater than for a 20–24-year-old woman. For the 40–44-year-old woman, the risk is 20.5 times greater. It is estimated that about one-half of embryos with trisomy 21 abort spontaneously.

The risk of recurrence in subsequent pregnancies is 1 in 100 until maternal age 35, after which the risk determined by age takes precedence. Other family members are not at increased risk of bearing children with this chromosomal abnormality.

CLINICAL PRESENTATION

Infants and children with trisomy 21 have a characteristic appearance (D$_x$ Box). They may be microcephalic, with flattening of both the occiput and face. The eyes have an upward slant, with prominent epicanthal folds, the ears are low-set and small, the nasal bridge is flattened, and the tongue appears large. The feet, hands,

Dx Trisomy 21

- Microcephaly, with flattening of both occiput and face
- Upward slant to the eyes with epicanthal folds
- Brushfield spots in eyes
- Small ears and mouth (therefore tongue appears large)
- Low-set ears
- Flat nasal bridge
- Broad, stocky neck, with loose skin folds at the nape
- Funnel-shaped or pigeon-breasted chest
- Small, stubby feet, hands, and digits, with brachyclinodactyly of the fifth digits
- Single transverse palmar crease on each hand
- Wide space between first and second toes
- Fair, mottled skin in newborns; dry skin in older children
- Hypotonia

and digits are small and stubby, and the fifth digit is slightly turned in (clinodactyly). A single palmar crease and a wide spacing between the first and second toes may be evident. After the newborn period, diffuse hypotonia and developmental delay are universally seen.

PATHOPHYSIOLOGY

All sources agree that in almost all cases (95%), Down syndrome is caused by nondisjunctional trisomy 21. The remaining cases are translocations (3–4%) and mosaics (1–2%). The translocations are unbalanced and usually occur with another acrocentric chromosome, usually 14/21 or 15/21. Approximately 75% of these are new mutations, and 25% are the result of a familial translocation. Therefore, if a child has a translocation, the parents must be evaluated for a balanced translocation. Mosaicism implies the presence of two cell lines: one normal and one with trisomy 21. As might be expected, children with Down syndrome as a result of mosaicism are affected less severely than those with nondisjunctional trisomy 21 or translocations.

EVALUATION

Routine health care maintenance for infants, children, or adolescents with trisomy 21 should cover the same issues in health education, prevention, and counseling that are discussed with other healthy patients and their families. In addition, specific medical as well as psychosocial issues pertinent to patients with trisomy 21 need to be addressed periodically.

NEWBORN PERIOD

Verification of the diagnosis of trisomy 21 is perhaps the single most important focus of the initial family visit. If trisomy 21 was unsuspected prenatally, and the diagnosis is based on the physical examination performed shortly after birth, a karyotype must be sent from the nursery. The results can be reviewed with the family when they return to the office for the one-to-two-week visit.

Several conditions that are associated with trisomy 21 are important to identify in the newborn period. They are congenital heart disease (risk: 30–50%), most commonly an endocardial cushion defect; GI malformations and obstructive disorders (risk: 12%) such as duodenal atresia, imperforate anus, tracheoesophageal fistula, pyloric stenosis, and Hirschsprung disease; congenital hypothyroidism (risk: 1%); congenital ocular anomalies (risk: 60%), including cataracts, strabismus, and nystagmus; hip dysplasias; and leukemoid reactions that resemble leukemia but resolve during the first month of life. Leukemia is more common in individuals with trisomy 21 than in the general population, but it still occurs rarely (< 1%).

History

Although associated conditions may not have been apparent in the newborn nursery, it is important to inquire about any symptoms that may indicate their current presence (Questions Box). In addition, the routine nutritional and developmental history should be documented. A detailed family and social history should also be obtained if this was not done in the hospital.

Physical Examination

All growth parameters (e.g., length, weight, head circumference) should be recorded and compared with those obtained at birth. Neonates with trisomy 21, like other term newborns, should regain birth weight by two weeks of life.

A complete physical examination must be performed on all neonates. In particular, the size of the fontanelles should be evaluated because of the increased incidence of congenital hypothyroidism. A bilateral red reflex and conjugate gaze should be documented to exclude congenital cataracts. A careful cardiac examination must be performed, noting any murmurs, irregular heart rates, abnormal heart sounds, or asymmetry of pulses. In addition to endocardial cushion defects, other associated cardiac malformations include ventricular septal defects, tetralogy of Fallot, and atrial septal defects. Cyanosis should also be evaluated. The abdomen should be palpated for organomegaly or any masses, and patency of the anus should be verified. An Ortolani test should also be performed for hip laxity. Finally, the

Questions: Trisomy 21

- Is the infant or child having any feeding problems?
- Does the infant or child appear to be gaining weight?
- Does the infant or child appear to hear?
- Does the infant or child vocalize? What words does the young child know?
- Does the infant or child appear to see?
- Does one eye ever wander or appear "lazy" by the end of the day?
- Has the infant or child had many ear infections?
- Is the infant or child constipated? If so, is the hair coarse and the skin dry?

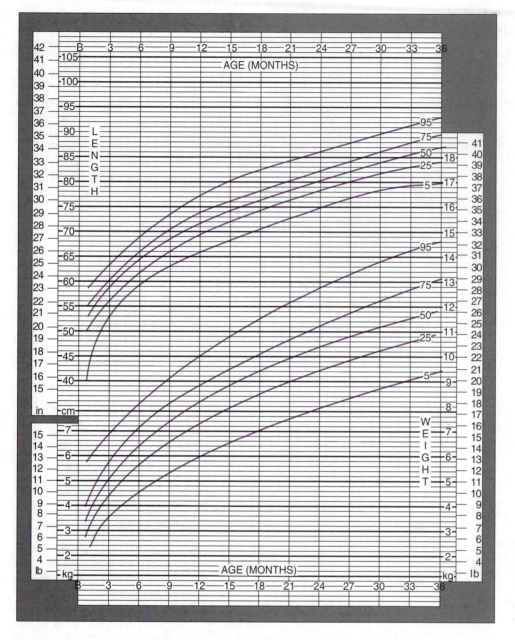

FIGURE 18–1. *Growth chart for boys with Down syndrome: 1 to 36 months. (Reproduced, with permission, from Cronk, C., et al. Growth charts for children with Down syndrome: 1 month to 18 years of age. Pediatrics 81:102–110, 1988.)*

neonate's tone should be evaluated; hypotonia is not an uncommon finding.

Laboratory Assessment

Prior to discharge from the nursery or when trisomy 21 is initially suspected based on clinical examination, a chromosomal karyotype should be performed to confirm the diagnosis. In addition, an ECG and a chest x-ray should be obtained in the nursery or shortly thereafter. Some physicians advocate including an echocardiogram in the initial evaluation of all infants for congenital heart disease, regardless of the findings on physical examination, ECG, or chest x-ray. Other laboratory tests that should be performed include a thyroid screen to check for congenital hypothyroidism, which may have been missed on the state neonatal screen; a CBC to look for a leukemoid reaction or polycythemia; and a brainstem

auditory evoked reponse (BAER) as a baseline study for hearing.

Anticipatory Guidance

Routine topics related to nutrition, growth, and development should be discussed in the newborn period. Other important issues to address include those pertaining to available resources for children and families such as early intervention programs and Down syndrome support groups in the community. Educational materials such as pamphlets and books may also be supplied at this time. Upcoming appointments with other physicians and allied health professionals should be reviewed. The schedule of health maintenance visits for infants and young children with trisomy 21 is essentially the same as that recommended by the AAP for other children.

INFANCY AND EARLY CHILDHOOD

History

Some additional historical issues to address at this time include a detailed developmental assessment focusing on progress made since the last visit. Inquiries regarding the development of any new conditions associated with Down syndrome such as hearing deficits or hypothyroidism should be made. Oropharyngeal problems such as sleep apnea secondary to the underdevelopment of the nasopharynx and enlarged tonsils should also be reviewed.

Physical Examination

All growth parameters (height, weight, and head circumference) should be measured at each visit and plotted on growth charts for children with Down syndrome (Fig. 18–1 through 18–4). Children with trisomy 21 are shorter than other children and may have poor weight gain in their first year. Later in life, obesity unrelated to the syndrome may become a problem, however.

As with routine well child visits in other infants and children, a complete physical examination should be performed at each patient encounter. Noteworthy aspects of the examination in infants and children with trisomy 21 are given in Table 18–1.

Laboratory Assessment

Infants with trisomy 21 should have all routine screening tests and immunizations. In addition, they should have their hearing monitored during the first year of life. A BAER with a tympanogram should be performed by eight months of age; hearing should be checked annually thereafter. Referral to an audiologist

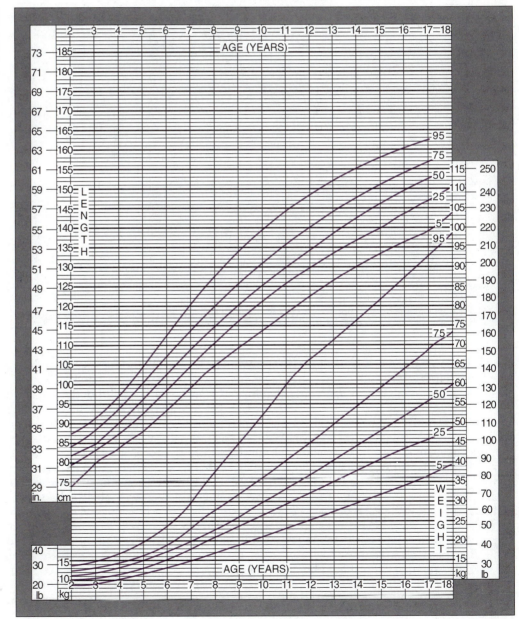

FIGURE 18–2. *Growth chart for boys with Down syndrome: 2 to 18 years. (Reproduced, with permission, from Cronk, C., et al. Growth charts for children with Down syndrome: 1 month to 18 years of age. Pediatrics 81:102–110, 1988.)*

FIGURE 18–3. *Growth chart for girls with Down syndrome: 1 to 36 months. (Reproduced, with permission, from Cronk, C., et al. Growth charts for children with Down syndrome: 1 month to 18 years of age. Pediatrics 81:102–110, 1988.)*

should be considered in any infants who appear to have a hearing deficit or significant speech delay. A history of recurrent otitis media may also warrant referral to an otolaryngologist.

Developmentally appropriate gross visual screening should be performed in infants between 6 and 12 months of age at each visit. Positive findings on physical examination or indeterminate visual assessments warrant referral to an ophthalmologist. Children's vision should continue to be checked annually in the office until 5 years of age, because there is a 30 to 50% risk of refractive errors between three and five years. A formal ophthalmology consult should occur at about four years.

Thyroid screening tests should be performed early in infancy, if not in the neonatal period. Current AAP recommendations include repeating these studies at 4 to 6 months of age, at 12 months, and then annually.

Lateral cervical radiographs to detect atlantoaxial instability or subluxation are recommended once in early childhood. Much controversy exists regarding whether neck films are an adequate screening tool for any potentially serious complication. Some authorities have suggested that these studies are more important in children who participate in contact sports or athletic activities (e.g., the Special Olympics) and in those who are symptomatic. Neck films should then be repeated at 3–4-year intervals.

A cardiac evaluation should be made early in infancy if it was not performed in the newborn period. The primary care practitioner may prefer to have a pediatric cardiologist complete this examination (depending on the practitioner's experience and comfort level).

A dental referral should be made by the age of four years or earlier if the children have any dental problems.

Anticipatory Guidance

Growth and developmental progress should be reviewed with parents at the end of each visit, and any concerns or unmet expectations should be addressed at this time. Often the developmental delay associated with trisomy 21 is not apparent to families until infants are four to six months of age and not achieving the expected milestones of rolling over or sitting. The diagnosis and associated conditions should then be reviewed once again. It should also be emphasized to families that the degree of mental retardation in trisomy 21 is quite variable, ranging from mild (IQ, 50–70) to moderate (IQ, 35–50) to severe (IQ, 20–35). Social function is not necessarily related to IQ. If the child is not already enrolled in an early intervention program, the positive role of such an experience should be addressed. The availability of support groups for parents and other family members should also be discussed.

In the early childhood years, plans for preschool attendance and future educational opportunities should be reviewed with families. The role of discipline and the presence of common behavioral problems such as temper tantrums and biting should be assessed in preparation for school entry and socialization. Developmentally appropriate safety issues such as toddler car seats and adult supervision while in the bathtub or pool should also be discussed. Some experts suggest that the advantages and disadvantages of reconstructive craniofacial surgery during early childhood should be reviewed.

OLDER CHILDHOOD AND ADOLESCENCE

History

Older, school-age children with Down syndrome should continue to visit their primary care physician at

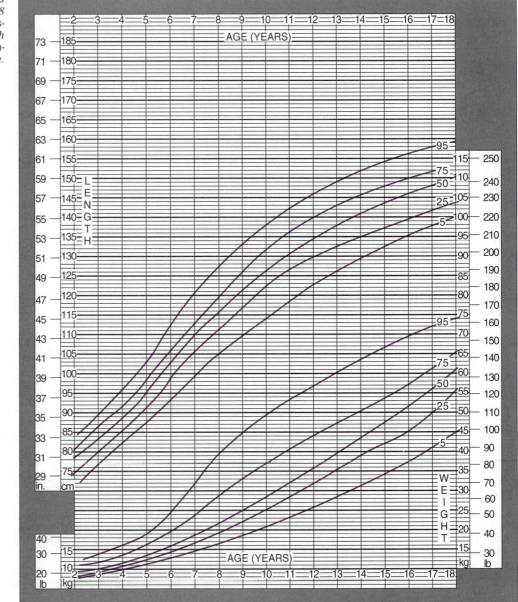

FIGURE 18–4. *Growth chart for girls with Down syndrome: 2 to 18 years. (Reproduced, with permission, from Cronk, C., et al. Growth charts for children with Down syndrome: 1 month to 18 years of age. Pediatrics 81:102–110, 1988.)*

TABLE 18–1. Aspects of the Physical Examination in Children With Trisomy 21

- Look for dry sensitive skin and alopecia, which develops in approximately 10% of children and resolves spontaneously.
- Monitor the size of the anterior and posterior fontanelles, since delayed closure may indicate hypothyroidism.
- Check for visual abnormalities, such as strabismus, nystagmus, cataracts, refractive errors, and blepharitis.
- Document recurrent serous otitis media. It is estimated that 40–60% of children with trisomy 21 have significant conductive hearing loss, and 20–30% have some degree of neurosensory loss.
- Examine the oropharynx carefully for delayed dentition, malocclusion, and caries.
- Perform a thorough cardiac examination, and note any evidence of previously unrecognized congenital heart disease.
- Palpate the abdomen for distention or organomegaly. Children with trisomy 21 have a slightly increased risk of developing acute nonlymphoblastic or acute lymphoblastic leukemia.
- Perform a rectal examination in infants or children with a history of constipation.
- Evaluate any musculoskeletal abnormalities such as overall hypotonia and joint laxity (most commonly in the knees and hips) that might contribute to overall gross motor delay.

least annually. Although this is not recommended in general, those children with trisomy 21 require visits for screening for the development of common medical conditions and for assisting families with educational planning. Specific medical issues to address during the history pertain to possible signs or symptoms of visual or hearing deficits; evidence of hypothyroidism, such as a decrease in activity, coarse, dry hair, and constipation; and skin or dental problems such as eczema and caries, which are not uncommon in patients with Down syndrome. A careful nutritional history should also be taken because of the propensity for obesity.

Physical Examination

A complete physical examination should be performed. Growth parameters should continue to be plotted, although head circumference is probably now less important. The skin should be examined closely for dryness or any evidence of acne during adolescence. The Tanner stage of both males and females should be noted and discussed with the parents. A pelvic examination is not indicated as a part of the routine visit unless there is concern about sexual abuse or an STD. A complete neurologic examination should also be performed in the patient participating in sports activities such as the Special Olympics to look for signs indicating impending atlantoaxial dislocation.

Laboratory Assessment

Annual thyroid screening (thyroid-stimulating hormone, T_4) is recommended for all school-age children and adolescents with trisomy 21, in addition to other routine screening tests. An audiologic evaluation should also occur at least once in older children and then annually thereafter. Because of the risk of keratoconus, an annual ophthalmology consultation should be arranged after the age of 10 years. In addition, children with trisomy 21 should be encouraged to continue annual dental visits because gingivitis, periodontal disease, and bruxism (teeth grinding) are common in these individuals.

Anticipatory Guidance

The major part of the visit with school-age and adolescent children should be spent on developmental, educational, and vocational anticipatory guidance. Educational placement and future goals should be both developmentally appropriate for the child and acceptable for the parent. Activities requiring socialization and the development of responsibility should continue to be encouraged; these can be very stressful for parents and other family members, however. Injury prevention should be highlighted as well, especially since older children are becoming more independent. In early adolescence, prevocational and vocational training within the school curriculum should be reviewed. In addition, brief discussions regarding independent living, group homes, and financial resources (e.g., community-supported employment for young adults) should begin during adolescence.

Puberty, fertility, and contraception are extremely important to address with adolescents and their parents. The patient's psychosocial development and physical sexual maturation should be discussed, including menstrual hygiene and any foreseeable problems with its management. Contraception and the potential for victimization must be addressed as well, particularly with female patients. Males with trisomy 21 are usually sterile.

TABLE 18–2. Health Supervision for Children With Down Syndrome

	Newborn Period	Infancy and Early Childhood*	Older Childhood and Adolescence†
History	X	X	X
Developmental Assessment (by test or report)		X	X
Physical Examination (including measurements)	X	X	X
Visual testing	X	X	X
Hearing	X	X	X
Laboratory Assessment			
Karyotype	X		
Annual thyroid screen	X	X	X
Echocardiogram	X		
Neck radiographs	X	X	X
Consultation			
Genetics	X		
Cardiology	X	X	X
Ophthalmology	X	X	X
Ear-nose-throat	X	X	X
Dental		X	X

*Visits should be scheduled every 2–3 months.
†Visits should be scheduled every 1–2 years.

TABLE 18–3.   Counseling the Family After a Prenatal Diagnosis of Down Syndrome

---

Review the data that established the diagnosis in the fetus.

Explain the mechanism of occurrence and risks for recurrence.

Review the manifestations of trisomy 21, commonly associated conditions, and the variable prognosis based on the presence of these conditions.

Discuss other modalities that confirm the presence of associated anomalies such as a fetal echocardiogram in the case of congenital heart disease.

Explore treatment options and interventions for associated conditions.

Offer resources to assist the family with decisions related to completing or terminating the pregnancy.

Refer the family to a clinical geneticist or genetics counselor.

MANAGEMENT

If a prenatal diagnosis of Down syndrome is made, and the general pediatrician is asked to participate in counseling the family, the points listed in Table 18–3 should be covered.

In addition to providing preventive health care during well child visits, the management of children with trisomy 21 is influenced by the presence of any associated conditions and the age at diagnosis. The primary goal should be to help affected infants and children reach their full potential. For example, if a newborn is found to have congenital heart disease and is clinically stable, then referral to a pediatric cardiologist is necessary but not emergent. However, suspected GI atresia or obstruction in a neonate is a medical emergency, and surgical consultation should be sought immediately.

Conditions such as congenital or acquired hypothyroidism should be treated aggressively with thyroxine and monitored closely during the first two years of life. Evaluation by a pediatric endocrinologist is warranted at the time of diagnosis and periodically thereafter. Other conditions associated with Down syndrome such as sensorineural hearing loss or refractive errors can be followed by the primary care practitioner in conjunction with the appropriate pediatric subspecialist.

PROGNOSIS

Individuals with trisomy 21 can be expected to live well into their sixties unless they are born with a congenital heart lesion. The major cause of morbidity and mortality is the development of symptomatic Alzheimer's disease, which occurs in approximately 15% of adults after the fourth decade. Fortunately, most adults with Down syndrome remain asymptomatic, despite histopathologic evidence of the disease.

Case Resolution

In the case described at the beginning of the chapter, the family should be encouraged by the healthy progress of their daughter. For this visit, anticipatory guidance should consist of a review of early intervention services, available resources, and general support services for the patient and her family. Medical screening should include vision and hearing, in addition to the routine hemoglobin or spun hematocrit that is performed in all healthy children. If the results are normal, the next visit should take place in three months.

Selected Readings

Carey, J. C. Health supervision and anticipatory guidance for children with genetic disorders (including specific recommendations for trisomy 21, trisomy 18, and neurofibromatosis I). Pediatr. Clin. North Am. 39:25–53, 1992.

Committee on Genetics, American Academy of Pediatrics. Health supervision for children with Down syndrome. Pediatrics 93:855–859, 1994.

Cronk, C., et al. Growth charts for children with Down syndrome: 1 month to 18 years of age. Pediatrics 81:102–110, 1988.

Hayes, A., and M. L. Batshaw. Down Syndrome. Pediatr. Clin. North Am. 40:523–535, 1993.

Levy, S. E., and S. L. Hyman. Pediatric assessment of the child with developmental delay. Pediatr. Clin. North Am. 40:465–477, 1993.

CHAPTER 19

WELL CHILD CARE FOR PRETERM INFANTS

Monica Sifuentes, M.D.

H$_x$ A 2½-month-old infant girl was discharged from the neonatal intensive care unit two weeks ago, where she had been since birth. She was the product of a 29-week gestation born via spontaneous vaginal delivery to a 32-year-old primigravida. The perinatal course was complicated by premature rupture of membranes and maternal amnionitis. Several aspects of the neonatal course were significant, including respiratory distress that required surfactant therapy and two weeks of endotracheal intubation; a grade II intraventricular hemorrhage on head ultrasound at one week of life; group B streptococcal bacteremia; hyperbilirubinemia, which was treated with phototherapy; several episodes of apnea, presumably associated with the prematurity; and a history of poor oral intake with slow weight gain.

The infant's parents have a few questions about her feeding schedule and discontinuing the apnea monitor, but they feel relatively comfortable caring for their daughter at home. She is feeding well (2 oz of formula every 2–3 hours) and is becoming progressively more alert according to the family.

The infant's weight gain has averaged 25 g/day. The rest of the physical examination is normal, except for dolichocephaly and a left esotropia.

Questions

1. What constitutes well child care in preterm infants?
2. What are the nutritional requirements of preterm infants in the months following discharge from the hospital?
3. What information must be considered in the developmental screening of preterm infants?
4. What immunization schedule is appropriate for preterm infants? Do they require any special immunizations?
5. What specific conditions or illnesses are more likely to affect preterm infants than term infants?

Preterm, or premature, infants are born at less than 36 weeks' gestation and often weigh less than 2500 grams. Providing primary care for these infants is an important and challenging task for general pediatricians and other allied health practitioners. Well child care for preterm infants often requires coordination of medical, developmental, and social services for multiple chronic conditions. Because preterm infants are at increased risk for both developmental and neurologic sequelae as a result of their prematurity, routine well child care must also include formal developmental assessments as well as the usual screening tests. In addition, more frequent, longer visits may be necessary to evaluate preterm infants' nutritional and developmental progress and to assess how families have adjusted to caring for infants at home. Primary care physicians must learn to manage these and many other complex issues while providing families with comprehensive anticipatory guidance.

EPIDEMIOLOGY

The number of preterm infants discharged from neonatal intensive care units (NICUs) has increased tremendously in the past 20 years. Improvement in both morbidity and mortality for infants weighing less than 1500 grams is quite impressive. For example, in the 1970s, less than 10% of extremely low-birth-weight infants (weight < 750 g) survived. Today, 40 to 50% of such infants may live. Infants who weigh 750 to 1000 grams have also shown a marked decrease in mortality from approximately 70% in the 1970s to less than 30% in the late 1980s. Similarly, the survival rate of infants who weigh between 1000 and 1500 grams is now 90%, a dramatic increase from 50% in the early 1970s.

Several factors have contributed to this improvement. Advances in technology, a better understanding of the physiology of preterm infants, important antenatal and perinatal interventions, and the development of specific medical treatments such as surfactant therapy are a few of these factors. In addition, these contributions have greatly affected the morbidity associated with prematurity, which may directly influence long-term outcome.

EVALUATION

The purpose of the health maintenance visit for preterm infants is the same as for other healthy children: to provide consistent preventive health care and education for patients and their parents. Prematurity, however, places the infants at risk for additional medical and neurodevelopmental conditions.

History

At the initial visit it is imperative to review the entire past medical history and hospital course with the family. Ideally, the NICU should provide a discharge summary that includes the following information:

1. Birth weight and significant prenatal and perinatal information.
2. An overview of the hospital course, including significant illnesses, events, and surgical procedures.

3. A list of current medications, including dosing intervals.

4. Immunizations given in the hospital or at the time of discharge.

5. Screening laboratory data.

6. Problems remaining at discharge.

Any significant complications or concerns should be discussed with the parents as soon as possible to assess their understanding of these issues as well as expectations for improvement.

Specifically, growth, nutrition, and developmental issues should be addressed at each visit (Questions Box). Adequate or desirable weight gain should be explained to the caregivers in terms of the infants' current weight versus the discharge weight. Infants under the age of six months should gain, on average, 20 to 40 g/day while at home. To ensure continued weight gain, many preterm infants are discharged from the NICU on a 24-hour feeding schedule, which requires that parents feed infants at least every three hours. The necessity for this practice should be reevaluated during the first few weeks following discharge after infants have demonstrated adequate weight gain.

The need for supplementation with iron, fluoride, and vitamins should also be addressed (see Management).

Probably the most important part of the preterm health maintenance visit is the developmental history. Parental expectations and observations should be noted and any developmental concerns should be evaluated. The adjusted developmental age should be calculated by subtracting the number of weeks the infant was born prematurely from the current chronologic age in weeks. The adjusted age should then be used for all formal and informal developmental assessments. The importance of correcting for prematurity until children are approximately 2½ years of age must be emphasized when discussing developmental progress and giving anticipatory guidance to parents.

Questions: Well Child Care for Preterm Infants

- How much did the infant weigh when discharged from the hospital?
- Is the infant breast-fed or bottle-fed?
- How often and how much does the infant feed?
- Does the infant have any feeding problems (e.g., colic, gastroesophageal reflux)?
- Does the infant take dietary supplementation of vitamins and minerals?
- Is the infant's development appropriate for the adjusted chronological age?
- What developmental milestones has the infant reached? Does the infant roll over? Smile? Sit up?
- Does the infant appear to hear and see?
- Who cares for the infant?
- Do the parents have any concerns regarding growth, development, or nutrition?
- Is the infant on an apnea monitor? Have there been any apneic episodes?

Physical Examination

A complete physical examination should be performed at each visit to monitor the status of associated medical conditions. All growth parameters (weight, height, and head circumference) should be plotted on the growth chart and adjusted for prematurity. Average daily weight gain in grams/day should also be calculated. In addition, blood pressure must be recorded, especially if an umbilical catheter was used during the neonatal period.

Some findings of the physical examination are consistent with prematurity, whereas others are signs of complications of prematurity. The size and shape of the head must be evaluated, especially if the infant has a history of intraventricular hemorrhage or hydrocephalus. In infants who have been treated neurosurgically for hydrocephalus, ventriculoperitoneal shunt and tubing may be palpated. Visual abnormalities such as strabismus must be carefully ruled out by examination as well as by history, because up to 20% of preterm infants may have an ophthalmologic problem (see Chapter 50, Strabismus). Oropharyngeal abnormalities such as a palatal groove, high arched palate, or abnormal tooth formation may occur as a result of prolonged endotracheal intubation. Discoloration of teeth may also result from exposure to high bilirubin levels. Baseline intercostal, substernal or subcostal retractions, wheezing, and tachypnea in former premature babies with moderate-to-severe bronchopulmonary dysplasia (BPD) should be documented (see Chapter 109, Chronic Lung Disease).

Chest scars secondary to the placement of chest tubes should be noted. Adult female breasts may be affected if scarring occurs on or close to breast tissue. The umbilicus may appear hypoplastic as a result of umbilical catheter placement and suturing. Multiple scars on the heels from blood sampling or on the distal extremities from intravenous catheters and cutdowns may be evident.

The genitalia of both male and female preterm infants should be examined closely for inguinal hernias. The male scrotum should be examined for cryptorchidism. A careful evaluation for congenital hip dislocation should be performed until children are ambulatory (see Chapter 71, Developmental Hip Dysplasia).

The most important part of the physical examination is probably the neuromuscular examination. Increased muscular tone, asymmetry, and decreased bulk should be noted along with the presence of any clonus or asymmetry of deep tendon reflexes. Inappropriate reflexes such as a persistent Moro or fisting beyond four months of age should also be documented. Other abnormalities (e.g., scissoring or sustained clonus) in the neurologic examination may become more apparent as infants become older. The detection of subtle early findings is important, so appropriate intervention, such as physical therapy, can be instituted as soon as possible.

Laboratory Tests

In addition to the standard screening tests performed on all healthy infants and children during health maintenance visits, several laboratory studies are particularly important in preterm infants. Such tests include a CBC and reticulocyte count to check for anemia; electrolytes in infants with BPD on diuretics to detect hypokalemia or alkalosis; and serum calcium, phosphorus, and alkaline phosphatase levels in infants with documented rickets or an increased risk for rickets (birth weight < 1000 g or prolonged history of total parenteral nutrition) to evaluate the need for specific vitamin and mineral replacement therapy. Therapeutic drug levels for commonly used medications such as phenobarbital, theophylline, or caffeine should also be measured if appropriate.

Results of screening tests performed before discharge should also be reviewed and repeated as indicated. This applies to auditory evaluations and ophthalmologic examinations. EEGs and pneumograms should be reserved for preterm infants with a history of seizures or apnea and bradycardia of prematurity, respectively. Pulse oximetry is indicated for infants with severe BPD receiving supplemental oxygen who are going to be weaned from therapy.

Imaging Studies

A head ultrasound should be repeated only if necessary. A baseline chest x-ray in infants with BPD is usually not warranted, because multiple films have already been taken in the NICU. A head CT scan may be considered in infants with a progressively abnormal neurologic examination and abnormal rate of head growth.

MANAGEMENT

Well child care in relatively healthy preterm infants has two components. One is the provision of routine health care maintenance for infants and appropriate developmental anticipatory guidance for parents, and the other involves the incorporation of treatment for chronic conditions into each visit. Health care maintenance should include nutrition counseling, developmental surveillance, immunizations, and assessment of vision and hearing, in addition to standard screening tests discussed above. Outside resources concerning developmental delay can be reviewed with parents (Table 19–1). Care related to chronic conditions includes adjusting medication doses such as diuretic therapy, weaning from supplemental oxygen, and discontinuing the apnea monitor.

TABLE 19–1. How to Provide Parental Support and Education

Understand parental expectations
Legitimize parental fears
Be a source of support and encouragement
Provide consistent, honest information
Assume the role of the overall "coordinator of care"
Provide referrals to outside resources, including respite care

---

Nutrition

According to the Committee on Nutrition of the AAP, most healthy preterm infants require 110 to 130 kcal/kg/day to achieve adequate growth. Physicians must keep in mind, however, that caloric requirements vary with individual infants depending on associated chronic conditions such as BPD and malabsorption. In cases of inadequate weight gain, the number of calories in each feeding may be raised either by increasing the volume or concentrating the formula, thus raising its caloric density. The introduction of solid foods is appropriate once infants have developed acceptable oral motor skills for swallowing solids.

Preterm infants require vitamin and mineral supplements. Breast-fed preterm infants should receive multivitamins as well as iron and fluoride supplements. Although formulas for full-term infants supply most vitamins and minerals needed by preterm infants, daily multivitamins can also be given. Additional vitamin D, calcium, and phosphorus are necessary only in infants who have documented rickets or are at high risk (i.e., < 1000 g birth weight) for the disease. Mature breast milk contains low levels of nutrients. A human milk fortifier alleviates the need for these supplements. Folate and vitamin E are usually no longer needed by the time infants weigh 2000 to 2500 g and are taking full feeds. Iron supplementation should be continued until infants are eating adequate iron-fortified solids. Daily fluoride should be given into adolescence.

Developmental Assessment

Both informal and formal developmental surveillance should include referral to an early intervention program, particularly in extremely low-birth-weight infants (Table 19–2; see Chapter 14, Normal Development).

Immunizations

Routine immunization schedules recommended by the Committee on Immunization Practices of the AAP should be followed. The administration of any vaccine is determined by the chronologic or postnatal age, not the gestational age. Standard doses and intervals should also be used (see Chapter 17, Immunizations). Several studies have shown an adequate serologic response despite a history of prematurity. Absolute and relative contraindications to specific vaccine components or to live vaccines for preterm infants are identical to published guidelines for term infants and children. Physicians should note that in preterm infants greater than six months of age with chronic lung disease, administration of influenza vaccine is recommended during the winter.

Assessment of Vision and Hearing

Specialized follow-up visits for visual and auditory sequelae of prematurity must be arranged at the health maintenance visit. An initial ophthalmologic screening

TABLE 19–2.   Guidelines for Developmental Surveillance

For pediatricians using developmental screening tests, the yielded score should be used to determine when to refer. For those who choose not to use standardized tests, the following guidelines are suggested. Be concerned if:

At 6 months adjusted age, the infant:
Is not sitting, even with support
Makes no effort to reach or bat at objects
Does not localize sound
Only momentarily grasps
Keeps hands fisted
Does not mouth objects

At 12 months adjusted age, the infant:
Is sitting but not crawling
Does not search for hidden objects
Does not vocalize consonant and vowel combinations
Does not attend to books
Does not respond to simple, familiar directions such as "pat-a-cake"

At 18 months adjusted age, the child:
Does not walk
Does not imitate sounds or motor actions
Cannot build a tower with blocks
Is most interested in putting toys in mouth at play
Knows fewer than eight words

At 24 months adjusted age, the child:
Does not put two words together in speech
Has play skills that remain primarily imitative
Has gross motor skills that are lacking in balance and control
Cannot complete a simple puzzle or shape sorter
Cannot identify basic body parts

At 36 months chronologic age, the child:
Does not follow simple commands, including "give me"
Does not use prepositions in speech
Cannot copy a circle
Has such poor articulation that it is impossble for others to understand
Does not jump with both feet off the ground

At 4 years, the child:
Still uses phrases instead of sentences
Does not know color names
Cannot give first and last name
Cannot pedal a tricycle

Modified, with permission, from Bernbaum, J.C., and M. Hoffman-Williamson. Primary Care of the Preterm Infant. St. Louis, Mosby-Year Book, 1991, p. 71.

examination should have been performed between five and seven weeks of age in infants less than 1500 g or less than 30 weeks' gestation, irrespective of oxygen exposure, and in infants between 1500 and 1800 g or between 30 and 35 weeks' gestation who have been exposed to oxygen. A repeat examination prior to discharge or one month later may also be required to detect the extent and progression of retinopathy of prematurity (ROP). Further follow-up is then dictated by the ophthalmologist. Preterm infants are also at increased risk for the development of strabismus and myopia (independent of ROP).

A BAER or a behavioral audiogram should be performed by three months of age but no later than six months of age. Referral to an audiologist should be made if infants "fail" the initial screening or if parents or practitioners have any concerns.

Other Possible Problems

Preterm infants with chronic lung disease are at increased risk for respiratory illness, especially during the winter. Parents should be informed of this risk and counseled about symptoms such as tachypnea and wheezing associated with simple URI. Practitioners should have a low threshold for considering a diagnosis of pneumonia in these infants in the appropriate clinical setting. Primary care providers should also keep in mind that preterm infants with BPD are at increased risk for SIDS.

Preterm survivors who were critically ill can be particularly at risk for developing the **vulnerable child syndrome,** because their parents often perceive them as fragile and vulnerable. Features of this syndrome include abnormal separation difficulties for both mother and child, sleep difficulties, parental overprotectiveness and overindulgence, lack of appropriate discipline, and excessive preoccupation with the infant's health. Serious behavioral problems may arise as a result of such parent-child interactions. Primary care providers must be cognizant of early signs of this syndrome and should try to prevent its occurrence by reassuring parents about the infant's well being. Every effort should be made to normalize the family's schedule once the infant is stable and to encourage parent-infant interactions unrelated to health care.

PROGNOSIS

No single risk factor successfully predicts the long-term prognosis for premature infants. Although some aspects of prognosis are indeed influenced by the complexity of the infant's hospital course, birth weight has been found to be one of the best predictors of mortality and morbidity. Large, comprehensive studies evaluating the morbidities associated with extremely low birth weight are only now being published, however. Thus most predictions made regarding the long-term outcome of premature infants, especially those who weigh less than 1000 grams, are incomplete. Research has shown that despite the decrease in respiratory distress syndrome in surfactant-treated infants, the incidence of other preterm complications such as intraventricular bleeds or ROP has not been reduced significantly. The implications of these findings on long-term development remain to be seen.

Prematurity does not seem to affect children's overall height significantly. Several studies have shown that preterm infants are smaller and thinner than their normal term peers in the first few years of life but often "catch up" by the time they reach middle childhood—about seven or eight years of age. Genetic factors continue to influence ultimate stature in these children.

Studies of developmental outcome are much more equivocal; the concept of "catch up" varies with each individual case. Vague definitions of developmental delay and what is appropriate for age make gathering data very difficult. In addition, reports about the incidence of moderate-to-severe handicapping conditions are conflicting, especially in extremely low-birth-weight infants. Regardless, neurodevelopmental impairment is a concern for physicians who care for preterm infants.

Case Resolution

In the case presented at the beginning of the chapter, the infant's current feeding schedule should be continued because appropriate weight gain has occurred. Iron, fluoride, and multivitamin supplementation should be given. The apnea monitor can be discontinued after the infant reaches 40 weeks' gestation and has a normal pneumogram. The first set of immunizations should be administered at this visit, and any questions that the family has should be answered. A follow-up visit with the general pediatrician should be scheduled in three to four weeks. Vision, hearing, and formal developmental testing should be arranged in one to two months.

Selected Readings

American Academy of Pediatrics, Committee on Nutrition. *Pediatric Nutrition Handbook*. Evanston, IL, American Academy of Pediatrics, 1993.

Aylward, G. P., et al. Outcome studies of low-birth-weight infants published in the last decade. J. Pediatr. 115:515–520, 1989.

Bernbaum, J. C., S. Friedman, and M. Hoffman-Williamson. Preterm infant care after hospital discharge. Pediatr. Rev. 10:195–206, 1989.

Bernbaum, J. C., and M. Hoffman-Williamson. *Primary Care of the Preterm Infant*. St. Louis, Mosby–Year Book, 1991.

Bregman, J., and L. V. S. Kimberlin. Developmental outcome in extremely premature infants: impact of surfactant. Pediatr. Clin. North Am. 40:937–953, 1993.

Casey, P. H., et al. Growth patterns of low-birth-weight preterm infants: a longitudinal analysis of a large, varied sample. J. Pediatr. 117:298–307, 1990.

Cunningham, C. K., J. A. McMillan, and S. J. Gross. Rehospitalization for respiratory illness in infants of less than 32 weeks' gestation. Pediatrics 88:527–532, 1991.

Gross, R. T. Day care for the child born prematurely. Pediatrics 91:189–192, 1993.

Hack, M., et al. School-age outcomes in children with birth weights under 750 g. N. Engl. J. Med. 331:753–759, 1994.

McCormick, M. C., et al. The health and developmental status of very low birth weight children at school age. J.A.M.A. 267:2204–2208, 1992.

Phelps, D. L. Retinopathy of prematurity. Pediatr. Rev. 16:50–56, 1995.

Siegel, M. D. Advances in neonatology: view from a practicing pediatrician. Pediatr. Clin. North Am. 40:1105–1114, 1993.

Volpe, J. J. Intraventricular hemorrhage and brain injury in the preterm infant: diagnosis, prognosis and prevention. Clin. Perinatol. 16:387–411, 1989.

C H A P T E R   2 0

NEEDS OF CHILDREN WITH PHYSICAL AND SENSORY HANDICAPS

Monica Sifuentes, M.D.

H$_x$ A six-year-old physically handicapped girl is brought to the office for a routine physical examination for school.

The girl was the full-term product of a normal pregnancy and delivery. The mother, who received regular prenatal care, was 25 years of age at the time. She used no illicit drugs, alcohol, or any other medications. At delivery, skin defects of the scalp, abdomen, and both knees were noted. The anterior fontanelle was enlarged. In addition, the infant had transverse, bilateral limb defects of both feet and fingers and short, dysplastic thumbs.

During the first year of life, the girl was admitted to the hospital several times for leakage of CSF from the calvarium defect. Although the skin defects have healed, a bony defect measuring 3 x 4 cm remains at the crown of the head.

The girl now attends special education classes and will be mainstreamed in the upcoming year. She uses prostheses for her legs and has undergone several procedures to give her better opposition in her primitive thumbs. She also wears a protective helmet at all times. Her growth and development are normal for age.

Questions

1. Why is early identification and intervention important for infants and children with disabilities?
2. What are the unique needs of infants and children with handicaps?
3. What role do primary care practitioners play in the care of children with handicaps?
4. What are the appropriate referrals and resources for families of children with handicaps?
5. What specific psychosocial issues should be addressed whenever children with handicaps visit their primary care practitioners?

Handicaps range from mildly to moderately disabling, depending on the nature and extent of the condition. For unprepared parents, however, the diagnosis of any handicap can be overwhelming and disappointing. Early identification of a disabling condition by physicians leads to appropriate, definitive treatment for certain disabilities. Where such treatment is not available, prompt identification improves children's long-term outcome and allows families to obtain appropriate resources for their children. Through early intervention, infants and children with irreversible conditions can be introduced to medical, educational, and psychosocial services available in the community. These services are crucial if children with handicaps are to reach their full potential.

EPIDEMIOLOGY

The prevalence of children in the United States with disabilities is difficult to assess. Recent studies report that approximately 17% of children under the age of 17 years have at least one disability, including deafness or trouble hearing, blindness, cerebral palsy, epilepsy, speech impediments, and other learning and behavioral problems. In addition, an estimated 30% of these children have more than one disability. A single sensory handicap such as deafness affects approximately 3.5% of children, and blindness occurs in 1% of children.

The presence of any disabling condition has a profound impact on the health and education of affected children. Studies show that children with disabilities have 1.5 times more doctor visits and spend 3.5 more days in the hospital than children without these conditions. Children with handicaps miss twice the number of school days and are twice as likely to repeat a grade compared to children without handicaps.

In addition, numerous associated conditions occur more commonly in children with disabilities. These include mental retardation, growth failure, nutrition problems, and behavioral and emotional disorders. Problems with dentition, respiratory infections, and bowel and bladder continence may also develop.

CLINICAL PRESENTATION

Children with handicaps can present in a variety of ways depending on age. They may be seen for a routine health maintenance visit, and delayed development is apparent on examination. Children can also present with specific complaints, such as poor vision or hearing,

D$_x$ **Children With Physical and Sensory Handicaps***
• Growth failure
• Microcephaly
• Abnormal neurologic examination, including hypertonicity, spastic diplegia or quadriplegia, and brisk deep tendon reflexes
• Developmental delay
• Speech or hearing deficit
• Visual deficit
————
* May not be present in all children.

or with more general concerns, such as growth failure (Dx Box). Behavioral problems or difficulties in school may be the reason for the initial visit.

PATHOPHYSIOLOGY

Disabilities include a variety of childhood conditions that are manifested as physical, sensory, psychological, or cognitive impairments. They may be acquired or congenital and static or progressive. Etiologies are often multifactorial.

Cerebral palsy, for example, is a collection of non-progressive disorders resulting from a CNS insult early in brain development. It is characterized by abnormal motor movements and posturing and may be accompanied by other disabilities. Causes of cerebral palsy include prematurity (i.e., low birth weight), asphyxia, prenatal abnormalities (e.g., placental insufficiency), congenital infections (e.g., toxoplasmosis, CMV), and biochemical abnormalities (e.g., severe hyperbilirubinemia). Other rarer causes are environmental toxins (e.g., alcohol [maternal alcoholism]) and genetic disorders (e.g., inborn errors of metabolism). Severe postnatal injuries can also lead to cerebral palsy; the classic example is meningitis. An estimated 25% of cases of cerebral palsy have no discernible cause, however.

DIFFERENTIAL DIAGNOSIS

Multiple conditions can lead to physical or sensory handicaps, the most common being cerebral palsy. Other etiologies include prematurity complicated by intraventricular hemorrhage, exposure to ototoxic drugs such as aminoglycosides, refractory seizures, congenital infections such as toxoplasmosis, and endocrine disorders such as poorly treated congenital hypothyroidism.

EVALUATION

History

When initially evaluating children with newly diagnosed handicaps, practitioners should first assess any primary parental concerns. A complete medical history should then be obtained, including information about the pregnancy and birth. General screening questions about development are also important to ask (see Questions Box) so that children's developmental progress can be assessed. Specific questioning is warranted if parents are concerned about delayed development or if any of their answers indicate that their children are not attaining age-appropriate developmental milestones.

In cases of children with known sensory or physical handicaps, families should be asked directly at each visit about daily activities. Because many children with disabilities are also on daily medication for either seizures or other chronic conditions, it is also important to ask about any potential side effects of drugs.

In addition, an overall assessment of family dynamics should be made. It is important to inquire about the relationships between children with handicaps and

Questions: Children With Physical and Sensory Handicaps

- Were there any perinatal complications, such as premature rupture of membranes or fetal distress?
- Was the infant born prematurely? If so, how long did the infant remain in the hospital and for what reasons?
- Was the infant exposed to any toxins in utero?
- Is there any history of infection during the perinatal period or infancy?
- What developmental milestones has the infant or child mastered?
- Is the child attending school or some type of early intervention program?
  - How does the child get there?
  - What does the child do upon returning from school?
- Who feeds and bathes the child?
- Can the older child use the toilet without assistance?
- How is the child sleeping? Does the child take naps at school and at home?
- Has respite care been arranged for the family?
- Does the caregiver appear overwhelmed or excessively tired, especially one who is caring for a child with multiple handicaps?
- Do other family members help care for the child?
- Is the extended family available to help with the siblings?
- Are there any other handicapped people in the family?
- Does the family receive any financial assistance for care of the child?

their siblings, as well as the impact of these children on the parents' marriage.

Physical Examination

In general, a complete physical examination, including a neurologic assessment, should be performed at each visit. The height, weight, and head circumference should be plotted on the growth chart and compared to previous measurements. A failure of adequate growth as measured by any of these parameters should be examined closely. For example, microcephaly, nutritional problems, and growth failure are not uncommon in children with cerebral palsy. Depending on the disability, the main part of the examination should then focus on physical findings associated with the particular handicap. For children with physical handicaps such as congenital or acquired amputations, for instance, assessment of the skin that comes in contact with prosthetic devices is a pertinent aspect of the physical examination. In children with sensory handicaps such as unilateral hearing loss, the evaluation of a middle ear effusion or infection in the unaffected ear should be a priority.

Overall, for most children with disabilities, the neurologic examination is extremely important. The following questions should be asked: Are primitive reflexes such as the Moro and rooting reflexes present in neonates? Have all primitive reflexes been extinguished in older children? Do infants appear to visualize and track objects appropriately? Are there any abnormal movements of the trunk or extremities at rest? Is the muscle tone normal? Is any hyper- or hypotonicity evident? Is any asymmetry of the upper and lower extremities apparent? Are the deep tendon reflexes normal and symmetric? Is the gait appropriate for age?

Laboratory Tests

The laboratory evaluation of infants or children with physical or sensory handicaps depends on the specific disability. Not all patients need a costly array of diagnostic procedures. A chromosomal karyotype using peripheral leukocytes is helpful in children with suspected genetic disorders (e.g., abnormal facies or a major anomaly and developmental delay). Routine testing for the fragile X syndrome in all mentally retarded boys remains controversial.

Metabolic screening for inborn errors should be performed on children with mental retardation and any of the following symptoms: intermittent vomiting or lethargy, loss of developmental milestones, or seizures. Such screening is not needed in the routine evaluation of children with developmental delay and no other symptoms.

A screening test for visual acuity (Snellen test) and hearing (audiogram) should be performed in all children suspected of having sensory deficits, even mild ones. For infants or toddlers, a BAER or behavioral audiogram is a more appropriate screening test for hearing. A visual evoked response (VER) can be performed to test vision.

Psychometric testing may be helpful in certain school-age children to assess intellectual function.

Imaging Studies

An EEG is indicated in all patients who have a history of seizures or seizurelike episodes. Other brain imaging studies, such as CT or MRI scans of the head, can be performed when intrauterine infection, intraventricular hemorrhage, or genetic disorders with associated developmental delays are suspected. An EMG can be used to differentiate cerebral palsy from a congenital myopathy.

MANAGEMENT

Caring for children with a single handicap or multiple handicaps can be both a rewarding and challenging task for primary pediatricians. Although all cases should be handled individually, general guidelines have been developed for the provision of pediatric services for infants and children with special health care needs. They include recommendations for medical services, suggestions for parental involvement, assistance from community agencies, and fulfillment of specific federal requirements for educational opportunities for children with disabilities. Pediatricians who care for children with handicaps should be familiar with these principles of care, which are published by the American Academy of Pediatrics, and should incorporate them into the overall treatment plan.

General Considerations

The major role of primary pediatricians who care for children with handicaps is threefold: (1) to make therapeutic decisions for patients and families, (2) to serve as an advocate and overall coordinator of care, and (3) to inform families of available community resources. The most difficult part of providing care for children with disabilities is initially establishing the diagnosis. Whether the diagnosis is blatantly apparent or completely unsuspected, physicians are placed in the awkward position of breaking the news to families. Parents should be informed of the diagnosis as soon as possible, but care should be taken to refrain from discussing the prognosis, especially if it is still unknown. The cause of the disability and the possible complications of the condition should also be reviewed. *The primary goal is to help children with handicaps reach their full potential.*

Health care providers are in a unique position to establish a treatment plan with families that includes medical, psychosocial, and educational services. A multidisciplinary team that includes the pediatrician, a member of the school system, a social worker, and a representative of an early intervention program should be identified. Federally funded, nonprofit, regional centers can provide an organized treatment plan and entry into an early intervention program to some children with handicaps. To qualify, children must be diagnosed with certain disorders such as cerebral palsy, epilepsy, autism, or global developmental delay. In addition, infants considered "at risk" for developing disabilities qualify for assistance (e.g., premature infants with bronchopulmonary dysplasia and intraventricular hemorrhage). For children who do not qualify, similar services can be coordinated on an individual basis by the physician's office or the school district.

Children with severe physical and sensory handicaps are often cared for by many medical subspecialists in addition to primary care pediatricians. Pediatric orthopedic surgeons, plastic surgeons, geneticists, ophthalmologists, otolaryngologists, child neurologists, and psychologists or psychiatrists may be necessary. In addition, speech and language therapists, occupational therapists, and physical therapists are often an integral part of the medical team. Initial and ongoing therapeutic services provided by each of these individuals must be monitored periodically to assess the progress and overall effectiveness of the treatment plan. Ideally, services should be coordinated so that children as well as parents miss a minimum number of school and work days (e.g., Saturday and after-school appointments, visits to several providers on one day).

All information from diagnostic studies and initial evaluations should be shared among each of the health care providers to determine the eligibility of individual children for special services such as Supplemental Social Security (SSI). The case worker can then assist families to apply for the appropriate services.

Specific Medical Conditions

A number of medical conditions commonly occur in children with moderate to severe handicaps. While providing children with comprehensive well child care, general pediatricians can also address and treat these conditions.

Problems with adequate nutrition, which usually result from insufficient caloric intake, are manifested by growth failure. Depending on the degree of disability and amount of oropharyngeal dysfunction, the placement of a nasogastric or gastrostomy tube may be necessary. Caloric needs are 10 to 50% higher than normal basal needs to ensure growth.

Respiratory illness is not uncommon among these children. Close observation and conservative treatment of viral illnesses are often necessary. Aspiration pneumonia is likely to occur, especially in children with severe developmental delay, because of poor handling of oral secretions or severe malnutrition. To help minimize respiratory infections, influenza vaccine should also be administered during the winter months.

Maintaining good oral hygiene is another challenge, because some children with handicaps do not clear secretions well and retain food in their mouths, predisposing to cavity development. In addition, many children are treated with anticonvulsants and antibiotics that can cause gingival and enamel dysplasias. Abnormal oromotor coordination, tone, and posturing also contribute to the development of oropharyngeal deformities such as high, arched palate and overcrowded teeth. As with other children, fluoride supplementation and consistent preventive dental care are recommended.

Bowel and bladder continence is important to attain for several reasons. It allows children to function in a socially acceptable fashion, provides independence, and prevents the development of complications such as recurrent UTIs, diaper dermatitis, and decubitus ulcers. Behavior modification techniques coupled with positive reinforcement are associated with complete or partial success for bowel training.

Community Resources

Optimal care for children with developmental disabilities depends on maximum utilization of community agencies and resources. An assessment of parental and patient needs should first be performed and prioritized. The appropriate resources should then be identified for individual children. Primary care physicians may need to help determine the appropriateness of specific services for patients and families. Emphasis should be placed on integrating each child into support services used by all patients and their families to avoid any feelings of isolation. Support groups for siblings as well as parents, respite care, and in-home health service programs should also be investigated. Physicians should act as liaisons between all agencies. Case conferences are occasionally necessary to review the progress of individual children with each member of the health care team.

Education

Every effort should be made to enroll children with handicaps in conventional schools and to provide opportunities for socialization at an early age. Although this may be difficult for families to accept initially, it is important to introduce the concept of structured independence and mainstreaming, the placement of disabled children in classes with nondisabled children.

Until mainstreaming is achieved, several different educational possibilities can be considered, and each case should be evaluated on an individual basis. Choices include special education classes in separate schools (full- or part-time), special education classes in regular schools (full- or part- time), or part-time special education classes and part-time regular classes. The decision can be facilitated through the development of an Individual Education Plan (IEP) by a multidisciplinary team at the school. Parents and primary physicians are encouraged to participate in this evaluation.

PROGNOSIS

The prognosis for children with physical and sensory handicaps depends on the underlying etiology, the severity and extent of the disability, and early participation in an intervention program that includes services such as physical and occupational therapy. The majority of affected children are able to lead productive, independent lives when they receive adequate early intervention and education.

Case Resolution

Although the girl's medical condition appears stable, the physician should inquire about any ongoing problems or concerns, A complete examination should be performed; head growth, skin healing, and callus formation as a result

of prosthetic devices should be assessed. Routine screening laboratory tests required for school entry should be obtained. Integration into the regular classroom should be addressed with both the child and the mother at this visit, and a follow-up phone call to the school should also be made.

Selected Readings

American Academy of Pediatrics, Committee on Children with Disabilities. Pediatric services for infants and children with special health care needs. Pediatrics 92:163–165, 1993.

American Academy of Pediatrics, Committee on Children with Disabilities. Screening infants and young children for developmental disabilities. Pediatrics 93:863–865, 1994.

Boyle, C. A., P. Decoufle, and M. Yeargin-Allsopp. Prevalence and impact of developmental disabilities in U.S. children. Pediatrics 93:399–403, 1994.

Diamond, M., and I. W. Zarafu. The role of the pediatrician in the care of the handicapped child. Pediatr. Ann. 17:738–744, 1988.

Eicher, P. S., and M. L. Batshaw. Cerebral palsy. Pediatr. Clin. North Am. 40:537–551, 1993.

Fewell, R. R. Child care for children with special needs. Pediatrics 91:193–198, 1993.

Menacker, S. J. Visual function in children with developmental disabilities. Pediatr. Clin. North Am. 40:659–674, 1993.

Newacheck, P. W. Adolescents with special health needs: prevalence, severity, and access to health services. Pediatrics 84:872–881, 1989.

Palfrey, J. S., et al. Early identification of children's special needs: a study in five metropolitan communities. J. Pediatr. 111:651–659, 1987.

Strax, T. E. Psychological issues faced by adolescents and young adults with disabilities. Pediatr. Ann. 20:507–511, 1991.

Torfs, C. P., et al. Prenatal and perinatal factors in the etiology of cerebral palsy. J. Pediatr. 116:615–619, 1990.

CHAPTER 21

REPRODUCTIVE HEALTH*

Monica Sifuentes, M.D.

Hx An 18-year-old female college student in good health comes in for a routine health care visit during her spring break. She is unaccompanied by her parents and has no complaints, stating that she just needs a checkup. She likes college, passed all of her fall and winter classes, and has some new friends. She denies tobacco use but says most of her friends smoke. She occasionally drinks alcohol and has tried marijuana once. Although she is not sexually active, she is interested in discussing oral contraception. Her last menstrual period (LMP), which occurred two weeks ago, was normal. She is taking no medications. Her physical examination is entirely normal.

Questions

1. What issues are important to discuss with adolescents at reproductive health maintenance examinations?

*This chapter is largely devoted to a discussion of the reproductive health of adolescent females. However, "Evaluation" is divided into two sections—one for females and one for males. The reader is referred to Chapter 69, Sexually Transmitted Diseases, for more information regarding male reproductive health.

2. What are the indications for a full pelvic examination?
3. Which patients should have Pap smears? How often should this procedure be performed?
4. What methods of contraception are most successful in adolescent patients? What factors regarding each method should be considered?
5. What are the legal issues involved in prescribing contraception to minors in the absence of parents?

Adolescent visits to primary care physicians are relatively few and infrequent by the time teenagers reach puberty. At most, healthy adolescent patients are seen once or twice during high school for preparticipation sports physicals. If adolescents are not athletic or if their schools do not require such assessments, these teenagers will probably never visit their health care providers again while in school. Therefore, it is extremely important to use any interactions with adolescents as opportunities for anticipatory guidance and health education, particularly reproductive health education.

Reproductive health can be defined as sexuality-related services, screening, and counseling. Such services should be included as a part of the routine health maintenance examination of both male and female adolescents, for several reasons. The current rise of STDs in teenagers and the risk of AIDS make reproductive health issues increasingly important. In addition, adolescents rarely schedule appointments with health care providers prior to the initiation of coitus. Experimentation with drugs and alcohol also contributes to early, unplanned sexual experiences (Box 21–1).

Aside from issues of sexual activity, adolescents may also have questions about their progression through puberty. Normal variants in body habitus or certain physical characteristics can be a source of unnecessary anxiety for unknowing teenagers. Health education to alleviate these fears is ideal. Adolescents who come for physical examinations should be allotted extra time so that topics such as puberty, sexual activity, STDs, and contraception can be discussed. In addition, during more acute, problem-oriented visits, adolescents should be encouraged to voice any other problems or concerns they may have. Depending on the nature of these issues, follow-up appointments can be scheduled.

NORMAL PHYSICAL DEVELOPMENT

Puberty begins during early adolescence with the development of secondary sexual characteristics. A sexual maturity rating scale or Tanner staging is used to describe breast and pubic hair development in females and genitalia and pubic hair progression in males (Fig. 21–1, 21–2, and 21–3). The average age of menarche in the United States is 12.5 years and menarche usually occurs between Tanner stages 4 and 5. On average, male ejaculation or "wet dreams" occur at 13 years of age; they are unrelated to pubic hair development. Full fertility is achieved by age 15 years, or midadolescence, in most boys and girls.

BOX 21–1. Reproductive Health: Sexual Activity

Statistics regarding sexual activity among adolescents in the United States are startling. One in four females and one in three males have had sexual intercourse by 15 years of age. Among adolescents from 15 to 19 years of age, more than half are sexually active, and only one-third of these teenagers use contraception. As a result, nearly one million adolescent females under 20 years of age, or one out of every ten, become pregnant each year. A large majority of these pregnancies are unintended and occur premaritally, especially among certain racial and ethnic minority groups. The outcome of these pregnancies in 15–19-year-olds varies. An estimated 40 to 50% of these pregnancies result in live births, 30 to 40% end in abortion, and 10% are miscarried or stillborn.

Unprotected sexual activity among adolescents has several adverse health consequences, the most obvious being teenage pregnancy. Of the adolescents who continue their pregnancies, prematurity (< 37 weeks' gestation) and low birth weight (< 2500 grams) are two of the most frequently reported neonatal complications. Long-term maternal psychosocial sequelae of adolescent pregnancy include poor education, limited vocational training and skills, economic dependency on public assistance, subsequent unwanted births, and high rates of separation and divorce among teenage couples.

In addition to unintended pregnancy, the risk of contracting an STD such as chlamydia, human papillomavirus (HPV), herpes, and HIV is increased. In cases of PID from either gonorrhea or chlamydia, future problems with fertility and an increased risk of ectopic pregnancy may occur. HPV, which has been associated with the development of cervical cancer, has a prevalence of up to 40% in adolescents. Other STDs are also on the rise. More alarming, however, is the relationship between acquired immunodeficiency syndrome in young adults aged 20 to 29 and probable exposure to HIV during adolescence.

Many factors have been associated with the initiation of early coitus in adolescents. They include male gender; race/ethnicity; poverty; a large, single-parent family; previous teen pregnancy in the household (either mother or sibling); poor academic achievement; discrepancy between the onset of physical puberty and cognitive development; peer group encouragement; and problem behaviors such as drug use. In addition, religious affiliation and cultural norms probably influence this decision. The role of hormonal changes during puberty and their influence on behavior has yet to be determined.

An estimated 6% of adolescents have limited normal functioning because of a chronic illness. However, a majority of these adolescents experience normal pubertal development and fertility because of advances in medical treatment for conditions such as diabetes and sickle cell disease. Like their healthy peers, many of these adolescents begin sexual intercourse at an early age. Pregnancy and childbirth can exacerbate some illnesses and increase risks significantly for both adolescents and fetuses. The genetic implications and specific patterns of inheritance of certain chronic conditions must also be considered. For this reason, attention to sexual issues is essential for adolescents with chronic medical illness.

EVALUATION

History

The history obtained at a reproductive health visit should include two parts: the medical history, which focuses primarily on the gynecologic history in females, and the psychosocial interview. Regardless of the type

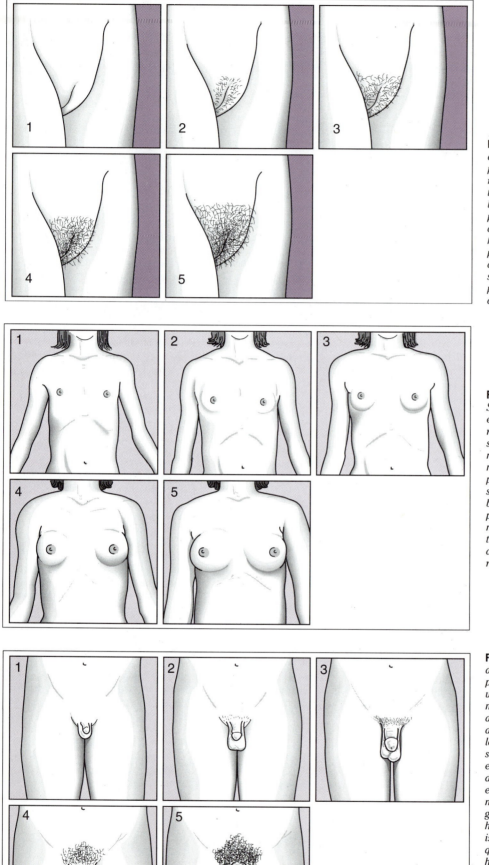

FIGURE 21–1. *Female pubic hair development. Sex maturity rating 1: prepuber-tal, no pubic hair; sex maturity rating 2: straight hair is extending along the labia and, between ratings 2 and 3, begins on the pubis; sex maturity rating 3: pubic hair is increased in quantity, is darker, and is present in the typical female triangle; sex maturity rating 4: pubic hair is more dense, curled, and adult in distribution but is less abundant; sex maturity rating 5: abundant, adult-type pattern; hair may extend on to the medial aspect of the thighs.*

FIGURE 21–2. *Female breast development. Sex maturity rating 1: prepubertal, elevations of papilla only; sex maturity rating 2: breast buds appear, areola is slightly widened and projects as small mound; sex maturity rating 3: enlargement of the entire breast with no protrusion of the papilla or of the nipple; sex maturity rating 4: enlargement of the breast and projection of areola and papilla as a secondary mound; sex maturity rating 5: adult configuration of the breast with protrusion of the nipple, areola no longer projects separately from remainder of breast.*

FIGURE 21–3. *Male genital and pubic hair development. Sex maturity rating 1: prepubertal, no pubic hair, genitalia unchanged from early childhood; sex maturity rating 2: light, down hair develops laterally and later becomes dark, penis and testes may be slightly larger, scrotum becomes more textured; sex maturity rating 3: pubic hair is extended across pubis, testes and scrotum are further enlarged, penis is larger, especially in length; sex maturity rating 4: more abundant pubic hair with curling, genitalia resemble those of an adult, glans has become larger and broader, scrotum is darker; sex maturity rating 5: adult quantity and pattern of pubic hair, with hair present along the inner borders of the thighs. The testes and scrotum are adult in size.*

Questions: Reproductive Health (both males and females)

For males and females:

- How is the adolescent feeling overall?
- Has the adolescent had any recent illnesses or conditions that the health care provider should know about?
- When was the last physical examination performed?
- Is the adolescent sexually active?
  - If so, when was the last episode of sexual intercourse?
  - Was the last episode of sexual intercourse protected or unprotected intercourse?
  - How old was the adolescent when he or she initiated coitus? Was it consensual?
  - How many sexual partners does the patient have? What gender are they (all contacts may not be heterosexual)?
- Is there any history of physical or sexual abuse?
- Has the adolescent or any of his or her partners ever been treated for an STD or tested for HIV?

Females only:

- What was the age at menarche?
- What was the date of the LMP and the duration and amount of flow?
- Are any symptoms such as cramping, bloating, or vomiting associated with menses?
  - Are any of these symptoms incapacitating? Do they cause the adolescent to miss school or work?
  - Do the mother or siblings have similar problems? If so, what do they do to manage them, if anything?

---

of visit scheduled, practitioners should take a few moments at the beginning to address routine health maintenance issues with adolescents (Questions Box: Reproductive Health). Physicians should find out whether female adolescents have ever had a pelvic examination. The gynecologic history should also be obtained from these patients.

In addition, current methods of contraceptive use, if any, should be reviewed (Questions Box: Contraceptive Use). If adolescent females take oral contraceptives, a review of the more emergent danger signs of birth control pills is warranted, especially at an initial visit. **ACHES** (**a**bdominal pain, **c**hest pain, **h**eadaches, **e**ye problems, **s**evere leg pain) is a useful acronym (Table 21–1).

The rest of the psychosocial history, otherwise known as the **HEADSSS** interview (**h**ome, **e**mployment and

Questions: Contraceptive Use

- What percentage of the time are condoms used?
- Is any other method also used, such as spermicidal foam or jelly?
- Is the adolescent female currently using oral contraceptives?
  - If so, what particular type is she taking, and how long has she been using this method of contraception?
  - How often does she forget to take the pill? *or* What does she do when she forgets to take the pill?
  - Does she experience common minor side effects such as breakthrough bleeding, nausea, weight gain, or acne?

TABLE 21–1. Danger Signs Associated With Oral Contraceptive Use

A	Abdominal pain (severe)
C	Chest pain (severe), shortness of breath
H	Headaches
E	Eye problems (visual loss or blur)
S	Severe leg pain (calf/thigh)

---

education, **a**ctivities, **d**rugs, **s**exual activity/sexuality, **s**uicide and depression, **s**afety), should be completed whether or not adolescents are currently sexually active (see Chapter 4, Talking to Adolescents). Risk factors for teenage pregnancy or multiple exposures to STDs should be kept in mind when formulating health care plans with adolescents.

Physical Examination

A complete physical examination should be performed on all adolescents, with particular attention paid to their Tanner stage.

Males

The genitalia should be examined closely for penile and testicular size, distribution of pubic hair, and presence of any ulcerative, vesicular, or wartlike lesions. Any urethral erythema or discharge should also be noted. Clinicians can use this opportunity to teach male adolescents how to perform a testicular self-examination.

Females

Prior to performing the physical examination, the physician should determine whether a full speculum examination is indicated (Table 21–2). Each decision should be made on an individual basis. Proper preparation of adolescents is imperative. This should include an explanation of the procedure and the physical sensations felt while the Pap smear and cervical cultures are being obtained, choice of who should be

---

TABLE 21–2. Indications for a Complete Pelvic Examination*

Part of contraceptive management
Pregnancy
Request by adolescent
Sexual activity
Partner with sexually transmitted disease (STD)
Previous history of STD
History of hepatitis B
Unexplained lower abdominal pain
Abnormal vaginal discharge
Unexplained vaginal bleeding
External venereal warts
Urinary symptoms

*Every adolescent female needs at least a visual examination of the external genitalia whether or not the above indications are met.

present during the examination (e.g., parent or friend who may have accompanied the patient), and a discussion of the desired positioning (i.e., supine versus semisitting). In addition, speculums and other equipment should be shown to adolescents. The goal is to minimize the adolescent's fears, anxieties, misconceptions, and discomfort regarding the examination.

A breast examination should be performed on female adolescents, and any breast tenderness, nodularity, or masses should be noted. Again, this portion of the examination can be used to educate patients about the purpose and importance of breast self-examinations.

The external genitalia should be examined in all adolescent females whether or not they are sexually active. The Tanner stage and any congenital anomalies such as an imperforate hymen should be noted. In sexually active adolescents, the external genitalia must be carefully examined for venereal warts, ulcers, and vesicular lesions. Any urethral erythema, edema, or discharge that may indicate an otherwise asymptomatic chlamydial infection should be noted. A vaginal discharge may be appreciated prior to inserting the speculum, but ideally, the cervix should be examined for cervical ectopy, friability, and any lesions or discharge from the os. The vaginal mucosa should also be inspected as the speculum is withdrawn.

During the bimanual examination, the cervix should be palpated for any cervical motion tenderness. Uterine size and position should be appreciated, and adnexal tenderness or masses should be noted. Because normal ovaries are approximately the size of almonds, they are often not palpated by the inexperienced clinician. A rectovaginal examination is necessary to rule out fistulas, especially in postpartum adolescents. If the practitioner is unable to perform a vaginal bimanual examination, a rectoabdominal examination can be done to assess uterine size and position and the presence of adnexal masses.

Laboratory Tests

A gonorrhea culture and a chlamydia rapid assay should be obtained in sexually active adolescents who have had unprotected intercourse or vaginal discharge or who have cervical friability noted on speculum examination. A saline and KOH wet mount should also be collected in symptomatic patients. A Pap smear should be performed in females who are sexually active or who have external genital warts, persistent vaginal discharge, or in utero exposure to DES. The Pap smear can also help detect *Trichomonas vaginalis* or the cytologic changes associated with human papillomavirus (HPV). Herpes simplex cultures should be done if painful vesicles are noted on examination.

Other laboratory tests include an RPR test for syphilis and an HIV test (after appropriate pretest counseling). Baseline CBC, liver function tests, cholesterol, and fasting glucose may be indicated before starting oral contraceptives but are not mandatory. A pregnancy test is warranted only in sexually active females if the practitioner chooses to begin oral contraceptives midcycle.

MANAGEMENT

Reproductive Health Education

All management plans during reproductive health visits should include a frank **discussion of puberty, sexuality, and STDs.** Ideally, preventive health care measures such as **breast and testicular self-examinations** have been reviewed during the physical examination. It is hoped that by encouraging adolescents' familiarity with these self-examinations, they will continue to perform them throughout their adult lives. The use of posters, plastic models, and written materials to support the discussion is greatly encouraged. The goal of education should be to assist adolescents in identifying and communicating their thoughts and feelings about sexual abstinence as well as sexual activity and to aid in the prevention of unintended pregnancies and STDs. Prevention programs offered by schools must be supplemented by open parental communication about sexuality in the home.

Legal Issues

The issue of **confidentiality** is important to consider when providing reproductive health care for adolescents. Parental involvement should be strongly encouraged, but health care practitioners are not required to disclose any information to parents except in cases of suicide or harmful intent to others. Contraceptive services can be provided to adolescents of any age without parental knowledge or consent. The complex issue of abortion varies from state to state.

Papanicolaou Smear

A Pap smear should be performed annually in all sexually active adolescent females. Although this is a conservative recommendation, it seems justified given adolescents' high rate of exposure to HPV and the association of certain types of HPV with the progression of cervical dysplasia. The general recommendation of the American Cancer Society and the American College of Obstetricians and Gynecologists is an annual Pap smear with the onset of sexual activity or at the age of 18 years (whichever comes first) until three or more consecutive smears are documented as normal. The Pap smear should be performed at least every two to three years thereafter. The increased rate of abnormal cervical cytology in recent years in younger women and the need for more frequent examinations are concerns with this approach.

Management following an abnormal Pap smear depends on the presence of atypia versus low-grade or high-grade squamous intraepithelial lesions. Further evaluation with colposcopy and cervical biopsy may be warranted. This decision should be made in consultation with the cytopathologist who reviewed the specimen and a gynecologist familiar with the management of cervical dysplasia in young women.

Contraceptive Methods

The appropriate method of contraception should be individualized. Barrier methods include condoms (male and female), diaphragms, contraceptive sponges, and cervical caps. Vaginal spermicides are available in a variety of forms (foams, jellies, creams, and suppositories) and can be used alone or can provide extra protection if used with a barrier method. Hormonal methods include oral contraceptives and long-acting progestin agents. Intrauterine devices are not used in teenagers because of the prevalence of STDs and risk of pelvic inflammatory disease (PID). The withdrawal method, or coitus interruptus, and natural family planning are ineffective methods for adolescents for protection against pregnancy.

Hormonal Contraception

Combined low-dose oral contraceptives are an effective means of birth control for adolescents. Monophasic pills contain a fixed dose of estrogen and progestin throughout the 21-day pill cycle. Biphasic preparations contain a lower dose of the progestin component during the first 10 days of the cycle. In the newest type of oral contraceptive, triphasic pills, the doses of both estrogen and progestin or the progestin component alone is varied. This contraceptive was created to decrease the overall progestin-related side effects such as hypertension, acne, and lipid abnormalities. Clear benefits associated with oral contraceptive use include prevention of pregnancy, protection against ovarian and endometrial cancers, decreased risk of functional ovarian cysts, and decreased menstrual symptoms such as dysmenorrhea. The potential risks, which include thromboembolic phenomena, hypertension, and changes in the lipid profile, are minimal compared to the morbidity and mortality associated with teenage pregnancy and childbirth.

The long-acting progestins, medroxyprogesterone acetate (Depo-Provera) and levonorgestrel (Norplant), have recently been approved for use in the United States. Depo-Provera, which is given intramuscularly every three months, inhibits ovulation for at least 14 weeks. Norplant provides continuous contraception for five years via six subdermal plastic rods inserted through a small incision in the upper, inner arm. Common side effects are irregular bleeding, especially in the first few months, and eventual amenorrhea with prolonged use of either method.

Nonhormonal Contraception

Numerous studies and clinical experience have shown that nonhormonal methods are less effective in adolescents. However, condoms in conjunction with a spermicide have become crucial as a method of contraception since the emergence of AIDS. They help prevent transmission of other STDs as well as HIV. A few moments, therefore, should be taken during the visit to explain and demonstrate proper use of condoms. Risks of condom use are minimal, except for allergic reactions to the spermicide, latex, or lubricants. The female condom, the most recent development in barrier contraception, has been heralded as a possible answer to teenage pregnancy and STDs because it is controlled by the female partner. Other nonhormonal methods should be reviewed with adolescents as needed.

Sexually Transmitted Diseases

All STDs should be treated according to specific guidelines published by the CDC based on current epidemiology. Readers should see Chapter 69, Sexually Transmitted Disease, for details regarding the diagnosis and management of STDs in adolescents.

Case Resolution

In the case scenario presented at the beginning of the chapter, a more detailed history should be obtained regarding the adolescent's menstrual history and daily activities (e.g., Who does she spend most of her time with?, What does she do in her spare time?). In addition, the indications for a pelvic examination should be reviewed. If they do not apply, the pelvic examination can be deferred until the next visit or when she becomes sexually active. A discussion should then follow regarding both barrier and hormonal methods of contraception and their role in the prevention of pregnancy and STDs.

Selected Readings

Centers for Disease Control and Prevention. Selected behaviors that increase risk for HIV infection among high school students—United States, 1990. M.M.W.R. 41:231–240, 1992.

Centers for Disease Control and Prevention. Sexual behavior among high school students. M.M.W.R. 40:885–888, 1992.

Emans, S. J., et al. Adolescents' compliance with the use of oral contraceptives. J.A.M.A. 257:3377–3381, 1987.

McAnarney, E. R., and W. R. Handee. Adolescent pregnancy and its consequences. J.A.M.A. 262:74–77, 1989.

McAnarney, E. R., and W. R. Handee. The prevention of adolescent pregnancy. J.A.M.A. 262:78–82, 1989.

Rauh, J. L. The pediatrician's role in assisting teenagers to avoid the consequences of adolescent pregnancy. Pediatr. Ann. 22:90–98, 1993.

Rosenfeld, W. D., and J. B. Swedler. Role of hormonal contraceptives in prevention of pregnancy and sexually transmitted diseases. Adol. Med. State Art Rev. 3:207–222, 1992.

Sikand, A., and M. Fisher. The role of barrier contraceptives in prevention of pregnancy and disease in adolescents. Adol. Med. State Art Rev. 3:223–240, 1992.

Schonberg, S. K., et al. Committee on adolescence, contraception and adolescents. Pediatrics 86:134–138, 1990.

Task Force on Pediatric AIDS. Adolescent and human immunodeficiency virus infection. The role of the pediatrician in prevention and intervention. Pediatrics 92:626–629, 1993.

CHAPTER 22

INJURY PREVENTION

Iris Wagman Borowsky, M.D., Ph.D.

H_x A three-year-old girl was brought to the emergency department with a BB in her right eye. The girl's 10-year-old brother inadvertently fired his BB gun, and a BB lodged in her right eye. The BB was surgically removed, but as a result of the injury, the girl is legally blind in that eye.

Questions

1. How extensive is the injury problem in children?
2. What are the different methods for injury prevention? How could this particular injury have been prevented?
3. What injury prevention program has been developed by the AAP?
4. What are some general guidelines for effective injury prevention counseling?

Traditionally, unintentional injuries have been called accidents. The problem with the term "accident," however, is that it implies unpredictability, carrying with it connotations of chance, fate, and unexpectedness. The perception that injuries are random, chance occurrences that cannot be predicted or prevented has been a major barrier to progress in injury prevention and the study and control of injury as a scientific discipline. According to the modern view of injury, "accidents" must be anticipated in order to be prevented. Specialists in injury prevention have tried to replace the word "accident" with "injury" and have developed the idea of "reducing injury risk." Thus, injuries are not random events at all; rather, they occur in predictable patterns determined by identifiable risk factors. For example, if a 10-year-old boy plays unsupervised with a "toy" BB gun, which is capable of expelling projectiles at velocities much greater than those required to penetrate the eye, the resulting injury can hardly be called an accident. On the contrary, the injury is entirely predictable.

EPIDEMIOLOGY

Injuries are the leading health problem among children in the United States. About 10,000 children under the age of 15 die from injuries each year. Injuries are the leading cause of death in individuals from the ages of 1 to 44 years, and motor vehicle crash injuries alone are the leading cause of fatalities from ages 1 to 34. After motor vehicle crashes, which account for about half of unintentional deaths from injuries in children, drowning is the second leading cause of such unintentional deaths in individuals from ages 1 to 24 years, and fires and burns are the third leading cause in children up to 15

years. Falls, poisoning, aspiration, suffocation, and firearms account for most of the remaining unintentional injury deaths in children. Deaths from intentional injury, homicide, and suicide are surpassed only by motor vehicle-related injuries as a cause of pediatric injury deaths.

Several epidemiologic factors are associated with higher death rates from unintentional injuries. These include male sex, low income, family stressors (e.g., death in the family, new residence, birth of a sibling), and residence in a rural area or a southern or mountain state. Injuries vary by race; Native Americans have the highest death rate from unintentional injuries and Asian Americans the lowest. The incidence of injuries varies seasonally, with July being the peak month.

Deaths from injury are only part of the problem. For every injury-related death, 34 children are admitted to hospitals for the treatment of injury; for every injured child admitted, 30 more are treated in emergency departments. Injury is a major cause of permanent disability and is associated with much unmeasurable grief and suffering. Overall, one of every five children in the United States receives medical attention for an injury each year.

STRATEGIES FOR INJURY PREVENTION

During this century, efforts to prevent injuries have shifted from changing the behavior of individuals to modifying the environments in which injuries occur. William Haddon, a medical epidemiologist, devised two useful frameworks for developing injury prevention strategies.

Haddon Matrix

This matrix relates three factors (host, vector, and environment) to the three phases of an injury-producing event (preevent, event, and postevent). The host, vector, and environment are viewed as elements that interact over time to produce injury. Table 22–1 shows a Haddon matrix of motor vehicle crash injuries. The precrash phase describes elements that determine whether a crash will occur; the crash phase, the variables that influence the nature and severity of the resultant injury; and the postcrash phase, the factors that determine the degree to which the injury is limited and repaired after the crash occurs. By describing the "anatomy" of an injury, the Haddon matrix illustrates the numerous characteristics that determine an injury and the many corresponding strategies for interfering with the production of an injury.

TABLE 22–1. The Haddon Matrix

Phase	Host (human)	Vector (vehicle)	Environment
Precrash	Driver vision Alcohol consumption	Brakes Tires Speed	Speed limit Road curvature Road signs
Crash	Use of safety belts Osteoporosis	Vehicle size	Median barriers Laws about use of safety belts
Postcrash	Age Physical condition	Fuel system integrity	EMS personnel training

Adapted, with permission, from Haddon, W. Advances in the epidemiology of injuries as a basis for public policy. Public Health Rep. 95:411–421, 1980. Originally adapted from Baker, O'Neill, and Karpf. The Injury Fact Book. Lexington, MA, 1989, and Haddon, W. Options for the prevention of motor vehicle crash injury. Isr. J. Med. 16:45–68, 1980.

Abbreviation: EMS, emergency medical service.

Haddon also developed a list of **10 countermeasures to prevent injuries** or reduce the severity of their effects. These 10 general strategies are:

1. Prevent creation of the hazard (e.g., stop producing poisons, toys with small parts, and nonpowder firearms; do not participate in dangerous sports).

2. Reduce the amount of the hazard (e.g., package drugs in smaller, nonlethal amounts; reduce speed limits).

3. Prevent the release of the hazard (e.g., use child-resistant caps for medications, toilet locks, and safety latches on cabinets and drawers).

4. Modify the rate or spatial distribution of release of the hazard (e.g., require air bags in cars, use child safety seats and seat belts, make poisons taste bad).

5. Separate people from the hazard in space or time (e.g., make sidewalks for pedestrians, bikeways for bicyclists, and recreation areas separated from vehicles).

6. Separate people from hazards with material barriers (e.g., use bicycle helmets and protective equipment for athletes; install fences around swimming pools; build window guards).

7. Modify relevant basic qualities of the hazard (e.g., place padded carpets under cribs, require guns to have safety locks).

8. Increase resistance to damage from the hazard (e.g., train and condition athletes, make structures more earthquake-proof, use flame-retardant sleepwear).

9. Limit the damage that has already begun (e.g., use syrup of ipecac or fire extinguisher; begin cardiopulmonary resuscitation).

10. Stabilize, repair, and rehabilitate injured individuals (e.g., develop pediatric trauma centers and physical rehabilitation programs).

Haddon's work served as a practical guide for thinking about ways to prevent injury. It emphasized the importance of considering injuries as a result of a sequence of events, with many opportunities for prevention. The shift of emphasis away from changing human behavior to prevent injury is particularly appropriate with regard to injuries in children, since inhibiting children's curiosity is impractical as well as undesirable.

Passive and Active Interventions

Interventions to prevent injuries can also be categorized as passive or active. **Passive or automatic strategies** protect whenever they are needed **without the action of parents or children.** An example is the automobile air bag. In a crash, the air bag automatically inflates to cushion the occupants. Other examples of strategies that work automatically are lowered water heater temperatures, not having guns in the home, and energy-absorbing surfaces under playground equipment. In contrast, **active interventions require action to become effective.** For example, nonautomatic safety belts are active strategies; every time protection is needed, individuals must "buckle up." Watching children continuously is a another example of an injury prevention strategy that requires constant activity.

Some strategies are partially automatic, requiring some action by individuals. Smoke detectors are one example. Functional smoke detectors can be very effective in preventing injury and death in house fires. Roughly one-third of smoke detectors, however, do not have working batteries. Batteries should be changed once a year, and, ideally, tested once a month. As might be expected, the greater the effort required for children to be protected, the smaller the chance that protection occurs. Therefore, whenever possible, passive measures are preferable because they are the most effective.

Several approaches have been used successfully to prevent childhood injuries, including education, legislation, enforcement, and engineering. Often these approaches can be effectively combined, as with child safety seats. Between 1977 and 1985 every state in the United States passed child restraint laws to protect infants and children by requiring that they be in an approved safety seat when riding in a motor vehicle. The car seat, an engineering intervention, is extremely effective when used correctly. Unfortunately, studies indicate that between one-third and two-thirds of car seats are used incorrectly. Education, an important factor in the passage of the child restraint laws, as well as strict enforcement of child safety seat laws, is essential to compliance. Parents must be urged to obtain and use the seats properly. Multifaceted efforts must continue because problems still exist. For example, there are illogical loop-holes in the laws, including exemptions when feeding, changing, or rocking a child to sleep; when an automobile has an out-of-state registration; or when an automobile is driven by someone other than a parent or legal guardian. Such exemptions reinforce parental misconceptions, particularly that the lap of an occupant (the "child crusher" position) is a safe position.

COUNSELING BY PEDIATRICIANS

Although the existence of significant gaps in parental knowledge about injury prevention has been clearly established, studies have shown that pediatricians spend surprisingly little time counseling parents about childhood safety. One study found that physicians spent an average of 12.4 seconds counseling parents of

6–11-month-old infants about injury prevention; the time was even less for children in other age groups. Some of the reasons for this limited discussion of safety issues may include lack of emphasis on preventive medical care in medical schools and pediatric training programs as well as absence of solid evidence showing that anticipatory guidance works. Recent research, however, suggests that educational efforts by pediatricians can make a difference in preventing injuries, particularly if they are combined with other prevention strategies. Parents report that they would listen to physicians much more than any other group regarding child safety.

The injury prevention program (TIPP) developed by the AAP is widely used for office safety counseling. The aim of TIPP is to firmly establish injury prevention as a standard of care for pediatricians. In its 1988 policy statement on injury prevention, the AAP suggested that pediatric providers focus their safety counseling on a few topics; other topics should be discussed depending on the injury risk factors that apply to each child (e.g., age, sex, location, season of the year, socioeconomic status of family). The AAP recommends that pediatricians advise parents of all infants and preschool children about (1) car seats, (2) smoke detectors (change batteries once a year), (3) safe hot tap water temperatures (water heater set at 120° F), (4) window and stairway guards or gates to prevent falls, and (5) syrup of ipecac. For all elementary school-age children, the AAP recommends that pediatric practitioners advise all patients and their parents about (1) seat belts, (2) bicycle helmets, (3) smoke detectors, and (4) pedestrian safety.

Injury prevention has been likened to immunizations. Because all children are at risk for injury, they all need a standard package of injury prevention counseling, just as all children need the standard immunizations to protect against infectious diseases. In addition, just as extra immunizations are given to certain high-risk children (e.g., pneumococcal and meningococcal vaccines for children with sickle cell disease), children who are at high risk for injuries need more injury prevention counseling, which should focus on the injuries that are most likely to occur.

Table 22–2 shows the age-specific counseling schedule of TIPP, which indicates the minimum topics to cover at each visit. Topics are scheduled for discussion before children reach a particular developmental milestone. For example, a discussion of falls is scheduled for the two- or four-week visit before infants normally begin to roll over, and a discussion of choking is scheduled for four months before they can grasp and put things in their mouths. Specific preventive measures should be also be reinforced at each visit. Other relevant topics include infant walkers, toy safety, safety around animals, poisonous plants, and guns. Suggested topics for safety counseling for teenagers are bicycle safety and helmet use, seat belt use, firearm use, water and sports safety, drinking, drug use and driving, and depression and suicide.

Some guidelines for health care professionals to keep in mind when counseling about injury prevention in

TABLE 22–2. The Injury Prevention Program (TIPP) Safety Counseling Schedule*

Visit	Introduce	Reinforce
Prenatal/newborn	Infant car seat, smoke detector, crib safety	
2–4 wk	Falls	Car seat
2 mo	Burns—hot liquids	Car seats, falls
4 mo	Choking	Car seat, falls, burns
6 mo	Poison Burns—hot surfaces	Falls, burns
9 mo	Water safety, toddler car seat	Poison, falls, burns
1 yr	Water safety, car seat	Poison, falls, burns
15 mo	Specific to need	Poison, falls, burns
18 mo	Specific to need	Poison, falls, burns
2 yr	Play equipment, tricycles, pedestrian safety	Car seat, poison, burns
3 yr	Play equipment, tricycles, pedestrian safety	Car seat, pedestrian safety, falls, burns
4 yr	Car seat, booster or seat belt	Pedestrian safety, play equipment, burns
5 yr	Bicycle safety, pedestrian safety	Fire and car safety
6 yr	Fire safety	Bicycle, pedestrian, and car safety
8 yr	Water safety	Bicycle and car safety
10 yr	Sports safety	Bicycle and car safety

*The adolescent age group is not included in TIPP. Suggested topics for counseling adolescents include bicycle, car, water, and sports safety; firearms; drugs and driving; and depression and suicide.

Adapted, with permission, from the Committee on Accident and Poison Prevention. TIPP: The Injury Prevention Program, A Guide to Safety Counseling in Office Practice. American Academy of Pediatrics, Elk Grove Village, IL, American Academy of Pediatrics, 1989.

children include involving parents and patients in educational efforts (e.g., have a bicycle helmet in the office for children to try on). Parents and children should be given simple, practical advice rather than general information (e.g., write the poison control number on the phone, buy a bottle of syrup of ipecac, never leave children unattended in a bathtub, wear a bicycle helmet). Objectives should be well defined and finite. Safety counseling probably will not be especially effective if parents are given a long list of hazards; most people have a limited attention span and memory. Two or three topics should be discussed per visit. Whenever possible, pediatricians should coordinate their educational efforts with current injury prevention efforts (e.g., bicycle helmet campaigns, handgun regulation) in the community.

PEDIATRICIANS AS ADVOCATES

Pediatricians can play a major role in injury prevention outside of the clinical setting. As advocates for child safety, health care professionals can contribute to community efforts in injury prevention either by starting a program or by providing support to ongoing programs.

Supporting legislation and regulatory intervention in injury prevention is another powerful advocacy role for pediatricians and other health care professionals. Dramatic reductions in injuries often follow safety legislation. After the Poison Prevention Packaging Act of 1970, deaths from ingestion of aspirin decreased by 65%. The Flammable Fabrics Act of 1967, the law mandating flame-resistant children's sleepwear, and child passenger safety legislation are other examples. Pediatric practitioners can heighten awareness among policy makers of the magnitude of the injury problem in children (e.g., telephoning or writing letters to legislators, testifying about the benefits of specific safety legislation). They can initiate injury prevention legislation individually or collectively (e.g., through the AAP). Pediatricians can also direct attention to hazardous products on the market; they can help initiate changes in the design of products and enact appropriate regulations (e.g., federal crib standards of 1974 mandating close spacing of vertical slats to reduce the risk of entrapment).

in the community, and the availability of emergency ophthalmologic services. Health care professionals have the opportunity to teach injury prevention to children and their parents as well as to influence the individuals who manufacture the products and pass the laws that affect children's risk of injury.

Case Resolution

Some of the factors that influenced the injury suffered by the girl in the case history are the ease with which BB guns are purchased, the marketing of BB guns as toys, the design of the guns, the recreational activities available to children

Selected Readings

Baker, S. P., et al. *The Injury Fact Book*. New York, Oxford University Press, 1992.

Childhood injuries. Am. J. Dis. Child. 144:625–731, 1991. (Entire issue.)

Committee on Accident and Poison Prevention. *TIPP: The Injury Prevention Program, A Guide to Safety Counseling in Office Practice.* Elk Grove Village, IL, American Academy of Pediatrics, 1989.

Haddon, W. Advances in the epidemiology of injuries as a basis for public policy. Public Health Rep. 95:411–421, 1980.

National Committee for Injury Prevention and Control. Injury prevention: meeting the challenge. Am. J. Prev. Med. 5(Suppl. 1), 1989.

Widome, M. Pediatric injury prevention for the practitioner. Curr. Probl. Pediatr. 21:428–468, 1991.

Wilson, M. H., et al. *Saving Children: A Guide to Injury Prevention*. New York, Oxford University Press, 1991.

CHAPTER 23

FOSTERING SELF-ESTEEM

Monica Sifuentes, M.D.

H$_x$ A four-year-old girl is brought to the office for a physical examination for preschool. Except for an episode of bronchiolitis at eight months of age, she has been healthy. Her mother expresses concern that her daughter is shy and does not always play well with other children. She has never participated in a day-care program; she spends most of her time with her mother, grandmother, and seven-year-old sister, with whom she gets along fairly well. Both parents work outside the home, her father full-time and her mother part-time.

The girl's medical history is unremarkable. She has reached all of her developmental milestones at appropriate ages, currently speaks well in sentences, is able to dress herself without supervision, and can balance on one foot with no difficulty.

The physical examination is entirely normal. However, numerous times during the visit, the mother tells her daughter to "sit up straight," "stop fidgeting," and "act your age."

Questions

1. What is self-esteem?
2. How do parents or other caregivers affect the development of their children's self-esteem both positively and negatively?
3. What observable warning signs in parent-child relationships negatively affect normal development of self-esteem?
4. What role does discipline play in the development of self-esteem?
5. What suggestions can primary practitioners give parents and other caregivers to help foster positive self-esteem in children?

Self-esteem can be defined as how one feels about oneself. According to educator Dorothy Briggs, the development of self-respect incorporates two basic concepts: "I am lovable" and "I am worthwhile." To children, "I am lovable" implies that they are valued and deserve to be loved. "I am worthwhile" means that children have something to offer others. Self-esteem is essential to children's health and well-being and influences the development of relationships during both childhood and adulthood.

As children develop into articulate and more social human beings, their interactions with others reflect their feelings of self-worth and security. This self-image is a product of several factors: individual personality, developmental stage, familial environment, degree of parental discipline, sibling and peer interactions, and school experiences. All parents hope that their children will develop a positive self-identity that will aid them throughout their lives. Primary care practitioners should offer parents useful suggestions to ensure this outcome. What parents and other adults can do to foster children's self-esteem is an important part of anticipatory guidance that is often not considered a critical part of the health care maintenance visit. Unfortunately, discussions related to self-esteem are usually held only as a result of a crisis or an observation noted by worried parents or teachers.

Parents should understand the difference between encouragement and pressure and should be introduced to the concept of positive communication. They should also understand the complex relationship between discipline and self-esteem. Pediatricians and other allied health professionals are in a unique position to offer specific recommendations for fostering self-esteem that may have a major impact on their patients' lives. Practitioners may also act as role models for parents by fostering children's self-esteem during health maintenance visits.

SELF-ESTEEM AND GROWTH AND DEVELOPMENT

Although some experts contend that self-esteem necessitates the development of certain cognitive functions, many professionals believe that parents and other caregivers can influence children early on in infancy. Crying newborns quickly adapt to the calming influence of a maternal figure. Infants who are three to four months of age often smile at all individuals for social interaction and protest being left alone. Once infants become more verbal and develop more advanced motor skills, they begin to respond consistently to both verbal and nonverbal cues from parents (e.g., laugh with parents, follow simple commands, are taken aback by a stern voice). If parental figures are warm and loving as well as supportive and consistent, infants learn to trust and enjoy these interactions.

By the time children are toddlers, they have developed a specific relationship with their caregivers and the rest of their environment. Presumably they have learned the meaning of "no" and have been reprimanded for going beyond the limits set by caregivers in their attempts at exploration. All children, regardless of temperament, exhibit negative behaviors such as temper tantrums and selfish behavior, which elicit some type of response from parents.

Preschool children become much more independent, and they spend more time away from primary caregivers. Despite this newly acquired independence, however, they still require attention from parents and often look to them for approval. They also enjoy playing alongside other children, although not necessarily in cooperative play (e.g., helping each other in addition to playing together).

Thus, from a very early age, children's concept of self-worth and competence is established and reinforced by those around them, especially their primary caregivers. This continues into the school years, with peers and teachers eventually assuming a more influential role in the continued development and reinforcement of self-esteem.

ENCOURAGEMENT VERSUS PRESSURE

To build positive self-esteem, children need encouragement at all levels of their development (Table 23–1). This can be in the form of verbal as well as nonverbal communication and should be distinguished from overt pressure. For example, infants should be allowed to explore new surroundings at their own pace rather than being overstimulated and forced to interact in an unfamiliar environment. They should be allowed to develop at their own rate and not coaxed into activities before they are ready.

Inadvertent pressure can also be detrimental to toddlers who are not yet ready to complete certain tasks. For instance, if parents wait to begin toilet training until toddlers are ready, the likelihood of success, and therefore a positive experience, is greater. Pressuring young children to give up pacifiers or another security object before they are emotionally ready may be quite anxiety-provoking.

Well-intentioned pressure may be equally harmful later in childhood. Forcing children to participate in rigid, structured play does not foster individual creativity or independence; children are merely doing what parents have arranged. Ideally, children should be encouraged to explore and occasionally take risks. Mistakes should be acceptable and even expected under these circumstances. They should be considered learning rather than humiliating experiences. Pressuring children to do things "right" or "perfectly" discourages normal, healthy, risk-taking behavior. In addition, it interferes with future efforts by children to participate in activities unless they are certain they can succeed.

TABLE 23–1. Understanding Discouragement and Using Encouragement

How to Discourage

Have negative expectations
Focus on mistakes
Expect perfection
Overly protect children

How to Encourage

Show confidence in children's abilities
Build on children's strengths
Value children as they are
Stimulate independence

COMMUNICATION THAT BUILDS SELF-ESTEEM

Specific ways to communicate that build self-esteem include active listening, use of positive language, discarding "labels," use of encouragement rather than pressure, and the use of the "I" method of communication (Table 23–2). The purpose of active listening is to hear the child's message and understand its meaning. Parents must be attentive, stop what they are doing, and look directly at children. Nonverbal cues such as body posture and facial expression should be appreciated. If children are having trouble understanding their feelings, the parent should repeat what they hear them saying ("It sounds like . . . ").

A nonjudgmental response is warranted if children have a question or concern. The basic message should be simple, clear, and directed specifically at the child. Words should be easily understood and spoken in a moderate tone, especially when discipline is necessary. Facial expression and body language should also be consistent with the message parents or caregivers are trying to convey.

Positive language should be used at all times, even when disciplining children. For instance, when children are playing kick ball in the house, most parents initially reprimand children by yelling, "Don't play ball in the house!" or "Haven't I told you before? No ball playing inside!" Instead of prefacing each sentence with "don't" or "no," parents or other adults should tell children what they can do, what the limits are, and the reason for these rules. For example, caregivers should say: "You may kick the ball outside in the backyard. If you kick it inside, you may break a window or hurt yourself or someone else." Communicating in this manner prevents normally active children from feeling as if they are always being reprimanded.

"Labels" such as "good" or "bad" should be avoided. If children repeatedly hear themselves referred to as "dumb-dumb" or "turkey," they begin to believe these phrases, no matter how innocuous they may initially seem to parents. Seemingly complimentary labels such as "smart" or "bright" may also create undue anxiety for children who then try to live up to these expectations continuously.

Parents should praise their children for successes and achievements. Failures should be minimized whenever possible, although the acknowledgment of mistakes can be important. For example, correcting a child's homework assignment for errors should be done in a nonthreatening manner. Parents should involve the child in the review process rather than simply marking up the paper with a red pen and telling the child to redo the assignment.

In addition, talents and abilities should be recognized and highlighted. Children should know that parents have confidence in their abilities and that any display of effort is appreciated. Small successes should be valued as much as large ones, no matter how seemingly insignificant they may be at the time. Parents and other caregivers should keep in mind that although extra positive reinforcement is never detrimental to children's self-esteem, lack of encouragement can hurt their self-image.

Many parenting courses teach primary caregivers to use the "I" method of communication, which requires that parents explain their feelings to children rather than blame them for their actions. This approach is believed to be less threatening and demeaning for children, especially in situations requiring discipline. The "I" method has four recommended steps:

1. Statement of behavior or situation to be addressed (e.g., "When you . . . ").
2. Statement in specific terms how one feels about the effect of the situation on oneself (e.g., "I feel . . . ").
3. Statement of reason (e.g., "because . . . ").
4. Statement of expectations (e.g., "I would like . . ." or "I want . . . ").

Using this approach, a parent's statement might be: "When you bite me, I feel pain because it hurts a lot. I would like you to please tell me what makes you angry instead of biting me."

DISCIPLINE AND SELF-ESTEEM

Ideally, parents or other adults should feel good about disciplining their children. Two general principles of discipline are to teach by example and to state expectations. Several different approaches to discipline have been adapted by various ethnic, cultural, religious, and socioeconomic groups. A discussion of each of these methods is beyond the scope of this chapter (see Chapter 27, Discipline). Parents and other caregivers should remember that certain methods of discipline can be very destructive to children's self-esteem. For instance, making an enuretic child "wear" the wet bedsheets or reprimanding a child with physical punishment (e.g., spanking) in public places can be demeaning.

TABLE 23–2. Communication That Builds Self-Esteem

Active listening
Use of positive language
Discarding "labels"
Use of encouragement
Use of the "I" method of communication

Case Resolution

In the case history the health maintenance visit is a good opportunity for fostering the child's self-esteem. The health care provider can begin by reassuring the girl and her mother that the child's overall health and development are normal. The shy child should be approached by inviting her to tell you some things about herself (e.g., "What do you like to do for fun?," "What is your favorite color?") and giving her some sincere general compliments (e.g., "What a pretty dress you are wearing!," "You have very pretty eyes"). The hope is that this approach will be repeated by the parent at home. In addition, the practitioner should offer concrete suggestions to the parent for positive communication, such as avoiding "don't" and "no" phrases.

Parents should be encouraged to think about the child's temperament when considering involvement in multiple school activities.

Selected Readings

Berman, B. D., et al. After-school child care and self-esteem in school-age children. Pediatrics 89:654–659, 1992.

Briggs, D. C. *Your Child's Self-Esteem*. New York, Doubleday, 1970.

Brooks, R. B. Self-esteem during the school years: its normal development and hazardous decline. Pediatr. Clin. North Am. 39:537–550, 1992.

Howard, B. J. Discipline in early childhood. Pediatr. Clin. North Am. 38:1351–1369, 1991.

Schmitt, B. D. Time-out: intervention of choice for the irrational years. Contemp. Pediatr. 10:64–87, 1993.

Sieving, R. E., and S. T. Zirbel-Donish. Development and enhancement of self-esteem in children. J. Pediatr. Health Care 4:290–296, 1990.

CHAPTER 24

SIBLING RIVALRY

Carol D. Berkowitz, M.D.

H$_x$ An eight-year-old boy is brought to the office for an annual checkup. During the course of the evaluation, his mother complains that her son and his six-year-old sister are always fighting. She says her son hits his sister and pulls her hair, and nothing she does prevents them from fighting. The boy is a B+ student and has no behavior problems in school. The past medical history and the physical examination are completely normal.

Questions

1. What is sibling rivalry?
2. What is the physician's role in counseling a family about sibling rivalry?
3. What is the role of anticipatory guidance in preparing older children for the birth of a new sister or brother?

Sibling rivalry refers to the rivalry between siblings based on the need for parental love and esteem. Historical examples of sibling rivalry include relationships between the biblical figures Cain and Abel, Joseph and his brothers, and Jacob and Esau. Sibling rivalry is also noteworthy in pairs of celebrities, such as actress Joan Fontaine and Olivia de Havilland.

Sibling rivalry, a universal phenomenon, results from a fear of displacement, dethronement, and loss of love that occurs with the birth of a new brother or sister. Older children fear they are not good enough and need to be replaced. Such feelings lead to a fear of abandonment. Jealousy also plays a role, and older children may be angry at younger siblings for displacing them within the family.

Sibling rivalry frequently has a negative effect on parents because it is hard for them to see one of their children hurt, even if it is by a sister or a brother. The challenge for parents is to know when and when not to intervene and what strategies to use to minimize conflicts. Physicians can help by offering anticipatory guidance to all parents and specific recommendations to parents with individual problems.

EPIDEMIOLOGY

Sibling rivalry is a universal phenomenon, and a number of factors influence its development. Time interval between children affects the degree of rivalry. Close spacing results in more problems, particularly when the children are less than two years apart. In such situations, older children still have dependency needs, often feel less secure, and experience a need for maternal attention. They stay closer to mothers, are less playful, and more tense. Closely spaced children engage in less spontaneous play, appear more angry, and issue sterner commands to their playmates.

Position in the family also influences sibling rivalry. Middle children experience what is referred to as "middle child syndrome;" they lack the prestige of older children or the privileges of younger ones. These children are often least secure and strive hardest to gain affection. Special difficulties may develop if middle children are the same sex as older ones. Middle children grow up to be flexible, adaptable, and good negotiators. In myths and folklore, youngest children are "favorites." They are often the ones defended by parents when there are bouts of fighting.

Twins rarely present a problem of sibling rivalry; instead they have a problem maintaining their individuality. However, sets of twins create problems for older siblings because they are not as unique as the pair of twins.

Step siblings also present a unique problem in sibling rivalry. Children of divorce frequently feel abandoned by one parent and in competition for the time and love of the custodial parent (see Chapter 102, Divorce). Competition with step siblings is especially difficult if the step siblings are in the same home.

CLINICAL PRESENTATION

Parental complaints related to sibling rivalry consist of fighting between siblings, including physical violence and verbal abuse; bickering; and regression to immature behavioral patterns. Although such immature behavior occurs most often following the birth of a new baby, it may also be apparent if one sibling is receiving more attention, such as during an illness or after a major accomplishment. Regressive behavior includes bed-wetting, drinking from a bottle, and wanting to be carried to bed. Substitution behavior, such as nail biting, in place of biting the new sibling, may occur after the birth of a new baby.

Before the birth of a new baby, parents may complain that their children exhibit temper tantrums, irritability, and solemnness. They may mimic the pregnancy by eating a lot and putting a pillow under their clothes. In addition, children may have psychosomatic complaints such as stomach aches or headaches.

DIFFERENTIAL DIAGNOSIS

Dilemmas concerning the correct diagnosis of sibling rivalry most often relate to the appearance of behavioral changes such as regressive or aggressive patterns after birth of a new sibling. For example, a child who was previously toilet-trained may become incontinent of urine. Although UTI may be considered in the diagnosis, a careful history concerning the birth of the sibling reveals the correct etiology.

EVALUATION

The evaluation of children with suspected sibling rivalry involves a history of the problem and parental strategies for dealing with the difficulties. The parent should be particularly queried about one-on-one opportunities between parents and individual children. The physical examination and laboratory assessment are noncontributory.

MANAGEMENT

The focus of management is to allow the parents to recognize the normalcy of sibling rivalry while helping them define the behaviors that are acceptable and not acceptable within the family context. Parents may not appreciate their child's fear of loss of parental love. They should be told that many children think, "If I am so good, why do I have to be replaced?" Physicians can also help parents deal with sibling rivalry by having them consider their treatment of children in terms of

uniformity versus uniqueness and quality versus inequality.

Birth of New Siblings

Parents may notice the behavioral changes in their children before the birth of the new sibling. These changes depend on the age of the children and the presence of other siblings. Children should be told about the upcoming birth. The timing depends on the children's age; younger children do not need much lead time. Some studies have evaluated the inclusion of older children in the birthing process. The results of these studies vary, but they suggest that children under the age of four need their mother for emotional support and are concerned about her physical exertion during the birthing process. Some older children may also want to distance themselves from the actual events.

Physicians should suggest that older children be involved in planning for the arrival of the new baby as a means of minimizing their feelings of exclusion. For example, they can help purchase clothes or prepare the baby's room. Physicians should also suggest that parents purchase a gift for older children that represents a present from the new baby. In addition, older siblings may be given a doll to serve as a baby they can care for. Parents should point out the advantages of being older with comments such as, "You can stay up later" or "You can walk and play with all these toys." Frequently, the birth of a new baby is met with regressive behavior in older siblings. Regressive behavior should be handled with tolerance and a realization that symptoms resolve with time.

Once the mother goes to the hospital, she should be advised to maintain contact with older children by writing or telephoning. At present, hospital stays are so brief that this period of separation is much shorter than previously. Household changes that may be necessitated by the birth of the new baby, such as room changes, the substitution of a bed for a crib, and entrance into nursery school, should be made before the arrival of the new baby.

Rivalry Between Older Children

Physicians need to consider individual parenting techniques when counseling parents of older children. Parents who compare one child to the other may foster contentious behavior, and those who strive to treat all children equally may inadvertently perpetuate rivalry. Children need to feel that they are unique rather than ordinary. For example, parents who buy both children the same presents may think they are preventing rivalry from developing, but they are actually depriving each child of a sense of uniqueness. The harder parents try to be uniform, the more vigilantly the children may look for inequality. Each child needs a parent's undivided attention, time alone together. The more agreeable a parent-child relationship, the more agreeable a sibling-sibling relationship, because each child has good self-esteem. Practitioners should rec-

TABLE 24–1.   Clues for Parents for Coping With Rivalry Between Siblings

Do
Allow children to vent negative feelings
Encourage children to develop solutions
Anticipate problem situations
Foster individuality in each child
Spend time with children individually
Compliment children when they are playing together
Tell children about the conflicts you had with your siblings when you were children
Define acceptable and unacceptable behavior

Don't
Take sides
Serve as a referee
Foster rivalry
Use derogatory names
Permit physical or verbal abuse between siblings

ommend uniqueness and quality in each parent-child relationship.

Parents sometimes have to deal with sibling rivalry between older children. Physicians should reassure parents that these older children should be allowed to vent their negative feelings toward each other. For example, if a girl refers to her brother by saying "I hate him," the parents should respond by validating these emotions and saying something like, "It sounds as if he's done something to really annoy you." Parents should also be advised not to take sides. They should examine how they usually respond to squabbling between siblings. Is one child's name always called first during a fight? Do they perpetuate sibling rivalry by using certain nicknames (e.g., "turkey brain") or other derogatory terms? Parents should assume that both parties are at least partially guilty and should not allow themselves to be drawn into the fight as referees. Parents can respond to a request for arbitration with a statement such as, "I wasn't here when things started, so I don't know who is right or wrong." The parents should also advise siblings

that they do not have to be friends with one another, but they should not hurt each other's feelings.

Anticipatory guidance helps parents anticipate conflictual situations such as long car rides and who sits where. Children should be allowed to work out a solution by themselves, with the stipulation that the parents will solve the problem if the children do not reach an agreement. Table 24–1 lists suggestions for parents who are seeking advice about fighting between children.

PROGNOSIS

Although sibling rivalry may last for years, most siblings become good friends as adults.

Case Resolution

In the case history presented at the beginning of the chapter, the mother should be advised not to serve as a referee. She should learn how to validate each child's feelings about the other. The physician can help her by talking to her son about his feelings. She should be advised to have a discussion with her children during which each child has the opportunity to define areas of conflict and the means to resolve them.

Selected Readings

Dunn, J. Annotation: sibling influences on childhood development. J. Child. Psychol. Psychiatry 29:119–127, 1988.
Hass, E., and P. Light. Talking about the new baby. Parents Magazine 58:68–70, October 1983.
Leung, A. K., and W. L. Robson. Sibling rivalry. Clin. Pediatr. 30:314, 1991.
Pakula, L. C. Sibling rivalry. Pediatr. Rev. 13:72–73, 1992.
Samalin, N., and P. McCormick. How to cure sibling fights. Parents Magazine 68:147–150, May 1993.
Schmitt, B. D. Sibling rivalry toward a new baby. Contemp. Pediatr. 7:111–112, 1990.
Schmitt, B. D. When siblings quarrel. Contemp. Pediatr. 8:73–74, 1991.

CHAPTER 25

TOILET TRAINING

Carol D. Berkowitz, M.D.

Hx   A two-year-old boy is brought to the office for a well child visit. His mother, who is about to begin toilet training her son, asks your advice. The mother says that by the time her daughter was two, she was already toilet trained, and

she wants to know if training her son will be any different. The boy was the product of a full-term pregnancy and a normal delivery. He has been in good health, and his immunizations are up to date. He is developmentally normal, has a 30-word vocabulary, and has been walking since the age of 13 months. His physical examination is normal.

Questions

1. When should physicians begin discussing toilet training with parents?
2. What factors help determine children's readiness to begin toilet training?
3. Is toilet training in boys different from toilet training in girls?
4. What are some of the methods used to toilet train children?

The age at which toilet training is carried out is culturally determined. Some cultures train children at a very early age. For example, in the East African Digo culture, some children between two and three months of age are conditioned to urinate or defecate when placed in certain positions. Similar conditioning practices are carried out in China. Chinese children are kept without diapers, and when caregivers who are holding them sense a change in their bodies in response to a need to eliminate, they place their children in an appropriate position. In addition, children are dressed in clothing that facilitates toileting. "Split pants," with the back and bottom portion missing, are used so that children can squat and eliminate without removing complicated clothing.

American culture has emphasized the learning aspects of toilet training as opposed to the conditioning aspects. This training focuses on the cognitive development of children and children's readiness to learn the complexity of the task.

Toilet training is potentially both a rewarding and frustrating experience for children and parents. Parents may have unrealistic expectations of children's capability or may be very intolerant of normal accidents that occur in the training process. It is important for physicians to introduce the topic of toilet training early on to prevent these unrealistic expectations. Children's refusal to toilet train is the second most common precipitant of fatal child abuse. It is recommended that the issue of toilet training be introduced and anticipatory guidance provided by the age of nine months.

EPIDEMIOLOGY

The age at which children are toilet trained varies depending on social considerations and social pressures. Prior to the 1920s, the American approach to toilet training was permissive. This attitude then changed, and the methods became more rigorous, requiring that children be trained at an earlier age. In 1947, only 5% of children were not trained by 33 months of age, but by 1975, this figure had increased to 42%.

As a general rule, girls are trained a bit earlier than boys. The large majority of children (80%) are trained simultaneously for bladder and bowel control. Approximately 12% are trained first for bowel control and about 8% for bladder control. Girls achieve nighttime continence at a younger age than boys.

PATHOPHYSIOLOGY

Toilet training involves the ability both to inhibit a normal reflex release action and then relax the inhibition of the involved muscles. For the process to be successful, a certain degree of neurologic and biologic development is essential. Myelinization of the pyramidal tracts and conditioned reflex sphincter control are necessary. Voluntary control is evidenced by myelinization of the pyramidal tracts by the age of 12 to 18 months. Conditioned reflex sphincter control occurs by nine months of age and voluntary cooperation between 12 and 15 months. In assessing the neurologic development of children, walking is viewed as one of the milestones that indicate motor readiness for toilet training.

Toilet training depends on both physiologic and psychological readiness. Cognitive development is assessed by children's ability to follow certain instructions.

Two years of age has been suggested as the appropriate age to initiate toilet training. As a rule, parents of clinic patients expect that their children will learn at an earlier age. Toilet training usually takes two weeks to two months to learn.

DIFFERENTIAL DIAGNOSIS

The differential diagnosis focuses on factors that contribute to a delay in acquisition of skills. Physicians should look for associated symptoms, such as dysuria, a weak urinary stream, constantly wet underwear, or fecal soiling, when assessing children who continue to manifest signs of either urinary or stool incontinence. In addition, it is important to determine if children are essentially toilet trained but are having intermittent accidents.

The most common cause of isolated daytime wetting in previously trained children is **UTI** (see Chapter 32, Enuresis). **Chemical urethritis** may also be associated with urinary incontinence. **Stress incontinence,** which has also been called giggle incontinence, may result in wetting. **Urgency incontinence** occurs when children delay going to the bathroom and then are unable to hold urine any longer. Some children have ectopic ureters, which can empty into the lower portion of the bladder, vagina, or urethra and cause a constant dribble of urine. **Labial fusion** may also be associated with daytime wetting. Urine pools behind the fused labia during voiding, and when children stand up, the urine exits. Children with **neurogenic bladders** may also have symptoms of daytime wetting.

Stooling accidents may be associated with chronic constipation and overflow incontinence or with Hirschsprung's disease. (See Chapter 33, Encopresis.)

EVALUATION

History, Behavioral Assessment, and Physical Examination

Toddlers who appear normal should be assessed for both their physiologic and psychological readiness to undertake this task. Physicians should provide anticipatory guidance to parents about toileting readiness. Affirmative answers should be obtained to the following three questions:

1. Do children exhibit bladder control as evidenced by (1) periods of dryness that last up to two hours and (2) facial expressions that show their physiologic response to the elimination process?
2. Do children have the motor skills necessary to get around? This essentially involves the children's ability to walk and remove their clothing.
3. Do children have the cognitive ability to understand the task at hand?

Cognitive ability can be assessed by giving children ten tasks to carry out and seeing if they are able to carry out at least eight of the ten tasks (Table 25–1).

Children who have had difficulties with toilet training need to undergo a similar assessment. In addition, a physical examination to rule out underlying problems such as spina bifida occulta, which may be associated with a neurogenic bladder, should be performed. A careful examination of the genitalia is important in children who are having urinary incontinence to determine if conditions such as labial fusion are evident. In children who are having stooling problems, physicians should check for an abdomen with feces-filled intestines, a sign of obstipation. In addition, a rectal examination should be performed to determine the presence of hard or impacted stools or any other abnormalities in the anal area.

Laboratory Tests

Although a laboratory assessment is not indicated in normal toddlers who are being toilet trained, diagnostic studies may be appropriate in children who are having problems with training. In older children, urinalysis may show evidence of a UTI.

TABLE 25–1.   Requests or Imperatives Used to Help Assess Toilet Training Readiness

Bring me the ball
Go to the door
Sit on the chair
Pick up the doll
Open the door
Give the pen to your Mom
Put the ball on the table
Put the doll on the floor
Take off your shoes
Open the book

MANAGEMENT

Physicians should help parents understand the appropriate approach to the toilet training process. Unfortunately, most parents do not obtain the necessary advice from physicians. In one report, no parents attending a clinic and only 7% of patients in a private practice received advice about toilet training from their physicians. Therefore, it is important for physicians to initiate the discussion early enough to prevent the development of any problems. Emphasis on the use of **rewards,** not punishments, is essential.

When toilet training children, parents should be advised to take the following approach:

1. Teach children the **appropriate vocabulary** related to the toilet training process. This could include words such as "pee," "poop," "dry," "wet," "clean," "messy," and "potty."
2. Tell children what the **purpose of the potty** is. In general, a child potty chair should be purchased. The potty chair has a number of advantages over the toilet. Children can sit on the potty and have their feet on the floor, which is more physiologically sound and gives them a greater sense of security.

Parents can encourage children to decorate the potty and put their names on it. The potty should be kept in a place where children spend a lot of time, such as the kitchen. Children should be allowed to sit on the potty with their clothes on for about a week before the process of toilet training begins. Then children should sit on the potty without their clothes on, but no attempt to catch either stool or urine should be made.

3. Encourage cleanliness and dryness by **changing children frequently.** Parents should ask their children whether they need to be changed using the appropriate vocabulary. This phase is important to continue as the toilet training process proceeds. Some parents mistakenly do not change their soiled children as a means of punishing them for having accidents. This gives children a confusing message about the need for cleanliness.

4. Explain the **connection between dry pants and going to the potty** to children. Children should understand that dry pants feel good and that they can keep their pants dry by going to the potty.

5. Help children understand the **physiologic signals** for using the toilet. Parents can facilitate this by observing children's behavior around the time of elimination and making comments such as, "When you jump up and down like that, Mommy knows you have to go to the bathroom."

6. Children must have the physiologic ability to postpone the "urge to go." This usually occurs when children have the ability to delay voiding for at least two hours. Parents then can initiate toilet training by taking children to the bathroom at two-hour intervals. In addition, children should sit on the toilet immediately after naps and 20 minutes after meals. Children should not be left on the toilet for more than five minutes and should be permitted to get up if they want. While sitting

on the potty, they can be entertained with reading a story or playing games.

Additional suggestions involve allowing children to have their clothes off and keep the potty chair near them during play. This facilitates using the potty and is reminiscent of the practice of using split pants in China.

Children who use the potty successfully should be rewarded. Rewards can be in the form of verbal comments such as "Mommy is so proud of you," hand clapping, or the use of candy, cookies, or star charts. Children can be consulted about what rewards they like. Punishment should not be used, particularly physical punishment. One report indicates that 15% of parents of clinic patients believe that spanking their children for accidents is acceptable. Parental disapproval of accidents can be articulated; however, parents should understand that accidents may continue to occur for months.

If children are trained on a potty chair, they can generally begin using a toilet between 2½ and 3½ years of age. Children can also use training pants, which are thickened underwear, or pull-ups, which are diaperlike underwear, rather than diapers.

If children demonstrate resistance to toilet training, the process should be delayed for one to two months. It is important for parents to avoid an aggressiveness-resistance struggle, because this then may become the source of future bowel problems, including constipation. Children who are regular, particularly those who have a bowel movement at the same time every day, are more easily toilet trained. Some children appear fearful of certain aspects of the toilet training process. These include fear of falling into the toilet (this is circumvented with the use of a potty) or fear of the loud noise of the flush. Allowing the child to flush the toilet without using it may dispel the fear. Some children become fascinated with flushing or rolling toilet paper, and parents have to prevent children from wasting water or paper.

One of the major components of toilet training children is **modeling.** Children should be allowed to enter the bathroom with the parents and even sit on the potty as one or the other parent sits on the toilet. Some children are very strong willed and independent. Strong-willed children, coupled with perfectionist parents, may have problems with toilet training.

Special considerations have to be made for children attending day care. Their teachers should be advised about the toilet training. Children should have "open bathroom privileges," which means that they should be permitted to leave the room to go to the bathroom without raising their hands or other reminders.

Medications have a limited role in toilet training. Some physicians recommend the use of drugs to increase bladder capacity. Although oxybutynin (Ditropan) increases bladder capacity and decreases the frequency of bladder contraction, it should not be used because it does not actually assist children with the toilet training process. However, children who are constipated may require stool softeners such as mineral oil or the addition of fiber bulk to their diet to facilitate the stooling process. Physicians should see children who appear to have toilet training problems on a weekly or biweekly basis until they show improvement. Parents can also be referred to the many books on toilet training, particularly if problems develop.

PROGNOSIS

All normal children are eventually toilet trained. The age when this occurs varies and is significant only if it restricts children from participating in school.

Case Resolution

The mother in the case history should be advised that this is a good time to initiate the toilet training process. She should be told that boys, as a group, are successfully toilet trained at a later age than girls. Her son can be assessed to see if he can follow at least eight out of ten instructions (see Table 25–1). If he can, the mother should be given the stepwise approach to initiating the toilet training process.

Selected Readings

Azrin, N. H., and R. M. Foxx. *Toilet Training in Less Than a Day*. New York, Simon & Schuster, 1974.

Christophersen, E. R. Toileting problems in children. Pediatr. Ann. 20:240–244, 1991.

Howe, A. C., and C. E. Walker. Behavioral management of toilet training, enuresis, and encopresis. Pediatr. Clin. North Am. 39:413–432, 1992.

Schmitt, B. D. Toilet training refusal: avoid the battle and win the war. Contemp. Pediatr. 3:32–50, 1987.

Schmitt, B. D. Toilet training without tears. Contemp. Pediatr. 8:47–49, 1992.

CHAPTER 26

CRYING AND COLIC

Geeta Grover, M.D.

H$_x$ The parents of a two-week-old infant bring their son to the emergency department because he has been crying persistently for the past four hours. He has no history of fever, vomiting, diarrhea, upper respiratory tract infection, or change in feeding. The infant is breast fed.

On physical examination, the infant appears well developed and well nourished. His weight is 7 lb, 7 oz—seven ounces more than when he was born. Although he is fussy and crying, he is afebrile with normal vital signs. The remainder of the physical examination is within normal limits.

Questions

1. What is the normal crying pattern in young infants?
2. What is colic?
3. What conditions are associated with prolonged crying in young infants?
4. What are key factors in the history of crying infants?
5. What laboratory tests are indicated in crying infants?
6. List a few of the management strategies that can be used by parents to soothe their crying or colicky infants.

EPIDEMIOLOGY

Qualitatively, **excessive crying** is any amount of crying that concerns or worries parents. Quantitatively, definitions of excessive crying have been based on the results of Brazelton's study of normal infants. This study found that the median daily crying time at two weeks of age is 1¾ hours; this time increases to a peak of 2¾ hours at six weeks of age and then decreases to less than one hour by 12 weeks. Apparently, more crying occurs during the evening hours, especially between the ages of three and six weeks.

Colic affects 10 to 20% of infants less than three months of age. It usually begins in the first few weeks of life. Colic is more specifically defined as crying that lasts for at least three hours per day for at least three days per week; episodes typically begin during the first three weeks of life and improve by three months. This definition is commonly referred to as the rule of threes.

CLINICAL PRESENTATION

Colicky infants are typically otherwise healthy infants under three months of age who cry or fuss inconsolably for extended periods of time, usually during the after-

Crying, an important method of communication between infants and caregivers, is nonspecific, and many stimuli can produce the same response (e.g., hunger, fatigue, pain). Parents report that they can discriminate among various types of cries in their infants. Crying can be divided into three categories: (1) normal or physiologic crying, (2) excessive crying secondary to distress (e.g., hunger) or disease, and (3) excessive crying without an apparent cause.

The difference between normal and excessive crying may be more qualitative than quantitative. Deciding whether crying is excessive varies with parents' expectations and thresholds. Expressed parental concern about extreme crying or fussiness requires attention. If parents complain that infants cry inconsolably or continuously as well as excessively, the crying may have an underlying organic etiology.

Colic, a poorly understood, benign, self-limited condition, falls into the third category. It manifests as unexplained crying or fussing in infants that usually occurs in the late afternoon or evening. During an episode of colic, infants cry and may either draw the knees up to the chest or rigidly stiffen the legs, flex the elbows, clench the fists, and turn red (Fig. 26–1).

FIGURE 26–1. *Colicky infant.*

noon or evening. The crying usually resolves within a few hours.

PATHOPHYSIOLOGY

Crying is a complex vocalization that changes during the first year of life as infants develop. In the first few weeks of life, crying is a signal that infants are experiencing a disturbance in homeostatic regulation (e.g., hunger, discomfort). As infants mature and begin to differentiate internal from external stimuli, crying may also be an indication of too little or too much environmental stimulation. During the second half of the first year, as infants mature neurologically and gain voluntary control over vocalizations, crying can be an expression of different affects (e.g., frustration, fear).

A variety of explanations for the etiology of **colic** have been proposed. Some authorities believe that colic may not be a pathologic entity but simply an extreme variant of normal crying. The condition may result from an allergy, cow's milk intolerance, abnormal intestinal peristalsis, or increased intestinal gas, which are some of the more frequently associated factors. Others have proposed that colic is caused by problems in the interaction between infants and their environment, specifically their parents. This interactional theory requires not only excessive crying on the part of the infant, but also an inability of the parents to soothe the crying infant. Whether maternal anxiety has any role in colic remains a controversial issue. More than one of these factors may contribute to the pathogenesis of colic.

DIFFERENTIAL DIAGNOSIS

An acute episode of excessive crying may be secondary to disease (e.g., fever, otitis media). An organic etiology should be suspected in infants who present with inconsolable crying of acute onset. Table 26–1 lists the most common causes. Some conditions occur in a more chronic or recurrent pattern, particularly if the condition is not treated.

The differential diagnosis of infants who experience recurrent episodes of excessive crying focuses more on behavior and temperament. Colic, persistent night awakening, difficult infant temperament (i.e., extreme fussiness, neonatal drug withdrawal) may cause recurrent crying. Persistent night awakening and difficult infant temperament are discussed in Chapter 12, Sleep, and Chapter 28, Temper Tantrums, respectively.

EVALUATION

A thorough history and physical examination usually provides clues to the diagnosis in instances of acute onset of crying.

History

The focus of the history should be on determining the presence of any associated symptoms. In addition, the circumstances surrounding the crying (e.g., oc-

TABLE 26–1. Most Common Causes of Acute Unexplained, Excessive Crying in Infants

Idiopathic*
Colic*
Infectious
  Otitis media
  Urinary tract infection
  Stomatitis
  Meningitis
Gastrointestinal*
  Constipation
  Gaseous distention
  Peristalsis problems
  Reflux
  Intussusception
Trauma
  Corneal abrasion
  Foreign body in the eye
  Hair tourniquet syndrome
Behavioral*
  Overstimulation
  Persistent night awakening
Drug Reactions
  Immunization reactions (most common: diphtheria-tetanus-pertussis vaccine)
  Neonatal drug withdrawal (narcotics)
Child Abuse
  Long bone fractures
  Retinal hemorrhage
  Intracranial hemorrhage
Hematologic*
  Sickle cell crisis
Cardiovascular
  Arrhythmia (supraventricular tachycardia)
  Congestive heart failure

*May present as acute or recurrent episodes of excessive crying.

currence during day or night) should be ascertained (Questions Box).

Physical Examination

A thorough physical examination is required for accurate diagnosis. Particular attention should be given to the following aspects of the examination:

1. Careful inspection of the skin after all clothing has been removed to look for any suspicious bruises or marks.
2. Palpation of all long bones to detect fractures.
3. Examination of all digits to check for "hair tourniquets" (single strands of hair wrapped around digits).
4. Examination of the retina to look for retinal hemorrhages (a sign of intracranial hemorrhage).

Questions: Crying and Colic

- Is this the first time the infant has cried inconsolably or does this happen on a recurring basis?
- Has the infant had a fever?
- Does the infant have any cold symptoms, vomiting, or diarrhea?
- Is the infant having any difficulty feeding? Is the infant formula- or breast-fed?
- Has the infant had a recent fall or accident?

5. Eversion of the eyelids to check for foreign bodies.

6. Fluorescein staining of the cornea to look for corneal abrasion.

Laboratory Tests

Except for urinalysis, most screening laboratory tests are probably not useful. Test selection can be guided by the history and physical examination (e.g., infants with fever without an apparent cause should have a septic workup, with an examination of blood, urine, and CSF). Urinalysis, which may provide clues to an underlying metabolic deficiency, is sometimes helpful. Even when the initial history and physical examination are nondiagnostic, infants who persist in crying inconsolably should be suspected of having a serious underlying condition (e.g., intracranial hemorrhage, drug ingestion). Such infants may warrant an extended period of observation or a more extensive workup that includes laboratory assessment.

Imaging Studies

Roentgenographic studies such as long bone x-rays may be necessary in some situations (e.g., infants with long bone pain on palpation, suspicion of child abuse). Infants with retinal hemorrhages should have a CT scan.

MANAGEMENT

Management and treatment depends on identification of the cause of the crying. Underlying organic conditions (e.g., UTI, fractures) should be treated. Management of colic depends on presumptions regarding its etiology. It is important for practitioners to reassure parents regarding the benign nature of colic and its resolution over time. Physicians should provide a caring and supportive environment in which the parents may express their concerns and frustrations. Reassurance along with practical suggestions regarding infant feeding and handling techniques (e.g., cuddling, swaddling, or rocking) may often suffice.

Management suggestions for colic should be customized for infants and families. The more common management techniques are listed in Table 26–2.

Changes in sensory input (e.g., soothing sounds or motions) may resolve crying and soothe colicky infants.

Prophylactic measures to prevent the passage of swallowed air through the pylorus can also be useful. Such techniques include feeding in an upright position and limiting the period of sucking at the breast or bottle to about 10 minutes (after this time, greater amounts of air are swallowed relative to the amount of milk ingested).

Methods to decrease intestinal spasm (e.g., abdominal massage, warm baths, avoidance of overfeeding) may be helpful. The use of suppositories or rectal thermometers to break up rectal spasm and thereby release retained gas should be discouraged.

Formula changes to eliminate possible allergens should be reserved for those infants with additional symptoms of allergy (e.g., wheezing, rash) or intolerance (e.g., vomiting, diarrhea, hematochezia, or weight loss).

Various drugs, including anticholinergics, motility-enhancing agents, barbiturates, laxatives, and antiflatulents, have limited success and are best avoided. Currently, antiflatulents (e.g., simethicone) are prescribed most commonly. Despite lack of scientific evidence to support their efficacy, parents indicate that they are effective.

As long as no adverse effects are evident, **folk remedies** (e.g., chamomile tea) can be supported if parents report satisfaction.

PROGNOSIS

Fortunately, the natural history of persistent crying during infancy is resolution over time. To date, no long-term sequelae of infantile colic have been identified except for a possible relationship with irritable bowel syndrome in childhood.

TABLE 26–2. Suggestions for the Management of Colic*

Parental reassurance
Alteration in techniques of infant feeding and handling
Alteration of sensory input to infant
Prevention of swallowed air from passing through pylorus
Dietary alterations
Medication
Folk remedies

*See text for further details.

Case Resolution

The infant described in the case history is experiencing an acute episode of unexplained crying. Despite a normal physical examination, he was observed for one hour in the emergency department because his crying persisted. Subsequently a septic workup was initiated, which revealed that a UTI was the source of the irritability.

Selected Readings

Barr, R. G. The normal crying curve: what do we really know? Dev. Med. Child Neurol. 32:356–362, 1990.

Brazelton, T. B. Crying in infancy. Pediatrics 29:579–588, 1962.

Carey, W. B. "Colic"—Primary excessive crying as an infant—environment interaction. Pediatr. Clin. North Am. 31:993–1005, 1984.

Hewson, P., F. Oberklaid, and S. Menahem. Infant colic, distress and crying. Clin. Pediatr. 26:69–75, 1987.

Metcalf, T. J., et al. Simethicone in the treatment of infant colic: a randomized, placebo-controlled, multicenter trial. Pediatrics 94:29–34, 1994.

Miller, A. R., and R. G. Barr. Infantile colic: is it a gut issue? Pediatr. Clin. North Am. 38:1407–1423, 1991.

Parkin, P. C., C. J. Schwartz, and B. A. Manuel. Randomized, controlled trial of three interventions in the management of persistent crying of infancy. Pediatrics 92:197–201, 1993.

Poole, S. R. The infant with acute, unexplained excessive crying. Pediatrics 88:450–455, 1992.

Taubman, B. A new answer to the old question of colic. Contemp. Pediatr. 8:44–63, 1991.

CHAPTER 27

DISCIPLINE

Carol D. Berkowitz, M.D.

H$_x$ A three-year-old boy is being threatened with expulsion from preschool because he is biting the other children. His mother states that he is very active and aggressive toward other children. In addition, his language development is delayed. She is at her wits end about what to do. The birth history is normal, and the mother denies the use of drugs or cigarettes, but she drank socially before she realized she was pregnant. The past medical and family histories are noncontributory, and the physical examination is normal.

Questions

1. What is the definition of discipline?
2. What strategies can parents use to discipline children?
3. What are the guidelines for using "time out"?
4. What is the relationship between corporal punishment and child abuse?

Discipline can be defined as an educational process in which children learn how to behave in a socially acceptable manner. It involves a complex set of interactions of attitudes, models, instructions, rewards, and punishments. Discipline is not synonymous with corporal punishment. The goal is to help children gain self-control and respect for others and to learn behavior that is appropriate for given situations.

PHYSICIAN-PARENT INTERACTIONS CONCERNING DISCIPLINE

Practitioners can assist parents by giving them guidelines for appropriate childhood discipline related to both routine and problem development. In particular, pediatricians can discourage corporal punishment as the major method of discipline. Frequently physicians fail to inquire about children's behavior. Unless the topic is brought up by parents, it is not discussed during the physician visit. On average, physicians spend only 90 seconds per visit on anticipatory guidance and counseling. However, one survey of mothers in a physician waiting room showed that up to 90% were concerned about one aspect of behavior. Sixty percent of mothers surveyed found physician intervention quite helpful.

Early in the physician-parent relationship, physicians may express their interest in behavioral problems by saying, "I am interested not only in your child's physical well being, but also in his (or her) growth and development and how he (or she) gets along with friends and family." They may then question parents about how children spend their days. During subsequent visits, pediatricians may say, "Parents of children of (child's name)'s age frequently worry about discipline. I wonder if you have any concerns."

PROBLEM BEHAVIORS

Behavioral problems can be placed in five major categories.

1. **Problems of daily routine.** Such problems refer to the refusal of children to go about their daily activities, such as eating, going to bed, awakening at a certain time, and toilet training.
2. **Aggressive resistance behavior.** This behavior is characterized by negativism and includes temper tantrums and aggressive responses to siblings and peers.
3. **Overdependent or withdrawal behavior.** Such behavior is typical of children who are very attached to their mothers. These clingy children find separation difficult, especially in a preschool setting.
4. **Hyperactivity or excessive restlessness.**
5. **Undesirable habits,** which include thumb sucking, nail biting, throat clearing, and playing with genitals.

Some of the behaviors listed above are age-appropriate, and physicians can help parents by counseling them about stage-related behavior, such as oppositional behavior in a two-year-old and independence-dependence problems in a 3–5-year-old. Parents may be more tolerant of a particular behavior if they understand what is normal at a given age. Just because something is normal, however, does not mean that it should be tolerated. Physicians can suggest to the parents ways of dealing with age-appropriate behavior (e.g., placing breakable objects out of reach of toddlers).

Certain behavioral problems reflect differences in childhood temperaments. Carey has compiled a series of temperament scales to assess children and adolescents of different ages. For example, some children are shy and have a hard time adjusting to new situations. If parents anticipate such problems, they are often less angry when difficulties arise.

Physicians can also be particularly helpful in detecting and advising parents about disparities in the achievement of different developmental skills. Some children acquire motor skills before verbal skills, yet parents expect their children to be equally versatile in speech and movement.

PSYCHOPHYSIOLOGY

All behaviors are modified by the responses and reactions of other individuals. The basic premise of discipline is to discourage unwanted behavior and to encourage desired behavior. This is accomplished by using techniques that are based on conditioning modalities.

Several factors contribute to an increased incidence of behavioral problems in children. Ten to fifteen percent of all preschool children are raised in grossly disturbed family situations. These homes are torn by divorce, death, separation, parental substance abuse, mental illness, or extreme poverty. Parental insecurity may also be a factor. In addition, families may have fewer social contacts than they once did because of greater mobility within society. As a result, they face greater social isolation.

DIFFERENTIAL DIAGNOSIS

Physicians must make two diagnostic decisions. First, they must determine whether a specific behavioral problem represents normal childhood behavior or an abnormality in behavior that warrants more specific intervention. Between 8 and 18% of behavioral disturbances may deserve physician intervention. More intensive management may be necessary for problems related to aggressive-resistant behavior and hyperactivity. Hyperactive behavior, which may exist as part of ADHD, may be a sign of a significant underlying problem that warrants one-on-one intervention or the use of neuropharmacologic agents (see Chapter 95, Attention Deficit/Hyperactivity Disorder).

Second, physicians must differentiate between acceptable corporal punishment and child abuse. Some individuals feel that any form of corporal punishment is unacceptable. The use of physical punishment is widely accepted in our society, however, and it is legally condoned in the home setting. Fractures and bruises are not acceptable, and physical abuse should be suspected in children who present with such injuries.

EVALUATION

History

The key component in the evaluation process is the assessment of the means parents use to discipline children (Questions Box). To obtain this information, physicians may simply ask parents, "How do you get your child to mind you?" This question is designed to lead to a discussion of how parents interact with their children. If parents have specific complaints, such as oppositional behavior, they should be questioned about the strategies they have used in their effort to discipline their children.

Physical Examination

Children's behavior should be assessed during the office visit. A general physical examination is useful to check for any signs of physical abuse as well as to evaluate children's well being. A developmental assessment is also helpful because it may delineate disparities in the achievement of certain skills. Some hyperactive children may warrant a more extensive psychodevelopmental assessment to look for findings consistent with ADHD. Behavioral checklists may be used to evaluate children's temperament.

Laboratory Tests

No specific laboratory or imaging studies are indicated for children with discipline problems.

MANAGEMENT

Physicians should assist parents in establishing appropriate guidelines for disciplining their children and reinforce the role of parents as the source of authority. It is important for parents to realize that total freedom results in uncontrollable anxiety.

Children mimic behavior, and **parents should act as role models.** If parents have temper tantrums when they are frustrated, their children may act in a similar manner. **Consistency** is also important. A system with a limited number of enforced rules is better than one with many different rules. In families where both parents are working, especially if they have overlapping time schedules, consistency is sometimes difficult to attain.

Physicians should emphasize to parents that it is best to **avoid power struggles.** Children engaged in a struggle often win because they have final control (e.g., refusing to eat). Children should always be given the opportunity to graciously back out of a situation and save face. It is easier to avoid situations that lead to head-on confrontations than to get out of them once the confrontation has occurred. Parents should be the source of information for physicians. This helps strengthen parents' egos and validates their ability to handle their children appropriately.

In the past, specific methods of dealing with children with discipline problems concerned the issues of permissiveness versus overpermissiveness and accommodation versus strict punishment. Overpermissiveness refers to the allowing of undesirable acts and may exacerbate anxiety and increase demands for privilege. Physicians should remind parents that preventing many behavioral disorders is easier than treating them. Discipline should not only discourage bad behavior but also reinforce good behavior.

Questions: Discipline

- What does the child do that the parents wish he or she would not do?
- What do the parents do to stop unwanted behavior?
- Does the child usually obey the parents?
- Where does most of the unwanted behavior occur?
- Which parent is responsible for disciplining the child?

The four types of discipline described below are used today.

Spanking

Spanking involves inflicting physical pain, which is usually successful in bringing about the immediate cessation or a decrease in problem behavior. Spanking tends to clear the air and get the punishment over with rather than producing a lingering guilt. To be truly effective, however, physical punishment must immediately follow the act. The "wait until Daddy comes home" approach is less effective because of the lack of temporal association. In addition, spanking tends to become situation-specific so that children associate a particular action with being spanked. This learning does not generalize to other situations.

Spanking may actually be damaging to the parent-child relationship. Differentiation of physical punishment from child abuse is often difficult. In general, punishment with the hands is acceptable, but punishment with objects and spanking on parts of the body other than the buttocks or thighs is unacceptable. Spanking may be an early precursor of later physical violence and subsequent abuse. Again, parents act as role models. Children should never be allowed to hit their parents. This makes children feel extremely insecure.

Scolding

Scolding involves the excess use of reasoning and explanations and is used by most parents as part of the discipline process. In families where communication or interaction is minimal, scolding may result in an initial increase in inappropriate behavior because this is the only way children receive any attention.

Ignoring

Ignoring represents the opposite of explaining and reasoning. This form of discipline is difficult to use successfully because parents must totally ignore children's behavior. If even the least flicker of recognition occurs, then activity increases. A brief initial increase in unwanted behavior, a so-called response burst, may occur with ignoring. This disciplinary method works better in younger children.

Time Out

"Time out," the most recommended form of discipline, refers to time out from positive reinforcement. Children are placed in a neutral or boring environment whenever they engage in inappropriate behavior. The time out technique can be used to discourage undesired habits. For example, parents may say, "You can suck your thumb, but you may only do it in such and such a room." This type of discipline is better than ignoring, especially if "ignored" children are receiving attention from siblings and peers. Children should understand the rules ahead of time and why the behavior is unacceptable. Once this is accomplished, time out may occur without any warning.

A timer should be used, and children should stay in the time-out area for one minute per one year of age. An appropriate area must be selected. This area should be fairly boring, so children's rooms are often not appropriate. A laundry room, a corner, or specific chair may be better. If children act unacceptably during the time out, the timer should be reset. If children have to go to the bathroom during time out, they are allowed one trip. After they return from the bathroom, the timer is reset.

The use of the time-out method is sometimes difficult. If the inappropriate behavior occurs in the morning when children are getting ready for school, time out just encourages children's desire to delay. "Beat the buzzer" is another idea that may be used in such situations. With "beat the buzzer," the timer is set. If children are dressed before the timer goes off, they may be rewarded for the behavior by being allowed to go to bed one half hour later. If the buzzer "beats" them, then they have to go to bed one half hour earlier.

Inappropriate behavior away from home presents the greatest difficulty. These situations can be dealt with in numerous ways, particularly if the behavior problem involves temper tantrums. When children are crying or screaming uncontrollably, it is best to remove them from the embarrassment of the situation. This "manual guidance" often occurs in a supermarket, where children select something that parents do not wish to buy. Parents can often circumvent this problem easily by walking into the supermarket and saying, "If you are a good boy (or girl) during the whole trip, then I will get you something at the checkout counter." If children still have temper tantrums, then they should be removed from the area and brought to a neutral place such as the automobile or a rest room and allowed to finish their crying and screaming. It has been said that a glass of cold water splashed in a child's face is sometimes very therapeutic. If the inappropriate behavior does not develop into a temper tantrum, then "marking" time out is helpful. This consists of putting a mark on the child's hand every time he or she engages in an inappropriate behavior. When the child returns home, the marks are totaled, and the time-out method is used.

Parents who complain about inappropriate behavior should be asked to keep a record of children's behavior for one or two weeks. This helps determine if the behavior is really inappropriate and what is motivating it. Parents should be encouraged to talk to their children in a reasonable manner and to verbalize what they think children are feeling. They might say something like this, "It's terrible to be three years old and get so upset. You feel that you can't get the things you want, but some day you will grow up and then you will be in charge. I am really sorry it is so hard for you right now." Physicians should tell parents that it is important to set limits for children and to avoid threatening, judging, and constantly criticizing children. Many parents have themselves been disciplined only with spanking and know no other means, and the advice that physicians offer is valuable.

Selected Readings

Carey, W. B. Pediatric assessment of behavioral adjustment and behavioral style. *In* Levine, M.D., W.B. Carey, and A.C. Crocker (eds.). *Developmental-Behavioral Pediatrics*, 2nd ed. Philadelphia, W. B. Saunders, 1992, pp. 609–612.

Carey, W. B. Temperament issues in the school-aged child. Pediatr. Clin. North Am. 39:564–584, 1992.
Christophersen, E. R. Discipline. Pediatr. Clin. North Am. 39:395–411, 1992.
Christophersen, E. R. Oppositional behavior in children. Pediatr. Ann. 20:267–273, 1991.
Howard, B. J. Discipline in early childhood. Pediatr. Clin. North Am. 38:1351–1369, 1991.
Rosenfeld, A., and D. Levine. Discipline and permissiveness. Pediatr. Rev. 8:209–215, 1987.
Schmitt, B. D. Discipline: rules and consequences. Contemp. Pediatr. 8:65–69, 1991.
Schmitt, B. D. Time-out: intervention of choice for the irrational years. Contemp. Pediatr. 10:64–71, 1993.
Schmitt, B. D. When a child hurts other children. Contemp. Pediatr. 7:81–82, 1990.
Socolar, R. R. S., and R. E. K. Stein. Spanking infants and toddlers: maternal belief and practice. Pediatrics 95:105–111, 1995.
Wissow, L. S., and D. Roter. Toward effective discussion of discipline and corporal punishment during primary care visits: findings from studies of doctor-patient interaction. Pediatrics 94:587–593, 1994.

CHAPTER 28

TEMPER TANTRUMS

Geeta Grover, M.D.

Hx   During a routine office visit, the parents of a three-year-old boy express concern about his recent behavior. They report that whenever he is asked to do something he does not want to do, he throws a "fit." He cries fiercely, falls to the floor, bangs his hands, and kicks his feet until his parents give in. He often displays such behavior at bedtime or mealtime if he is asked to turn off the television or eat foods that he does not want. He has two to three such episodes per week. The parents state that their home life has not changed, and the boy's teacher reports that he displays no such behaviors at preschool.

Questions

1. At what age are temper tantrums most common in children?
2. How do parents' reactions encourage or discourage temper tantrums?
3. What appropriate management strategies may help control such oppositional behavior?
4. What factors or aspects of such oppositional behavior indicate underlying pathology?

Temper tantrums are common, normal, age-related behaviors in young children. To a certain degree, oppositional behaviors such as negativism, defiance, and tantrums are part of the normal progression toward self-reliance and independence. Toddlers need to assert their freedom and explore their environment, which often puts them at odds with the limitations imposed by society and well-meaning parents. Young children cannot appreciate that rules and limitations have been established in the interest of their own safety and well being. They see only that their own desires have been thwarted, and they may react to this disappointment with intense emotions. Children are not simply upset because they cannot have their way. They are angry and frustrated, and they lose control over their emotions. During tantrums children cry and scream uncontrollably. They may fall to the floor, bang their heads, kick their feet, pound their hands, and thrash about wildly. Some children may throw things, try to hit one another, or destroy property.

Such intense displays of anger may be a terrifying experience for both children and parents. Some children use tantrums to gain attention, whereas others use them to achieve something or to avoid doing something. Recurrent temper tantrums may strain relationships among parents, children, and other family members.

EPIDEMIOLOGY

Temper tantrums are noted most often in children who are two to three years of age, but they may occur any time between the ages of 12 months and 5 years. Parental surveys reveal that about 20% of two-year-olds, 18% of three-year-olds, and 10% of four-year-olds have at least one tantrum per day. Boys and girls are affected equally. Although temper tantrums are unusual in school-age children, they often reappear in the form of verbal tantrums during adolescence when autonomy and independence once again become developmental issues.

BEHAVIORAL PATHOPHYSIOLOGY

Appreciation of children's level of maturity and the developmental tasks normally associated with the toddler and preschool years, when temper tantrums occur most often, facilitates an understanding of tantrum behavior. Young children who are exploring the world and developing a sense of autonomy think primarily in egocentric terms. They view reality from their own perspective and are unable to appreciate the perspective of other individuals. Only as they mature and enter school do they learn to recognize the position of others and begin to develop a sense of morality, of right and wrong. Toddlers may become frustrated or angry because of their lack of control over the world, inability to communicate, or limitations of their cognitive and motor abilities, which do not allow them to accomplish desired tasks. Unlike adults who have the ability to verbalize frustrations or simply walk away from unpleasant situations, young children have neither the sophisticated ability to articulate their feelings nor the freedom to walk away. Therefore, they may react to disappointments with temper tantrums.

Temper tantrums may be classified as normal or problematic based on their cause, frequency, and characteristics. Normal tantrums can simply be demands for attention or signs of frustration, anger, or protest. In the interval between tantrums, the child's disposition and mood are normal. The well-behaved three-year-old boy who has an occasional tantrum following the birth of a sibling, the two-and-one-half-year-old girl who throws a tantrum to express frustration because no one understands what she is trying to say, and the two-year-old boy who cries uncontrollably because he cannot complete the puzzle he has started or run fast enough to keep up with his four-year-old brother are all examples of normal tantrums. A typical reason for an avoidance-type tantrum is not wanting to go to bed at bedtime. All types of tantrums are more common when children are tired, ill, or hungry, because their ability to cope with disappointment and frustration is limited under these circumstances.

Frequent tantrums (> 5 per day) or tantrums that result in destruction of property or physical harm to the child or others are signs of problematic tantrums (Table 28–1). These tantrums result from factors that are beyond the child's control such as parental problems, school difficulties, or health-related conditions (Table 28–2). For example, the child with unrecognized hearing loss may be performing poorly at school and resort to tantrum behavior in frustration. Marital discord or domestic violence may create anxiety for a

child, which may manifest as frequent or destructive tantrums.

EVALUATION

Thorough history taking is essential (Questions Box). The frequency of the temper tantrums, circumstances that provoke them, a description of actual tantrums, and parental reaction must be ascertained. In some instances, this reaction may provide insight as to why the tantrums recur. In addition, parental expectations should be assessed. Expectations that are inappropriate for children's age and developmental maturity may create unnecessary tensions between parents and children and lead to tantrum behavior. Factors associated with problematic tantrums should also be assessed (see Table 28–1).

Tantrums that are frequent (> 5 per day), severe, or persist after the age of five years may be a sign of underlying conditions such as depression or low self-esteem. Frequent tantrums may also be associated with ADHD. Children with a history of impulsivity, hyperactivity, and inattention that are inappropriate for age should be evaluated for ADHD. Children who hurt themselves or others or destroy property during tantrums may have significant emotional problems. Peer pressure may inhibit tantrum behavior; if tantrums occur frequently at school, the presence of learning disabilities or speech and hearing deficits should be considered.

It is important to remember that physicians usually see children whose tantrums are frequent, severe, or cannot be controlled by parents. First, pediatricians must determine whether any underlying pathology may

---

Questions: Temper Tantrums

- How often does the child have temper tantrums?
- What circumstances provoke the tantrums?
- How does the child behave during the tantrums? What does the child do?
- How does the child behave in the interval between tantrums?
- How do the parents react to the child during the tantrums? What do they do or say?
- Are parental expectations consistent with the child's developmental stage?
- Have there been any changes at home or school (e.g., birth of a sibling, new school)?
- Is the child having any other behavioral problems (e.g., enuresis, sleep difficulties)?

TABLE 28–1.   Features of Problematic Tantrums

Tantrums that persist or get worse beyond 5 years of age
Frequent tantrums (> 5 per day)
Persistent negative mood or behavior in intervals between tantrums
Recurrent tantrums at school
Destruction of property during tantrums
Harm to self or others during tantrums
Other behavioral problems (e.g., sleep disorders, aggressive behaviors, enuresis)

TABLE 28-2. Underlying Causes of Problematic Tantrums

Parent-Related Factors

Marital discord
Abusive behavior toward children
Domestic violence
Substance abuse
Depression
Inappropriate parental expectations

Child-Related Factors

Health problems
    Chronic or recurrent illnesses
    Unrecognized illnesses (e.g., otitis media, sinusitis)
Disabilities
    Hearing loss
    Speech and language difficulties
    Learning disabilities
Emotional problems (e.g., low self-esteem, depression)
Attention-deficit/hyperactivity disorder (ADHD)
Temperament

Data from Needlman, R., B. Howard, and B. Zuckerman. Temper tantrums: when to worry. Contemp. Pediatr. 6:12–34, 1989.

be contributing to the behavior and, if so, what parental or child factors may be provoking it. Second, they must differentiate between normal tantrums and problematic tantrums. Identification and remediation of the cause of problematic tantrums are the first steps toward cure. Children with suspected underlying conditions such as ADHD or mood disturbances should be referred to the appropriate specialist for further evaluation.

MANAGEMENT

Punishment is not the solution to temper tantrums (see Chapter 27, Discipline). Health maintenance visits are an ideal time to provide **anticipatory guidance** regarding tantrums and discuss strategies to prevent or minimize this behavior. Parents typically report that their children become defiant and difficult to manage during the "terrible twos." At the 12- and 15-month visits, physicians should alert parents that this period is approaching and remind them that it is a normal part of development. Preventive strategies such as **child proofing** the home to minimize unnecessary conflicts should be discussed. In addition, parents can give young children **frequent opportunities to make choices** (e.g., which color shirt to wear or which of two foods to have for lunch). These opportunities allow children to exercise independence and autonomy in a positive rather than a negative manner. Physicians can provide **reassurance** that this unpleasant stage will pass; children will eventually become more cooperative and agreeable.

Parents should be told that helping children learn self-control and how to handle anger are keys to management. To expect that children will never get angry is unrealistic. Children should be taught how to

vent their anger and frustration in an acceptable manner (e.g., articulating their feelings, or hitting a designated punching bag or pillow). As children mature, their ability to verbalize their feelings increases, but even young toddlers can say "me angry."

Physicians should emphasize that it is **important for parents to remain calm** during children's temper tantrums. Shouting and spanking indicate to children that parents are also out of control. Children feel more secure if the adults around them are calm and in control.

Different types of temper tantrums may require specific treatment and management strategies. Parents should **be supportive** of children who are having tantrums resulting from frustration or fatigue by letting the children know that they understand. Children's energy should be redirected into activities they can do well. Parents should be encouraged to **praise positive behavior** (e.g., completing tasks properly, handling anger in an acceptable fashion). They should **ignore some tantrums,** such as those for purposes of attention seeking or wanting something. If children have no audience, they have no need to perform. **Time outs** may also be used in such situations (see Chapter 27, Discipline). Parents should not give in to children's wishes; this may reinforce tantrum behavior. **Physical movement** of children to where they belong may be necessary if they are refusing to do something (e.g., bed for the child who is refusing to go to sleep at bedtime) or in danger of hurting themselves. **Holding children** who are raging may give them a sense of security and help calm them. If temper tantrums occur outside the home, it may be necessary to accompany children to a **quiet, private place** such as an automobile until they calm down.

Case Resolution

The child in the case scenario appears to be having normal, age-appropriate tantrums. The boy's tantrums occur when he is asked to do something that he does not want to do. In these situations the parents should try to ignore the tantrums as much as possible and not give in to the child's wishes.

Selected Readings

Christophersen, E. R. Oppositional behavior in children. Pediatr. Ann. 20:267–273, 1991.

Cruikshank, B. M., and L. J. Cooper. Common behavior problems. *In* Greydanus, D. E., and M. L. Wolraich (eds.). *Behavioral Pediatrics.* New York, Springer-Verlag, 1992.

McIntosh, B. J. Spoiled child syndrome. Pediatrics 83:108–114, 1989.

Needlman, R., B. Howard, and B. Zuckerman. Temper tantrums: when to worry. Contemp. Pediatr. 6:12–34, 1989.

Schmitt, B. D. Temper tantrums. *In Your Child's Health,* rev. ed. New York, Bantam Books, 1991.

CHAPTER 29

BREATH-HOLDING SPELLS

Geeta Grover, M.D.

H$_x$ A 15-month-old girl is brought to the office because of parental concern about seizures. In the last month she has passed out momentarily three times. Each episode seems to be precipitated by anger or frustration on her part. Typically she cries, holds her breath, turns blue, and passes out. Each time she awakens within a few seconds and seems fine. The medical history and family history are unremarkable, and the physical examination is entirely within normal limits.

Questions

1. What are breath-holding spells (BHS)?
2. What is the differential diagnosis of BHS?
3. What, if any, laboratory studies are indicated in the evaluation of BHS?
4. What measures can be taken to prevent BHS? Are anticonvulsants necessary?
5. What, if any, are the long-term sequelae of BHS?

Breath-holding spells (BHS) are a benign, recurring condition of childhood in which anger or pain produce crying that culminates in noiseless expiration and apnea. The frequency of BHS, an involuntary phenomenon, is variable and ranges from several episodes a day to only several episodes per year. Although the spells are innocuous, they usually provoke parental fear and anxiety, because children often turn blue and become limp. The diagnosis can usually be made on the basis of a characteristic history and description of the episode, but the possibility of seizures should be considered.

EPIDEMIOLOGY

BHS occur in about 5% of all children between the ages of six months and six years, but they are most common in children between 12 and 18 months of age. The vast majority of children have experienced their first episode by 18 months and virtually all by two years of age. Although BHS have been described in children under six months of age, occurrence in such young infants is uncommon. Boys and girls are affected equally. A positive family history is found in about 25% of cases.

CLINICAL PRESENTATION

The typical clinical sequence of the two major types of BHS is described later in the chapter (see Pathophysiology and D$_x$ Box). After the spells, children may experience a short period of drowsiness.

PATHOPHYSIOLOGY

BHS may be classified as one of the nonepileptic paroxysmal disorders of childhood. These recurrent conditions, which have a sudden onset and no epileptiform focus, resolve spontaneously. Other disorders in this heterogeneous group include syncope, migraine, cyclic vomiting, benign paroxysmal vertigo, paroxysmal torticollis, sleep disorders (narcolepsy, night terrors, somnambulism), and shudder attacks.

Types of Breath-Holding Spells

The two major types of BHS are **cyanotic** and **pallid.** The cyanotic type is more common. Approximately 60% of children with BHS have cyanotic spells, 20% have pallid spells, and 20% of affected children have both types. Most commonly, affected children experience several spells per week.

Cyanotic episodes are more often provoked by an upsetting event, anger, frustration, or scolding rather than by injury or fear. Children usually cry or scream loudly. The cries becomes noiseless as children open their mouths and hold their breath in expiration. After approximately 30 seconds of apnea, a color change is apparent as children become cyanotic. The spell may terminate at this point, or children may proceed to lose consciousness and become limp. Some physicians refer to attacks that terminate prior to the loss of consciousness as simple BHS, whereas others do not classify such episodes as BHS at all. Rarely, loss of consciousness may be followed by a few seconds of rhythmic clonic jerking of the extremities, mimicking seizure-like activity, or rigid opisthotonic posturing of the body. The entire attack lasts less than one minute. Children generally resume full activity within a few minutes. Unlike the postictal period of epileptic seizures, prolonged periods of lethargy or drowsiness following spells are uncommon.

D$_x$ Breath-Holding Spells

- Identifiable precipitating event or emotion
- Brief duration
- Color change, if present, prior to loss of consciousness and rhythmic jerking of extremities
- Rapid restoration of full activity
- Normal neurologic examination

Pallid spells are similar to cyanotic BHS with some exceptions. Pallid episodes are more commonly provoked by minor injury, pain, or fear rather than frustration or anger; the initial cry is minimal prior to apnea and loss of consciousness; and children become pale rather than cyanotic. In pallid BHS, children often lose consciousness or tone after only a single gasp or cry, whereas in the cyanotic form, the period of apnea prior to loss of consciousness is much longer.

Etiology

Although the spells are triggered by identifiable stimuli, they are involuntary phenomena. It is believed that loss of consciousness in both the cyanotic and pallid forms is caused by cerebral anoxia. The actual mechanisms of the two types of BHS are different. The processes involved in cyanotic BHS are not clear. Proposed mechanisms include centrally mediated inhibition of respiratory effort and altered lung mechanics, which may inappropriately stimulate pulmonary reflexes, thus resulting in apnea and hypoxia. In the pallid form, the pale coloration and loss of tone are thought to result from vagally mediated severe bradycardia or asystole. Pallid spells have been spontaneously induced in the EEG laboratory using ocular compression to trigger the oculocardiac reflex. Vagally mediated bradycardia or asystole lasting more than two seconds has been produced by this maneuver.

DIFFERENTIAL DIAGNOSIS

The differential diagnosis primarily includes seizures and syncope secondary to cardiac arrhythmia or a vasovagal episode. Although vasovagal syncope, like BHS, may be provoked by fear or pain, it is uncommon in children under 12 years of age. Three factors may help differentiate BHS from true epileptic seizure activity. First, spells are usually provoked by some upsetting event or emotion, unlike seizures, which generally do not have a recognizable precipitating event. Second, episodes are brief in duration and followed by rapid restoration of full activity. Third, color change precedes loss of consciousness and rhythmic jerking of the extremities, whereas in the typical epileptic seizure, convulsive activity and loss of muscular tone usually precede

Questions: Breath-Holding Spells

- What happened before the episode?
- Was the child crying?
- What was the child's color before and during the episode?
- Was the child lethargic after the episode?
- Does the family have a history of breath-holding spells?

change in color. See Table 29–1 for the differential diagnosis of BHS.

EVALUATION

History

The history alone may be diagnostic (Questions Box). A family history of BHS should be obtained. It is essential to record a detailed history of the suspected breath-holding episode. The sequence in which the events occurred may help differentiate BHS from epileptic seizures.

Physical Examination

Children should have a complete physical examination, including a thorough neurologic evaluation. Focal neurologic signs or evidence of structural lesions such as meningomyelocele or hydrocephalus may lead the physician away from a diagnosis of BHS.

Laboratory Tests

If the history is consistent with BHS and the physical examination is normal, laboratory evaluation is usually unnecessary. An EEG may be performed if the physician is concerned about the possibility of epileptic seizures. In both forms of BHS, the EEG shows generalized slowing followed by flattening (a pattern characteristic of cerebral anoxia) during attacks, although it is unusual to record the EEG during BHS. The interictal EEG is normal in children with BHS, whereas it may often be abnormal in children with epilepsy. An ECG may be obtained if there is any question about cardiac arrhythmia.

MANAGEMENT

Management of BHS includes **parental support and reassurance.** BHS may be extremely frightening for parents to witness, especially if the episodes are routinely associated with loss of consciousness or seizure-like activity. Parents should be told about the involuntary nature of the attacks and be cautioned against reinforcing the spells by giving in to the child's wishes. They should be advised to avoid unnecessary discipline. Similarly, it is impossible to ensure that the child will never be frustrated or injured. Instead, they should be encouraged to handle the episodes in a "matter-of-fact" manner and continue age-appropriate discipline. They should be reassured that the long-term prognosis is excellent.

TABLE 29–1.   Differential Diagnosis of Breath-Holding Spells

Epileptic seizures
Syncope
  Cardiac arrhythmia
  Vasovagal
  Orthostatic
Benign paroxysmal vertigo
Cataplexy (transient loss of muscle tone associated with narcolepsy; rare before adolescence)
Occult or overt brainstem lesions (causing dysfunction within the pontomedullary area)
Central or obstructive apnea

Pharmacologic therapy is usually not necessary, but atropine sulfate may be considered in the management of children with frequent pallid BHS because of atropine's anticholinergic action. Anticonvulsants are not effective. Referral to a neurologist or psychiatrist may be considered at the family's request if the episodes are frequent and associated with loss of consciousness or if there is uncertainty regarding the diagnosis or management.

PROGNOSIS

BHS resolve spontaneously in the vast majority of children by five to six years of age. About 50% of cases resolve by the age of four years. Neither pallid nor cyanotic BHS are associated with an increased risk of development of epilepsy, although children with pallid BHS do have an increased incidence of developing syncopal attacks during adulthood.

Case Resolution

The child presented in the opening case scenario has a history and physical examination suggestive of BHS. The girl's episodes are consistent with cyanotic BHS. The episodes are preceded by an identifiable emotion, are brief in duration, and are followed by a rapid recovery of normal consciousness and activity.

Selected Readings

DiMario, F. J. Breath-holding spells in childhood. Am. J. Dis. Child. 146:125–131, 1992.

Golden, G. S. Nonepileptic paroxysmal events in childhood. Pediatr. Clin. North Am. 39:715–725, 1992.

Gordon, N. Breath-holding spells. Dev. Med. Child Neurol. 29:811–814, 1987.

Lombroso, C. T., and P. Lerman. Breath-holding spells (cyanotic and pallid infantile syncope). Pediatrics 39:563–581, 1967.

Nathanson, L. W. Breath-holding spells. *In The Portable Pediatrician for Parents*. New York, Harper Collins, 1994.

CHAPTER 30

FEARS AND PHOBIAS

Carol D. Berkowitz, M.D.

Hx A five-year-old girl is brought into the office by her mother, who complains that her daughter has been frightened of sleeping alone since the occurrence of an earthquake. The house did not sustain any significant damage, but the entire family was awakened. The mother says that the girl has become more timid. As nighttime approaches, she becomes particularly fearful. She will not stay in her bed, and she is comforted only by sleeping with her parents. In addition, the girl has had some bed-wetting accidents since the earthquake, and the mother wonders whether she should put her daughter in diapers. The physical examination, including the vital signs, is normal, except for the observation that the child is very clingy and whiny.

Questions

1. What are normal childhood fears?
2. When do these fears commonly occur?
3. What strategies are used to deal with these fears?
4. What are phobias?
5. What is school phobia and how is it best handled?

Fears are normal feelings that cause emotional, behavioral, and physiologic changes that are essential for survival. Fears are associated with psychological discomforts such as a negative, unpleasant feeling. Children may develop fears in response to actual events (e.g., earthquakes) or as a result of the temporal association of two events (e.g., seeing a scary movie on a rainy day and then becoming afraid of rain). Some fears appear to be innate, and others seem to be developmental. Children fear different things at different ages. For example, school phobia is sometimes particularly problematic in young, school-age children.

Phobias are overwhelming, intense, highly specific, and often irrational fears. When these fears are combined with avoidance behavior, they may be incapacitating. Anxiety refers to fear without a definable source. It is a vague feeling of uneasiness, apprehension, and foreboding of impending doom.

Different strategies are useful for dealing with different fears. It is important for parents not to trivialize these fears but to empower children to deal with them.

It is also important to realize that the parents sometimes foster fears by using threats with children such as "the doctor will give you a shot unless you eat your spinach" or "the boogie man will get you." By fostering fears, the parents are also fostering dependency. Parents lack the imagination that children have and find it difficult to understand the degree of fear that children experience.

FEARS CHARACTERISTIC OF CHILDREN OF VARIOUS AGES

Fears follow a developmental pattern. Neonates are believed to have no fear, although young infants whose faces are covered with a blanket struggle to toss off the blanket. Infants who are six months of age exhibit what is known as **stranger anxiety** in response to unfamiliar persons, places, or objects. To combat this anxiety, infants seek refuge with a parent. Stranger anxiety becomes equated with separation anxiety and reaches a peak at two years of age. Children between six months and two years of age are also frightened by loud noises and falling or quickly moving objects.

Children between the ages of two and five years are in what is termed the **"age of anxiety."** They fear many things, including animals, abandonment, loud noises, and darkness. Children in this age group are particularly fearful of physicians, hospitals, and getting hurt. Young children are afraid of the physically handicapped, who represent bodily injury, and monsters and scary movies. They sometimes displace their anger onto monsters and witches and attribute to these imaginary characters the bad feelings they are experiencing. Children in this age group have strong imaginations, which makes it difficult for them to differentiate fantasy from reality.

School-age children between six years of age and adolescence tend to have more abstract thoughts, and their fears are less relevant to physical immediacy. These children are afraid of the death of their parents or the burning of their home. They also fear war, growing up (expressed as "How will I know what to do?"), going into the next grade, being alone or being kidnapped, and the divorce of their parents. Children in this age group are often reluctant to bother their parents with their fears, and they can easily misinterpret parental concerns when they overhear parental conversation.

Separation anxiety, which may appear as school phobia, may also be evident in school-age children. Affected children develop physical complaints (e.g., stomach aches) on school days. The mother-child relationship is often disturbed, and the child is fearful of leaving the parent alone. The prevalence of school phobia is reported to be less than 5%. Childhood school phobia and parental history of panic attacks and agoraphobia may be associated.

Fears during adolescence relate to social functioning such as public speaking or talking to members of the opposite sex. Older children are also concerned about school failure and physical injury. They have many of the same fears expressed by younger school-age children, although phobias are uncommon. Phobias, which occur in less than 1.7% of the general population, are reported in 13% of disturbed children.

PATHOPHYSIOLOGY

Fear has its basis in a series of psychophysiologic reactions, which are mediated through a series of neurotransmitters. Elevated levels of certain transmitters such as gamma-aminobutyric acid and norepinephrine are associated with feelings of anxiety. Excess serotonin has also been related to anxiety disorders. Patients with panic attacks and anxiety disorders have disturbances in neurotransmitter regulation.

DIFFERENTIAL DIAGNOSIS

The challenge for physicians is to assess the etiology of the fear and to differentiate normal fears from those which may be signs of unusual stresses or signs of psychopathology. Appropriate fears represent a real reaction to a real danger. As a rule, children are more resilient than adults and recover more rapidly from traumatic events. On the other hand, children are prone to inappropriate fears, which may develop for a number of reasons.

Inappropriate fears may occur because of operant conditioning, in which a conditioned stimulus becomes associated with another object. Fear for the other object becomes reinforced through this association. True phobias represent neuroses and may occur in more than one family member.

School phobia, also called school refusal, may occur under three distinct conditions. Not uncommonly, young children who are entering school for the first time are frightened. This fear is a normal component of separation anxiety, which usually resolves within a few days of starting school. In contrast, older children may experience school phobia because they are truly afraid of a school situation. They may fear a teacher, violence, or a bully. To avoid the problem, children may actually request to change classrooms or schools. It is important to talk to children to find out what is behind their fear of school.

On the other hand, some children who appear fearful of school are actually concerned about parental separation (i.e., separation anxiety). Frequently these children enjoy school and miss attending it. Absences occur when feelings of separation from parents are so intense that they do not allow children to function well in school settings. This separation anxiety may result from parental illness or parents' fostering dependency in children. Children then see parents as vulnerable and are uncomfortable about leaving them alone.

School refusal is the third leading cause of school absenteeism after transient illness and truancy. Fifty percent of children with school refusal have other problems, including depression (28%), tantrums (18%), sleep disturbances (17%), obsessive-compulsive behavior (11%), other fears (10%), enuresis (3%), and learning disabilities (3%). Overall, school refusal has a good prognosis, although adolescents do not do as well as younger children, and individuals with a higher IQ have a poorer outcome. Twenty percent of parents of children with school refusal have a diagnosable psychiatric disorder. Issues of mother-child dependency are often a concern.

Another type of childhood fear concerns physicians and hospitals. Children have many concerns about what happens to them at the doctor's office. They are particularly fearful of needles. To children, needles represent possible mutilation. When asked to represent needles in drawings, children often portray needles as larger than themselves and very pointed. They comment that needles are sharp (e.g., "needles can make you pop, just like a balloon"; "needles can also take out all your blood until you die"). In addition, children are preoccupied with what happens to their blood. One youngster commented, "They check out your blood to see if it's good or bad, and if your blood is bad, then it means that you need to have more tests."

Hospitalization raises other issues concerning parental separation as well as painful procedures. As children adjust to hospitalization, they progress through three stages: protest, during which they complain about the hospital and cry; despair, during which they have given up hope that their parents will return; and detachment, during which they seem to be adjusting but actually have distanced themselves from their parents.

EVALUATION

Physicians should explore the area of childhood fears and phobias at routine health maintenance visits, even if parents do not have specific concerns. Sometimes parents are embarrassed by children's fears (e.g., the fear of an older child to sleep without a night light). Parents may not report children's fears unless these fears seem to be unusually intense. Practitioners may ask children, "What is the scariest thing you can think of?" If children are having difficulty providing details, physicians may ask them to name things that other children fear or to complete the sentence, "I feel afraid when _____." Alternatively, practitioners may suggest things that other children may fear: "Do the kids you know seem to be worried about kidnapping?"

History

The evaluation of children with specific fears demands a careful history that provides information about situations in which children are fearful (Questions Box). Physicians should consider fears within a developmental context, because many childhood fears are normal and experienced by all children. It is also important to look at changes in the family situation. Children sometimes develop what appear to be fears but

> **Questions: Fears and Phobias**
> - What fear does the child have? Exactly what does the child fear?
> - Under what circumstances was the fear originally expressed? Did any changes in the child's life occur around the time that the fear appeared?
> - Under what conditions is the fear currently expressed?
> - How long has the child had the fear?
> - How does the fear affect the daily living of the child and family?

in fact are behaviors designed to manipulate other family members. For instance, young children who sense marital discord may insist on sleeping with their parents as a way of ensuring that the parents are together rather than separate.

Physical Examination

A routine examination is warranted, but findings are usually normal.

Laboratory Tests

As a rule, laboratory tests are not required. Consultation with a child psychologist or psychiatrist may be useful.

MANAGEMENT

The management of the fear or phobia is determined by the degree to which children are incapacitated. As a general rule, **children should be empowered to conquer their fears.** Children's books that address the issues of certain fears can help achieve this empowerment. Books such as *The Berenstain Bears in the Dark* (Random House, 1982) discuss specific worries such as fear of lightning and thunder. These books often explain the basis of such natural phenomena in easy-to-understand terms. The books also normalize particular fears and show how one character is fearful. Parents can also re-create some of the sounds that children fear. For example, children who are afraid of the noise the wind makes are shown a teakettle where the hot steam blows through the whistle, creating the same noise as the wind. For fears about nuclear war, empowering children to become active, such as joining a nuclear protest group, may be useful.

Parents may feel helpless because they do not know how to deal with children's fears. Physicians should give them the necessary information. Children's fears should not be trivialized. Even if the **fears** are unfounded, they **should be validated.** In general, children should be questioned about whether they are fearful about a situation. The following two examples illustrate the proper handling of fears in children.

If children are visiting the dentist for the first time, it is appropriate for parents to ask, "Are you afraid?" If children reply, "Yes, a little bit," parents can say, "Almost everybody is afraid. Tell me what it is you're afraid of. Fear is a normal emotion, and I'm glad you told mc about it."

Parents of children who express fear of imaginary characters can reassure children that they do not exist. In addition, parents can tell children what the parents would do if such characters did exist. For instance, the father of a little girl who was afraid of witches told her, "There are no such things as witches. But if there were, and they came into your room, I would punch them in the nose and punch them in the stomach and beat them up, and then there would be no more witches to hurt you." By doing this, parents establish the reality of the situation and then also create a plan to deal with the problem should it actually happen.

Parents can also help to limit or reduce children's fears by **minimizing** their **exposure to fear-provoking situations** such as television shows or scary movies. These programs can be particularly frightening for some children, who should not watch them without adult supervision.

When dealing with children who have school phobia because of problems in school, it is important to determine if a change in school would be appropriate to facilitate their school attendance. This may be particularly appropriate in children whose schools are plagued with violence.

If, on the other hand, children's refusal to attend school is linked to separation anxiety, then a program of **desensitization** is recommended. Desensitization may involve the participation of mothers in the classroom for a period of time. When children acclimate and can tolerate some separation, mothers move to another area in the school such as the principal's office. Next they go outside the school grounds. As children reestablish a sense of well-being in spite of the separation, the mothers gradually move farther and farther away. This solution is somewhat problematic for mothers who work outside the home. Children with significant school refusal may need the assistance of child psychologists or psychiatrists.

Phobias may be treated using the concept of **flooding,** which consists of rapid, prolonged exposure to the feared item. For example, a child who is afraid of dogs is exposed to a friendly, docile, small dog while in the company of his or her parents. Alternatively, systematic desensitization, during which children are exposed to the feared objects over a series of weeks, coupled with relaxation techniques, is also utilized. Phobias usually require the help of mental health specialists.

Children who must undergo hospitalization benefit from a prehospital visit, when possible. This visit familiarizes the child with the facilities and explains proposed procedures. Many hospitals have child life specialists who ease the adjustment of children to their hospital stay.

PROGNOSIS

Most childhood fears resolve with time, nurturing, and reassurance. Most fears last only several weeks, and then new fears develop. As a rule, specific fears should not last longer than two years, and the younger the child, the shorter the duration of the fear.

Prognosis is good for children with true phobias, with 100% resolution of monosymptomatic phobias.

Case Resolution

In the case scenario, the girl's fear of sleeping in her bed was triggered by a significant environmental event. Although earthquakes are uncontrollable, the girl can be empowered to deal with manageable aspects of an earthquake as much as possible. She should be assured that in the same situation, many adults probably would also fear sleeping alone. The parents should stock a box with shoes, flashlight, radio, and water and place the box under the child's bed. In addition, they may also have their daughter get into her bed and then shake it, simulating the jiggling that she would experience during an earthquake. The girl should also practice getting out of bed and standing in the doorway. To combat the child's fear of separation during times of natural disaster, the parents should reassure their daughter that they will all be together.

Selected Readings

PHYSICIANS

American Psychiatric Association. *Diagnostic and Statistical Manual of Mental Disorders,* 4th rev. ed. Washington, DC, American Psychiatric Association, 1994.

Klein, R. G., H. S. Koplewicz, and A. Kanner. Imipramine treatment of children with separation anxiety disorder. J. Am. Acad. Child Adolesc. Psychiatry 31:21, 1992.

Klein, R. G, and C. G. Last. *Anxiety Disorders in Children.* Newbury Park, CA, Sage Publications, 1989.

McMenamy, C., and R. C. Katz. Brief parent-assisted treatment for children's nighttime fears. J. Dev. Behav. Pediatr. 10:145–148, 1989.

Sarafino, E. P. *The Fears of Childhood.* New York, Human Sciences Press, 1986.

Scholwalter, J. E. Fears and phobias. Pediatr. Rev. 15:384–388, 1994.

PARENTS AND CHILDREN

Berenstain, S., and J. Berenstain. *The Berenstain Bears and the Bully.* New York, Random House, 1993.

Berenstain, S., and J. Berenstain. *The Berenstain Bears in the Dark.* New York, Random House, 1982.

Berenstain, S., and J. Berenstain. *The Berenstain Bears Visit the Dentist.* New York, Random House, 1981.

Ziefert, H. *Nicky's Noisy Night.* New York, Penguin Books, 1986.

THUMB SUCKING AND OTHER HABITS

Carol D. Berkowitz, M.D.

H$_x$ A five-year-old boy is brought to the office because of thumb sucking. His mother claims that she has tried nearly everything, including tying his hands at night and using aversive treatments on his thumbs, but nothing has worked. She reports that her son has been teased at school and has few friends. He is in good general health, and his immunizations are up to date.

His growth parameters are at the 50th percentile. Except for a callus on the right thumb, the physical examination is normal.

Questions

1. What are common habits in children?
2. What is the significance of transitional objects?
3. What are the consequences of the common habits in children?
4. What are strategies used to break children of habits?

Habits are defined as somewhat complicated, repetitive behaviors. They are different from tics, which are rapid, repetitive muscle twitches involving the head, face, or shoulders. Tics are also referred to as habit spasms (see Chapter 88, Tics). Children have many socially unacceptable habits, including thumb sucking, nail biting, hair pulling (trichotillomania), rocking, biting other children, and teeth grinding (bruxism). Some habits, such as pica, are potentially harmful. Children engage in most of these habits because of their soothing potential.

One third of children use transitional objects such as thumbs for comfort. Blankets or favorite toys are traditional transitional objects that represent an age-appropriate coping mechanism. Most transitional objects are strokable, and the stroking often occurs in association with thumb sucking. Transitional objects sometimes present a problem because children experience distress if these objects are lost, misplaced, or need cleaning.

EPIDEMIOLOGY

Thumb sucking probably represents the most common habit of children. A reported 50 to 87% of children engage in this habit. The median age for the onset of hand sucking is 54 minutes of life, and 90% of newborns show hand sucking behavior by the age of two hours. Forty percent of children between the ages of one and three years, 33% of children between the ages of three and five, and 25% of children at the age of five still suck their thumbs. Some children suck their fingers rather than thumbs.

Other oral behavior may involve lip sucking, lip biting, and toe sucking. Lip sucking and biting begin at about five to six months of age and occur in about 90% of infants. It is unusual for these actions to persist as habits. Toe sucking is noted in infants who are six to seven months of age, and it is reported in 80% of normal infants.

Trichotillomania is a disorder once believed to be uncommon but now thought to affect eight million Americans (about five per thousand). The term, first coined in 1889, refers to alopecia from compulsive hair pulling. Hair pulling may involve hair from the head, eyebrows, eyelashes, or pubic area. Although trichotillomania appears to peak during early childhood and adolescence, the disorder is reported from infancy to adolescence. In young children, boys and girls are equally affected, but in older children and adolescents, females outnumber males.

Rhythmic habits are stereotypic, repetitive behaviors that usually occur in infants under the age of one year. These habits are reported in 15 to 20% of the population. Rhythmic habits include rocking (about 19% of infants), when infants rock back and forth; jouncing (5–10%), when they move up-and-down on their hands and knees so that the whole crib rocks; head rolling (8%); and head banging (5%). Rhythmic habits are seen more commonly in boys; the male-female ratio is 3:1. These habits usually occur with a frequency of 60 to 80 movements per minute, often when infants are tired, and last for less than 15 minutes before they fall sleep.

Rhythmic movements have been equated with **sleep tics.** These tics are reported in 20% of children, most often between the ages of six and ten years. As a rule, tics are three times more common in boys than in girls. They tend to be noted with increased frequency in children who are shy, overly self-conscious, or have obsessive-compulsive tendencies. Tics usually occur when children are under stress.

Biting, an aggressive habit noted in toddlers, may be related to teething. It occurs more often in children with slow verbal skills.

Nail biting (onychophagia) is usually believed to be a sign of internal tension. The disorder affects 10 to 40% of children. Nail biting begins between the ages of three and six, and the peak age is 13 years. One third of adolescents bite their nails, but 50% of these adolescents break the habit by the time they reach adulthood. Nail biting in adults is regarded as a sign of emotional and social immaturity and regression. The family history for nail biting is often positive.

Identical twins are concordant for the condition in 66% of cases. In contrast, the incidence in dizygotic twins is 34%.

Pica, which is not a normal behavior, is defined as the ingestion of nonfood products. The peak incidence of pica is between the ages of one and three years. The incidence is increased in children from lower socio-economic levels, and the behavior occurs in 10% of children who present with lead poisoning.

Teeth grinding (bruxism) is reported in 5 to 15% of children. Boys are more commonly affected than girls, and the disorder appears to regress later in life. It is reported with increased incidence among mentally retarded children. The cause is unknown.

CLINICAL PRESENTATION

Children with common habits, such as thumb sucking or rhythmic movements, may be brought to the physician with these particular complaints because the parent wants advice about stopping the behavior. Other children may present with consequences of habits, such as alopecia (trichotillomania), paronychia (nail biting), or lead intoxication (pica) (D_x Box).

PSYCHOPHYSIOLOGY

Children engage in habits to reduce stress and provide comfort. Thumb sucking is related to nonnutritive sucking. Although the initial purpose of sucking is nutritional, the pleasure associated with sucking reinforces the behavior. Infants who are served from a cup from birth develop no interest in sucking. Humans and other primates spend more time in nonnutritive than in nutritive sucking. Monkeys use a five-point hold, with two hands, two feet, and mouth (holding on to their mother's nipple) for attachment. Universal thumb sucking is noted even in orphan monkeys, and sucking is thought to be an important aspect of environmental adaptation. Nonnutritive sucking occurs even in the absence of fatigue, hunger, or discomfort, and has a purpose in itself—to provide comfort and be self-soothing. The maximum intensity of sucking occurs at seven months.

In bottle-fed infants, thumb sucking appears to commence when feeding stops. Some infants, described as "type A," seem to be satisfied only when their thumb is in their mouth. As infants spend more time engaged in motor activity, they spend less time thumb sucking.

Placid infants who cry less also do less sucking. Some studies have shown that thumb sucking is less common in breast-fed infants, and that thumb suckers as a group feed less frequently (every 4 hours rather than 3 and for 10 minutes rather than 20).

Nail biting is related to thumb sucking, a form of oral gratification, and children may progress from thumb sucking to nail biting. The pattern of nail biting usually involves placement of the hand in the vicinity of the mouth, tapping of the fingers along the teeth, quick spasmodic bites with the fingers around the central incisors, and the removal and inspection of the hands. Other oral habits, such as pencil gnawing, gum chewing, lip biting, nose picking, and nail picking are related activities. The cause of teeth grinding is unclear.

Rocking habits are believed to be kinesthetically pleasing and soothing and a means of autostimulation. The etiology of hair pulling is less apparent. In recent years, investigators have linked trichotillomania to disorders of serotonin reuptake and placed it in the category of obsessive-compulsive behavior. Some individuals who engage in trichotillomania have abnormal head positron emission tomography. Pica, which is also considered abnormal, may be associated with mental retardation, environmental deprivation, or inadequate nutrition, particularly iron deficiency.

DIFFERENTIAL DIAGNOSIS

The differential diagnosis of most habits is not difficult. Tics or habit spasms should be differentiated from Tourette's syndrome. This syndrome, which is reported in 1 in 3000 children, is a neurologic disorder characterized by severe, frequent, and multiple tics. These tics are also often vocal and consist of sounds such as hissing, barking, grunting or coprolalia, and repetitive profanities. Some of the rhythmic habits may be mistaken for seizures but can be easily distinguished because of the stereotypic, repetitive nature of the behavior.

Trichotillomania usually has a classic physical appearance that has been referred to as the "tonsure Friar Tuck" pattern baldness, with baldness around the vertex of the head. The differential diagnosis of trichotillomania includes alopecia areata, tinea capitis, syphilitic alopecia, and androgenic alopecia (see Chapter 90, Disorders of the Hair and Scalp). Alopecia secondary to trichotillomania is usually characterized by broken hairs of variable length. Other disorders in the differential diagnosis include traction alopecia, related to tight braids or hair brushing; atopic eczema; seborrheic dermatitis; hypothyroidism; SLE; and dermatomyositis.

EVALUATION

Habits must be evaluated in the context of the child's developmental level and home situation. Children who present with thumb sucking, nail biting, and teeth grinding usually do not require an assessment other than a routine health maintenance history and physical examination. However, children who present with movements that resemble tics should be carefully questioned about the frequency and duration of the tics, the effect

---

D_x Childhood Habits

- History of a habit
- Callus on thumb or fingers
- Short, chewed nails
- Alopecia
- Lead intoxication
- Iron deficiency anemia

of the tics on their behavior, and whether coughing is associated with the tics (sign of Tourette's syndrome). The occurrence of obsessive-compulsive mannerisms should also be noted.

Children with trichotillomania should be evaluated for the disorders listed above. An easy evaluation process for trichotillomania involves shaving the hair in the middle of the area of baldness. The growth of these small hairs is uniform because children are unable to pull them out. Disorders such as syphilis and collagen vascular diseases can be ruled out using appropriate laboratory studies. Fungal infections can be differentiated by the use of appropriate cultures.

Children who present with pica should be evaluated for the presence of iron deficiency anemia and lead poisoning.

MANAGEMENT

The management of childhood habits should be directed at the specific symptoms. The issue of thumb sucking versus the use of pacifiers can be addressed by anticipatory guidance. **Pacifiers,** which were initially discouraged, are now believed to have some advantages over thumb sucking. With pacifiers, the risk for dental disturbances is lower, because the pacifiers are softer and are accompanied by a plastic shield that puts counter pressure on the teeth. Pacifiers are also detachable and cleanable.

Pacifiers can be lost, however. Parents should be advised not to attach a pacifier to the child's shirt with a string because of risk of strangulation. For children who are pacifier-dependent and are unable to go back to sleep if they lose their pacifier at night, multiple pacifiers can be placed in the crib to make finding one easier. For infants who desire pacifiers because they complete their feeding in under 20 minutes, a nipple with a smaller hole can be used or the cap can be screwed on the bottle more tightly to prolong the time spent in nutritive sucking.

It is suggested that parents do not try to stop thumb sucking behavior until children have reached the age of four years. Dental problems in late thumb suckers include anterior open bite, increased overjet (protruding upper incisors), intruded and flared upper incisors, lingually flipped lower incisors, and warped alveolar ridge. The physician should reassure parents that children who stop sucking their thumb prior to the onset of the secondary dentition are not at risk for poor dentition.

Numerous devices have been proposed to help with the cessation of thumb sucking, but reported success has been variable. The use of arm restraints, particularly at night, is not recommended and may result in rumination. Bitter paints such as Stop Zit seek to reduce thumb sucking by subjecting children to a bitter, aversive taste. This medication consists of 49% toluene, 19% isopropyl alcohol, 18% butyl acetate, 11% ethylcellulose, and 0.3% denatonium benzoate. A three-quarter ounce bottle is toxic if ingested in its entirety. The principle of retraining, where thumb sucking becomes a duty and children are required to suck all ten fingers, one at a time, has also been recommended. Some recommend that elastic bandages be put on the hand of nocturnal thumb suckers. Problems associated with thumb sucking include sore thumbs, calluses and candidal infections. Dentists may fashion a reminder appliance, making it difficult for children to suck their thumbs.

Encouragement works better than nagging, as a rule, and a **reward system** is particularly useful in children who are five to six years of age. Parents may be referred to books such as *Danny and His Thumb* (K.F. Ernst; Prentice-Hall, Englewood Cliffs, NJ, 1973) and encouraged to talk to their children about how good it feels not to suck their thumb. A star chart and diary are also useful. Sometimes telling children something like, "Mommy would be so proud of you if you didn't suck your thumb now that you're such a big girl or a big boy" is effective. In addition, the pressure to stop thumb sucking becomes greater during the school years. Children who suck their thumbs are regarded by their peers in first grade as less intelligent, less happy, less likable, and less desirable as friends.

In children who suck their thumbs and twirl their hair at the same time, the hair twirling stops once the thumb sucking ends. Hair pulling in young children seems to often resolve spontaneously but is more problematic in adolescents and adults. In children, behavior modification, including putting socks on the hands and the use of time out for hair pulling, in addition to extra attention for not pulling the hair, is recommended. In older individuals, hair pulling may be related to obsessive-compulsive disorders. Trichotillomania may lead to the presence of bezoars (hairballs) from swallowed hair. The results of treatment with agents such as isocarboxazid, amitriptyline, clomipramine, and fluoxetine are more successful in adults than in children.

Nail biting also often responds to behavior modification. Olive oil may be put on the nails to make them soft so there are fewer jagged edges to bite.

Rhythmic habits are less easy to modify. For the most part, reassurance is all that is available. The use of metronomelike devices has had no demonstrable effect. Children over the age of three years who disturb the family's sleep with their rhythmic habits may be given mild sedatives such as diphenhydramine. Other maneuvers involve placing the crib or bed on carpeting to decrease the amount of noise from movement.

Children who engage in biting behavior should be managed with behavior modification, including praising of good behavior and time out for inappropriate behavior.

Iron deficiency resulting from pica requires iron supplementation. Lead intoxication should be managed with chelation and environmental manipulation.

PROGNOSIS

Most habits are not harmful to children's health. The major problem is social acceptability. Parents should be encouraged to stop a habit before it becomes ingrained. This can often be done by praising good behavior and encouraging activities during which the unwanted behavior does not appear. Habits that do not respond to parental influence often resolve spontaneously under peer pressure.

Case Resolution

In the case history presented at the beginning of the chapter, it is important for the physician and the mother to empower the boy to stop thumb sucking before he finds himself ostracized by his classmates. He might be allowed to suck his thumb at certain times and in certain places (e.g., "You can suck in your room after school for fifteen minutes"). Books geared at children and parents to help stop the thumb sucking are recommended, and the boy is rewarded for times when he is not sucking his thumb.

Selected Readings

Blum, N. J., V. J. Barone, and P. C. Friman. A simplified behavioral treatment for trichotillomania: report of two cases. Pediatrics 91:993–995, 1993.

Brazelton, T. B. Sucking in infancy. Pediatrics 17:400–404, 1956.

Dimino-Emme, L., and C. Camisa. Trichotillomania associated with the "Friar Tuck sign" and nail biting. Cutis 47:107–110, 1991.

Friman, P. C., and B. Schmitt. Thumb sucking in childhood: guidelines for the pediatrician. Clin. Pediatr. 28:438–440, 1989.

Friman, P. C., et al. Influence of thumb sucking on peer social acceptance in first-grade children. Pediatrics 91:784–786, 1993.

Peterson, J. E., and P. E. Schneider. Oral habits: a behavioral approach. Pediatr. Clin. North Am. 38:1289–1307, 1991.

Schmitt, B. Helping the child with tics (twitches). Contemp. Pediatr. 8:31–32, 1991.

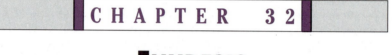

CHAPTER 32

ENURESIS

Carol D. Berkowitz, M.D.

H$_x$ A nine-year-old boy who is in good general health is evaluated for a history of bed-wetting. He is the product of a normal pregnancy and delivery and achieved his developmental milestones at the appropriate time. The boy was toilet trained by the age of three years, but he has never been dry at night for more than several days at a time. Enuresis occurs at least three to four times a week even if he is fluid-restricted after 6 PM. The boy never wets himself during the day, has normal stools, and is an average student. His father had enuresis that resolved by the time he was 12 years old.

The boy's physical examination is entirely normal.

Questions

1. What conditions account for the symptoms of enuresis?
2. What is the appropriate evaluation of children with enuresis?
3. What is the relationship between enuresis and emotional stresses or psychosocial disorders?
4. What management plans are available for enuresis?
5. How do physicians decide which management technique is appropriate for which patients?

Enuresis is defined as involuntary urination in children whose age and development suggest achievement of bladder control. Urinary continence is reached earlier in girls than in boys, and the diagnosis of enuresis is reserved for girls over the age of five years and boys over the age of six. Diurnal enuresis is wetting that occurs during the day. Nocturnal or sleep enuresis refers to involuntary urination that occurs during the night. The term **primary enuresis** is used when children have never achieved sustained dryness, and **secondary enuresis** is used when urinary incontinence recurs after three to six months of dryness.

Physicians can be particularly helpful by routinely questioning parents about bed-wetting during health maintenance visits. Many families are otherwise reluctant to bring up this embarrassing complaint, because enuresis is viewed as socially unacceptable. It poses particular difficulties if children wish to sleep away from home.

EPIDEMIOLOGY

Enuresis, one of the most common conditions of childhood, affects 10 to 20% of first-grade boys and 8 to 17% of first-grade girls. By age 10 years, 5 to 10% of boys have enuresis (1% of army recruits are enuretic). Seventy-four percent of affected children have nocturnal enuresis, 10% diurnal enuresis, and 16% both. Primary enuresis affects the large majority (75–80%) of children with enuresis. Although the overall incidence of secondary enuresis is lower (20–25%), it increases with age; secondary enuresis makes up 50% of cases of enuresis in children 12 years of age.

- Bed-wetting
- Old enough to be toilet trained
- Precipitating problem such as diabetes or UTI
- Encopresis
- ADHD
- Family history of enuresis

Several epidemiologic factors have been associated with enuresis, including low socioeconomic level, large family size, single-parent family, low birth weight, short height at 11 to 15 years of age, immature behavior, relatively low IQ, poor speech and coordination, and encopresis (fecal incontinence; 5–15% of cases). Enuresis occurs more often in institutionalized children. Enuresis has a familial basis, and as many as 77% of children are enuretic if both parents were similarly affected. Concordance for enuresis is reported in 68% of monozygotic twins and 48% of dizygotic twins.

CLINICAL PRESENTATION

A history of enuresis may be obtained as a presenting complaint or elicited by physicians during a health maintenance visit. Medical complaints such as encopresis or ADHD may be associated with the enuresis (D$_x$ Box). The physical examination is usually normal.

PATHOPHYSIOLOGY

Delayed control of micturition has several possible causes (Table 32–1).

1. **Faulty toilet training.** Faulty toilet training may perpetuate both diurnal and nocturnal enuresis but is not expected to selectively perpetuate the latter. Parental expectations are believed to play a role in the toilet training experience. Parents who allow children to sleep in diapers may be delaying the achievement of nighttime dryness, but it is unlikely that the use of diapers causes nocturnal enuresis.

TABLE 32–1.   Causes of Enuresis

Primary Enuresis
Faulty toilet training
Maturational delay
Small bladder capacity
Sleep disorder/impaired arousal
Allergens
Nocturnal polyuria/relative vasopressin deficiency

Secondary Enuresis
Urinary tract infection
Diabetes mellitus
Diabetes insipidus
Nocturnal seizures
Genitourinary anomalies
Sickle cell anemia
Medication use
Emotional stress

2. **Maturational delay.** The development of the inhibitory reflex of voiding may be delayed in some children, which may contribute to enuresis until the age of five years. It is unlikely that maturational delay persists as a cause of enuresis beyond this age. Experts believe that maturational delay is not a reasonable explanation if children can achieve dryness in the daytime but not at night.

3. **Small bladder capacity.** Evidence suggests that some children with enuresis have smaller bladder capacities. Bladder capacity in ounces is estimated as the age in years plus two. For example, five-year-old children have a bladder capacity of 7 ounces (210 mL). Adult bladder capacity is 12 to 16 ounces (360–480 mL).

4. **Sleep disorder/impaired arousal.** It has been suggested that children with enuresis are in "deep sleep" and do not sense a full bladder. However, studies have shown that enuresis occurs during all stages of sleep, particularly in the first one third of sleep and in transition from non-REM stage 4 to REM sleep. During this period body tone, respiratory rate, and heart rate increase, and erection and micturition occur. Children with enuresis do not appear to sleep more deeply than other children.

5. **Allergens.** No evidence confirms the notion that exposure to certain foods (e.g., food additives, sugar) contributes to enuresis. However, some parents believe that bed-wetting is decreased if certain foods such as sodas and sweets are eliminated from the diet.

6. **Nocturnal polyuria/relative vasopressin deficiency.** Research has shown that although nonenuretic children exhibit a diurnal variation in vasopressin secretion, this rhythm is disturbed in some children with enuresis, resulting in nocturnal polyuria.

DIFFERENTIAL DIAGNOSIS

Primary nocturnal enuresis is usually related to the conditions discussed in Pathophysiology. An organic problem is rarely the cause. However, secondary enuresis frequently results from an organic problem, such as UTI, diabetes mellitus, diabetes insipidus, nocturnal seizures, genitourinary anomalies (e.g., ectopic ureter), sickle cell anemia, medication (e.g., diuretics, theophylline), or emotional stress. When primary enuresis is both diurnal and nocturnal, some of these conditions should also be considered.

EVALUATION

History

A thorough history should be obtained when evaluating children with enuresis (Questions Box).

Physical Examination

A general physical examination should be performed, with particular attention to certain areas. The pattern of growth should be plotted. Blood pressure should be obtained. The abdomen should be assessed for evidence of organomegaly, bladder size, and fecal impaction. A rectal examination should be performed to evaluate rectal tone.

If possible, physicians should watch children void. Practitioners should determine whether children can start and stop micturition and whether the stream is forceful. Dribbling in girls may indicate an ectopic ureter. The appearance of the genitalia should be assessed. Labial fusion in girls may trap urine, allow reflux into the vagina, and lead to dribbling. Epispadias, hypospadias, or cryptorchidism may be present in boys. Any of these conditions suggests a possible underlying genitourinary anomaly.

The neuromuscular integrity of the lower extremities should be evaluated. This may provide a clue to a disorder such as spina bifida occulta. The presence of some anomaly in the sacral area, such as a sacral dimple or a tuft of hair, may also be a sign of this condition.

Laboratory Tests

Only a minimal laboratory evaluation is indicated in most children with primary enuresis. Urinalysis, including specific gravity, and a urine culture is indicated. A CBC, hemoglobin electrophoresis, serum electrolytes, and BUN should also be considered. Studies such as urine culture and blood glucose are more often indicated in cases of secondary enuresis.

Diagnostic Studies

In cases in which the urinalysis is abnormal, the culture is positive, or genitourinary anomalies are apparent on physical examination, a renal ultrasound and vesicoureterogram may be warranted. Vertebral x-rays are appropriate in the diagnosis of spina bifida. An EEG is indicated if nocturnal epilepsy is suspected.

MANAGEMENT

Primary Enuresis

Family counseling about enuresis should be part of all management plans. Issues related to psychosocial stress should be explored, particularly in cases of secondary enuresis. Families should be advised that the wetting is not intentional and that punishing children for accidents is inappropriate. However, children may take some responsibility for the consequences of their actions, such as removing soiled bedding or helping with the laundry. They should be rewarded for "dry" nights. Star charts, in which a sticker or gold star is applied to a calendar for each dry night, have traditionally been used. The exclusive use of these charts without other interventions has limited success, however, and suggests that the enuresis may have a volitional component. Star charts should be used in conjunction with other management strategies.

Two treatment modalities are acceptable for managing enuresis. Most studies do not support the use of fluid restriction as a reliable means of controlling enuresis.

Conditioning therapy involves the use of an alarm that is triggered when children void during the night. Children are awakened by the sounding of the alarm, and further urination is inhibited. Eventually bladder distention is associated with inhibition of the urge to urinate. When conditioning therapy is used for four to six months, it is associated with a success rate of 70%. If the alarm is used for four more weeks with sustained dryness, relapses are uncommon.

Because patient cooperation is needed with the alarm system, its use is reserved for children over the age of seven years. A newer system is a transistorized version of the original device that contains a small sensor in the underwear and an alarm on the wrist or collar.

Pharmacologic agents include tricyclic antidepressants (TCAs) and desmopressin. TCAs, especially imipramine, have been successfully used to treat nocturnal enuresis, although the mechanism of action is uncertain. The antidepressant action of the drug, its effect on sleep and arousal, and its anticholinergic properties may all play a role. The bladder capacity of individuals with enuresis may be increased by 34%, which indicates that the anticholinergic effects of the drug may be the most significant.

Imipramine should not be prescribed for children under the age of six or seven years because of potential adverse effects. The recommended dosage is 0.9–1.5 mg/kg/d. In general, children under the age of eight years are given 25 mg one to two hours before bedtime, and older children are given 50–75 mg. Beneficial results usually occur within the first few weeks of therapy. Medication is usually continued for three to six months to prevent relapses, which are reported in up to 75% of cases. The drug should be tapered by reducing the dose or using an alternate-night regimen. Side effects are rare and include insomnia, nightmares, and personality changes. Acute overdoses are potentially fatal secondary to cardiac complications.

Desmopressin (DDAVP), an analog of vasopressin, the antidiuretic hormone, is a newer pharmacologic agent used for enuresis. DDAVP probably works to decrease nocturnal urine production. Most patients respond rapidly to DDAVP and become dry within one to two weeks of the initiation of therapy. The medication is sprayed into the nostril. The initial dose, which can be doubled if patients fail to respond, is one puff (10 mg) in each nostril. Complications, such as epistaxis, nasal pain, congestion, and headache, may occur at higher doses. Severe hyponatremia has also been reported with DDAVP in the face of high fluid intake. If patients achieve a two-week period of dryness, the dose can be tapered at two-week intervals.

Treatment of enuresis in children with small bladder capacities includes bladder retention training. Such children are fluid loaded and asked to delay voiding for five to ten minutes. This strategy is generally reserved for children with diurnal enuresis.

Secondary Enuresis

The management of secondary enuresis should focus on the treatment of the causal disorder, such as a UTI or diabetes mellitus.

PROGNOSIS

The prognosis for children with enuresis is good. The spontaneous cure rate is 15% per year. Medical management results in a reduction in symptoms in over 70% of affected children.

Case Resolution

The boy in the case scenario has primary nocturnal enuresis. The history of childhood enuresis in the father is significant. Two management options, behavior modification and treatment with DDAVP or imipramine, can be discussed with the family. The child's symptoms will probably spontaneously improve over time.

Selected Readings

Moffat, M. E., et al. Desmopressin acetate and nocturnal enuresis: how much do we know? Pediatrics 92:420–425, 1993.

Norgaard, J. P., S. Rittig, and J. C. Djorhous. Nocturnal enuresis: an approach to treatment based on pathogenesis. J. Pediatr. 114:705–710, 1989.

Rappaport, L. The treatment of nocturnal enuresis—where are we now? Pediatrics 92: 465–466, 1993.

Treatment of childhood enuresis. Clin. Pediatr. 32: 1993. (Entire issue.)

Rushton, H. G. Nocturnal enuresis: epidemiology, evaluation and currently available treatment options. J. Pediatr. 114:691–696, 1989.

Warady, B. A., U. Alon, and S. Hellerstein. Primary nocturnal enuresis: current concepts about an old problem. Pediatr. Ann. 20:246–255, 1991.

CHAPTER 33

ENCOPRESIS

Carol D. Berkowitz, M.D.

H$_x$ A seven-year-old boy presents with the complaint of soiling his underpants. His mother states that he has never been completely toilet trained, and that stooling accidents occur at least two to three times a week, mainly during the day. The boy rarely has a spontaneous bowel movement without assistance. He sits on the toilet for just a few minutes and has small pelletlike stools. His mother has never sought medical care before for this problem.

The boy is very fidgety during the physical examination. The vital signs are normal and the child's height and weight are at the 25th percentile. His abdomen is soft but distended, with palpable loops of stool-filled bowel. A small amount of stool is present around the anus and in the boy's underpants. Digital examination of the rectum reveals hard stool. The rectal tone is normal as is the rest of the physical examination.

Questions

1. What is the definition of encopresis?
2. What is the difference between retentive and nonretentive encopresis?
3. What are some physiologic conditions that contribute to encopresis?
4. What conditions may be mistaken for encopresis?

Encopresis is the repeated passage of stool, either voluntary or involuntary, in children who should be toilet trained on the basis of age and developmental level and who have no primary organic pathology. The term "encopresis," which was originally used for children with psychogenic soiling, is similar to enuresis. Now encopresis is used in a broader sense to refer to all types of fecal incontinence.

Retentive encopresis occurs in the face of constipation (obstipation) in which chronic rectal distention leads to the seepage of liquid stool around hard, retained feces. Sometimes this is called overflow soiling. The onset of symptoms is usually about four years of age. Approximately 95% of cases of encopresis are retentive. **Nonretentive encopresis** is characterized by the passage of soft stool without colonic distention or retention of stool. Primary encopresis occurs when children have never been completely toilet trained. Secondary encopresis occurs in children who have had a period of complete continence of stool. The majority of encopretic children have secondary encopresis.

EPIDEMIOLOGY

Encopresis is reported in approximately 2% of eight-year-old boys and about 0.7% of eight-year-old girls, making the condition three times more prevalent in boys than in girls. This sex ratio reverses in the elderly, in which the prevalence of encopresis is twice as high in females as in males. An association between encopresis, enuresis, and ADHD is sometimes present. About 15% of children with enuresis also have encopresis. Family history for encopresis may also be positive; 16% of affected children have one affected parent, usually the father. An association between encopresis and child sexual abuse has been reported in a small number of children.

CLINICAL PRESENTATION

Children with encopresis have a history of staining of the underpants, which may be hidden in drawers or under beds by embarrassed children. Occasionally

Encopresis

- Incontinence of stool
- Constipation
- Hyperactivity
- Distended abdomen
- Stool-filled loops of bowel
- Lax rectal tone

parents are unaware of the problem. Stooling accidents occur more frequently at home than in school. Some children have a history of constipation (D$_x$ Box).

PATHOPHYSIOLOGY

A history of constipation, often with painful defecation, is associated with retentive encopresis. With time, the colon distends and liquid feces seep around impacted stool (Fig. 33–1). In 30 to 50% of children, anal spasm, referred to as animus, occurs. In another 40%, rectal hyposensitivity is apparent so that the children are unaware of the presence of the stool. Some children have an evacuation release disorder, in which the presence of the stool does not result in relaxation and stool evacuation. In such cases, the rectum is chronically

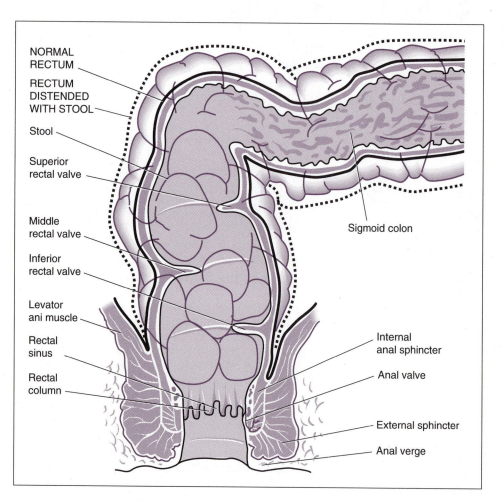

NORMAL RECTUM
RECTUM DISTENDED WITH STOOL
Stool
Superior rectal valve
Middle rectal valve
Inferior rectal valve
Levator ani muscle
Rectal sinus
Rectal column

Sigmoid colon

Internal anal sphincter
Anal valve
External sphincter
Anal verge

FIGURE 33–1. *Diagram of the rectum, anal canal, and sigmoid colon distended with stool.*

distended by stool. Water is absorbed and the stool becomes harder and drier. The distended rectum fails to sense the presence of the stool. When evacuation is attempted, the process is painful, leading to further retention (see Chapter 82, Constipation).

Encopresis has been associated with a short attention span and a high level of motor activity. Affected children are unable to sit on a toilet for more than a few minutes and do not adequately attend to the task of stool evacuation. As a result, they get off the toilet after the incomplete evacuation of only small amounts of stool. In some toddlers, constipation is related to the struggle of toilet training and an unwillingness to sit on the toilet (see Chapter 25, Toilet Training).

The pathophysiology of nonretentive encopresis appears to be psychogenic. Some children who have been chronically sexually abused have lax anal tone, which may contribute to the fecal incontinence.

DIFFERENTIAL DIAGNOSIS

The differential diagnosis of encopresis focuses on organic conditions associated with chronic constipation. These conditions include Hirschsprung's disease, disorders of intestinal motility (e.g., pseudo-obstruction), disorders of anal tone and anal anatomy (e.g., imperforate anus with fistula), disorders of the lumbosacral spine (e.g., meningomyelocele), and previous surgeries (e.g., repair of imperforate anus). Congenital anorectal anomalies, which are reported in 1 in 5000 live births, are rare.

Most of these conditions can be ruled out on the basis of a careful history and physical examination. In some cases, specific testing such as anal manometry or rectal biopsy may be necessary to exclude a particular disorder.

EVALUATION

History

The age of onset of the problem should be determined. In general, affected children are four years of age and older. A detailed history of the stooling pattern should be obtained (Questions Box). The frequency and consistency of stools as well as quantity of stools should also be noted. In addition, the presence of nocturnal episodes of encopresis should be determined. In cases of secondary encopresis, the duration of fecal continence and the occurrence of any events such as the birth of a sibling or the start of school

---

Questions: Encopresis

- Does the child have spontaneous bowel movements (without enemas or suppositories)? If so, how frequently?
- Does the child have large, dry, hard stools that clog the toilet?
- Does the child have a history of enuresis or ADHD?
- What is the pattern of encopresis (i.e., is the encopresis primary or secondary)?
- What happens to the child's stained underwear?

---

that may have precipitated the episodes of encopresis should be noted. Some children experience the onset of encopresis when they start school. Because of "toilet phobia," they are unwilling to use the public toilet in the school setting.

Physical Examination

The next step involves the performance of a comprehensive physical examination, paying particular attention to the abdomen to check for the presence of distended, stool-filled loops of bowel. The rectal area should be assessed for rectal tone and the presence of hard stool. Children with retentive encopresis have normal or tight anal tone on rectal examination because they are frequently contracting their external anal sphincter to prevent the seepage of the liquid stool.

Abnormalities around the anus such as fistula should also be noted. The underpants should be evaluated for the presence of stool, mucus, or pus. A sensory and motor examination of the lower extremities helps determine if any signs of spinal cord dysfunction are evident. An evaluation of the skin over the spinal area may reveal abnormalities such as sacral dimples or tufts of hair.

Children who do not exhibit abdominal distention may have soft stool on rectal examination, which indicates nonretentive encopresis. If patulous anal tone is noted, spinal cord abnormalities or prior child sexual abuse should be suspected.

Diagnostic Tests

Most children with encopresis require few laboratory studies. Anorectal manometry, which may be used to measure the pressure generated by the anal sphincter, may also reveal abnormalities of anal tone or evidence of aganglionosis. The Child Behavioral Checklist is useful to determine if certain behavior problems exist. Such problems may either potentiate the encopresis or result from it.

Imaging Studies

In most encopretic children, imaging studies are not necessary. If x-rays of the abdomen are taken in children with retentive encopresis, distended, stool-filled bowel may be noted. A barium enema is useful if Hirschsprung's disease is to be ruled out. EMG to determine whether the innervation of the external anal sphincter is intact is recommended for children with encopresis who fail to respond to routine treatment.

MANAGEMENT

The management of encopresis focuses on patient education and counseling. **Dietary manipulation** is important. Parents should be told that children require a high-fiber diet with decreased milk (≤ 16 oz per day) and fruit juices such as pear or peach. It has been suggested that a "team and coach" approach is the most successful route, and that bowel training be likened to "fitness training."

The **pharmacologic management** of retentive encopresis involves an adequate cleanout of retained stools using mineral oil and laxatives. The decision about which laxatives to use depends on the degree of constipation. If the degree of fecal retention is mild, a high-fiber diet and stool-bulking agents or oral laxatives such as senna derivatives or bisacodyl may be used in association with stool softeners or lubricants such as mineral oil. The amount of mineral oil may be titrated up to ensure success. Some practitioners recommend that mineral oil be given until it oozes from the rectum. The amount may then be titrated back to a lower level.

If the degree of retention is more severe, suppositories or enemas may be needed. Occasionally, children have to be disimpacted manually. Alternative methods to manual disimpaction include two to three sodium phosphate enemas over one to two days or eight ounces of mineral oil a day for four days. Once the fecal accumulation has been relieved, every effort should be made to keep children regular. This can be accomplished with the combined use of toilet retraining, stool softeners or laxatives, and enemas or suppositories.

The toilet retraining process requires that children sit on the toilet at least two or three times a day, usually after meals, for about 10 minutes or until they have had a bowel movement. Some practitioners recommend the use of an egg timer to ensure that children spend the appropriate amount of time on the toilet. Children should be requested to maintain a diary of their evacuation, which may take the form of a star chart. Stars or other rewards are given for successful bowel movements in the toilet. Spontaneous bowel movements should be rewarded with stars or other acknowledgments.

If children skip a day between bowel movements, they may be treated with a suppository, such as a glycerin or a bisacodyl suppository. If they still have not succeeded in having a bowel movement, then an enema may be appropriate. This sequence should be maintained until children are having bowel movements in the toilet and not soiling for at least one month. In general, stool softeners are required for at least three to six months. The regimen may have to be modified, particularly in younger children.

Behavior modification and biofeedback are two other modalities that can be used to help manage encopresis. Consultation with specialists such as pediatric gastroenterologists may be required.

Thirty percent of children with encopresis may need psychological consultation. Children with evidence of child sexual abuse or nonretentive encopresis should be referred to a psychologist early in the course of therapy. The underlying psychosocial problems of children with nonretentive encopresis must be adequately addressed before their condition can improve.

PROGNOSIS

The prognosis for children with retentive encopresis is reportedly good with appropriate intervention. It is estimated that about two thirds of affected children experience long-lasting remission within six months of the initiation of medical management, and another 30% are considerably improved.

The prognosis for children with nonretentive encopresis is less predictable and highly dependent on the underlying psychopathology.

Case Resolution

In the case scenario, the boy exhibits typical manifestations of retentive encopresis. His condition should be managed with the use of laxatives, stool softeners, and toilet retraining with a star chart. The possible ADHD should be addressed separately but may be contributing to his inability to attend to the task of toileting.

Selected Readings

Howe, A. C., and C. E. Walker. Behavioral management of toilet training, enuresis, and encopresis. Pediatr. Clin. North Am. 39:413–432, 1992.

Loening-Baucke, V. Modulation of abnormal defecation dynamics by biofeedback treatment in chronically constipated children with encopresis. J. Pediatr. 116:214–222, 1990.

Madoff, R. D., J. G. Williams, and P. F. Caushaj. Fecal incontinence. N. Engl. J. Med. 326:1002–1007, 1992.

Nolan, T., and F. Oberklaid. New concepts in the management of encopresis. Pediatr. Rev. 14:447–451, 1993.

Partin, J. C., et al. Painful defecation and fecal soiling in children. Pediatrics 89:1007–1009, 1992.

Schmitt, B. D. Soiling with constipation in the school-age child. Contemp. Pediatr. 9:75–78, 1992.

Schmitt, B. D. Soiling without constipation. Contemp. Pediatr. 9:69–70, 1992.

Schmitt, B. D., and R. D. Mauro. Twenty common errors in treating encopresis. Contemp. Pediatr. 9:47–65, May 1992.

ACUTE AND EMERGENT PROBLEMS

CHAPTER 34

FEVER AND BACTEREMIA

Geeta Grover, M.D.

H$_x$ An eight-month-old girl is brought to the emergency department with a two-day history of fever and increased fussiness. She is irritable but consolable by parents. On examination, she has a rectal temperature of 103.1° F (39.5° C). The rest of the physical examination is within normal limits, and no source for the fever is apparent.

Questions

1. How does the height of fever influence the evaluation and management of infants and young children with fever?
2. What, if any, laboratory studies are required in the evaluation of infants with fever?
3. What are the management options for children with fever of unknown source? How does clinical appearance affect management?

Normothermia, which is equivalent to a body temperature of 98.6° F (37.0° C), is the result of the delicate balance of heat gain and heat loss that allows the body to maintain a constant core temperature. Mean body temperature exhibits a diurnal variation, with a peak in the early evening (approximately 6 PM) and a nadir in the early morning (approximately 6 AM). With fever, the central thermostat of the body increases to a new "set point," and heat loss and heat gain are again balanced at this higher temperature. Fever is not a disease but a nonspecific symptom of some underlying condition or process that involves inflammation. Although there is no consensus regarding the exact temperature that denotes fever, it is generally accepted that a rectal temperature of at least 100.4° F (38.0° C) represents a fever.

Bacteremia is the presence of bacteria in the blood. **Occult bacteremia** is bacteremia in children with a benign clinical appearance and no apparent source of serious infections (e.g., pneumonia, UTI). **Septicemia** is the presence of microorganisms in the blood with localized or systemic disease in an ill-appearing child.

EPIDEMIOLOGY

Children in the first two to three years of life have approximately six to ten infectious illnesses each year. Thus fever is one of the most common presenting complaints seen in children. Up to one third of outpatient visits by children to both emergency departments and private practitioners are for fever. By some estimates, 20 to 30% of after-hours calls to pediatricians concern fever.

The risk of serious bacterial illness (SBI) in infants under three months of age with fever is generally believed to be higher than in older infants with fever. For the purposes of this discussion, SBIs include meningitis, bacteremia, UTI, osteomyelitis, septic arthritis, pneumonia, bacterial gastroenteritis, and serious skin and soft tissue infections (e.g., cellulitis, adenitis). In febrile infants (rectal temperature ≥ 100.4° F [38.0° C]) under three months of age, the prevalence of SBI is approximately 5 to 9%, whereas the prevalence of occult bacteremia is about 3 to 4%. Historical, physical, and laboratory criteria may help to identify infants at low risk for SBI (Table 34–1). The organisms commonly implicated in SBI in this age group are presented in Table 34–2. Although group B streptococci and *Escherichia coli* account for the vast majority of infections, other pathogens such as *Salmonella* spp. are important after the first month of life.

The risk of occult bacteremia in children 3 to 36 months of age with fever without localizing signs (FWLS) is approximately 3 to 5%. Occult bacteremia occurs with about the same frequency both in children with FWLS and in children with fever who are the same age and have common childhood infections that are usually treated on an outpatient basis (e.g., otitis media, pharyngitis). Factors increasing the risk of bacteremia are young age, high fever, and high WBC count. Authorities estimate that approximately 10% of children with temperatures over 102.2° F (39.0° C), WBC counts over 15,000/μL, and no focus of infection have bacteremia. Hyperpyrexia (temperature > 106.0° F [41.1° C]) has been associated with an increased incidence of bacteremia and meningitis. *Streptococcus pneumoniae*

TABLE 34–1. The Rochester Criteria for Evaluation of Febrile Infants Aged 60 Days or Less*

Low Risk Factors for SBI

Infant appears generally well
Infant has been previously healthy
   Born at term (≥37 weeks' gestation)
   Did not receive perinatal antimicrobial therapy
   Was not treated for unexplained hyperbilirubinemia
   Had not received and was not receiving antimicrobial agents
   Had not been previously hospitalized
   Had no chronic or underlying illness
   Was not hospitalized longer than mother
No evidence of skin, soft tissue, bone, joint, or ear infection
Laboratory values
   Peripheral WBC count: 5000–15,000/μL
   Absolute band count: ≤1500/μL
   Urinalysis WBC count: ≤10/hpf on microscopic examination of a spun urine sediment
   Stool WBC count: ≤5/hpf on microscopic examination of a stool smear (only for infants with diarrhea)

*Rectal temperature ≥100.4° F (38.0° C).
Abbreviations: SBI, serious bacterial infection; hpf, high-power field; WBC, white blood cell.
Reproduced, with permission, from Jaskiewicz, J.A., et al. Febrile infants at low risk for serious bacterial infection—an appraisal of the Rochester Criteria and implications for management. Pediatrics 94:390–396, 1994.

accounts for 70 to 90% of cases of occult bacteremia. *Haemophilus influenzae* and *Neisseria meningitidis* cause about 5 to 20% and 5% of cases, respectively (see Table 34–2).

CLINICAL PRESENTATION

In some febrile children fever may be the only complaint, and these children otherwise look fine and behave normally. Other children with fever may appear less interactive, quieter, and less energetic than children of the same age without fever. Appetite decreases, and children may become more fussy. Because young children, especially infants under three months of age, have fewer and more subtle behavioral signs when febrile, physicians must maintain a high index of suspicion for SBI even in the absence of localizing signs. Physical findings associated with fever include flushed cheeks; hot, dry skin; shivering (uncommon in young infants); cool distal extremities; tachycardia; and tachypnea (D$_x$ Box). Occult bacteremia, by definition, has no additional abnormal physical manifestations.

TABLE 34–2. Organisms Implicated in Serious Bacterial Infection/Occult Bacteremia in Children

Infants Less Than 3 Months of Age

Group B streptococcus
Escherichia coli
Listeria monocytogenes
Salmonella species (infants > 1 month of age)
*Haemophilus influenzae** (infants > 1 month of age)

Children Between 3 and 36 Months of Age

Streptococcus pneumoniae
H. influenzae type B (Hib)*
Neisseria meningitidis

*The incidence of Hib disease is decreasing significantly with the wide use of conjugate Hib vaccines, which began in 1987.

D$_x$ Serious Bacterial Illness

- Lethargy, irritability, or change in mental status
- Tachycardia disproportionate to the degree of temperature elevation
- Tachypnea or labored respirations
- Bulging or depressed anterior fontanelle
- Nuchal rigidity
- Petechiae
- Localized erythema, pain, or swelling
- Abdominal or flank pain
- Fever

PATHOPHYSIOLOGY

Fever is an elevation in the thermoregulatory set point of the body. The thermoregulatory center is located in the preoptic region of the anterior hypothalamus, and an elevation in the hypothalamic set point above the normal body temperature initiates the physiologic changes that lead to fever. Exogenous pyrogens (e.g., bacteria, viruses, antigen-antibody complexes) stimulate host inflammatory cells (e.g., macrophages, polymorphonuclear cells) to produce endogenous pyrogens (EPs). Interleukin-1 is currently regarded as the prototypical EP. EPs cause the hypothalamic endothelium to increase intermediary substances such as prostaglandins and neurotransmitters, which then act on the preoptic neurons of the anterior hypothalamus to produce an elevated set point. The body uses physiologic mechanisms (e.g., peripheral vasoconstriction, shivering) and behavioral actions (e.g., bundling up, drinking hot tea) to increase body temperature to reach and maintain this higher set point, thus producing fever (Fig. 34–1).

In contrast, the thermoregulatory set point of the body is normal in hyperthermia. Due to abnormal physiologic processes, heat gain exceeds heat loss, and the body temperature rises in spite of efforts to return to the control set point.

DIFFERENTIAL DIAGNOSIS

In the vast majority of cases, the duration of fever in children is short, and signs and symptoms are localized. FWLS is an acute episode of fever that lasts one week or less in children in whom history, physical examination, and preliminary laboratory tests fail to find a source. The majority of children with FWLS are eventually found to have acute, generally self-limited, infectious illnesses. Occult bacteremia is a major concern in young children with FWLS, primarily in infants less than 36 months of age. High-risk factors for occult bacteremia are presented in Table 34–3. Fever of unknown origin (FUO) is fever of at least eight days' duration in infants or children in whom routine history, physical examination, and laboratory assessment fail to reveal a source.

The differential diagnosis of children with an acute febrile illness is primarily infectious (Table 34–4), in-

FIGURE 34–1. *Pathophysiology of fever production. Antipyretics work by blocking the synthesis of PGE₂.*

cluding both benign, generally self-limited illness such as URI, and less common, more serious illness such as meningitis and osteomyelitis. Occasionally, a child with FWLS turns out to have a noninfectious illness such as a collagen vascular disease or neoplasia. By comparison, the differential diagnosis of children with FUO is quite broad (Table 34–5) and contains both infectious and noninfectious disorders.

EVALUATION

History

The medical history can provide a great deal of valuable information in the evaluation of children with

---

TABLE 34–3. Risk Factors for Occult Bacteremia

Age ≤ 36 months
Temperature ≥ 103.1° F (39.5° C)
White blood cells ≥ 15,000/μL or ≤ 5000/μL
Total band cells ≥ 500/μL
Erythrocyte sedimentation rate ≥ 30 mm/hr
Underlying chronic disease (malignancy, immunodeficiency, sickle cell disease, malnutrition)
Clinical appearance (irritability, lethargy, toxic appearance)

TABLE 34–4. Common Infectious Causes of an Acute Episode of Fever in Children

Upper Respiratory Tract
Upper respiratory infection (common cold)
Otitis media
Sinusitis

Pulmonary
Bronchiolitis
Pneumonia

Oral Cavity
Gingivostomatitis
Pharyngitis
Dental abscess

Gastrointestinal Tract
Acute gastroenteritis (bacterial or viral)
Appendicitis

Genitourinary Tract
Urinary tract infection
Pyelonephritis

Musculoskeletal
Septic arthritis
Osteomyelitis

Central Nervous System
Meningitis

Miscellaneous (including noninfectious causes)
Bacteremia
Immunization reaction
Viral exanthems (e.g., chickenpox, measles)
Neoplasia
Collagen vascular disease

TABLE 34–5. Common Causes of Fever of Unknown Origin (FUO) in Children*

Infectious Diseases
Bacterial
  Localized infection: mastoiditis, sinusitis, pneumonia, osteomyelitis, pyelonephritis, abscess (e.g., abdominal, pelvic)
  Systemic disease: tuberculosis, brucellosis, salmonellosis, leptospirosis, tularemia
Viral
  Hepatitis viruses
  Cytomegalovirus
  Epstein-Barr virus (infectious mononucleosis)
  Human immunodeficiency virus
Fungal
  Disseminated coccidioidomycosis
  Disseminated histoplasmosis
Miscellaneous
  Malaria
  Rocky Mountain spotted fever
  Syphilis
  Lyme disease

Neoplasia
Leukemia
Lymphoma
Hodgkin's disease
Neuroblastoma

Collagen Vascular Diseases
Juvenile rheumatoid arthritis
Systemic lupus erythematosus
Rheumatic fever

Miscellaneous
Inflammatory bowel diseases
Kawasaki disease
Thyroiditis
Drugs
Factitious fever

*For a complete discussion of FUO, the reader is referred to Lorin, M.I., and R.D. Feigin. Fever of unknown origin. *In* Feigin, R.D., and J.D. Cherry (eds.). *Textbook of Pediatric Infectious Diseases*, 3rd ed. Philadelphia, W.B. Saunders, 1992, pp. 1012–1022.

fever (Questions Box). The history should focus on the duration and severity of the fever. The presence of associated symptoms that may be signs of specific organ system involvement should also be noted.

Physical Examination

Vital signs provide important diagnostic clues. The effect of fever on the heart and respiratory rates should be noted. The heart rate increases by 10 beats per minute for each degree Fahrenheit of temperature elevation above normal (98.6° F). Tachycardia disproportionate to the degree of temperature elevation may suggest dehydration or sepsis. Tachypnea, which is often the only sign of a respiratory infection, may also be seen in response to metabolic acidosis (most commonly secondary to sepsis or shock). These changes may be clues to an occult focus.

Observation of the overall hydration and well-being of children is extremely important. An attempt should be made to determine whether children are behaving and responding in an age-appropriate fashion. Physicians should look for spontaneous movements, negative responses to adverse stimuli, and positive responses to pleasant stimuli.

In addition, all febrile children should receive a complete physical examination. This is important even when the history may suggest involvement of one organ system. For example, in young children, vomiting and fever may often be the only signs of a UTI, and the problem is not necessarily gastroenteritis, as suggested by the history. The condition may go undiagnosed unless a thorough examination, including evaluation of the urine, is performed.

Growth parameters should be measured. Weight loss, although nonspecific, can be an important finding.

The anterior fontanelle should be palpated. It may be normal, bulging as a result of CNS infection or congestive heart failure, or depressed secondary to dehydration. The ears should be examined carefully; pneumatic otoscopy should be used. Careful inspection may reveal

the source of fever, especially in children under the age of three years. The occurrence of otitis media should not preclude further workup for invasive bacterial disease in children who do not appear well. The oropharynx should also be examined. Dry or "tacky" mucous membranes may provide clues to dehydration. Enlarged, inflamed, or exudative tonsils often signal the presence of a group A streptococcal infection, especially in children who are 5 to 10 years of age. Epstein-Barr and adenoviral infections should also be considered in such cases. Respiratory symptoms such as labored respirations, retractions, nasal flaring, stridor, rales, rhonchi, or wheezing may all be clues to respiratory tract infections. Enanthems on the buccal mucosa, or exanthems on the skin, are often signs of viral infections.

The presence of petechiae in association with fever indicates serious underlying infection. Children with such conditions should receive a comprehensive evaluation. Localized areas of pain, erythema, swelling, or all of these signs may point to cellulitis, septic arthritis, or osteomyelitis. Nuchal rigidity, if present, can be an important clue to the presence of meningitis. Because it is rarely present in infants under two years of age, physicians must maintain a high index of suspicion for meningitis in children of this age.

Two groups of children require special attention: (1) infants under three months of age and (2) infants and young children 3 to 36 months of age with FWLS. Determining the cause of fever in young infants can be diagnostically challenging. Nonspecific signs and symptoms such as irritability, increased fussiness, feeding intolerance, or mild respiratory distress may be the only clues to the presence of SBI. Elevated rectal temperatures in children in this age group should not be attributed to overbundling.

The evaluation of children 3 to 36 months of age with FWLS should be guided by clinical appearance and the criteria for occult bacteremia (see Table 34–3). Neither the infants' response to antipyretics nor improvement in clinical status after defervescence helps in predicting bacteremia.

Thorough and repeat physical examinations are important in the evaluation of children with FUO. For these reasons, children with FUO are often hospitalized for workup. Significant weight loss may be suggestive of a chronic illness such as inflammatory bowel disease. Joint pain or rashes may be signs of collagen vascular disease. A rectal examination should be performed to look for tenderness, which may be indicative of an abdominal or pelvic abscess.

Laboratory Tests

Infants less than three years of age with fever should receive a thorough laboratory assessment, including a CBC, blood culture, urinalysis and urine culture, and lumbar puncture. If bacterial gastroenteritis is suspected, a stool smear should be examined for the presence of WBCs. At present, no single laboratory test can accurately predict the likelihood of bacteremia in febrile children.

Older infants and children may be classified as either low or high risk for SBI or occult bacteremia based on overall clinical impression, history, and physical examination. Routine laboratory assessment may not be required for low-risk children, but high-risk children should at least have a CBC and blood culture. The CBC provides additional information that can aid in the decision of whether or not to obtain further laboratory or imaging studies.

A focus of infection in an ill-appearing child should not prevent further workup. In addition, the laboratory assessment of children with fever and petechiae should be aggressive, because the incidence of invasive bacterial disease is 8 to 20% and the incidence of meningococcal meningitis or sepsis is 7 to 10%.

All children with FUO should have a CBC. Other appropriate initial screening laboratory studies include tuberculin skin testing, blood and urine cultures, chest radiograph, ESR, or C-reactive protein and liver enzymes.

Imaging Studies

Routine imaging studies, except for chest radiography, are not usually necessary. Chest radiographs should be performed in febrile infants under three months of age with respiratory symptoms. In older infants and children, chest radiographs should be obtained if lower respiratory tract signs (e.g., wheezing, rales) of pulmonary disease are present. Other imaging studies, such as bone or gallium scans, may be performed if indicated.

MANAGEMENT

Management of children with fever includes both controlling the fever and treating the underlying process causing the fever. There is no evidence that fever itself is harmful. To the contrary, animal studies have suggested that fever may have some survival advantage.

Despite the possible beneficial effects of fever, febrile children may still feel uncomfortable. Fever should be reduced to relieve the associated discomfort and malaise. **Antipyretics** such as acetaminophen and ibuprofen can be used. Aspirin should be avoided in children because of the association with Reye's syndrome and viral illnesses. **Sponging** or **bathing** with tepid water and **unbundling** children aid in fever reduction. Ice water or alcohol baths should be avoided.

Some authorities have argued that fever should be reduced in an effort to prevent febrile seizures. However, the occurrence of such seizures is related more to the rapidity of rise in temperature than the height of the temperature itself. In addition, febrile seizures usually occur at the onset of a febrile illness before the need for antipyretics is even realized (see Chapter 35, Febrile Seizures).

Any focal bacterial infection should be treated with appropriate antimicrobial therapy. In the absence of a focal infection, management of febrile children depends on age. Infants under one month should be hospitalized for observation and administered **intravenous antibi-**otics pending culture results. Infants between one and three months can be managed safely at home if they satisfy the following criteria: (1) they do not have symptoms of serious infection, (2) results of their laboratory tests are within normal limits, and (3) reliable follow-up is assured.

Ill-appearing children between 3 and 36 months of age with FWLS who are suspected of having an SBI should be hospitalized for repeat assessments and intravenous antibiotics. However, if children appear well but have a risk for SBI based on high-risk factors (see Table 34–3), empiric outpatient **ceftriaxone** therapy (50 mg/kg intramuscularly) can be considered. Individual assessment of risk for bacteremia is necessary. Such therapy is not an alternative to hospitalization for children who appear clinically ill. Before administering ceftriaxone, a minimal laboratory workup, including CBC, blood culture, and urinalysis and urine culture should be performed. A lumbar puncture is highly recommended, especially in infants under one year of age. A chest radiograph may be performed if clinically appropriate.

In febrile children over the age of 36 months, expectant antibiotics are generally not indicated. Children of any age who are at high risk for SBI include those with fever and petechiae, immunocompromised children (e.g., children with HIV, malignancy, sickle cell disease) and children with some types of congenital heart disease (e.g., cyanotic lesions). These children require an intensive evaluation and often the institution of expectant antibiotic therapy before a pathogen is isolated.

PROGNOSIS

Occult bacteremia may resolve without therapy and have no sequelae, but it may persist or produce localized infections such as meningitis or septic arthritis. In bacteremic children who do not receive antimicrobial therapy, the risk of persistent bacteremia is approximately 20%, and the risk of meningitis is about 10%. These risks vary depending on which organism is isolated from the blood. In general, the risk of developing serious sequelae is greater with bacteremia caused by *H. influenzae* compared to *S. pneumoniae* (25% vs. 6%).

Case Resolution

The infant presented in the case history is irritable and has a high fever of unknown source. She should receive a thorough history and physical examination in addition to a complete laboratory assessment, including a lumbar puncture. Management should be based on reassessment after all laboratory data are available. If laboratory assessment reveals a focus of infection such as a UTI, she should be managed with antibiotics. If laboratory assessment fails to reveal a source for the fever, she can receive an intramuscular injection of ceftriaxone as expectant management for occult bacteremia and be reevaluated in 24 hours or be managed without antibiotics.

Selected Readings

Baraff, L. J., et al. Practice guidelines for the management of infants and children 0 to 36 months of age with fever without source. Pediatrics 92:1–12, 1993.

Dinarello, C. A., and S. M. Wolff. Pathogenesis of fever in man. N. Engl. J. Med. 298:607–612, 1978.

Grover, G., et al. The effects of bundling on infant temperature. Pediatrics 94:669–673, 1994.

Jaskeiwicz, J. A., et al. Febrile infants at low risk for serious bacterial infection—an appraisal of the Rochester Criteria and implications for management. Pediatrics 94:390–396, 1994.

Kluger, M. J. Fever revisited. Pediatrics 90:846–850, 1992.

Lorin, M. I., and R. D. Feigin. Fever of unknown origin. *In* Feigin, R. D., and J. D. Cherry (eds.). *Textbook of Pediatric Infectious Diseases*, 3rd ed. Philadelphia, W. B. Saunders, 1992, pp. 1012–1022.

Nizet, V., R. J. Vinci, and F. H. Lovejoy. Fever in children. Pediatr. Rev. 15:127–135, 1994.

Powell, K. R. (ed.). Management of febrile infants and children. Pediatr. Ann. 22:459–504, 1993. (Collection of articles on fever.)

CHAPTER 35

FEBRILE SEIZURES

Kenneth R. Huff, M.D.

H$_x$ A 20-month-old girl is brought to the emergency department by paramedics because she is having a seizure. She is unresponsive and hypertonic, with arched trunk and extended arms and legs that are jerking rhythmically. Her eyes are open, but her gaze is directed upward. She has bubbles of saliva around her lips as well as circumoral cyanosis. Her vital signs are respiratory rate, 60/min; heart rate, 125 beats/min; blood pressure, 130/78; and temperature, 105.8° F (41.0° C). Her respirations are grunting. An assessment of her respiratory status discloses that she is moving air in all lung fields, and there is no evidence of upper airway obstruction.

The paramedics inform you that the girl has been convulsing for approximately six minutes. A Dextrostix reveals a normal serum glucose. Blood samples for other blood tests are sent to the laboratory, and urine is collected. An intravenous line is started, and the girl is given lorazepam by intravenous push. Within two minutes, her movements cease, and her respirations become slow and even. Her physical examination shows no signs of trauma. Her only abnormality other than her unresponsive mental status is an inflamed and bulging right tympanic membrane.

The girl's parents tell you that she has had a mildly stuffy nose for two days, but has been afebrile and has seemed to be her usual self. While she was playing, she became cranky, and her parents put her in her crib for her nap. Thirty minutes later they heard grunting noises, found her in the midst of a seizure, and called the paramedics. The girl has never had a seizure before. Her father recalls that his mother once told him that he had several "fever seizures" as an infant.

Questions

1. What are the characteristics of simple febrile seizures?
2. What is the appropriate evaluation of children with febrile seizures, whether it is the first one or a recurrence?
3. What is the risk of recurrence of nonfebrile seizures following a febrile seizure?
4. What are the treatment options for children with febrile seizures?

Febrile seizures are easily recognized, dramatic, generalized convulsions. These seizures are associated with the presence of a fever (often sudden) from a source outside the nervous system; age of less than five years; and absence of chronic brain pathology, including developmental delay; and the absence of acute or chronic chemical or structural aberrations of the brain. Frequently, familial predisposition to such seizures plays a role. Despite the relatively uniform presentation of the seizure, individual clinical variables and social factors may affect the treatment and prognosis.

EPIDEMIOLOGY

Febrile seizures occur in children between the ages of six months and five years but are more common in those who are less than three years of age. Some studies indicate that as many as 5% of all children experience at least one febrile seizure. The recurrence rate is 30 to 50% in children less than one year of age, but drops to 25% between one and three years, and is only 12% after three years. Seizures usually occur with an increase in fever, and often so suddenly that the febrile illness is not recognized by the family before the seizure. Frequently the febrile illness is eventually diagnosed as a URI. The multigenerational familial history that is often seen suggests an autosomal dominant form of genetic transmission.

Dx Febrile Seizures

- Sudden unresponsiveness, tonic posturing, and generalized rhythmic jerking
- Fever source outside nervous system
- Age six months to five years
- Normal neurodevelopmental history

TABLE 35–1. Simple Versus Complex Febrile Seizures

Feature	Simple	Complex
Onset of clonic movements	Generalized	Focal
Duration	< 15 minutes (usually < 90 seconds)	> 15 minutes
Number of seizures/ febrile illnesses	1	Repetitive
Interictal neurologic examination	Normal	Abnormal
Subsequent EEG result	Normal	Abnormal
Family history	Positive for febrile seizures	Positive for afebrile seizures
Developmental history	Normal	Variable

CLINICAL PRESENTATION

Febrile seizures are characterized by generalized, symmetric, tonic posturing and clonic movements of a few minutes' duration that occur suddenly in children whose developmental progress is normal. Fever is present, although it may not have been recognized before the seizure, and its source is outside the nervous system. Within a few hours of the seizure, children become neurologically well (Dx Box).

PATHOPHYSIOLOGY

The susceptibility of young children to febrile seizures may be related to an increased incidence of sudden high fevers in this age group, a developmental genetic factor that may lower the seizure threshold, or both. A sudden increase in temperature to a sufficiently high level can provoke seizures regardless of age. Seizures occur more frequently with fever in many seizure-prone patients who have epilepsies of different etiologies. Perhaps circulating pyrogens interact with a brain cellular circuitry mechanism, causing hypersynchronous depolarization and a seizure. Both the definition of the genetic marker and the mechanism of generalized seizures are not yet fully understood.

DIFFERENTIAL DIAGNOSIS

When a young child presents with a fever and a seizure, the possibility that the seizure is symptomatic of meningitis, encephalitis, or (rarely) subarachnoid hemorrhage must be ruled out. Signs of meningeal irritation may not be reliable in children less than 18 months, and these and other signs of the illness may be obscured in the postictal period. The fever may be coincidental to a seizure of different etiology such as trauma, toxic ingestion, metabolic derangement, degenerative or neurocutaneous disorder, or stroke. It should be determined whether children in the appropriate age range have had a true febrile seizure or a "seizure with fever," which may be an early fever-provoked episode of a nonfebrile seizure disorder. The length of a seizure with fever is greater than 15 minutes. In contrast, most febrile seizures last less than 90 seconds, although a significant number of episodes that otherwise satisfy the definition of "febrile seizure" present as status epilepticus. In children with otherwise typical febrile seizures, the presence of any of the following four factors leads to the diagnosis of "complex febrile seizure" (Table 35–1): (1) more than one febrile seizure during the same infectious illness, (2) abnormal interictal EEG, (3) history of a focal onset or presence of focal neurologic signs following a febrile seizure, and (4) presence of an abnormal neurodevelopmental history or examination before the seizure or abnormal neurologic examination or brain imaging study after the postictal period.

EVALUATION

History

After the seizure has been controlled and the child has been stabilized, a more detailed history relating to the circumstances of the seizure should be obtained (Questions Box).

Physical Examination

Children should be examined completely. Physicians should look for bruises, fractures, retinal hemorrhages, or other signs of trauma. The presence of dysmorphic features, enlarged organs, or bony changes should be noted. The skin should be examined for abnormal, pigmented spots. Lateralized signs of tone or strength should be assessed. An appropriate evaluation to determine the etiology of the fever should be performed (see Chapter 34, Fever and Bacteremia).

Questions: Febrile Seizures

- What were the child's symptoms a few days before the seizure?
- Where was the child and what was he or she doing just before the seizure?
- Were there any pregnancy-related or perinatal complications?
- Has the child's development been normal or similar to that of siblings?
- Have any other family members had seizures of any kind, including any when they were infants?

Laboratory Tests

If the seizure is prolonged or children still appear ill after the postictal period, metabolic and toxicologic laboratory studies on blood and urine should be performed. Appropriate metabolic blood tests may include glucose, electrolytes, and ammonia levels. If children recover rapidly, however, these tests have a low yield of abnormality. An examination of the CSF is necessary in cases of suspected meningitis. In cases of a first-time seizure, this diagnosis almost always needs to be suspected.

Imaging Studies

An EEG can be useful for prognosis, although some clinicians have not recommended this test in patients with uncomplicated febrile seizures. CT and MRI scans have a low yield of abnormal results in patients who previously have been neurodevelopmentally normal and have had a febrile seizure.

MANAGEMENT

If children are still convulsing on presentation and have been for at least five minutes, then they should be managed as for status epilepticus (see Chapter 113, Seizures and Epilepsy). The airway must be secure, blood tests drawn and sent to the laboratory, an intravenous line started, and lorazepam administered in the appropriate dose to stop the seizure.

If children are not in status epilepticus, management decisions are made on a more long-term basis. Whether to recommend **anticonvulsant prophylaxis** for children who have experienced febrile seizures is **controversial.** Factors that must be considered include (1) the benign, age-limited nature of the condition; (2) the morbidity of the anticonvulsant treatment; (3) the chance of recurrence of febrile or nonfebrile seizures; (4) the risk of overmedication during an acute recurrence; and (5) the family's reaction and social disruption caused by the seizures. Daily doses of phenobarbital or valproic acid are effective prophylactic anticonvulsants. Diazepam may be administered on an intermittent basis at the time fever is recognized (Table 35–2). The most commonly used regimen is daily phenobarbital, but its potential side effects include hyperactive behavior disorder and depressed cognition. Valproic acid may provoke acute liver dysfunction in children under the age of two years who are taking other medications.

Recommendations for prophylactic anticonvulsant treatment are often individualized. Anticonvulsants are reserved for those children who present with status epilepticus, respiratory compromise, or complex febrile seizures. Children who have frequently recurring seizures may also warrant anticonvulsant therapy if the seizures are extremely disruptive for the family and deleterious to parent-child interactions despite educational efforts by medical caretakers.

Intermittent anticonvulsant therapy depends on recognition of the fever before the seizure. Studies show

SIDE EFFECTS [margin annotation]

TABLE 35–2. Treatment Options for Febrile Seizures

Cooling measures during febrile illness (antipyretics or bathing in tepid water)
Family reassurance and education
Diazepam, 0.3 mg/kg PO q8h (during febrile illness only)
Phenobarbital, 3–5 mg/kg PO daily, for prophylaxis
Valproic acid, 30 mg/kg PO divided twice daily, for prophylaxis

that rigid fever control does not have a significant prophylactic effect on seizures, perhaps because of the dependency on awareness. In addition, fever control measures may subsequently reduce other symptoms of illness.

PROGNOSIS

The risk of recurrence of febrile seizures is higher in infants less than one year of age and lower in children over three years. Children who have febrile seizures are three to six times more likely to develop nonfebrile seizure disorders or epilepsy later in life. Many of these children have had complex febrile seizures, however. The prognosis for children with simple febrile seizures is generally good; they have no other neurologic episodes later in childhood.

Case Resolution

In the case history presented at the beginning of this chapter, the girl had a somewhat prolonged simple febrile seizure, a diagnosis supported by the positive family history. Her family is educated about treatment options. They became comfortable with a decision to use intermittent therapy with diazepam for her subsequent febrile illnesses, realizing that a fever may not be recognized before the seizure.

Selected Readings

Autret, E., et al. Double-blind, randomized trial of diazepam versus placebo for prevention of recurrence of febrile seizures. J. Pediatr. 117:490–494, 1990.

Berg, A. T., et al. Predictors of recurrent febrile seizures: a meta-analytic review. J. Pediatr. 116:329–337, 1990.

Farwell, J. R., et al. Phenobarbital for febrile seizures—effects on intelligence and on seizure recurrence. N. Engl. J. Med. 322:364–369, 1990.

McKinlay, I., and R. Newton. Intention to treat febrile convulsions with rectal diazepam, valproate, or phenobarbital. Dev. Med. Child Neurol. 31:617–625, 1989.

Nelson, K. B., and J. H. Ellenberg. Predictors of epilepsy in children who have experienced febrile seizures. N. Engl. J. Med. 295:1029–1033, 1976.

Nelson, K. B., and J. H. Ellenberg. Prognosis in children with febrile seizures. Pediatrics 61:720–727, 1978.

Rosman, N. P. A controlled trial of diazepam administered during febrile illnesses to prevent recurrence of febrile seizures. N. Engl. J. Med. 329:79–84, 1993.

CHAPTER 36

RESPIRATORY DISTRESS

James S. Seidel, M.D., Ph.D.

H$_x$ A six-month-old boy has been coughing and breathing fast for the past day. This morning he refused his bottle and has been irritable. On examination, the infant is fussy. He has a respiratory rate of 60 breaths/min, a pulse of 140/min, and a normal blood pressure and temperature. In addition, he has nasal flaring, intercostal and supraclavicular retractions, and occasional grunting.

Questions

1. What are the causes of respiratory distress in infants and children?
2. What are the signs and symptoms of respiratory distress in infants and children?
3. What are the signs and symptoms of impending respiratory failure in infants and children?
4. What are the critical interventions for infants and children in respiratory distress?

Respiratory distress and respiratory failure may cause significant morbidity and mortality in infants and children. The signs and symptoms of respiratory compromise may be subtle, particularly in small infants. Decompensation may occur rapidly if ventilation or oxygenation is inadequate. Respiratory distress is defined as increased work of breathing, and it usually precedes respiratory failure. Respiratory failure occurs when ventilation or oxygenation is not sufficient to meet the metabolic demands of the tissues. Thus oxygenation of the blood is inadequate or carbon dioxide is not eliminated. This may be caused by diseases of the airway or poor respiratory effort (Table 36–1).

EPIDEMIOLOGY

Primary care physicians frequently care for children in respiratory distress in both offices and emergency departments. In 1990 there were 701,000 hospital admissions for respiratory disease, many of which were in young infants with infections. Other admissions were for reactive airway disease (asthma).

CLINICAL PRESENTATION

Increases in respiratory rate and work of breathing are the most common signs of respiratory disease. Tachycardia is often present, although bradycardia may be a sign of impending cardiopulmonary failure. Signs of poor oxygenation include alterations in mental status, head bobbing, and change in skin color. Cyanosis is often a late sign; it occurs when the amount of unsaturated hemoglobin is at least 5 g/dL. Children may first appear dusky or pale. If children are anemic, cyanosis may not be evident, although the oxygen saturation is low (D$_x$ Box).

PATHOPHYSIOLOGY

The adequacy of respiration depends on effective gas exchange and the ability to move an adequate volume of gas in and out of the airways. Infants and children generally breathe with minimal effort. In very young children, the diaphragm and abdominal musculature are used for respiration, and the tidal volume is approximately 6–8 mL/kg. If the tidal volume is decreased because of obstruction, children compensate by increasing the res-

---

TABLE 36–1. Causes of Respiratory Distress in Infants and Children

Infection
  Bronchiolitis
  Pneumonia
  Croup
  Epiglottitis
Congenital anomalies
Foreign body aspiration
Reactive airway disease (asthma)
Submersion injuries
Pneumothorax
Smoke inhalation
Toxin exposure
Heart disease
Metabolic disease
Neuromuscular disease

D$_x$ Respiratory Distress

- Increased respiratory rate
- Changes in tidal volume or minute ventilation
- Presence of retractions: intercostal, substernal, diaphragmatic, or supraclavicular
- Nasal flaring
- Decreased or absent breath sounds
- Changes in inspiratory-expiratory ratio
- Production of sounds with respiration (e.g., gurgling, stridor, rhonchi, grunting)
- Alterations in mental status
- Inability to speak in sentences
- Presence of pale or cyanotic skin
- Presence of central cyanosis

BOX 36–1. Comparison of Respiratory Systems in Children and Adults

- The head in children is proportionally larger and has less muscular support.
- The tongue in children is larger in relation to the mouth and can cause airway obstruction.
- The airway diameter is smaller in children. Reductions in size due to secretions or inflammation cause greater resistance to air flow.
- The larynx is higher and more anterior in children, which makes visualization of the vocal cords more difficult.
- The narrowest part of the airway in children is at the cricoid ring, unlike in adults, where the narrowest point is at the vocal cords.
- The trachea in children is short. In newborns it is 4 cm long, and in 18-month-old infants, 7 cm. In adults, it is 12 cm.
- The major muscle of respiration in children is the diaphragm. Any interference with diaphragmatic motion in young children impedes respiratory function. Intercostal muscles are immature in children.
- Children have less pulmonary reserve volume.
- Normal respiratory rates are higher in children and vary by age.

piratory rate, thus attempting to maintain an adequate minute ventilation (minute ventilation = respiratory rate × tidal volume). If the minute ventilation is still insufficient for adequate gas exchange, or children can no longer sustain the increased work of breathing, then respiratory failure ensues. Respiratory failure may progress to cardiopulmonary arrest.

Infants and children are more prone than adults to respiratory distress because of the differences between their respiratory systems (Box 36–1).

EVALUATION

History

A brief history should be taken (Questions Box).

Physical Examination

Before a complete assessment can proceed, critical interventions that may change children's clinical status should be made. Children should be placed in a position of comfort, and oxygen should be applied. Both ventilation and oxygenation should be assessed.

Respiratory and heart rates should be determined for a period of at least 30 seconds. In infants, abdominal excursions should be counted, and in older children,

Questions: Respiratory Distress

- For how long has this problem been occurring? Has a similar problem ever occurred before?
- Did the problem begin while the child was eating?
- Has the child had any recent infections?
- Are any members of the household ill?
- Is the child taking any medications?

TABLE 36–2. Vital Signs by Age

Age	Respiration (breaths/min)	Pulse (beats/min)	Blood Pressure (Systolic)
Newborn	30–60	100–160	50–70
1–6 wk	30–60	100–160	70–95
6 mo	25–40	90–120	80–100
1 yr	20–30	90–120	80–100
3 yr	20–30	80–120	80–110
6 yr	18–25	18–25	80–110
10 yr	15–20	15–20	90–120

chest excursions should be counted. Respiratory rates in children are higher than in adults; infants may breathe 40 times per minute, one-year-olds 25 times per minute, and 10-year-olds 18 times per minute (Table 36–2). These rates vary with age and changes of activity, emotion, and illness. Abnormal respiratory rates are defined as being faster than normal (tachypnea), slower than normal (bradypnea), or absent (apnea). Neonates may exhibit periodic breathing, with periods of regular respirations alternating with irregular breathing. This is a normal variant for age. True apnea (cessation of respiration) is accompanied by change in skin color or altered level of consciousness.

The depth of respiration should be noted. Whether breaths are deep, gasping, or shallow should be determined. Rapid, shallow respirations may not provide enough inspiratory time for adequate gas exchange. The heart rate may also reflect respiratory compromise.

Breath sounds should first be listened to in the axillae and then at the bases and apices. The absence of breath sounds may be an ominous sign. Children's breath sounds are usually well transmitted across the thorax because of the thin chest wall. It is not uncommon to hear upper airway noises when auscultating the lungs.

Abnormal sounds are caused by turbulent air passing through a narrowed airway. Resistance to flow through a hollow tube increases exponentially. Thus the smaller the airway, the greater the resistance to flow generated by even small changes in the radius (e.g., as with edema, secretions, or foreign bodies). The nature of the sounds produced depends on the location of the narrowing in the airway. Gurgling and stridor come from the upper airway, and rhonchi and wheezing from the lower airway. If no abnormal sounds are evident, and breath sounds are absent or decreased, the airways may be totally obstructed. Grunting is caused by turbulent air coming in contact with a partially closed glottis. Children who grunt are generating their own Valsalva maneuver, which results in the partial obstruction of the upper airway and the production of positive end-expiratory pressure.

The physician should also observe the effort children expend in breathing. Increased work of breathing occurs when intercostal, subcostal, or supraclavicular retractions are present, the accessory muscles of respiration are used, breathing is abnormally noisy, or nasal flaring is seen.

In addition, the physician should observe the inspiratory-expiratory ratio while assessing the work of breathing. The ratio is approximately 1:1 in most patients. Prolonged expirations are most often seen with reactive airway disease.

Laboratory Tests

Although the physical examination is the most important tool for assessing children in respiratory distress, laboratory tests such as complete and differential blood counts, ESRs, and blood cultures may help in the diagnosis of infection. It should be remembered that meningitis and metabolic derangement may present with tachypnea not associated with increased work of breathing. Arterial blood gases should be reserved for patients in impending respiratory failure.

Peak expiratory flow or forced expiratory volume in one second (FEV_1) determinations can be helpful in assessing children with reactive airway disease.

Imaging Studies

Chest radiographs can aid in assessing children in respiratory distress but should not be routinely performed in patients with known reactive airway disease unless children have a fever or are in status asthmaticus.

MANAGEMENT

All infants or children in respiratory distress should be managed emergently. In such situations, assessment and intervention often occur simultaneously. All children in respiratory distress should be placed on a cardiac monitor and assessed frequently. The highest possible oxygen concentration should be delivered. Children should never be forced to use an airway adjunct, because this may cause increased anxiety and distress. Patients with clear airways can be maintained with simple interventions such as oxygen blown by the face or given by mask or nasal prongs. More advanced airway management (bag-valve-mask ventilation or endotracheal intubation) may be necessary for children who need assisted ventilation, airway protection, or hyperventilation.

Position

Children in respiratory distress who are alert and breathing spontaneously should be allowed to choose a position of comfort. Small infants who are incapable of positioning themselves are best placed upright with care taken not to flex or extend the neck. Children and their caregivers should be kept together to reduce anxiety.

The proper position for unconscious children is the "sniffing position," with the neck slightly flexed and the head extended to open the airway. This can be facilitated by placing a towel under the occiput of the head. If simple positioning does not relieve an obstruction, then the airway should be opened using the chin lift or jaw thrust. If spinal trauma is a possibility, only the jaw thrust should be used.

Oxygen Administration

Oxygen should be delivered by any method tolerated by children.

Nasal Prongs

Nasal prongs have two advantages; they are noninvasive and allow maintenance of a constant gas flow even when talking and eating. The concentration of oxygen delivered is limited, however, and irritation and drying of the mucous membranes may result.

Oxygen Masks

Masks deliver a higher concentration of humidified oxygen. Disadvantages include obstruction of children's visual field, potential for carbon dioxide retention, and anxiety because the face is covered. Various types of masks can be used.

The **simple mask** can deliver 35 to 65% oxygen concentration at flow rates of 6–10 L/min. Room air is drawn into the mask through the exhalation ports in the side of the mask.

A **partial rebreathing mask** is desirable when higher concentrations of oxygen (50–60%) are required. During exhalation, oxygen flows into the reservoir bag along with one third of the exhaled gas. Entrapment of room air is minimized when patients breathe oxygen from the reservoir bag.

A **nonrebreathing mask** has valves that allow only oxygen to flow from the reservoir bag to the patient on inhalation and additional valves on the exhalation ports of the mask that prevent entrapment of room air.

The **face tent** is a soft plastic bucket shaped to the chin that is well tolerated by children. The face tent allows high-flow oxygen to be delivered, and it has the advantage of allowing access to the face and mouth (Fig. 36–1).

FIGURE 36–1. *Use of a face tent.*

A **Venturi mask** is rarely used in children but has the advantage of precisely titrating the oxygen concentration to be delivered from 24 to 60%.

Assisted Ventilation

Children with potential respiratory failure require assisted ventilation with bag-valve-mask devices or endotracheal intubation. Masks of the proper size should be used. The upper edge of the mask should fit snugly over the bridge of the nose without touching the eyes. The lower edge should rest directly on or just above the mandible. An oropharyngeal airway should be inserted in unconscious children to prevent the tongue from obstructing the upper airway. Endotracheal intubation is indicated in those children who require control of the airway, who need airway protection, or who require hyperventilation.

PROGNOSIS

Respiratory failure and resulting cardiopulmonary arrest are preventable in most infants and children if their condition is carefully assessed and appropriate critical interventions are made. Careful attention to ventilation and oxygenation of patients usually results in a good outcome.

Case Resolution

The fussy infant discussed in the case history has obvious signs of respiratory distress, including tachypnea, tachycardia, grunting, nasal flaring, and retractions. The differential diagnosis includes foreign body, infection, and reactive airway disease. It is important to place the infant in a position of comfort and provide supplemental oxygen before any diagnostic studies, such as chest x-ray, are performed. Pulse oximetry should be monitored. The clinical status of the infant should be reassessed periodically to prevent further deterioration.

Selected Readings

American Heart Association. Guidelines for cardiopulmonary resuscitation and emergency cardiac care: pediatric basic life support. J.A.M.A. 268:2251–2261, 1992.

Chameides, L., and M. F. Hazinski (eds.). *Textbook of Pediatric Advanced Life Support.* Dallas, American Heart Association, 1994.

Downes, J. J., Fulgencio, and R. C. Raphaely. Acute respiratory failure in infants and children. Pediatr. Clin. North Am. 19:423, 1972.

Seidel, J. S. Respiratory emergencies and cardiopulmonary arrest. *In* Barkin, R. (ed.). *Pediatric Emergency Medicine: Concepts and Clinical Practice.* St. Louis, Mosby–Year Book, 1992, pp. 73–83.

CHAPTER 37

STRIDOR AND CROUP

James S. Seidel, M.D., Ph.D.

H$_x$ A two-year-old boy has been breathing noisily for one day. For the past week he has had a "cold," with a runny nose, fever (temperature: up to 100.4° F [38° C]), and a slight cough. The cough has gradually become worse and now has a barking quality.

On examination, the child is sitting up, has a respiratory rate of 48 breaths/min with marked inspiratory stridor, and an occasional barking cough. His other vital signs include heart rate, 100 beats/min, and temperature of 101.1° F (38.4° C). He has intercostal retractions, his breath sounds are slightly decreased bilaterally, and his skin is pale. The remainder of the examination is normal.

Questions

1. What are the common causes of stridor?
2. What is the pathophysiology of viral croup?
3. How are children with stridor managed?

Noisy breathing is a common symptom that often accompanies respiratory infections in children. The presence of **stridor,** a crowing sound, often concerns children's caregivers. Some parents try home remedies to alleviate the symptoms, whereas others immediately seek help in the office or emergency department setting. **Croup,** a type of noisy breathing, is an inflammation of the larynx, trachea, and upper bronchioles (laryngotracheobronchitis). It is one of the most common causes of barking cough in children.

EPIDEMIOLOGY

Croup most commonly affects children between six months and three years of age, generally in the fall or early winter. Children less than one year of age make up 26% of cases. The condition is more common in boys than girls; two-thirds of all hospitalized children with croup are boys.

Noisy respiration, which may be indicative of croup, may also be a sign of epiglottitis. The incidence of this condition in children has been dramatically reduced in the past five years because of immunization against *Haemophilus influenzae*. Many young children are incompletely immunized, however, and epiglottitis should be considered in toxic-appearing children with rapid onset of symptoms of upper airway obstruction. Prior to *H. influenzae* type b immunization, the ratio of cases of epiglottitis to croup was 1 to 100.

PATHOPHYSIOLOGY

Stridor

Stridor is generally caused by obstruction of the airway between the nose and the larger bronchi. Obstruction at the level of the nose or pharynx may produce snoring or gurgling sounds. The level of the obstruction determines the quality of the sounds produced by turbulence of airflow across a narrowed airway. Turbulence of airflow in the laryngeal area or upper trachea causes the crowing sound characteristic of stridor. Edema and inflammation at the cords and subglottic areas result in inspiratory stridor, whereas obstruction below the cricoid cartilage may lead to both inspiratory and expiratory stridor.

Some of the more common causes of stridor are listed in Table 37–1. The sounds produced at various levels of obstruction can give the primary care provider clues as to the etiology of the problem. The most common cause of stridor that begins shortly after birth is tracheomalacia, a condition secondary to the immaturity of the cartilage of the trachea. Laryngomalacia, which is caused by floppy supraglottic structures, resolves after several months.

The upper airway of infants and children is more susceptible to obstruction as a result of anatomic differences between children and adults. The tongue of children is relatively large, and the epiglottis is floppy and shaped somewhat like the Greek letter omega (Ω). The angle between the epiglottis and the glottis is more acute in children, which makes direct visualization of the airway more difficult. Cartilaginous structures are less rigid in infants. During inspiration, negative intraluminal pressure is generated below the level of obstruction, which leads to narrowing of the airway and turbulence of the air flow. This occurs more often in children because the tracheal rings are not well formed. In addition, the smaller size of the airway in children makes resistance to air flow greater when obstruction is present.

The smaller the airway, the greater the resistance to flow (resistance increases exponentially). Alterations in the diameter of the airway are most often caused by edema and inflammation from a variety of conditions, including congenital anomalies, infection, allergic and anaphylactic reactions, cysts, tumors, and trauma. Even localized areas of airway narrowing in infants and children can lead to respiratory distress because the airway is so small, particularly at the cricoid ring, which is the narrowest portion of the airway in children.

Croup

Croup is most often caused by an infection with parainfluenza virus (type I or II), respiratory syncytial virus, or influenza virus. Particularly severe disease may be associated with influenza A infection. Infection occurs via droplets spread from other infected individuals.

The virus first attacks the nasopharynx and subsequently spreads to the larynx and upper trachea. The infection causes inflammation and edema of the airway that often involves the vocal cords, producing the typical barking cough, hoarseness, and inspiratory stridor. In severe cases the lower airways also may be involved, leading to impaired alveolar ventilation. In some children, bacterial infection may occur with bacterial tracheitis or extension of infection to the lower airway. Airways of infants are small and particularly susceptible to obstruction because of the narrow subglottic region and the laxity of the cartilaginous structures.

Spasmodic croup, which occurs at night, may be recurrent. It is characterized by the sudden onset of hoarseness, barking cough, and stridor. This condition may resolve when children are exposed to humid air. The etiology is unknown but is probably either a reaction to a viral infection or an allergic phenomenon.

DIFFERENTIAL DIAGNOSIS

The differential diagnosis of stridor is presented in Table 37–2.

TABLE 37–1.   Causes of Stridor

Congenital Anomalies

Tracheomalacia
Laryngomalacia
Choanal atresia
Laryngeal web
Laryngocele
Subglottic stenosis
Vascular ring
Macroglossia (Beckwith's syndrome)
Tracheal web or cyst

Inflammatory Lesions

Viral croup
Epiglottitis
Abscess (retropharyngeal, peritonsillar, parapharyngeal)
Tracheitis
Bronchitis
Severe tonsillitis
Angioneurotic edema
Infectious mononucleosis
Diphtheria

Trauma

Direct trauma to the upper airway
Postintubation subglottic stenosis

Foreign Body
Neoplasm
Neurogenic

Laryngeal paralysis
Poor pharyngeal muscle tone

TABLE 37–2.   Differential Diagnosis of Stridor

Data	Viral Croup	Spasmodic Croup	Epiglottitis	Foreign Body
Age	3–36 months	3–36 months	1–8 years	All ages
Prodrome	URI symptoms; onset over 2–5 days	None; sudden onset at night	Usually none; rapid onset over several hours	None; sudden onset
Fever	Low-grade	None	Usually above 39° C	None
Cough	Barking	Barking	None or dry	May or may not be present
Respiratory distress	Present	Present	Present	Usually present
White blood cell count	Normal or slightly elevated	Normal	Elevated	Normal
Blood culture	No growth	No growth	*H. influenzae*	No growth
Radiograph	Subglottic narrowing; steeple sign	Subglottic narrowing (±)	Swollen epiglottis	Air trapping; may show a foreign body

EVALUATION

History

A complete history should be obtained (Questions Box).

Physical Examination

It is important to assess the degree of respiratory distress and to place children in a position of comfort; monitor heart rate, ventilation, and oxygenation; and deliver oxygen (see Chapter 36, Respiratory Distress). The stridorous sounds produced are usually inspiratory but may be inspiratory and expiratory if the disease progresses to the lower airway. The presence of stridor at rest or with sleep should be assessed. Breath sounds may be decreased bilaterally, and severe tachypnea, with respiratory rates from 40 to 80 breaths/min, may occur. The peripheral or central cyanosis associated with severe disease should be noted.

Laboratory Tests

Laboratory tests such as a CBC and blood culture are rarely helpful unless the physician is concerned about bacterial infection. The WBC count may be normal or mildly elevated, and the differential count may show a predominance of polymorphonuclear cells. If epiglottitis is being considered, no blood should be drawn until the airway has been visualized and secured.

Imaging Studies

Radiographs of the soft tissues of the upper airway are often helpful. In children with croup, lateral neck films may reveal ballooning of the hypopharynx, a normal epiglottis, and narrowing of the subglottic area (Fig. 37–1). The frontal view shows the classic "steeple sign" of the subglottic area where the airway narrows like a steeple or pencil tip. Radiographic studies should not delay the management of children with suspected epiglottis. Widening of the epiglottis (thumb-shaped

FIGURE 37–1. *Lateral neck radiograph of viral croup. Note the ballooning of the hypopharynx and the narrowing in the subglottic area. (Courtesy of Dr. J.S. Seidel, Division of General and Emergency Pediatrics, Harbor-UCLA Medical Center.)*

Questions: Stridor and Croup

- Did the child have an antecedent respiratory infection?
- Does the child have a fever? If so, how high is the temperature?
- Was the onset of stridor abrupt?
- Does the child have any ill contacts?
- Does the child have any associated symptoms such as vomiting, diarrhea, or rash?
- Is the child feeding normally?
- Is the child drooling?

rather than pinky-shaped) may be seen on lateral neck films in such patients if radiographs are obtained.

Other imaging studies, such as a barium swallow or CT scan of the thorax, are helpful in diagnosing congenital anomalies (e.g., vascular ring).

MANAGEMENT

Most children with croup and stridor can be managed as outpatients. Care givers should be given careful instructions so that they understand the course of the illness, know what to expect, and realize when emergency care is needed. Children with a prolonged history of stridor may require consultation with a head and neck specialist. If a specific cause of stridor, such as a foreign body, is identified, appropriate management should be instituted.

Children with croup should be treated with gentleness and should not be upset. Agitation and crying increase respiratory distress and oxygen demand. Procedures should be kept to a minimum.

Cool mist should be provided by "blow by" or mask. Airway adjuncts that cause increased agitation should not be used. **Humidified oxygen or air,** which decreases the viscosity of secretions and reduces the edema of the airway, is the most important therapy for croup. Management of spasmodic croup requires only humidified air, and symptoms usually resolve within six hours of the onset.

The heart rate, respiratory status, and oxygen saturation should be monitored. Pulse oximetry should be used.

Treatment with **drugs** is controversial. Some steroids have been shown to be effective. One or two doses of intramuscular dexamethasone are used by some institutions. Continuous or long-term therapy with steroids does not seem to alter the clinical course of the disease or the period of hospitalization. Treatment with antibiotics is not indicated unless infection with bacteria is evident.

Use of racemic epinephrine is also controversial. Several studies have shown that there was no difference in the long-term outcome between those children who were treated with epinephrine and those who received a placebo. Other studies have clearly demonstrated an acute effect of the drug when given via nebulizer. "Rebound" respiratory distress after the drug effects have worn off has been reported in the literature.

Hospitalization should be considered for children in severe respiratory distress, those who are unable to eat, and those whose parents are unable to cope with the tasks required to manage children at home. It is always indicated for children with a bacterial infection such as epiglottitis or tracheitis.

About 10% of infants and children with croup may need **controlled ventilation with endotracheal intubation.** The indications for intubation include severe respiratory distress, hypoxia, and hypercapnia. A major complication of endotracheal intubation in children with croup is subglottic stenosis, which develops because the endotracheal tube may traumatize the inflamed airway, leading to permanent damage. Patients should be extubated as soon as possible.

Direct laryngoscopy may be necessary in some children where the etiology of the stridor is not clear. This procedure should be done by a practitioner who is experienced in managing the airway.

PROGNOSIS

Stridor is a serious sign, which is indicative of upper airway obstruction and potential respiratory compromise. Although it has many causes, the prognosis is usually determined by the rapidity of diagnosis and the institution of appropriate therapeutic measures, particularly stabilizing the patient and ensuring patency of the airway. Certain conditions such as croup often resolve spontaneously within a few days, although some children require hospitalization and, rarely, assisted ventilation. Other conditions, such as foreign bodies or tumors, necessitate aggressive intervention to prevent death from airway obstruction.

Case Resolution

In the case history at the beginning of this chapter, the two-year-old with the antecedent infection and stridor has the classic signs of croup. First, adequate ventilation and oxygenation should be ensured. As soon as the assessment and management of airway, breathing, and circulation are completed, other diagnostic studies and specific therapy, such as racemic epinephrine, can be considered.

Selected Readings

Cherry, J. D. Croup, laryngotracheitis, spasmodic croup and laryngotracheobronchitis. *In* Feigin, R. D., and J. D. Cherry (eds.). Pediatric Infectious Diseases, 3rd ed. Philadelphia, W. B. Saunders, 1992, pp. 209–220.

Cressman, W. R., and C. M. Myer III. Diagnosis and management of croup and epiglottitis. Pediatr. Clin. North Am. 41:265–276, 1994.

Latourneau, M. A., S. Schuh, and M. Gausche. Respiratory disorders. *In* Barkin, R. M. (ed.). Pediatric Emergency Medicine: Concepts and Clinical Practice. St. Louis, Mosby-Year Book, 1992, pp. 969–1033.

Super, D. M., et al. A prospective double-blind study to evaluate the effect of dexamethasone in acute laryngotracheitis. J. Pediatr. 115:323–329, 1989.

CHAPTER 38

SIDS AND APNEA

Carol D. Berkowitz, M.D.

H$_x$ A four-month-old male infant is brought to the emergency department by paramedics after being found blue and not breathing by his mother. He had previously been well except for a mild upper respiratory infection. His mother fed her son at 2:00 AM, and when she checked on him at 6:00 AM, she found him blue and lifeless. Although the mother smoked cigarettes during pregnancy, the pregnancy and delivery were otherwise normal. The infant received the appropriate immunizations at two months of age.

Questions

1. What factors are associated with SIDS?
2. How are SIDS and apnea related?
3. What is the appropriate evaluation of infants who present with apnea or have a history of apnea?
4. What services are available to families who have lost infants to SIDS?

Sudden infant death syndrome (SIDS), also referred to as crib death, is defined as the sudden, unexplained death of infants or young children that is not adequately explained by history, a thorough postmortem examination, or a death scene examination. The term SIDS was officially designated in 1963 to describe the syndrome of sudden, unexpected death of infants less than one year of age in whom no pathologic etiology could be determined after a careful autopsy. The syndrome has been known since biblical times; parents were advised not to lie with their children for fear of suffocating them. SIDS is the second leading cause of death of infants between the ages of one month and one year, second only to congenital anomalies. Most of the recent SIDS research has sought to determine the etiology of the disorder, define the relationship between SIDS and apnea, and determine patient and environmental risk factors.

SIDS-like events associated with successful resuscitation were once described as near-miss SIDS or aborted crib death. The term that is now used is apparent life-threatening event (ALTE). ALTE episodes are characterized by some combination of apnea, color change, marked change in muscle tone, and choking or gagging. Infants who experience ALTEs may appear to have died, which makes the events frightening to observers.

EPIDEMIOLOGY

SIDS accounts for 5000 to 10,000 deaths per year in the United States, with an overall incidence of slightly under

TABLE 38–1. Risk Factors for Sudden Infant Death Syndrome

Lower socioeconomic class
Maternal youth
Unmarried mother
Maternal smoking
Maternal substance abuse
Prematurity
Bronchopulmonary dysplasia

---

2 per 1000. SIDS affects boys more commonly than girls and occurs more often in the winter months. This seasonality may be related to infection with respiratory syncytial virus. The frequency of SIDS differs in different populations in both the United States and other countries. The disorder is reported less frequently in Asian Americans, with an incidence of 0.51 per 1000, and more often in Native Americans, with an incidence of 5.93 per 1000.

Numerous epidemiologic, maternal, and infant factors have been associated with SIDS, including prematurity and intrauterine growth retardation (Table 38–1). Infants with bronchopulmonary dysplasia (BPD) are particularly at risk for SIDS. One study has reported that approximately 11% of premature infants with BPD subsequently died of SIDS. A disproportionate number of infants with SIDS come from lower socioeconomic groups, although this is true for infants dying from all causes. Mothers of children with SIDS are frequently young and unwed; smoke cigarettes or use drugs, such as heroin, methadone, or cocaine; and have had fewer doctor visits during the prenatal and postpartum periods.

CLINICAL PRESENTATION

Victims of SIDS present in cardiopulmonary arrest, with a history of previous good health or antecedent URI. Infants who have experienced an ALTE may appear pale, cyanotic, hypotonic, lethargic, and have bradycardia (D$_x$ Box). If resuscitation is successful, infants may look normal and be fully alert.

PATHOPHYSIOLOGY

The exact cause of SIDS is unclear. More than 70 different theories have been proposed. The relationship between SIDS and apnea engendered a great deal of interest in the 1970s and 1980s. Studies assessed ventilatory response of infants with ALTE to different conditions (e.g., hypoxia) as well as the appearance of

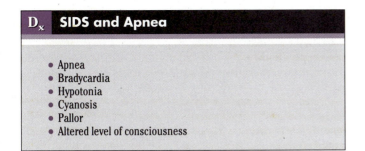

Dx SIDS and Apnea

- Apnea
- Bradycardia
- Hypotonia
- Cyanosis
- Pallor
- Altered level of consciousness

postmortem tissue from SIDS victims. The postmortem tissue has often shown evidence of long-standing hypoxia such as brainstem gliosis. Other changes initially observed on autopsy such as thickening of smooth muscle and small blood vessels in the lungs, hypertrophy of the right ventricle, and hematopoiesis in the liver have not been borne out by subsequent studies.

Research concerning the relationship between apnea and ventilation suggests that three separate components are associated with respiratory abnormalities in some infants who have experienced ALTEs. First, central apnea, which may be associated with immaturity, infection, or congenital anomalies, results from primary failure of the respiratory control center. Affected infants fail to respond appropriately to hypercarbia and hypoxia. Second, airway obstruction may be associated with apnea. Obstructive apnea is noted in infants with craniofacial anomalies and Down's syndrome. Obstructive apnea contributes to ALTE an estimated 5% of the time. Infants with obstructive apnea demonstrate increased chest wall movement in the face of decreasing heart rate and decreasing oxygen levels (pO_2). Third, expiratory apnea may play a role. Infants with expiratory apnea experience sudden atelectasis, ventilation perfusion inequalities, hypoxia, and marked cyanosis, which occurs in 5 to 10 seconds. Expiratory apnea is often associated with sudden death. Cardiac arrhythmias or anomalies do not appear to be causative in SIDS.

Recent studies have implicated sleeping in the prone position with an increased incidence of SIDS. Researchers have examined the relationship between the worldwide incidence of SIDS and infant sleep positions. No association between aspiration and sleeping in the supine position in normal infants apparently exists. A number of mechanisms have been postulated linking SIDS to sleeping in the prone position. Sleeping in the prone position may be associated with upper airway obstruction, rebreathing of expired air, or hyperthermia. Because of the link between sleeping in a prone position and apnea, the American Association of Pediatrics recommends a supine or side sleeping position for normal infants.

The association between SIDS and fatal child abuse has also received attention. The evaluation of the home environment of SIDS victims, referred to as death scene investigations, may reveal accidental causes of death for some of these children. Alternatively, such investigations may reveal that children died from inflicted injuries. A comprehensive autopsy should include an assessment for long bone fractures as well as intracra-

nial hemorrhage, which establish inflicted trauma as the cause of the sudden death. In some municipalities, child fatality boards review each case of reputed SIDS to determine whether an etiology other than SIDS is present. Infants with Munchausen's syndrome by proxy may present with SIDS or ALTE. Such infants are suffocated by the parents until they become apneic or die.

DIFFERENTIAL DIAGNOSIS

The major challenge for physicians who care for children with SIDS or ALTE is to determine if any underlying condition may have caused the symptomatology (Table 38–2). Sepsis, seizures, gastroesophageal reflux, inborn errors of metabolism, cardiac anomalies, and child abuse should all be considered. The circumstances surrounding ALTEs suggest which of these conditions is suspect. A sepsis evaluation is particularly warranted in children who have symptoms such as fever, vomiting, or diarrhea. Infants with abnormal movements or ALTEs when awake may be experiencing seizures. The apnea may represent the seizure or a postictal event. Apnea may also accompany gastroesophageal reflux. In general, affected infants have a history of eating, regurgitating, and then developing apnea. As previously noted, child abuse, particularly with intracranial hemorrhage, may result in apnea or SIDS.

Inborn errors of metabolism are reported in 4 to 8% of cases of ALTE. They should be considered in infants with other symptoms, such as vomiting or failure to thrive, or in the context of a positive family history. Rarely, cardiac arrhythmias, most notably prolonged QT interval or Wolff-Parkinson-White syndrome, are associated with apnea or sudden episodes of bradycardia.

EVALUATION

History

The history may provide the clue to the etiology of SIDS or ALTE (Questions Box).

Physical Examination

A complete examination should be conducted. If infants are floppy and have poor color or have required either mouth-to-mouth resuscitation or vigorous stimulation, significant events are likely. Physicians should check for the presence of bruises, dysmorphic features,

TABLE 38–2. Differential Diagnosis of Sudden Infant Death Syndrome (SIDS)/Apparent Life-Threatening Event (ALTE)

Sepsis
Seizures
Cardiac arrhythmias/anomalies
Gastroesophageal reflux
Inborn errors of metabolism
Child abuse
Intracranial hemorrhage

Questions: SIDS and Apnea

- What were the events leading up to the episode?
  - Was the child awake and eating, indicating that gastroesophageal reflux should be considered?
  - Was the child awake and did the eyes roll back or the body stiffen or jerk, suggesting that a seizure may have occurred?
- How serious was the event? Did breathing resume spontaneously or did cardiopulmonary resuscitation have to be initiated?
- Have similar events occurred in the past?
- Is the infant basically well? Has the infant been ill recently?
- Do the siblings have a history of SIDS or ALTE that would suggest the presence of a familial disorder or child abuse?
- Were there any problems with the pregnancy or delivery?
- Is there a history of maternal drug use during pregnancy?

growth impairment, abnormal neurologic or developmental findings, which may suggest an alternative etiology.

Laboratory Tests

In general, the laboratory workup is guided by the findings of the history and physical examination (Table 38–3). A sepsis evaluation, including a CBC, blood culture, lumbar puncture, and urine culture, is appropriate to rule out sepsis in toxic-appearing infants. Serum electrolytes and glucose are important to check because they may indicate an inborn error of metabolism or other abnormalities (e.g., hypoglycemia), which may be associated with apnea with or without the presence of a seizure. When a metabolic etiology is suspected, a test for serum ammonia level should be performed. Hypotonic infants should be evaluated for infantile botulism by sending a stool specimen for testing. All infants with a history of apnea or ALTE should be admitted to the hospital for observation, workup, and monitoring.

Imaging Studies

A chest x-ray should be performed to rule out pneumonia if sepsis is suspected. If the history and physical examination suggest other etiologies, an EEG, CT, and barium swallow may also be ordered.

MANAGEMENT

In addition to the diagnostic workup, other evaluation to determine if infants are at risk for repeated episodes of apnea, bradycardia, or upper airway obstruction is warranted. Infants who have not been fully resuscitated in the field should be resuscitated, stabilized, and admitted. Any identifiable conditions such as sepsis or seizures should be appropriately managed. In most cases, no etiology for the apneic episodes can be determined. The majority of children who succumb to SIDS have not had a previous episode of apnea or an ALTE.

The administration of **xanthine derivatives** such as caffeine, 5–7.5 mg/kg/day, or theophylline, 6–9 mg/kg/day to a serum level of 5–15 mg/dL, may be used to manage infants who have experienced ALTEs. These medications stimulate the respiratory center and prevent central apnea. The efficacy of xanthine derivatives in the management of apnea other than that associated with prematurity has not been established, however.

A second treatment method involves **home apnea monitoring.** A 1986 consensus statement of the National Institutes of Health described three groups of infants who should be candidates for home monitoring: term infants who have unexplained apnea of infancy, which is usually manifested by an ALTE or an abnormal pneumogram; preterm infants who have experienced apnea of infancy beyond 40 weeks postconception; and subsequent siblings of two or more SIDS victims. Apnea monitoring involves an apparatus that measures both chest wall movement and heart rate. Parents must be instructed in equipment maintenance, alarm interpretation, and cardiopulmonary resuscitation. In general, monitoring equipment is distributed by companies who provide 24-hour service to ensure that the equipment is functioning. The cost of evaluating infants with ALTE is $3000 to $5000, and the monthly rental and maintenance costs of monitoring devices are $150 to $300. Whether monitoring has made any difference in the incidence of SIDS in infants who have experienced an ALTE is unclear. Monitoring may be discontinued if infants have had no periods of apnea that require stimulation or resuscitation for a minimum of two to three months. Underlying neurologic problems should be adequately addressed and corrected before monitoring is discontinued.

In addition to managing infants with ALTE, physicians must provide care to families whose infants have succumbed to SIDS. In most jurisdictions, cases of SIDS must be reported to the coroner's office. Some coroners maintain a Child Death Review Board that further investigates each case, sometimes initiating a death scene investigation. The diagnosis of SIDS can only be reached following a full autopsy. It is important for physicians to tell families when they think the cause of death is SIDS even before definitive autopsy results are available. Parents of children who have succumbed to SIDS should be referred to support groups and agencies

TABLE 38–3. Laboratory Studies to Consider in Evaluating Infants with Apparent Life-Threatening Event (ALTE)

Often Indicated

Complete blood count
Blood culture
Lumbar puncture
Urine culture
Chest x-ray
Serum electrolytes
Blood sugar
Serum ammonia

Sometimes Indicated

Electroencephalogram
Computed tomographic scan
Barium swallow

to help them deal with the loss of their children. Information about these organizations can be obtained from the National Foundation for Sudden Infant Death, 101 Broadway, New York, NY, 10036.

PROGNOSIS

The prognosis for children who have experienced an ALTE varies and depends on predisposing conditions. Bronchopulmonary dysplasia and abnormal neurodevelopmental conditions are generally associated with a poor prognosis.

Case Resolution

The infant presented in the case history succumbed to SIDS. In spite of resuscitative efforts by the paramedics, he could not be revived. The mother is advised of the diagnosis of SIDS and referred to the appropriate agency. The coroner is notified about the case and the presence of any associated physical findings such as bruises.

Selected Readings

American Academy of Pediatrics Task Force on Infant Position and SIDS. Positioning and SIDS. Pediatrics 89:1120, 1992.

Bass, M., R. E. Kravath, and L. Golass. Death-scene investigation in sudden infant death. N. Engl. J. Med. 315:100, 1986.

Carroll, J. L., and G. M. Loughlin. Sudden infant death syndrome. Pediatr. Rev. 14:83, 1993.

Chiodini, B. A., and B. T. Thatch. Impaired ventilation in infants sleeping face down: potential significance for sudden infant death syndrome. J. Pediatr. 123:686–692, 1993.

Emery, J. L. Child abuse, sudden infant death syndrome, and unexpected infant death. Am. J. Dis. Child. 147:1097–1100, 1993.

Goyco, P. G., and R. C. Beckerman. Sudden infant death syndrome. Curr. Probl. Pediatr. 20:229–346, 1990.

Haas J. E., et al. Relationship between epidemiologic risk factors and clinicopathologic findings in the sudden infant death syndrome. Pediatrics 91:106–112, 1993.

Posonby, A-L., et al. Factors potentiating the risk of sudden infant death syndrome associated with the prone position. N. Engl. J. Med. 329:377–382, 1993.

CHAPTER 39

APPROACH TO THE TRAUMATIZED CHILD

Jill M. Baren, M.D.

H$_x$ A 6-year-old boy is brought to the emergency department after being struck by an automobile while crossing the street. He was found unconscious at the scene. Initial evaluation shows that the boy has an altered level of consciousness; shallow respirations; ecchymosis across the upper abdomen; and a deformed, swollen left thigh. The pediatric emergency physician is called on to discuss an initial assessment and management plan for the injured child with the trauma surgeon.

Questions

1. What are the most common mechanisms of injury responsible for trauma in children?
2. What are some of the physiologic differences between adults and children that make children more susceptible to certain types of injuries?
3. Which areas of the body are most likely to be injured in a typical automobile-versus-pedestrian crash?
4. What are the components of a primary survey in pediatric trauma patients?
5. What radiographic and laboratory studies should be performed in children with multiple injuries?

Trauma is often referred to as the neglected disease of modern society. Childhood trauma, in particular, is poorly understood. Death from trauma is higher in pediatric patients than in adults. Mechanisms of injury may be similar in adults and children, but children have particular physiologic and psychologic responses to injury. Health care professionals should realize that children have unique anatomic and physiologic features (Box 39–1); they are not just small adults. Evaluation and management of traumatized children may require specialized equipment. Recognition of such facts, coupled with expertise in the performance of emergency procedures, should improve the outcome of children who sustain major injuries.

EPIDEMIOLOGY

More than 50% of the deaths of children who are 1 to 14 years of age are caused by traumatic injuries. Approximately 1.5 million pediatric injuries result in 500,000 hospitalizations, and 15,000 to 25,000 deaths (1.5%) occur each year. The magnitude of the problem becomes even more evident when morbidity is considered. Between 50,000 and 100,000 children per year become permanently disabled as a result of their injuries. Such disabilities have an enormous impact on society; they result in financial and emotional losses for families and many years of lost productivity for individuals.

Blunt trauma, which is more common than penetrating injury in children, represents about 87% of all childhood injuries. In certain age groups (e.g., 13–18-year age group), however, penetrating injury accounts for a higher percentage of the total, especially among minority populations in urban areas. Causes of trauma, listed in order of frequency, are motor vehicle crashes (>40%), falls (15–20%), homicide (13%), and suicide (10%). Included in the remainder are drowning, bicycle crashes, and automobile-versus-pedestrian crashes. Male children are injured twice as often as females. Different mechanisms of injury predominate in different age groups; the figures given above refer to overall causes of trauma.

CLINICAL PRESENTATION

Children who sustain severe trauma present with multiple organ system injury manifested by shock, respiratory failure, or altered mental status (singly or in combination). Those with mild to moderate injury may present in this way or simply with localized signs and symptoms in the injured area.

PATHOPHYSIOLOGY

Patterns of injury are important to identify to develop strategies for injury prevention. One common pattern in the United States is the triad of injuries that results from an automobile-versus-pedestrian crash (Waddell's triad) (Fig. 39–1). Multisystem injury is the

rule rather than the exception in children. Internal injury should not be ruled out, even if no evidence suggestive of external trauma is apparent. Because children are anatomically and physiologically different from adults, they are more susceptible to different types of injury (see Box 39–1). The most striking physiologic differences between adults and children concern responses to acute blood loss.

Hypovolemic shock secondary to acute blood loss is the most common cause of shock in pediatric trauma patients. In general, hemorrhagic shock is a clinical state where the cardiac output is unable to meet the metabolic demands of the tissues for oxygen and nutrients; it is not defined by any absolute blood pressure value.

Acute blood loss stimulates peripheral and central receptors and results in an increased production of catecholamines and adrenocorticoids. The body responds by increasing peripheral vascular resistance, stroke volume, and heart rate. Children are able to tolerate increases in heart rate and peripheral vascular resistance very well at first, and they exhibit normal blood pressure in the presence of hypovolemic shock. By the time their blood pressure falls, they have probably already lost 20 to 25% of their circulating blood volume. In adults, blood pressure tends to decline after a less significant blood loss and therefore may be recognized sooner (Fig. 39–2). Another obstacle to the recognition of shock in children is the lack of knowledge on the part of many health professionals of age-

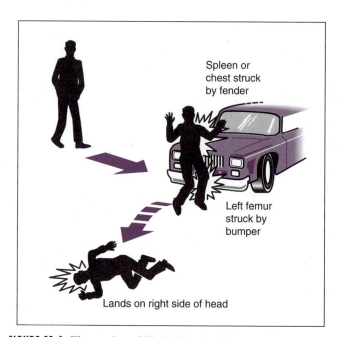

FIGURE 39–1. *Illustration of Waddell's triad. Femur, abdominal, and contralateral head injuries (Waddell's triad) should be expected to result from automobile-versus-pedestrian crashes in the United States. An automobile traveling on the right side of the road strikes a child crossing the street on the left side of the body. The left femur is likely to be injured by the bumper, and the abdomen or chest strikes the grille as the child is lifted into the air and lands on the opposite side of the head, sustaining blunt head trauma. Waddell's triad illustrates the necessity of having a high degree of suspicion for a complex of injuries based on a well-known mechanism.*

FIGURE 39–2. *Graph showing cardiovascular response to hypovolemia in children.* Blood pressure does not begin to decline until the volume deficit is more than 25% because of the compensatory increase in vascular resistance. Cardiac output drops earlier and is manifested clinically as skin signs (delayed capillary refill; cool, clammy skin), tachycardia, and so on.

appropriate vital signs, particularly blood pressure. Table 39–1 gives the normal blood pressure ranges for children of different ages.

Three stages of shock correspond to the progression of volume loss. In the first stage, **compensated shock,** mechanisms for preserving blood pressure are still effective. Decreased capillary refill, diminished pulses, cool extremities, and tachypnea may be apparent, and blood pressure is normal and accompanied by tachycardia. Unrecognized, untreated compensated shock rapidly progresses to **uncompensated shock.** Examination reveals decreased level of consciousness, pallor, reduced urine output, and lower blood pressure with weak, thready pulses and tachycardia. Despite therapy, uncompensated shock becomes **irreversible shock,** resulting in irreparable organ damage.

Shock has several causes, and it is important to emphasize that shock should never be attributed solely to head trauma. The pathways resulting in decreased blood pressure in patients with head trauma are present only at the terminal stages. Therefore, the possibility of blood loss from internal organs should be pursued promptly. Children with spinal cord injuries may have spinal shock, but this tends to be a rare occurrence. Spinal shock may be distinguished from hypovolemic shock by its manifestation of decreased blood pressure together with decreased heart rate secondary to decreased sympathetic tone.

EVALUATION AND MANAGEMENT

Because of the high potential for serious morbidity and mortality in trauma patients, evaluation and management are performed simultaneously. This care is best handled using an organized, multidisciplinary team approach, with preestablished criteria for activation of the trauma team. For example, the entire team responds for all falls greater than 10 feet. The types of subspecialists that make up a trauma team are decided by individual institutions.*

Several approaches to the assessment of trauma patients have been developed by professional organizations. The Advanced Trauma Life Support (ATLS) course of the American College of Surgeons and the Basic Trauma Life Support (BTLS) course of the American College of Emergency Physicians are two such approaches. Both the ATLS and the BTLS methods stress the importance of a primary evaluation, or primary survey, to identify and treat life-threatening injuries and a more detailed regional examination, or secondary survey, after stabilization. In addition, they both adhere to the principles of serial examination and reassessment after each intervention. The reader should understand the rationale for the trauma examination and its parts. (See Selected Readings for textbooks of pediatric emergency medicine that explain the rationales for trauma examination and provide detailed descriptions of evaluation and management techniques.)

Physical Examination

The **primary survey** begins with an assessment of level of consciousness, patency of the airway, and quality of breathing. When evaluating injured patients, physicians should always assume that the cervical spine has been injured and should use in-line immobilization to secure it. Basic airway maneuvers for positioning should be performed. The safest method is the jaw thrust or chin lift to avoid moving the cervical spine (Fig. 39–3). The oral cavity should be examined for foreign bodies, blood, or secretions; the most common form of airway obstruction in children is a posteriorly displaced tongue, which is relieved by good airway positioning. Advanced airway maneuvers (bag-valve-mask ventilation or endotracheal tube intubation) are performed in the primary survey if children have apnea, significant respiratory distress or head trauma, or an airway that cannot be maintained with basic techniques. All trauma patients are given supplemental oxygen by mask or nasal cannula at a concentration of 100%.

TABLE 39–1.   Normal Vital Signs for Children of Different Ages

Age	Respiration (breaths/min)	Pulse (beats/min)	Blood Pressure (Systolic)
Newborn	30–60	100–160	50–70
1–6 wk	30–60	100–160	70–95
6 mo	25–40	90–120	80–100
1 yr	20–30	90–120	80–100
3 yr	20–30	80–120	80–110
6 yr	18–25	18–25	80–110
10 yr	15–20	15–20	90–120

---

*Most institutions have trauma teams composed of pediatric emergency and critical care specialists, anesthesiologists, trauma surgeons, neurosurgeons, emergency nurses, respiratory therapists, and x-ray technicians.

FIGURE 39–3. *Correct method for positioning the head with chin lift or jaw thrust.*

After adequate ventilation has been secured, circulatory status is assessed. All pediatric trauma patients require placement of the largest bore intravenous catheter obtainable for that patient. In life-threatening situations, peripheral vascular access is attempted either three times or for 90 seconds, whichever comes first. If peripheral attempts fail, then intraosseous infusion or central venous access should be used. A bolus of 20 mL/kg of an isotonic fluid (normal saline or Ringer's lactate) should be given. This may be repeated, if necessary, to treat hypovolemic shock. After 80 mL/kg, administration of blood or other crystalloid products should be considered, and the likelihood of surgical exploration is high. Acutely exsanguinating wounds are treated using direct pressure bandages.

A brief neurologic assessment is also performed during the primary survey. This examination includes level of consciousness, pupillary size and reactivity, and in some cases, a Glasgow Coma Scale score or Children's Coma Scale score.

Once life-threatening conditions are stabilized, more information can be collected. The **secondary survey** involves a head-to-toe examination of children, fully exposed, to identify additional injuries. It also includes an **AMPLE** history (**a**llergies, **m**edications, **p**ast history/hospitalizations/surgeries, **l**ast meal, **e**vents preceding trauma) (Table 39–2). A detailed history of events pre-

ceding trauma should ensure that injuries are consistent with the causal mechanism. Health care professionals should be prepared to consider abuse when specific diagnoses do not correlate with either the history given by the care giver or the developmental ability of the child. Measurement of vital signs should occur, and other devices such as Foley catheters or nasogastric tubes should be placed at this time. Every time an intervention is performed, repeat assessments that incorporate the elements of the primary survey are made.

Laboratory Tests

Most institutions have a standardized trauma panel (CBC with differential, electrolytes, BUN, creatinine, glucose, amylase, PT, PTT, and blood typing and cross-matching). In addition, drug and alcohol screens may be performed because increasing numbers of children are using these substances.

Imaging Studies

When multiple trauma is suspected, radiographs of at least the chest, pelvis/abdomen, and cervical spine should be obtained. This prevents practitioners from missing injuries in children who may be unconscious and who had life-saving procedures performed during resuscitation, such as cardiopulmonary resuscitation or intubation, thus obscuring an area of injury from examination. Additional radiographs may be indicated when other areas of injury are detected on secondary survey. Children are often initially distracted from one injury because of the presence of a more painful stimulus.

PROGNOSIS

The highest survival rates for seriously injured children have been found among those who are brought to the operating room for treatment within one hour of the injury. Definitive care for trauma takes place in the operating room, and initial stabilization takes place in the emergency department. An organized, preestablished, multidisciplinary approach to care is essential if this is to remain true. Health care professionals who treat children should not only become adept at the recognition and initial stabilization of injuries, but should also serve as advocates for injury prevention and coordinated prehospital care services in the community.

TABLE 39–2. AMPLE History

A	Allergies
M	Medications
P	Past history/Hospitalizations/Surgeries
L	Last meal
E	Events preceding trauma

Case Resolution

The 6-year-old boy in the case history sustained multiple trauma from an automobile-versus-pedestrian crash. He presents with altered level of consciousness; respiratory failure (shallow respirations); potential internal organ injury, which may lead to shock; and probable fracture of the left femur, which may also contribute to the development of shock. These injuries are identified by performance of a primary and secondary survey. Proper management includes stabilization of the cervical spine, airway management, aggressive early shock treatment with fluid replacement, and a vigilant search for additional injuries. Continued reassessment is also an integral part of emergency department stabilization.

Selected Readings

Chameides, L., and M. F. Hazinski (eds.). Textbook of Pediatric Advanced Life Support. Dallas, American Heart Association, 1994.

Fitzmaurice, L. S. Approach of multiple trauma. In Barkin, R. M. (ed.). Pediatric Emergency Medicine Concepts and Clinical Practice. St. Louis, Mosby-Year Book, 1992, pp. 173–183.

Inaba, A. S., and P. N. Jeward. An approach of pediatric trauma: unique anatomic and pathophysiologic aspects of the pediatric patient. Emerg. Med. Clin. North Am. 9:523–548, 1991.

McCulty, D. L., and J. S. Surpure. Pediatric trauma: initial evaluation and stabilization. Pediatr. Ann. 19:584–596, 1990.

Ruddy, R. M., and G. R. Fleisher. An approach to the injured child. In Fleisher, G. R., and S. Ludwig (eds.). Textbook of Pediatric Emergency Medicine, 3rd ed. Baltimore, Williams & Wilkins, 1993.

Schafemeyer, R. Pediatric trauma. Emerg. Med. Clin. North Am. 11:187–205, 1993.

Schiffman, M. A. Nonoperative management of blunt abdominal trauma in pediatrics. Emerg. Med. Clin. North Am. 7:519–535, 1989.

Ziegler, M. M., and J. M. Templeton. Major trauma. In Fleisher, G.R., and S. Ludwig (eds.). Textbook of Pediatric Emergency Medicine, 3rd ed. Baltimore, Williams & Wilkins, 1993.

CHAPTER 40

ABDOMINAL TRAUMA

Jill M. Baren, M.D.

H$_x$ An 8-year-old boy who is riding a bicycle at a speed of 20 miles per hour accidentally crashes into a tree. On arrival at the trauma center, the paramedics report that the bike handlebars rammed into the child's stomach, "knocking the wind out of him." The boy complains of dizziness and vomits several times. Initial vital signs show a heart rate of 135 beats/min and a respiratory rate of 24 breaths/min. The abdomen is flat but tender to palpation in the midepigastric region and left upper quadrant.

Questions

1. What are the most frequent types of intra-abdominal trauma in children?
2. What are the early recognizable signs of shock in children?
3. What are the basic components of the treatment of shock?
4. What is a simple rule for establishing the lower limit of normal blood pressure in children?

Although head injuries are responsible for the majority of traumatic deaths in children, abdominal trauma is the leading unrecognized cause of fatal injury, specifically because early shock is not recognized. Death results when the extent and nature of abdominal injuries are neither appreciated nor appropriately managed, fluid replacement is inadequate, and airway maintenance is not implemented soon enough. Clinicians should be knowledgeable about mechanisms of injury that result in abdominal trauma and the methods for aggressive treatment of hemorrhagic shock.

EPIDEMIOLOGY

Twenty-five percent of children who sustain multisystem trauma have significant abdominal injury. When both head and abdominal injury occur simultaneously, the risk of death is higher than when either occurs alone. Blunt force mechanisms are responsible for almost 95% of abdominal injuries; the remainder are a result of penetrating force. Examples of blunt force, presented in order of frequency, are motor vehicle crashes, pedestrian versus automobile collisions, falls, sports injuries, and direct blows from both abuse and assault. Injuries to the liver and spleen predominate; injuries to the kidney, bowel, and pancreas occur less often. In multiple injuries, the incidence of trauma involving pelvic organs (bladder, ureter, iliac vessels) is also high, especially when pelvic fractures occur. A straddle injury (e.g., fall that occurs when climbing over a fence) can also result in abdominal and pelvic trauma.

CLINICAL PRESENTATION

Pain, distention, and ecchymoses tend to be more reliable signs of pathology, whereas the absence of bowel sounds is less consistent as a marker for injury. (See D$_x$ Box for signs and symptoms suggestive of abdominal trauma.) No particular sign, however, is completely reliable.

Dx Abdominal Trauma

- Pain
- Tenderness
- Distention
- Peritoneal signs (absent or diminished bowel sounds, rebound tenderness)
- Ecchymoses
- Tire tracks
- Seat belt marks
- Urine, stool, or nasogastric aspirate positive for blood
- Unexplained hypotension or other signs of hypovolemic shock

PATHOPHYSIOLOGY

Blunt trauma largely involves injury to solid, not hollow, intraabdominal organs (i.e., liver and spleen rather than small bowel) for a variety of reasons. First, the rib cage is flexible in children. Therefore, rib fractures are less likely to occur, reducing the potential for penetration of abdominal organs by broken ribs. Second, children have less well developed abdominal musculature and less adipose tissue than adults, and thus blunt force is transmitted to abdominal organs more easily. Third, because the diaphragm is oriented more horizontally in children than in adults, the liver and spleen lie more anteriorly and caudally within the abdomen.

It is important to emphasize that abdominal injury may lead to excessive blood loss. The pathophysiology of hemorrhagic shock is discussed in detail in Chapter 39, Approach to the Traumatized Child. The liver and spleen are highly vascularized organs that bleed profusely when lacerated. Even the accumulation of subcapsular hematomas without rupture may cause a profound drop in hematocrit. Because intraabdominal organs are not directly visible when a patient is examined, signs and symptoms of injury are not always obvious. Therefore, hemorrhagic shock should always be suspected with abdominal trauma. Likewise, large volumes of blood can accumulate in the pelvis, and because of its proximity to the abdomen, the pelvis should always be considered as a reservoir for hemorrhage in abdominal as well as pelvic trauma.

DIFFERENTIAL DIAGNOSIS

Physicians should be familiar with the most common patterns of abdominal injury, and they should consider the possibility of specific injuries. Any abdominal organ can be injured by any mechanism, either blunt or penetrating. The spleen is the most common intraabdominal organ injured by a blunt force. **Hepatic injuries** are the most common fatal abdominal injuries, although they are less frequent than splenic injuries. The right lobe of the liver is injured more frequently than the left lobe.

Injuries to hollow viscera such as the stomach and intestines, which represent only about 5 to 15% of injuries from blunt forces, are difficult to diagnose. Three mechanisms lead to injuries of hollow structures:

(1) "crush" between the anterior wall of the abdomen and the vertebral column; (2) deceleration, which causes shearing of the bowel from its mesenteric attachments; and (3) "burst," which occurs when an air-filled or fluid-filled loop of bowel is closed at both ends at the time of impact. Peritonitis may develop in 6 to 48 hours secondary to fecal spillage (soiling) or devascularization as a consequence of any of these mechanisms. Occasionally, a diagnosis of hollow viscera injury is made incidentally or may be delayed more than 48 hours, highlighting the need for serial examination. Duodenal and pancreatic injuries are examples of potentially delayed diagnoses that can have grave consequences. Leakage of bile and enzymes may activate autodigestion of the pancreas and result in sepsis.

EVALUATION

Determining which organ or organs may be injured from abdominal trauma is difficult. Physicians tend to focus on injuries to the extremities, pelvis, face, or chest that are painful and distracting to children and more clinically obvious to the examiner. Initial clinical impressions may be incorrect, causing delay in diagnosis or unnecessary surgical exploration.

History

The history should focus on the mechanism of injury and the physiologic response of the child, especially in the prehospital setting (e.g., initial hypotension, tachycardia, cyanosis) (Questions Box). A poor history concerning the circumstances of the injury may contribute to a delayed diagnosis.

Physical Examination

An abnormal physical examination may not always be indicative of pathology. Clinicians should avoid relying on physical examination alone as a predictor of abdominal injury. Studies have demonstrated that patients with and without proven injuries often showed no significant differences with respect to physical findings.

Vital signs should be monitored. In children, the range for normal heart rate, respiratory rate, and blood pressure is age dependent. A simple rule for calculating the lower limit of normal systolic blood pressure is $70 + (2 \times \text{age in years})$. Physicians should always remember that a drop in blood pressure is a late sign in the development of shock (see Chapter 39, Approach to the Traumatized Child).

Serial abdominal examinations increase the likelihood of detecting a previously missed condition. Inspection

Questions: Abdominal Trauma

- How was the child injured?
- How long ago did the injury occur?
- What parts of the body were injured?
- Has the child received any treatment prior to coming to the hospital?

of the abdomen to look for ecchymosis, distention, tire tracks, penetrations, or paradoxical motion should occur first. Auscultation for bowel sounds follows this inspection, and palpation should come last. Palpation should be done in all four quadrants to elicit tenderness, rebound, and guarding. If a hepatic or splenic injury is initially suspected, palpation should be minimized to avoid further hemorrhaging.

Laboratory Tests

Laboratory evaluation should be guided by the history and physical examination. A urinalysis to look for hematuria and check for associated genitourinary injuries is helpful. Elevated serum transaminases, amylase, and alkaline phosphatase may be indicative of injury, but normal values do not exclude pathology.

Diagnostic Studies

Diagnostic peritoneal lavage (DPL) is used in some institutions for the evaluation of abdominal trauma. An invasive procedure with a high overall accuracy for detecting injuries, particularly those of the pancreas and bowel, DPL has been replaced to some extent by CT scanning of the abdomen in most institutions. DPL does have an advantage over CT scanning for unstable patients because DPL is performed in the emergency department, which is fully equipped for resuscitation. Most CT scanning areas are not ideal for the critically injured patient because they may lack the proper personnel and equipment to provide ongoing care in a deteriorating patient. In an unstable child with a severe head injury who must undergo immediate craniotomy, DPL is an effective, rapid way to determine if an abdominal injury is also present, and the procedure can be performed simultaneously in the operating room.

Imaging Studies

As with laboratory tests, the use of these techniques depends on the history and examination. Plain radiographs of the pelvis are useful for identifying fractures. The presence of pelvic fractures should increase suspicion for both genitourinary and abdominal injuries. Although plain radiographs of the abdomen are less helpful for defining injuries, they may show fluid accumulation and displacement of bowel or free air from a perforated loop of bowel.

CT of the abdomen is the gold standard for the evaluation of abdominal trauma in spite of the few disadvantages outlined above. It has an accuracy of over 97% for identifying an abdominal injury if one is present. Injuries most likely to be missed by CT are pancreatic and bowel injuries, but the use of both oral and intravenous contrast during the study minimizes this risk. Overall, many specialists in pediatric trauma prefer abdominal CT to DPL for two reasons: (1) CT is less invasive and (2) CT provides excellent, comprehensive diagnostic information. The images can also be extended to include the pelvis if associated pelvic trauma is suspected.

MANAGEMENT

Management of abdominal trauma in children occurs simultaneously with evaluation. The stabilization of children with abdominal trauma, especially in the context of multiple trauma, requires a multidisciplinary team approach that includes surgeons, pediatricians, and emergency physicians. A discussion on the approach to trauma management can be found in Chapter 39, Approach to the Traumatized Child.

Hypovolemic shock, if present, is the primary complication of abdominal trauma on which to focus, because the leading unrecognized cause of death in affected children is profound blood loss. **Airway problems** and **breathing difficulties** should be addressed initially, followed by **vascular access** and **fluid replacement.** No more than three attempts at peripheral vascular access should be made (in 90 seconds or less) before moving on to more invasive procedures.

The intraosseous route should be used for the next vascular access attempt in children who are less than six years of age. The flat, medial portion of the proximal tibia is most commonly used for the procedure, which is performed with an intraosseous, bone marrow, or spinal needle (Fig. 40–1). Fluids and medications, delivered into the marrow cavity, then flow into the venous circulation. Intraosseous cannulation is rapid, simple, and may be life saving. It is limited by low flow rates (approximately 30 mL/minute), which can be augmented either by using pressure on the intravenous bag or by pushing fluid by hand through a syringe. Complications associated with intraosseous line placement are rare. All physicians who care for pediatric trauma patients should be familiar with this technique.

A variety of central venous access sites, such as femoral, subclavian, and internal jugular, may be used in

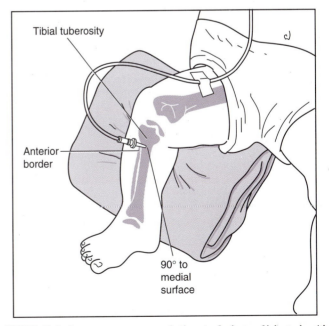

FIGURE 40–1. Intraosseous cannulation technique. (Adapted, with permission, from Chameides, L. (ed.). Textbook of Pediatric Advanced Life Support. Dallas, American Heart Association, 1994.)

PEDIATRICS: A PRIMARY CARE APPROACH

TABLE 40–1. Signs and Symptoms of Hemorrhagic Shock in Children

Tachycardia
Increased capillary refill (> 2 seconds)
Cool and mottled skin, pallor
Respiratory distress
Anxiety, irritability, decreased responsiveness
Thirst
Orthostatic fall in blood pressure, supine hypotension (late sign)

older children. Upper and lower saphenous vein cutdowns are also possible access sites. The Seldinger technique, with insertion of a large-bore catheter over a guidewire, is often used. A description of these procedures is beyond the scope of this book but may be found in many other texts, including the Textbook of Pediatric Advanced Life Support published by the American Heart Association (see Selected Readings).

Fluid replacement begins with a 20–40-mL/kg bolus of crystalloid solution, either normal saline or Ringer's lactate. If no improvement in circulation occurs, additional 10–20-mL/kg boluses may be given, and type-specific blood should be considered. Frequent hematocrits or hemoglobins should be determined to monitor ongoing blood loss. Vital signs should be repeated frequently. Serial examinations, which detect the signs and symptoms of shock (Table 40–1), are the most important gauge of hemodynamic recovery and stability. All children require close hospital observation, preferably in a pediatric trauma center and intensive care unit.

If hemodynamic stabilization is not achieved after appropriate vascular access and fluid resuscitation, the trauma surgeon will most likely perform an exploratory laparotomy. If children have been stabilized with initial airway and circulatory support, diagnostic procedures such as CT scans can be performed as part of the emergency department evaluation. Once identified, specific organ injury can be managed.

PROGNOSIS

Morbidity and mortality related to abdominal trauma depend on the specific organ injury and the style of management. More than 40% of patients with major liver injuries die in the prehospital setting. However, a large number of minor liver injuries can be managed nonoperatively. Currently, an increasing number of injuries to the spleen and liver are managed with observation in the pediatric intensive care unit. Surgical exploration and repair is performed only if patients become hemodynamically unstable. Reduction in anesthetic-related mortality, postsplenectomy sepsis, and a decrease in other postoperative complications have resulted from this shift in practice style. Without surgical intervention, however, an injury such as complete splenic rupture has a 90 to 100% mortality rate.

Case Resolution

The boy in the case scenario sustained isolated abdominal trauma. Initial presenting signs and symptoms are consistent with internal organ injury, specifically splenic hematoma, internal hemorrhage, and compensated shock (e.g., tachycardia, tachypnea). The child should undergo initial resuscitation with attention to the airway, breathing, and circulation, especially fluid repletion. Serial hemodynamic measurement and hematocrits, if stable, permit diagnosis of specific injuries by CT scanning. Surgical consultation with expectant observation is the likely management choice. If the child deteriorates, surgical intervention would ensue. Trauma to the small intestine, particularly a duodenal hematoma, must also be suspected because of the mechanism of injury.

Selected Readings

Abdominal trauma. In Barkin, R. M. (ed.). Pediatric Emergency Medicine Concepts and Clinical Practice. St. Louis, Mosby-Year Book, 1992, pp. 173–183.
Chameides, L. (ed.). Textbook of Pediatric Advanced Life Support. Dallas, American Heart Association, 1994.
Inaba, A. S., and P. N. Seward. An approach to pediatric trauma; unique anatomic and pathophysiologic aspects of the pediatric patient. Emerg. Med. Clin. North Am. 9:503–548, 1991.
Schafermeyer, R. Pediatric trauma. Emerg. Med. Clin. North Am. 11:187–205, 1993.
Schiffman, M. A. Nonoperative management of blunt abdominal trauma in pediatrics. Emerg. Med. Clin. North Am. 7:519–535, 1989.

CHAPTER 41

HEAD TRAUMA

Jill M. Baren, M.D.

Hx A 2-year-old girl is playing on a window ledge unsupervised. She pushes the screen out and falls onto the concrete sidewalk below, striking her head. A neighbor reports that she is unconscious for 10 minutes. When paramedics arrive, the girl is awake but lethargic. She is transported to the emergency department. Her vital signs are normal. A scalp hematoma is present, and a depressed area of cranial bone is palpated.

Questions

1. What are the priorities in the initial stabilization and management of pediatric head trauma?
2. What is the difference between primary and secondary brain injury?
3. What are the common structural injuries sustained by children with head trauma?
4. What are the various modalities available for treatment of increased intracranial pressure (ICP)?
5. Name and briefly describe the scoring systems used in the evaluation of mental status in children with head trauma.

Although the vast majority of childhood head injuries are minor and can be treated on an outpatient basis, it is important for clinicians to become adept at recognizing and managing more severe forms of head injury. The various clinical presentations of pediatric head trauma range from simple scalp lacerations to intracranial hematomas. Familiarity with techniques for assessment of mental status and control of ICP can help reduce morbidity from traumatic brain injury. Furthermore, health care providers can help lower mortality from head trauma by actively promoting injury prevention to patients and communities.

EPIDEMIOLOGY

Head injury is the leading cause of morbidity and mortality in pediatric trauma patients. About 250,000 children per year sustain head trauma; 150,000 suffer injury to the brain tissue itself, and 20% of these injuries result in permanent neurologic sequelae. Overall mortality from isolated head trauma is believed to be 6 to 35% but increases in the presence of other injuries. In children with trauma to multiple parts of the body, 70% of the deaths that occur within 48 hours of hospitalization are the result of trauma to the head. Major causes of head trauma in children are motor vehicle crashes (45% of cases) and falls (38%). The remainder of cases are due to bicycle accidents, sports injuries, assault, and child abuse.

CLINICAL PRESENTATION

Children who have sustained head trauma may present with a history of an antecedent event (e.g., fall or collision with another child) or signs and symptoms related to the injury. These include external bruises or lacerations; alterations in the level of consciousness (LOC); and neurologic findings, including seizures. Vital signs may be altered; in particular, deep or irregular respiration, hypertension, or bradycardia may be apparent (Dx Box). These changes are indicative of elevated ICP.

PATHOPHYSIOLOGY

The mechanism of injury that produces head trauma varies with age, but motor vehicle crashes are the first or second leading cause in all age groups. Severe head injury in children less than one year of age is usually the result of abuse. Other physical findings on examination such as retinal hemorrhages substantiate the abuse. Younger children tend to fall, school-age children have pedestrian or bicycle accidents as well as falls, and adolescents can be the victims of assault or motor vehicle crashes.

Compared to adults, children have a higher center of gravity, an increased head-to-body ratio, and weaker

Dx **Head Trauma***

- LOC
- Somnolence
- Pallor
- Emesis/nausea/anorexia
- Irritability
- Lethargy
- Seizure
- Ataxia
- Weakness
- Pain
- Parasthesias
- Amnesia
- Headache
- Visual changes
- Confusion/altered mental status

---

*All of these symptoms may not be present in head trauma.

neck muscles that predispose the head to injury. Children also have other anatomic disadvantages such as thinner cranial bones and less myelinated brain tissue, which increases the risk of injury to brain parenchyma.

Normally, blood flow to the brain is maintained at a constant rate, a process known as autoregulation. With severe brain injury, autoregulation is lost and blood flow to the brain is equal to cerebral perfusion pressure (CPP). CPP is the difference between mean arterial pressure (MAP) and ICP. A CPP that is either too high or too low can be detrimental.

Control of CPP after head injury in children is challenging. Focal hematomas, which are seen more often in adults, can be evacuated surgically to relieve pressure. In contrast, children tend to develop diffuse cerebral edema that requires management. However, children have a greater capacity for recovery despite these initial difficulties. This is especially true in very young children, whose open sutures and fontanelles permit expansion of the skull from edema and blood.

In the area of head trauma, it is important to understand the difference between primary and secondary brain injury. Primary injury is the structural damage that occurs to the head and its various structures at the time of the injury. Secondary injury is damage to the brain tissue after the initial event. Such damage may result from hypoxia, hypoperfusion, hypercarbia, hyperthermia, and altered glucose or sodium metabolism. It is imperative that the overall goal of management involve the prevention of secondary brain injury; primary brain injury can be prevented only through education and safety.

DIFFERENTIAL DIAGNOSIS

Head trauma can result in a wide variety of clinical syndromes with different degrees of severity. Often the signs and symptoms of one type of injury overlap with another. Figure 41–1 illustrates the anatomic location of various head injuries.

Scalp lacerations may be either superficial or deep to the galea. They are caused by both blunt and penetrating mechanisms. Penetration of the skull table by a lacerating object (e.g., knife, bullet) is associated with a vast potential for damage and a poor outcome. Soft tissue injuries include abrasions, scalp hematomas, subgaleal hematomas, and cephalhematomas. These injuries are readily managed.

The majority of skull fractures are simple and linear. When fractures cross the path of a blood vessel or venous sinus, the potential for complications related to hemorrhage is increased. Other fracture types are compound, diastatic, base-of-skull, and depressed. Base-of-skull fractures usually present with hemotympanum, blood or CSF in the ear canal, Battle's sign (postauricular ecchymosis), raccoon eyes (periorbital ecchymosis), or cranial nerve palsies. Depressed skull fractures often require operative management to lift the depressed fragment away from the underlying brain.

Head injury may result in a concussion or concussive syndrome, which is defined as a transient LOC with amnesia with no abnormality detected on CT scan of the

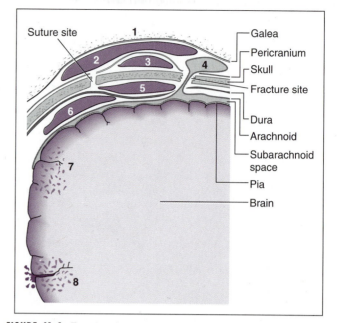

FIGURE 41–1. *Functional anatomy of brain and surrounding structures with sites of pathology. 1, caput succedaneum; 2, subgaleal hematoma; 3, cephalhematoma; 4, porencephalic cyst or leptomeningeal cyst; 5, epidural hematoma; 6, subdural hematoma; 7, cerebral contusion; 8, cerebral laceration. (Redrawn, with permission, from Tecklenburg, F.W., and M.S. Wright. Minor head trauma in the pediatric patient. Pediatr. Emerg. Care 7:40–47, 1991.)*

brain. Neurologic examination is usually normal, but patients may experience headache, vomiting, and other minor symptoms. Concussions can also have minor and subtle neurologic sequelae, such as dizziness or headache, for months following the injury (postconcussive syndrome).

A cerebral contusion occurs with a more severe injury such as a high-speed motor vehicle crash. A coup-contrecoup injury may be produced when the brain strikes the skull, anteriorly bruising the frontal lobe and then posteriorly bruising the occipital lobe. Clinical manifestations depend on the location of the contusion. Bleeding and swelling of surrounding tissue are major concerns in the acute setting.

Epidural hematomas are collections of blood that accumulate between the skull bone and the tough outer covering of the brain (dura). They are often the result of tears in the middle meningeal artery caused by skull fractures. Classically, patients have initial LOC followed by a lucid interval and then rapid deterioration secondary to brain compression. On CT scan an epidural hematoma appears as a large collection of blood with convex borders next to the skull (Fig. 41–2A). Surgical evacuation is required in the majority of cases.

Subdural hematomas, which are five to ten times more common than epidural hematomas, accumulate between the dura and the underlying brain tissue. They are associated with both skull fractures and contusions. On CT scan they appear to have crescent-shaped borders (Fig. 41–2B). Large subdural hematomas usually require surgery for evacuation.

FIGURE 41–2.
A. *Epidural hematoma, marked by the asterisk. Note convex borders and midline shift.*
B. *Subdural hematoma. Note crescent shape.*
C. *Diffuse axonal injury. Note ground-glass appearance and tightly compressed ventricles.*
(Reproduced, with permission, from Harris, J.H., Jr., W.H. Harris, and R.A. Norelline. The Radiology of Emergency Medicine, 3rd ed. Baltimore, Williams & Wilkins, 1993. pp. 15, 16, 17.)

The initial force that results in severe head trauma may produce a shearing or tearing effect on the axonal white matter of the brain known as diffuse axonal injury (DAI) (Fig. 41–2C). As a result of DAI, cerebral edema and elevated ICP occur, maximally within 24 to 48 hours postinjury. It is difficult to predict which patients will recover from this diffuse damage. Children have a better prognosis than adults.

EVALUATION

In children with acute head injuries, especially when other organ system trauma is present, assessment and management occur simultaneously. A primary survey is performed with attention to airway, breathing, circulation (ABC), and cervical spine immobilization as well as a rapid, gross neurologic assessment of responsiveness and pupillary size and reactivity (see Chapter 39, Approach to the Traumatized Child, for more information about treating trauma patients). Cervical spinal injuries are less common in children than head injuries. However, all children with altered LOC; painful, distracting injuries; inability to communicate; focal neurologic deficits; or localized pain, swelling, or ecchymosis of the cervical spine require careful evaluation.

History

Historical data are obtained during the secondary survey or reassessment phase of evaluation. Prehospital health care providers or witnesses to the injury should be asked about details of the event (Questions Box).

Physical Examination

Secondary survey actions include palpation and inspection of the scalp for soft tissue swelling, irregularity, lacerations, and fullness of the fontanelle. Facial bones should be tested for stability. Other clues to possible head trauma include presence of a septal hematoma, draining fluid from the nose or ears, and malocclusion of the mandible. (See Chapter 39, Approach to the Traumatized Child, for more information on primary and secondary survey of trauma patients.)

A comprehensive neurologic examination is the most important part of the secondary survey. This examination should include mental status, cranial nerves, deep tendon reflexes, muscle tone, muscle strength, sensation, cerebellar function, and funduscopic evaluation if possible. When describing mental status, imprecise terms such as "altered," "lethargic," and "obtunded"

Questions: Head Trauma

- What was the mechanism of injury (motor vehicle crash, ejection from motor vehicle, fall, assault)?
- What was the shape of the object(s) striking the head?
- What was the velocity of object(s) striking the head?
- What was the height of the fall?
- What was the type of impact surface?
- What was the child's immediate status after injury?
- What changes in status occurred before arrival at the hospital?
- Did the child lose consciousness? If so, for how long?

TABLE 41–1.   Children's Coma Scale

I. Ocular response	
a. Pursuit	4
b. Extraocular muscles intact, pupils reactive	3
c. Fixed pupils, extraocular muscles impaired	2
d. Fixed pupils, extraocular muscles paralyzed	1
II. Verbal response	
a. Cries	3
b. Spontaneous respirations	2
c. Apneic	1
III. Motor response	
a. Flexes and extends	4
b. Withdraws from pain	3
c. Hypertonic	2
d. Flaccid	1
Maximum score	11

should be avoided. Several widely used scoring systems are available for mental status assessment of children who have suffered head trauma. A number of scales exist for assessment of the level of coma. The Children's Coma Scale (CCS) is used by some clinicians for children up to the age of 4 years. The Glasgow Coma Scale (GCS) is used universally in children over the age of five, and the modified Glasgow Coma Scale is used in children under the age of five.

Each scoring system has three components: eye opening to various stimuli, verbal responses, and motor responses. Scores should be tabulated when children first present to establish a baseline. They can then be used for reassessment on an hourly basis until patients have stabilized or returned to normal mental status. Use of these scores helps promote consistent and accurate communication among health care providers. Tables 41–1 and 41–2 show how to calculate the CCS and GCS scores. Classification of mild, moderate, or severe head trauma, based on the GCS score, is illustrated in Table 41–3.

TABLE 41–2.   Glasgow Coma Scale

I. Eye opening	
a. Spontaneous	4
b. To command	3
c. With pain	2
d. No response	1
II. Verbal response*	
a. Oriented, communicative (oriented)	5
b. Disoriented, confused (words)	4
c. Inappropriate (vocal sounds)	3
d. Incomprehensible (cries)	2
e. No response (no response)	1
III. Motor response	
a. Obeys commands	6
b. Localizes pain	5
c. Flexes with pain	4
d. Flexes abnormally with pain	3
e. Extensor response	2
f. None	1
Maximum score	15

*Assessment of verbal response is modified in children.

TABLE 41–3.   Definitions of Head Injuries in Children Secondary to Initial Glasgow Coma Scale (GCS) Score

Head Injury	Initial GCS		Duration of LOC
Mild	13–15	and	<20 minutes
Moderate	9–12*		
Severe	≤8	or	Coma ≥ 6 hours

*Denotes no deterioration below that range.

Adapted, with permission, from Goldstein, B., and K.S. Powers. Head trauma in children. Pediatr. Rev. 15:213, 1994.

Laboratory Tests

The most useful laboratory tests are a CBC, serum electrolytes, serum glucose, and possibly a toxicologic screen, if appropriate. These tests do not help establish a diagnosis but help guide management.

Imaging Studies

Several diagnostic modalities are available to assess the extent of head injuries. Although plain radiographs of the skull may be useful for identifying fractures, they are generally not justified. CT scans provide much more comprehensive information. Noncontrast CT scans are adequate in the setting of acute trauma and detect skull fractures, soft tissue swelling, cerebral contusions, intracranial hematomas, diffuse cerebral edema, compression, midline shift of brain structures, and ventricular enlargement or compression.

All patients classified as having moderate to severe head trauma (GCS < 13) should have a head CT scan performed on arrival at the emergency department. For minor head trauma (GCS = 13–15) with varying degrees of LOC, the decision to perform a CT scan is based on historical data, physical findings, physician experience, and the psychosocial situation of patients and their families. A list of suggested criteria for obtaining a CT scan for mildly injured patients can be found in Table 41–4.

Although MRI may be superior to CT for identifying diffuse axonal injury and certain types of hemorrhage, MRI has limited use for severely injured patients in the acute phase of injury. In general, MRI takes longer (30–60 minutes) to complete, and the scanners are often not in the vicinity of the emergency department.

TABLE 41–4.   Indications for CT Scans in Children with Head Trauma

Alteration in level of consciousness, waxing and waning or deteriorating mental status
Glasgow Coma score ≤ 14
Focal neurologic deficits on examination
Palpation of a depressed skull fracture
Posttraumatic seizures
Persistent vomiting, headache, lethargy
Trauma to multiple areas of the body
Associated facial or neck trauma
Age less than 2 years

MANAGEMENT

The ABCs are the initial management priorities for children with head injuries, as they are in other trauma patients. The primary goal of management of acute head trauma is the prevention of all possible mechanisms of secondary brain injury. Prompt neurosurgical consultation should be obtained for all children with head trauma except those with very minor injuries.

Obtaining control over the airway is of paramount importance in patients with head trauma. Hyperventilation is one way to reduce ICP. Hyperventilation lowers arterial carbon dioxide (pCO_2), leading to cerebral vasoconstriction and decreased cerebral blood flow. The bag-valve-mask technique should be used initially, followed by rapid sequence intubation to minimize hypoxic and hypercarbic insult. Rapid sequence intubation often involves agents such as lidocaine and thiopental that either reduce ICP or blunt the rise in ICP that occurs during intubation. Care must be taken not to lower the pCO_2 too much, because this may deprive the brain of needed blood flow; the target range for pCO_2 is 27 to 32 mm Hg.

Circulation and MAP should be aggressively supported with fluids to prevent hypoperfusion to the brain. Hypovolemia or hypotension should never be assumed to result from head trauma alone. Children should be examined carefully for evidence of internal organ injury (see Chapters 39, Approach to the Traumatized Child, and 40, Abdominal Trauma, for more detailed information concerning management of traumatized children).

Because CPP is determined by both MAP and ICP, increases in ICP may impede blood flow to the brain and exacerbate ischemic injury. Administration of diuretics and osmotic agents such as mannitol and elevation of the head of the bed to 30 degrees to promote venous drainage are examples of methods used to reduce ICP. Paralytic agents and sedatives may be needed to prevent agitation, which also leads to increased ICP. To assist in monitoring for sudden increases in ICP and to provide drainage of excess CSF, intraventricular pressure catheters can be placed.

Hyperthermia should be avoided, and alterations in serum electrolytes should be minimized. Patients with head injuries should be monitored closely for the development of diabetes insipidus or syndrome of inappropriate secretion of antidiuretic hormone. Prophylaxis with anticonvulsants is still controversial, but any seizure activity must be rapidly recognized and treated.

Children with minor head injuries (GCS = 13–15 or CCS = 11) with no LOC or a brief witnessed period of LOC, no focal deficits on neurologic examination, no high-risk skull fractures, and no persistent vomiting, who demonstrate improvement and normal mental status (GCS = 15 or CCS = 11) after four to six hours of observation can be discharged with written instructions if they have adequate transportation back to the hospital and a telephone. Children should be admitted if these criteria cannot be reliably fulfilled. Younger children (< 4 years of age) are more difficult to assess accurately and consistently; therefore, admission should be strongly considered if their mental status is not completely normal or at baseline. Physicians should be wary of discharging children whose conditions have not improved to baseline following minor injuries even if their CT scans are normal.

More moderate head injuries (initial GCS = 9–12) necessitate a longer period of evaluation, probably in a monitored setting with neurosurgical consultation. Severe head injuries (GCS < 8) require aggressive stabilization in the emergency department with the measures described above and admission to a pediatric intensive care unit.

PROGNOSIS

Age is the most important prognostic factor in outcome. Younger children tend to do better than older children. It is still difficult to predict the outcome of any individual patient, however. Scalp lacerations, most skull fractures, and concussions are low-risk injuries. Intracranial hemorrhage, specific skull fractures, head injury secondary to child abuse, and trauma accompanied by diffuse cerebral edema are high-risk injuries.

If untreated, severe head injury may lead to death from herniation. Herniation results when cranial contents are too large for the space inside the skull, and the brain is compressed down through openings of the skull. Herniation can occur at several locations, such as through the foramen magnum or by compression against the cerebellar tentorium. Depending on the area being stretched or compressed, different clinical syndromes are produced.

Other complications from severe head trauma are posttraumatic seizures, requiring lifelong treatment with anticonvulsants; hydrocephalus, necessitating a ventriculoperitoneal shunt catheter; and persistent vegetative or severely impaired mental states. Sequelae such as postconcussive syndrome may result from less severe head trauma. Some of the characteristics of this syndrome include dizziness, headache, irritability, memory deficits, impaired behavior, and impaired cognitive development. These may persist for months after the head injury.

Case Resolution

The case scenario involves a young child with a significant mechanism of injury; brief LOC; and a depressed, altered mental status. Initial physical findings prompt suspicion of a depressed skull fracture and overlying soft tissue injury. Appropriate diagnostic tools after evaluation of the ABCs are a cranial CT scan followed by admission for observation, monitoring, and serial neurologic examination. Operative repair of the skull fracture may be necessary.

Selected Readings

Bruce, D. A. Head trauma. *In* Fleisher, G. R., and S. Ludwig. Textbook of Pediatric Emergency Medicine, 3rd ed. Baltimore, Williams & Wilkins, 1993.

Dolan, M. Head trauma. *In* R. M. Barkin (ed.). Pediatric Emergency Medicine Concepts and Clinical Practice. St. Louis, Mosby-Year Book, 1992.

Goldstein, B., and K. S. Powers. Head trauma in children. Pediatr. Rev. 15:213–219, June 1994.

Graneto, J. W., and D. F. Soglin. Transport and stabilization of the pediatric trauma patient. Pediatr. Clin. North Am. 40:365–380, 1993.

Inaba, A. S., and P. N. Seward. An approach to pediatric trauma. Emerg. Med. Clin North Am. 9:523–548, 1991.

Sampson, J. H., E. R. Rossitch, and W. J. Oakes. Initial management of pediatric head trauma. Am. Fam. Physician 45:2621–2628, 1992.

Schafermeyer, R. Pediatric trauma. Emerg. Med. Clin. North Am. 11:187–205, 1993.

Tecklenburg, F. W., and M. S. Wright. Minor head trauma in the pediatric patient. Pediatr. Emerg. Care 7:40–47, February 1991.

CHAPTER 42

INCREASED INTRACRANIAL PRESSURE

Kenneth R. Huff, M.D.

Hx A 7-year-old boy has a two-week history of recurrent vomiting. No fever, abdominal pain, or diarrhea has accompanied the vomiting, and the boy's appetite has decreased only slightly. The vomiting, which has had no particular relationship to meals, has been gradually increasing in frequency and is occurring every night. Yesterday, there were four episodes. The boy's parents have noticed that their son is generally less active; he spends more time playing on the floor of his room and does not want to ride his bicycle or play with neighborhood friends. Some unsteadiness in the boy's gait has developed in the last few days. His parents attribute this to weakness from the vomiting.

The child's vital signs are normal except for a blood pressure of 130/80. Although the boy is somewhat pale and uncomfortable, he does not appear to be in acute distress. His abdominal examination is unremarkable. His speech is grammatically correct but sparse and hesitant, and he seems inattentive. On lateral and upgaze the boy has some nystagmus, and upgaze is somewhat limited. Some diplopia on left gaze is apparent, with slight failure of left eye abduction. The left eye does not blink as much as the right eye. Fundal examination discloses elevated disks with indistinct margins. No upper extremity weakness is evident. The right foot is slightly weaker than the left, ankle tone is bilaterally increased, and three to four beats of clonus on the right and bilateral, positive Babinski reflexes are present. Some tremor occurs in both arms with finger-to-nose testing. The boy walks with shuffling, small steps; his gait has a slight lurching character, and he veers to the right.

Questions

1. What clinical situations are associated with increased ICP?
2. What is the pathophysiologic process leading to ICP?
3. What studies are used to evaluate children with ICP?
4. What measures are used to treat children with ICP?

The problem of increased intracranial pressure (ICP) can be understood in terms of the intracranial volume, which has three primary components: brain parenchyma, CSF, and blood. Except during the first two years of life, before most of the cranial sutures are fused, the skull and dura form a rigid compartment; any increase in one of the three components of intracranial volume occurs at the expense of the other two. Decreased volumes lead to increased pressure, which may damage brain parenchyma, cause hydrocephalus, or reduce arterial perfusion of the brain.

ICP is normally lower in neonates. In older children pressures above 13 mm Hg (180 mm H_2O) are abnormal, and levels above 20 mm Hg may become symptomatic. Although normal mental function is possible at pressures of up to 40 mm Hg, the ICP becomes dangerous when the perfusion pressure is compromised. This occurs as the ICP approaches 40 mm Hg below the mean arterial pressure (the mean of pressures measured continuously in a major artery). Decreased perfusion produces swollen, damaged tissue that further exacerbates the pressure-volume problem in a "snowballing" fashion.

EPIDEMIOLOGY

Head trauma is a leading cause of increased ICP. Infants may be victims of nonaccidental trauma; older children may be stricken pedestrians or bicycle riders, the occupants of motor vehicles, or victims of falls; and adolescents may be victims of penetrating trauma such as gunshots. Such trauma is a major source of morbidity in children and requires careful monitoring and management of ICP.

Brain tumors are the most common solid tumors in children and frequently lead to increased ICP either by direct mass effect or blockage of CSF flow. Ischemic brain damage resulting from a difficult delivery, a submersion incident, or major cerebral vessel thrombosis is a more common source of increased ICP. Some cytotoxic causes of brain swelling, such as lead intoxication and fatty liver failure in Reye's syndrome, cause increased ICP less commonly now than previously.

Benign intracranial hypertension or pseudotumor cerebri may also lead to increased ICP. When an association with clinical circumstance is present, this condition is seen most frequently in obese adolescent females and the following situations: thrombosis of a lateral venous sinus following complicated otitis media, treatment with high doses of vitamin A or tetracycline, and after withdrawal of steroid therapy.

CLINICAL PRESENTATION

Children with ICP may present with a history of recurrent vomiting, headache that awakens them from sleep, and lethargy. Physical findings may include elevated optic disk, failure of upgaze, hypertonicity of the extremities, and depressed consciousness. Localized findings on neurologic examination may point to a lesion indicative of a space-occupying intracranial mass, which contributes to increased ICP (D$_x$ Box). A prior history of trauma, ischemia, or intoxication may also raise suspicions of these conditions in the child with compatible findings.

PATHOPHYSIOLOGY

Changes in any of the three components making up the intracranial volume may result in increased ICP in several ways. First, the brain parenchyma component may be directly increased by mass lesions such as neoplasms, abscesses, or hemorrhages. Edema may also increase the brain parenchyma (volume). Fluid may accumulate because of vascular leakage due to cytokines. Brain edema also results from cytotoxic damage, cell death, and necrosis. Cytotoxic mechanisms include swelling of intact cells; cell rupture, producing increased osmotic pressure; and inflammation in an attempt to repair damaged cells. Cytotoxic brain edema may be caused by a number of cellular insults such as hypoxemia; ischemia; toxins, including neuronal excitotoxins; and absence of needed energy substrates. These cellular insults may be a consequence of a diversity of local or diffuse brain problems, including major vessel thrombosis, trauma (e.g., local contusion or diffuse axonal injury), anoxia from cardiac arrest, hyperten-

sion, encephalitic infection, or metabolic poisoning.

Second, the pressure of the CSF component of intracranial volume (ventricles or subarachnoid spaces) may increase in hydrocephalus. Hydrocephalus can result in two ways: (1) from a discrepancy in the rate of formation of CSF relative to absorption, and (2) an obstruction between the point of formation in the lateral ventricles and the site of absorption at the arachnoid granulation. An obstruction can occur with a congenital malformation, parenchymal or CSF mass such as a cyst or neoplasm, or CSF inflammatory cells from meningitis, ventriculitis, or hemorrhage. The small passageways connecting the ventricular system, the foramina of Monro and the aqueduct of Sylvius, the exits of the ventricular system, the foramina of Magendie and Luschka, and the cisterns surrounding the brain stem are particularly vulnerable sites of obstruction.

Third, ICP may rise because the blood component may increase. One process that leads to this increase is venous outflow obstruction, such as occurs with lateral sinus thrombosis, a cause of pseudotumor cerebri. Other processes that raise jugular venous pressure may also increase ICP. In addition, the intracranial arterial vascular volume is affected by carbon dioxide partial pressure. It not only increases with hypercarbia but also decreases with hypocarbia, which allows for iatrogenic lowering of ICP by hyperventilation.

The body tries to maintain adequate brain perfusion in the face of increasing ICP by increasing the mean arterial pressure, a condition referred to as the Cushing reflex. Although the relationship may not be direct and universally reliable, this rise in systemic pressure can be a useful sign of increased ICP.

Acute or subacute changes in pressure in an intracranial compartment may produce a pressure gradient, which may precipitate a brain herniation syndrome (Fig. 42–1). An ominous sign of transtentorial temporal lobe herniation is loss of pupillary light reflex. This herniation often leads to irreversible brain stem damage as well as new perfusion deficiencies and additional edema. An ill-advised lumbar puncture, which lowers the spinal compartment pressure acutely and increases the pressure gradient from the posterior fossa, can lead to compression of medullary centers. Eventually, apnea and death may occur.

DIFFERENTIAL DIAGNOSIS

Conditions increased ICP, including seizures, metabolic derangements, and complicated migraine, sometimes have a similar clinical presentation. In children with neurologic signs who are not fully responsive, distinguishing an ictal or postictal state from a condition that may be producing increased ICP is often difficult. Findings that suggest an electrical disturbance include clear, rhythmic, clonic movements or lightning myoclonic jerks; rapid, intermittent changes of tone or posturing that differ from irreversible decerebrate posturing; abrupt, fluctuating changes of autonomic function (e.g., heart rate, blood pressure, pupillary size); saliva production without swallowing; and history of prior seizures. Sometimes, however, only

---

D$_x$ Increased ICP

- Loss of appetite, nausea, vomiting, headache, or lethargy
- Inattention, decreased arousability, papilledema, upgaze paresis
- Increased tone, positive Babinski reflex
- Focal signs and history compatible with an intracranial mass
- Mass lesion, cerebral edema, or enlarged ventricles in an imaging study

FIGURE 42–1. *Depiction of the anatomy of several potential herniation syndromes caused by intracranial compartment pressure gradients related to a mass (hematoma, neoplasm, or acutely necrotic brain tissue) in a cerebral hemisphere. 1, trans-falxine herniation; 2, uncal herniation; 3, contralateral tentorial-midbrain damage; 4, central herniation and foramen magnum pressure cone. These syndromes often lead to further brain ischemia and additional increases in ICP. The drawing on the left depicts a normal brain.*

direct EEG and ICP monitoring are able to distinguish ongoing seizure activity from increased ICP as the cause of change in level of responsiveness.

In some cases, diffuse brain dysfunction from a toxic or metabolic etiology mimics a lesion, producing increased ICP. Examples of toxic-metabolic problems include medication intolerance, electrolyte or blood chemistry aberrations, and systemic infections. With toxic-metabolic disorders, difficulty paying attention is often accompanied by a confusional state with disorientation, incoherency, and sometimes agitation. In contrast, with increased ICP, inattention is frequently associated with slowness of thought, perseveration, impaired gait, and decreased mental activity.

The symptoms and signs of complicated migraine sometimes also mimic those of increased ICP. At the initial headache presentation or with a short headache history, however, the complicated migraine diagnosis may be one of exclusion. If children display focal neurologic signs along with some symptoms of increased ICP, imaging studies to rule out space-occupying lesions and

laboratory confirmation of normal pressure by lumbar puncture manometry may need to be performed.

EVALUATION

History

A thorough neurologic history should be taken (Questions Box). Headache, nausea and vomiting, drowsiness, and intermittent changes in visual acuity are important historical factors.

Physical Examination

Vital signs and head circumference should be noted. When increased ICP is suspected, a careful neurologic examination is warranted. Particular attention should be paid to the mental status and level of responsiveness of patients. Specific joint muscle tone and strength as well as gait should be evaluated in cooperative patients. The funduscopic appearance of papilledema and the integrity of the cranial nerves, motor responses, and breathing pattern should be assessed for brain stem level localization of the lesion. Particularly in comatose children, findings should be reassessed at frequent intervals to follow a potentially rapid process such as impending tentorial or central brain stem herniation, which necessitates immediate intervention.

Useful assessment instruments for initial, rapid evaluation and subsequent monitoring are the Glasgow and Children's (ages 4 years and below) Coma Scales (Table 42–1). However, these scales do not contain adequate information for all clinical decisions related to patients with increased ICP.

Questions: Increased ICP

- How long has the child been vomiting?
- When does the vomiting occur?
- Is the vomiting related to meals?
- Do the headaches awaken the child?
- Has there been a progressive decline in activity level or loss of developmental skills?
- Does the child display weakness or change in gait?
- Does the child have a recent history of trauma or lack of oxygen?

TABLE 42–1. Glasgow and Children's Coma Scales*

Glasgow		Children's	
Eye opening	Points	*Ocular Response*	Points
Spontaneous	4	Pursuit	4
To command	3	Extraocular muscles intact; pupils reactive	3
With pain	2	Extraocular muscles impaired; pupils fixed	2
No response	1	Extraocular muscles paralyzed, pupils fixed	1
Verbal Response	Points	*Verbal Response*	Points
Oriented, communicative	5	Cries	3
Disoriented, confused	4	Spontaneous respirations	2
Inappropriate	3	Apneic	1
Incomprehensible	2		
No response	1		
Motor Response	Points	*Motor Response*	Points
Obeys command	6	Flexes and extends	4
Localizes pain	5	Withdraws from pain	3
Flexes with pain	4	Hypertonic	2
Flexes abnormally with pain	3	Flaccid	1
Extensor response	2		
No response	1		

*Glasgow Scale from Teasdale, G., and B. Jennett. Assessment of coma and impaired consciousness: a practical scale. Lancet 2:81–84, 1974. Children's scale from Raimond, A.J., and J. Hirschauer. Head injury in the infant and toddler: coma scoring and outcome scale. Child's Brain 11:12–35, 1984.

In infants, a unique collection of signs—bulging, raised fontanelle, frontal bone bossing with prominent venous distention, "sunset sign" (inability to look up and lid retraction from midbrain tectal pressure), hypertonicity, and hyperreflexia—may be secondary to increased ICP from hydrocephalus. Papilledema is not present, perhaps related to greater compliance of the infant skull.

Laboratory Tests

If mental status changes are suggestive of a toxic or metabolic aberration, appropriate laboratory screens should be performed. These may include electrolytes, toxicologic screen, liver function and kidney function tests, and CSF examination if signs of meningeal irritation or infection without lateralized signs of altered tone or strength are present.

Diagnostic Studies

A CT or MRI scan should be performed whenever children's signs or symptoms indicate the possibility of increased ICP. Intravenous contrast should be done if disruption in the blood-brain barrier (e.g., infection, inflammation, neoplasia) is suspected and patients are not hypersensitive and have adequate kidney function.

MANAGEMENT

Management should first be directed to treating the lesion producing the increased ICP, if possible. If a single mass lesion is present, **neurosurgical craniotomy** may be necessary. If an inflammatory process is present, **anti-inflammatory agents** and **antibiotics** may be required. **Mineralocorticoids** are useful in situations in which the pressure is produced by a component of vasogenic edema, such as that surrounding neoplasms. Following directed specific treatment of the underlying lesion, increased ICP may resolve spontaneously. If hydrocephalus is present after initial therapy due to ongoing blockage of CSF pathways, **ventriculoperitoneal shunting of CSF** may be necessary.

Patients with ICP that is severely elevated or likely to rise rapidly require treatment in an intensive care unit. As in any emergent physiologic situation, the airway, breathing, and circulation must be secured first. ICP is quantitated on an ongoing basis to direct interventions to maintain brain perfusion. Neurosurgically placed devices such as the cranial "bolt," which fixes to the cranium and measures ICP without penetrating the subarachnoid space, and the intraventricular catheter (ventriculostomy) are commonly used. Ventriculostomy also allows for therapeutic CSF drainage to relieve increased ICP. Pressors are used to maintain systemic pressure. If acute lowering of ICP is necessary, hyperventilation reduces the intracranial arterial blood volume most effectively but must be limited to prevent decreased brain perfusion and ischemia production.

Pharmacologic agents may be used. **Diuretic agents such as mannitol also reduce brain water volume,** but care must again be taken because they eventually cross the blood-brain barrier and can draw more fluid into the brain if used too frequently. These agents are often used to counter ICP waves or increased pressure with endotracheal suctioning or other procedures. EEG monitoring of cerebral electrical activity is often useful in patients with decreased or fluctuating level of responsiveness. **Anticonvulsants** are indicated if seizures are present. In severe, refractory increased pressure due to an acute focal process, **barbiturates** such as pentobarbital or **benzodiazepines** such as midazolam can be given intravenously with appropriate monitoring

TABLE 42–2. Management Interventions in Increased ICP

Maintain serum osmols at 300–320 mOsm
Keep head elevated to 30 degrees
Maintain normal blood pressure
Controlled hyperventilation to $PaCO_2$ at 30–32 mm Hg
Supplemental O_2 and PEEP as needed to keep $PaO_3 > 90$ mm Hg and $FiO_2 < 50\%$
If ICP progressively rises, pressure waves higher than 20 mm Hg last longer than five minutes, or any pressure in first 24 hours is higher than 30 mm Hg, then give mannitol, 1 g/kg IV
If mannitol needs repeating in less than four hours or osmolality is greater than 320 mOsm:
  Give pentobarbital, 5 mg/kg IV, then 2 mg/kg/hr IV monitoring to blood level of 25–35 µg/mL, burst-suppression pattern with 10 seconds between bursts on EEG, and cardiac index greater than 2.7 L/min/m^2
  or
  Give midazolam by titrating the dose starting at 0.1 mg/kg/hr IV to the same EEG criteria and limited by the same cardiac index criteria

of brain electrical activity, serum levels, and systemic and brain perfusion pressures (Table 42–2).

PROGNOSIS

Patients may recover fully from increased ICP if brain perfusion pressure is adequately maintained and the underlying brain lesion generating the increased pressure can be resolved. Ultimately the prognosis depends on the nature of the lesion; its propensity to generate ICP that may be refractory to treatment, leading to brain damage or death; and its reversibility, permanence, or recurrence potential.

Case Resolution

The boy in the case history has focal signs and symptoms referable to the brain in the posterior fossa of the intracranial cavity as well as symptoms of increased ICP. An emergent CT scan shows subacute hydrocephalus due to obstruction of CSF flow produced by a large mass in the cerebellum and brain stem on the left side. He begins taking dexamethasone. Two days later the mass is surgically excised and is found to be malignant. Because the ICP remains high, a ventriculoperitoneal shunt is subsequently required for the hydrocephalus. The boy's recovery is otherwise uneventful, and he begins evaluation for further brain tumor therapy.

Selected Readings

Adams, R. D., and Victor, M. Principles of Neurology, 4th ed. New York, McGraw-Hill, 1991.

Bruce, D. A. Head injuries in the pediatric population. Curr. Probl. Pediatr. 20:61–107, 1990.

Fishman, R. A. Cerebrospinal Fluid in Diseases of the Nervous System, 2nd ed. Philadelphia, W.B. Saunders, 1992.

Nussbaum, E., and S. P. Galant. Intracranial pressure monitoring as a guide to prognosis in the nearly drowned, severely comatose child. J. Pediatr. 102:215–218, 1983.

CHAPTER 43

ACUTE RENAL FAILURE

Sudhir K. Anand, M.D.

Hx A ten-month-old girl has a two-day history of fever, vomiting, and watery diarrhea. The child has previously been healthy. Her diet has consisted of Similac with iron, baby food, and some table food. Since the onset of her illness, she has not been drinking or eating well, and she has thrown up most of what she has eaten. Her mother has tried to give her Pedialyte and apple juice on several occasions but has had limited success. The child has had 8 to 10 watery stools without blood or mucus each day. Her temperature has varied between 98.6 and 101.8° F (37.0 and 38.8° C); her mother has given her daughter acetaminophen, which she has vomited. The girl's four-year-old brother and her parents are doing well and have no vomiting or diarrhea.

The physical examination reveals a severely dehydrated (15%), listless infant. Her weight is 9.4 kg, her height is 74 cm, her temperature is 101.1° F (38.4° C), her heart rate is 168 beats/min, her respiratory rate is 30/min, and her blood pressure is 72/40 with an appropriately sized cuff. Capillary refill is two to three seconds. The skin appears dry, but no rash is present. Head and neck, chest, heart, and abdominal examination are normal. Until the results of routine blood studies are available, an intravenous fluid bolus of 180 mL D5 normal saline (20 mL/kg) over one hour is administered. The girl is catheterized to obtain urine and determine the flow rate over the next several hours. Urinalysis is performed.

Questions

1. What are the three categories of acute renal failure?
2. What is the etiology of acute renal failure in children?
3. What tests distinguish the three types of acute renal failure?
4. What is the appropriate management for children with acute renal failure? What are the indications for dialysis?

Acute renal failure (ARF) is the sudden decrease in kidney function with accumulation of nitrogenous waste products (e.g., creatinine, BUN). Most children with ARF have oliguria (urine volume < 400 mL/m^2/day or < 25% of daily recommended fluid intake for age). In some children, however, urine output may remain normal (nonoliguric ARF). Unlike many other organ failures, ARF is often completely reversible. Although ARF is still associated with considerable morbidity, with appropriate management, including use of dialysis, mortality due to renal failure itself is now minimal in children.

EPIDEMIOLOGY

ARF may occur in children with a wide variety of medical or surgical conditions, especially in children who are critically ill. The exact incidence of ARF in children is not known, but ARF is often observed in pediatric intensive care units (ICUs). The incidence of ARF is about 10 to 20% in neonatal ICUs.

CLINICAL PRESENTATION

Most children with ARF initially present with the clinical findings of the primary condition that led to the renal problem. Other findings, such as decreased urine output, edema, and heart failure (with administration of excessive fluids), result from ARF (D_x Box). Hyperkalemia with cardiac arrhythmia, hyperventilation due to acidosis, and nausea and vomiting due to uremia may occur as renal failure progresses.

ETIOLOGY AND PATHOPHYSIOLOGY

The causes of ARF are usually grouped into three categories: prerenal, intrinsic renal, and postrenal disorders (Table 43–1). This classification helps with diagnosis and formulation of the initial treatment plan.

Prerenal Disorders

In these disorders, decreased total or "effective" circulating blood volume caused by such conditions as dehydration, heart failure, or third spacing leads to decreased renal perfusion. The resulting decrease in the glomerular filtration rate (GFR) in early stages can be easily reversed by improving renal perfusion. If hypoperfusion is prolonged, however, ischemic damage to the kidney occurs and intrinsic renal failure develops (see below).

Postrenal Disorders

Urinary obstruction due to posterior urethral valves or other lesions occasionally leads to ARF, especially during infancy.

D_x Acute Renal Failure

- Decreased urine output
- Hematuria
- Edema
- Elevated serum creatinine
- Elevated BUN
- Elevated fractional excretion of sodium

TABLE 43–1.   Etiology of Acute Renal Failure in Children

Prerenal Causes
Decreased plasma volume
  Dehydration, hemorrhage, third spacing of plasma volume in burns, sepsis, bowel obstruction
Other causes of renal hypoperfusion
  Shock, hypoxia, congestive heart failure, hepatorenal syndrome, bilateral renal artery stenosis, cardiac surgery
Postrenal Causes
Bilateral obstruction
  Posterior urethral valves, trauma to urethra, neurogenic bladder, bilateral ureteropelvic obstruction
Obstruction of only functioning kidney
  Ureteropelvic obstruction, stone
Intrinsic Renal Causes
Vascular
  Renal artery or vein thrombosis, disseminated intravascular coagulation
Glomerular
  Severe (rapidly progressive) glomerulonephritis from any etiology, hemolytic-uremic syndrome
Interstitial
  Interstitial nephritis due to allergic reaction to drugs (e.g., methicillin), sepsis
Tubular (acute tubular necrosis [ATN])
  Ischemia due to prolonged hypoperfusion: all causes listed in prerenal category; if sufficiently prolonged, it will lead to ATN
  Nephrotoxins: aminoglycoside antibiotics, indomethacin, radiocontrast agents, ethylene glycol, methanol, heavy metals
  Pigments: myoglobinuria, hemoglobinuria
  Uric acid: hyperuricemia, tumor lysis syndrome
Congenital renal anomalies (especially in newborns and young infants)
  Bilateral cystic dysplastic kidneys, reflux nephropathy, polycystic kidneys, oligomeganephronia

Intrinsic Disorders

Intrinsic renal failure occurs because of injury to the vascular, glomerular, interstitial, or tubular components of the kidney (see Table 43–1). ARF resulting from renal tubular lesions is called acute tubular necrosis (ATN), although in many patients with ATN, necrosis of tubular cells is minimal. Certain histologic changes that characterize ATN include loss of brush border microvilli in tubular cells, detachment of epithelial cells from basement membrane, and cast formation from cellular debris and protein.

Children with prolonged shock due to trauma (hemorrhage), sepsis, or dehydration often develop ATN. This is the most frequent type of intrinsic ARF observed in children. Hemolytic-uremic syndrome (HUS) is another common cause of ARF in young children. In newborns and young infants, ARF may result from or be superimposed on a preexisting congenital renal disorder, especially if a child has previous abnormal urinary findings or delay in physical growth.

The pathogenesis of ATN in humans is controversial, and no single mechanism completely explains the sequence of events that lead to ATN. Ischemic and toxic ATN result from a complex interplay of hemodynamic, nephronal, and cellular changes. These include hypoperfusion of glomeruli, resulting in reduced GFR; injury to cortical and medullary tubules with their cellular debris, leading to tubular obstruction; and increase in intratubular pressure and further decrease in GFR. At the renal cellular level, decreased production of high-energy phosphates (ATP, ADP) contributes to damage to cell membranes and cell cytoskeletons, alterations in cell polarity, and entry of increased amounts of calcium, intracellular free radicals, and phospholipids. These changes lead to altered function and cellular swelling and eventually result in cell death. It is hoped that with better understanding of the pathophysiology of ARF, innovative, improved ways to both prevent and treat the disease will be developed.

DIFFERENTIAL DIAGNOSIS

The diagnosis of ARF is established by the demonstration of sudden increase in serum creatinine or BUN. Presence of decreased urine output is also helpful. Identification of the clinical disorder that led to ARF is often obvious, but at other times, extensive evaluation to discover the etiology of the primary disorder may be necessary. It should be determined whether children have chronic renal failure or superimposition of ARF on a preexisting renal condition.

EVALUATION

Laboratory and radiologic tests are more helpful diagnostically than history and physical examination.

History

Possible development of ARF should be anticipated in all critically ill children. A history of decrease in urinary volume, hematuria, dysuria, and nausea and vomiting should be sought in all such patients. The presence of previous urinary disorders and delayed growth may point to preexisting kidney conditions (Questions Box).

Physical Examination

Evaluation of physical growth, presence or absence of hypotension or hypertension, arrhythmia, dehydration, or edema should be made. Examination of the flank area for renal enlargement or tenderness and of the bladder for distention is necessary to help determine the etiology of ARF.

Laboratory Tests

The following laboratory tests are recommended in all children with ARF: CBC, with red blood cell morphology

---

TABLE 43–2. Diagnostic Indices in Acute Renal Failure*

Test	Prerenal	Intrinsic Renal
Urinalysis	Normal, occasional granular casts	Renal epithelial cells; pigment casts
Urine osmolality (mOsm/kg H_2O)	> 600	< 400
Urine specific gravity	> 1.020	<1.015
Urine sodium (mEq/L)	< 15	> 40
U/P creatinine†	> 40	< 20
Fractional excretion of sodium (FENa)‡	< 1%	> 2%

*Values in patients with nonoligouric acute renal failure often overlap and fall between prerenal and renal values. In addition, values in newborn infants differ from those in children beyond one year of age (see Anand in Selected Readings for values in newborns)

†U/P creatinine = urinary-plasma creatinine ratio (mg/mg).

‡$FENa = \dfrac{UNa}{UCr} \times \dfrac{PCr}{PNa} \times 100$

UNa = urine sodium (mEq/L)
UCr = urine creatinine (mg/dL)
PCr = plasma creatinine (mg/dL)
PNa = plasma sodium (mEq/L)

---

and platelet count; serum sodium, potassium, and bicarbonate; BUN; creatinine, uric acid, calcium, and phosphorus; glucose; total protein and albumin concentration; urinalysis and urine culture; and spot urinary sodium and creatinine concentration and osmolality. If children are not voiding frequently, catheterization of the bladder is advisable temporarily (4–6 hours) to obtain urine for analysis. Residual volume should also be assessed, and the urinary flow rate (especially the response to initial fluid therapy) and presence of an outflow obstruction should be determined. All infants should have an ECG.

The diagnosis of ARF can easily be established by laboratory tests and determination of urinary output over a specific time. Oliguria is defined as urine output less than 400 mL/m²/day or less than 1 mL/kg/hour in infants less than one year of age, less than 0.75 mL/kg/hour in children two to six years of age, and less than 0.5 mL/kg/hour in children more than six years of age. Urinalysis, urine specific gravity or osmolality, urine creatine: plasma creatinine ratio, urinary sodium concentration, and fractional excretion of sodium help differentiate prerenal from intrinsic ARF (Table 43–2).

Tubular epithelial cells and brown pigmented casts are often seen in patients with ATN. Evidence of hematuria or proteinuria signifies glomerular disease, especially glomerulonephritis or HUS. Presence of blood on dipstick but absence of RBCs on sediment examination suggests hemoglobinuria or myoglobinuria as the basis of ATN.

Although urinary indices are helpful in differentiating prerenal from intrinsic ARF, a simple clinical method to distinguish between the two can be used. A therapeutic trial of volume expansion with 20 mL/kg of D5 normal saline is administered intravenously over one hour (after the possibilities of congestive heart failure and urinary obstruction are excluded). If oliguria persists at the end of one hour, furosemide, 2 mg/kg, is given. If urinary output does not increase following furosemide administration, intrinsic ARF should be suspected and fluid administration reduced. Some physicians believe that by increasing urinary output, furosemide may help

---

Questions: Acute Renal Failure

- How frequently is the child passing urine?
- Is the amount of daily urine decreased, increased, or unchanged?
- Does the child have hematuria or dysuria?
- Does the child have nausea or vomiting?
- Has the child had any previous urinary problems?
- (Older children) Does the child have a history of enuresis or nocturia?
- Is the child's physical development normal or delayed?
- Does the child have a history consistent with the primary condition that may have led to the ARF?

prevent imminent ARF or may transform oliguric into nonoliguric ARF. Its effectiveness has not been established, however. Once intrinsic ARF has developed, repeated administration of high-dose furosemide has few benefits and can cause toxicity, especially hearing loss.

Imaging Studies

All infants and children with ARF should have a chest x-ray. Renal ultrasonography is the most useful test for differentiating between intrinsic ARF and postrenal ARF or identifying congenital anomalies. Renal ultrasound can detect the presence or absence of kidneys, enlarged kidneys, dilated pelvocalyceal system, or a distended bladder. Other investigative tests such as voiding cystourethrography, renal scans, angiography, CT, MRI, or renal biopsy may occasionally be necessary but are generally not indicated in children with ARF.

MANAGEMENT

Currently, no treatment leads to recovery of renal function in humans with established intrinsic ARF. Certain drugs, such as ATP-MgCl2, thyroxine, and atrial natriuretic hormone, have been used in experimental animals with variable results. The goal of therapeutic management of intrinsic ARF is maintenance of normal body homeostasis while awaiting spontaneous improvement.

After dehydration is corrected, **daily fluid intake** is limited to replacement of insensible water loss (about 30% of daily recommended fluid intake for age), urinary losses, and fluid losses from nonrenal sources (e.g., nasogastric drainage). Overhydration should be avoided in patients with ARF because it can cause edema, congestive heart failure, hypertension, hyponatremia, encephalopathy, and seizures.

Patients with complete anuria require no sodium intake. **Sodium** losses should be replaced daily in patients with urinary output, however. Preferably, the amount of sodium required should be determined by measuring daily urinary sodium losses.

Once ARF is suspected, **potassium** intake from all sources should be restricted. Severe hyperkalemia can often be avoided early in the course of the disease with strict adherence to potassium restriction. The level of serum potassium as well as ECG changes should be closely monitored. Patients with mild hyperkalemia may be treated with ion exchange resins; sodium polystyrene sulfonate (Kayexalate) may be given orally every four to six hours or by retention enema every one to two hours. Dialysis is more effective for treating hyperkalemia and may be warranted if serum potassium has been rising slowly over several days and dialysis is indicated for other reasons (see below).

Hypocalcemia and hyperphosphatemia are common in ARF, and small alterations in levels of **calcium** and **phosphorus** require no treatment. For serum phosphate greater than 8 mg/dL, phosphate binders such as calcium carbonate may be used. If serum calcium is less than 8 mg/dL, intravenous or oral calcium should be given to prevent tetany.

Mild metabolic acidosis is common in ARF and requires no treatment. If blood pH is less than 7.2 or serum bicarbonate is less than 12 mEq/L, sodium **bicarbonate** may be administered.

Adequate nutrition is important in ARF because it prevents excessive tissue breakdown. If renal failure is expected to be short in duration (3–4 days), most calories may be provided as carbohydrates. If ARF is expected to last longer, adequate calories in the form of carbohydrates along with daily protein intake of 1 g/kg should be provided.

Many children with ARF can be managed by the conservative measures described above. If renal failure lasts more than seven days or if complications develop, however, **dialysis** should be performed. The usual indications for dialysis include uncontrollable hyperkalemia or acidosis, volume overload with potential for pulmonary edema or congestive heart failure, and progressive uremia with BUN greater than 120 mg/dL or creatinine greater than 6 mg/dL. In children, peritoneal dialysis is usually preferred over hemodialysis. If peritoneal dialysis is contraindicated, continuous hemodiafiltration is another option.

ARF can often be prevented by anticipating its possible occurrence in children with high-risk conditions, such as dehydration, trauma, sepsis, and shock, or after cardiac surgery. Prompt recognition of prerenal failure and its aggressive management with volume expanders, inotropic agents, or judicious use of diuretics may prevent the development of intrinsic ARF. Nephrotoxic agents such as gentamicin should be avoided in high-risk patients if possible. When these drugs are used, they should be monitored meticulously, with frequent measurement of blood levels.

PROGNOSIS

The duration of oliguria in ARF may be short (1–2 days) or long (a few weeks). Recovery is usually first indicated by an increase in urinary output. BUN and creatinine may rise during the first few days of diuresis before beginning to return to normal. During diuresis, large quantities of sodium and potassium may be lost in the urine. Serum electrolytes should be closely monitored, and adequate replacements should be made to prevent hyponatremia or hypokalemia.

In children with ARF, outcome largely depends on the primary condition, the severity of damage to other organs, and the expertise in managing ARF. Nonoliguric ARF is consistently associated with a shorter clinical course and better prognosis than oliguric ARF. Most children with ATN recover completely. However, children with more severe kidney involvement (cortical necrosis) may have residual renal impairment or chronic renal failure.

Case Resolution

In the case scenario, a series of diagnostic studies are performed. The laboratory results are: hemoglobin, 13.8

g/dL; hematocrit, 41%; WBC count, 12,400/µL; neutrophils, 58%; band forms, 6%; lymphocytes, 32%; monocytes, 3%; and eosinophils, 1%. The platelet count is 277,500/µL. Serum sodium is 136 mEq/L; potassium, 5.1 mEq/L; chloride, 110 mEq/L; bicarbonate, 10 mEq/L; BUN, 84 mg/dL; creatinine, 2.8 mg/dL; and glucose, 68 mg/dL. The specific gravity is 1.015, the specimen is protein trace, blood, WBC and nitrite negative, and the sediment has many epithelial cells, one to two RBCs, and many granular and pigmented casts. Spot urinary sodium is 65 mEq/L, creatinine is 39 mg/dL, and the fractional excretion of sodium is 3.4%.

These results are most consistent with the diagnosis of intrinsic renal failure because the fractional excretion of sodium is increased. Recovery may take a few days to a few weeks.

Selected Readings

Anand, S. K. Acute renal failure (in the newborn infant). *In* Taeusch, W., R. Ballard, and M. E. Avery (eds.). Diseases of the Newborn, 6th ed. Philadelphia, W. B. Saunders, 1991, pp. 892–897.

Anderson, R. J. Prevention and management of acute renal failure. Hosp. Pract. 28:61–75, 1993.

Gaudio, K. M., et al. Acute renal failure: clinical aspects. *In* Holliday, M. A., T. M. Barratt, and E. D. Avner (eds.). Pediatric Nephrology, 3rd ed. Baltimore, Williams & Wilkins, 1994, pp. 1186–1203.

Sehic, A., and R. W. Chesney. Acute renal failure: diagnosis. Pediatr. Rev. 16:101–106, 1995.

Siegel, N. J., et al. Acute renal failure: pathophysiological mechanisms. *In* Holliday, M. A., T. M. Barratt, and E. D. Avner (eds.). Pediatric Nephrology, 3rd ed. Baltimore, Williams & Wilkins, 1994, pp. 1176–1186.

Weinberg, J. M. The cell biology of ischemic renal injury. Kidney Int. 39:476–500, 1991.

HEAD, NECK, AND RESPIRATORY SYSTEM

CHAPTER 44

CRANIOFACIAL ANOMALIES

Carol D. Berkowitz, M.D.

H_x A 3500-gram boy is born by normal spontaneous vaginal delivery to a 28-year-old gravida III para III mother after an uncomplicated full-term gestation. The Apgar scores are 9 and 10. On physical examination, the infant is well but has an incomplete, left-sided unilateral cleft of the lip as well as of the palate.

No other family members have such a deformity, but the mother and father are distantly related. The mother had prenatal care. During the pregnancy she had no illnesses, took vitamins but no other medications, and did not smoke, drink alcohol, or use illicit drugs.

The mother is planning to feed the infant with formula and wonders if she should do anything special. She is also wondering if her son's lip deformity can be repaired before she takes him home from the hospital. Except for the cleft, the physical examination is normal.

Questions

1. What craniofacial anomalies are common in children?
2. What are feeding considerations in infants with cleft lip or palate?
3. What is the appropriate timing of surgery for the more common craniofacial anomalies?
4. What are the major medical problems that children with craniofacial anomalies, particularly clefts of the lip or palate, experience?

The most frequently seen major craniofacial anomalies in children are cleft lip and cleft palate. Other common craniofacial problems include microtia, craniosynostosis, and facial asymmetry.

EPIDEMIOLOGY

The overall incidence of cleft lip with or without cleft palate is 1 in 1000, and that of isolated cleft palate is 1 in 2500. The sex distribution varies with the type of cleft. Isolated clefts of the palate occur twice as frequently in girls, but clefts of the lip with or without clefts of the palate appear twice as often in boys.

The type of cleft, the sex of the child, and whether parents or other siblings are similarly affected influence the risk for recurrence of clefts in subsequent offspring. In general, the risk for recurrence of clefts is 4 to 7% for cleft lip with or without cleft palate and 3% for isolated cleft palate.

Clefts may occur either as isolated findings or as part of syndromes such as Pierre Robin sequence, where they are associated with micrognathia and glossoptosis. In Van der Woude's syndrome, clefts of the lip or palate are associated with lip pits. This condition is inherited in an autosomal dominant manner.

CLINICAL PRESENTATION

Most craniofacial anomalies are readily apparent (see D_x Box). Some anomalies, such as cleft lips or microtia, are noted immediately in the delivery room. Other anomalies, such as craniosynostosis, develop over time. Because the onset of craniosynostosis may be gradual, parents may fail to recognize the condition, which usually appears as asymmetry of the face or skull.

Children with craniofacial anomalies may also have medical problems that occur secondary to the deformity. Infants with cleft palate may present with FTT because of difficulty feeding. Older infants and children may experience recurrent otitis media, speech impairments, or psychosocial stress. Nasal regurgitation of liquids may occur in children with obvious palatal clefts or more subtle deformities, such as submucous clefts of the soft palate.

D_x **Craniofacial Anomalies**

- Cleft of the lip or palate
- Small, atretic, or malformed ear
- Asymmetry of the face
- Misshapen skull
- Recurrent otitis media
- Speech impairment

PATHOPHYSIOLOGY

Clefts of the lip and palate (Fig. 44–1) are believed to develop as a result of an interruption in the merging of the middle and lateral portions of the face during the sixth to seventh week of gestation. The palate normally closes with an anterior to posterior progression. Any interference with this progression (e.g., tumor or encephalocele in the roof of the mouth) leads to a cleft. A vascular disruption may also result in ischemia in the involved areas.

The presence of a cleft palate affects normal oropharyngeal functioning, including sucking and speech. Children may exhibit hypernasal speech due to the escape of air through the nose and have articulation problems. Recurrent otitis media appears to be related to dysfunction of the eustachian tube.

Microtia, a small atretic pinna of the ear, results from failure of development of the pinna and portions of the external auditory canal. It is most likely caused by a vascular accident during the twelfth week of gestation. Similar anomalies have been created in laboratory animals by ligature of the stapedius artery.

Craniosynostosis refers to the premature closure of the sutures, which should remain open until two to three years of age. What initiates this pathologic ossification is unclear. Any or all of the sutures can be affected, and the closure may result in asymmetry of the skull or microcephaly. Premature closure of all sutures is often associated with diseases of the central nervous system with failure of the brain to grow.

Microcephaly may result from premature closure of some or all of the sutures as a primary event or from impairment of the brain and its growth related to some other problem, such as hypoxic encephalopathy or congenital infection.

Fusion of individual sutures prevents growth of the skull in the direction of that suture, and skull expansion proceeds in an axis parallel to that of the suture (Fig. 44–2). If the sagittal suture fuses prematurely, the head is long and narrow, a condition referred to as **scaphocephaly** (boat head). If the coronal sutures fuse too soon, the head is flattened; this condition is called **brachycephaly.** Premature closure of the metopic suture results in the triangular-shaped head characteristic of **trigonocephaly.**

Premature closure of the lambdoidal sutures leads to **plagiocephaly** (flat head) (Fig. 44–3). Plagiocephaly may also result from malpositioning in utero or after birth. Malar and contralateral occipital flattening related to preferential positioning by infants are characteristically seen in affected infants. Torticollis, often related to injury to the sternocleidomastoid muscle at birth (see Chapter 77, Disorders of the Spine) and abnormal positioning after birth, may cause plagiocephaly.

DIFFERENTIAL DIAGNOSIS

In general, the differential diagnosis of clefts of the lip and palate presents few problems. However, submucous clefts may be more difficult to diagnose. Children with such clefts may present with recurrent otitis media or hypernasal speech. Physical examination may reveal a bifid uvula and occasionally a notch at the junction of the hard and soft palates.

Determining whether any physical finding represents an isolated anomaly or is part of a genetic syndrome may be challenging. Any associated anomalies (e.g., syndactyly or atrial septal defect) suggest the possibility of a genetic problem (Tables 44–1 and 44–2).

Microtia does not present a diagnostic dilemma. The anomaly usually appears sporadically as an isolated condition, although, like a cleft, it may be part of some other syndrome. Microtia is associated with midfacial hypoplasia and antimongoloid slant to the eyes in Treacher Collins syndrome. Microtia may also occur in Goldenhar's syndrome, which is characterized by several associated findings, including hemifacial microsomia (one side of the face smaller than the other), epibulbar dermoids, hemivertebrae, microphthalmia, and renal and cardiac anomalies.

Craniosynostosis may also be an isolated finding or associated with a condition such as Apert's syndrome,

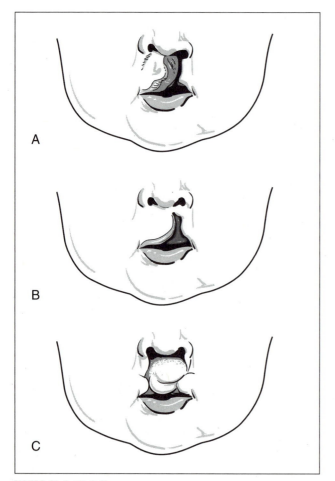

FIGURE 44–1. Cleft lips.
A. *Unilateral, complete cleft lip.*
B. *Unilateral, incomplete cleft lip.*
C. *Bilateral, complete cleft lip.*

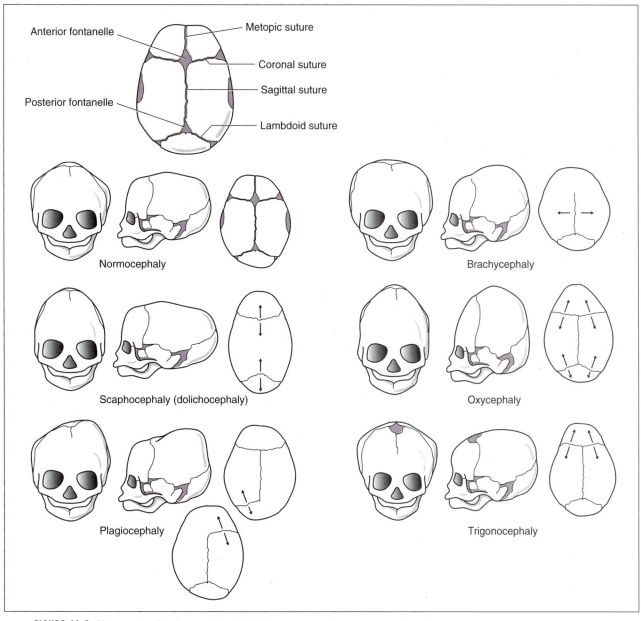

FIGURE 44–2. Changes in the shape of the skull when sutures fuse prematurely. *Growth occurs parallel to the fused suture.*

in which clefts of the palate are also seen. A careful neurodevelopmental assessment helps determine the cause of microcephaly. Plagiocephaly may present a diagnostic dilemma: Is the condition related to unilateral craniosynostosis or to torticollis and malpositioning after birth? A careful assessment of the neck for masses frequently helps differentiate between these two possibilities.

EVALUATION

Care must be taken to assess children and determine if the anomalies are isolated findings or components of a syndrome. This information is important both in terms

of patient care and genetic counseling for parents regarding the likelihood of having future offspring with similar anomalies.

History

A medical, family, and psychosocial history should be obtained (Questions Box). Whether the condition appeared at birth or some time later is particularly significant in lesions affecting the skull, such as craniosynostosis. Maternal use of certain medications, such as diazepam, phenytoin, and isotretinoin (Accutane), and alcohol is associated with an increased incidence of clefts of the lip and palate.

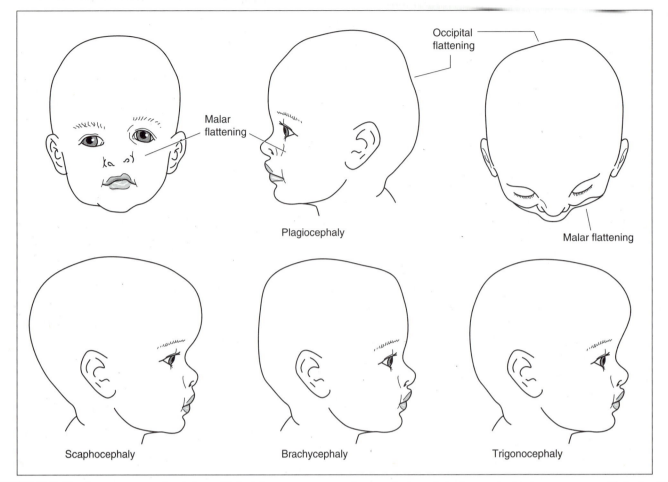

FIGURE 44–3. Classic appearance of an infant with facial asymmetry secondary to plagiocephaly (top row); classic appearance of infants with craniosynostosis (bottom row).

Physical Examination

Height, weight, and head circumference should be measured and plotted at each visit. Head circumference is especially important in children with craniosynostosis or facial asymmetry. The growth of children with craniofacial anomalies must be carefully monitored. Problems with adequate weight gain are frequently experienced by infants with clefts.

The physical examination should focus on defining the extent of the anomaly and determining if associated abnormalities are present. Such abnormalities may involve the face or other parts of the body, including the skeleton. Cardiac murmurs may be noted in children with clefts, and these murmurs should be carefully evaluated.

Children with clefts should be carefully assessed for the presence of otitis media at each visit. Periodic hearing assessments should be carried out in children with clefts or microtia. Speech and development should also be evaluated.

Laboratory Tests

Routine laboratory tests are not indicated in most children with craniofacial anomalies. Chromosomal

TABLE 44–1. Genetic Syndromes Associated with Clefts

Apert
Ectodactyly, ectodermal dysplasia
Goldenhar
Meckel
Optiz
Popliteal pterygium
Stickler
Treacher Collins
Van der Woude

TABLE 44–2. Anomalies Associated with Cleft Lips and Palates

Nasal glioma or meningoencephalocele	Aniridia
Persistent buccopharyngeal membrane	Cleft larynx
Congenital neuroblastoma	Polydactyly
Congenital heart disease	Anencephaly
Thoracopagus twins	Foot deformities
Congenital oral teratoma	Oral duplication
Forearm bone aplasia	Spina bifida
Lateral proboscis	Aplasia of trochlea
Sacral agenesis	Laryngeal web

Questions: Craniofacial Anomalies

- Did the child suffer any injuries at birth?
- Was the child born in an abnormal position?
- Have the findings been present since birth, or did they appear later?
- Has the anomaly led to any changes in the child's health, such as recurrent ear infections or speech difficulties?
- Does the child have any family history of craniofacial anomalies?
- Does the mother have a history of illness during pregnancy?
- Was the mother exposed to any medications, particularly teratogenic agents, during pregnancy?
- Did the mother use alcohol during pregnancy?
- Is the child experiencing difficulties in school (e.g., teasing)?
- How is the child performing in school?
- Is development progressing normally? What are the child's milestones?
- Is the child's speech understandable?

studies are indicated if a genetic disorder is suspected.

Imaging Studies

X-rays and imaging studies may be indicated in children with facial asymmetry, micro- and macrocephaly, and craniosynostosis. Renal ultrasound may be necessary in children with microtia because of the association between ear and renal anomalies.

MANAGEMENT

The management of children with craniofacial anomalies usually requires the expertise of a multidisciplinary team, including a pediatrician, plastic surgeon, ear-nose-throat specialist, speech pathologist, social worker, psychologist, orthodontist, and prosthodontist. Primary care physicians who are not part of the team can receive information regarding appropriate patient care and follow-up. It is important for primary care physicians to be familiar with the appropriate nomenclature to be able to communicate with consultants. In brief, clefts of the lip are unilateral or bilateral and complete or incomplete. A complete cleft extends into the nares (see Fig. 44–1). Clefts of the palate may involve the entire palate or be confined to the secondary or soft palate.

Routine **well child care,** including monitoring of growth and administration of immunizations, is most important in the management of children with craniofacial anomalies. Some infants with clefts are slow feeders. Mothers should be told that although breastfeeding can be carried out, it is often slow and difficult. Some formula-fed infants require the use of special nipples or feeders. A specific cleft palate feeder, which consists of a plastic bottle that allows for compression of the unit during feeding, is available. A soft, premature-type nipple can also be obtained. Long nipples, such as lamb's nipples, which are used to feed infant lambs, are not routinely recommended because they cause infants to gag. Infants who gain weight slowly may need to be given concentrated formulas (see Chapter 98, Failure to Thrive).

Hearing and speech should be monitored. Chronic prophylactic **antibiotics** or the insertion of **pressure equalization tubes** may be needed to manage recurrent otitis media (see Chapter 46, Otitis Media). Speech problems require the expertise of a speech pathologist and placement of children in **speech therapy** in either the community or school.

Surgical correction is indicated for many anomalies. Clefts are usually repaired as staged procedures during the first two years of life. Repair of the cleft lip, the first procedure, is scheduled when infants weigh 10 pounds, are 10 weeks of age, and when their hemoglobin is 10 (rule of tens). Appropriate weight gain is therefore critical to ensure timely surgery. Repair of the cleft palate, the second procedure, is usually undertaken when infants are between 12 and 18 months of age. Surgical correction of clefts does not alter children's propensity to otitis media. This condition improves as children get older, however. Refinement of the cosmetic results, including rhinoplasty, occurs throughout childhood. Orthodontia is frequently a key component to achieve a cosmetically acceptable result and appropriate occlusion of the dentition for speech and chewing.

Children with isolated unilateral microtia often hear, and surgery is recommended for cosmetic purposes. Surgical correction of microtia is usually initiated when children are five years of age, before they start school. At this time the ear has achieved 90% of its growth, and children are spared the potential embarrassment of their deformity in the school setting.

Craniosynostosis can be corrected surgically, although the procedure is major and has significant risks. A controversy about whether neurodevelopmental problems are related to craniosynostosis or whether they represent a preexisting condition has arisen. In developmentally normal children with evidence of closure of all the sutures, surgical repair is believed to be warranted. In other cases, the procedure is thought to be reconstructive because it normalizes the appearance of children with a deformation.

In children with plagiocephaly, where the deformation is believed to be related to torticollis, **passive stretching of the neck** five to six times a day (with each diaper change) is used to manage the condition. In addition, it is recommended that bright objects such as mobiles be placed over children's cribs to encourage head turning.

Psychologic counseling should be available to affected children and their families to help them adjust to the anomalies and the reactions of society. Parents may be referred to community agencies such as the Cleft Palate Guild to help them cope with the potential stress related to giving birth to children with this anomaly.

PROGNOSIS

Most anomalies can be surgically corrected, leaving little residual evidence of the deformity. School success and psychological well-being may be more resistant to remediation, and are highly dependent on the supportiveness of the family and their emotional resources.

Children who grow up in settings where the deformity is thought to be embarrassing have long-term problems with low self-esteem.

follow-up appointment in about two weeks should be arranged. Weight gain can be monitored, and the adjustment between the mother and the infant should be assessed.

Case Resolution

The infant in the case history has a cleft of the lip and palate. The mother is advised that the infant can be given formula, and she is given a supply of special feeders. She should have the opportunity either to meet other parents of children with similar anomalies or to view pictures of children who have undergone a repair.

The mother should also be advised about the timing of surgery. She should be told that the surgery cannot be scheduled until the infant is approximately 10 weeks old. A

Selected Readings

Berera, G. Index of suspicion: submucous cleft palate. Pediatr. Rev. 14:191–192, 1993.

Fields, H. W. Craniofacial growth from infancy through adulthood. Pediatr. Clin. North Am. 38:1053–1125, 1991.

Kaufman, F. L. Managing the cleft lip and palate patient. Pediatr. Clin. North Am. 38:1127–1147, 1991.

Marion, R. W. Craniosynostosis. Pediatr. Rev. 16:115–116, 1995.

Suslak, L., and F. Desposito. Infants with cleft lip/cleft palate. Pediatr. Rev. 9:331–334, 1988.

Throkelsson, T., F. Mimouni, and W. S. Ball, Jr. Sagittal and lambdoidal craniosynostosis. Am. J. Dis. Child. 146:1311–1312, 1992.

CHAPTER 45

COMMON ORAL LESIONS

Geeta Grover, M.D.

H$_x$ A seven-year old girl is brought to the office for evaluation of a swelling on the inside of her lower lip of four to six weeks' duration. Her mother reports that it increases and decreases in size. The girl says that the swelling is not painful, and she cannot remember hurting her lower lip. On examination, a raised, bluish, nontender, 1 x 1 cm swelling is apparent along the mucosa of the lower lip.

Questions

1. What is the differential diagnosis of lip masses?
2. What laboratory or radiographic tests are useful in the evaluation of oral lesions?
3. What management strategies are used to treat cystlike oral lesions?
4. When should children with oral lesions be referred to subspecialists?

Primary care physicians are often required to evaluate lesions in the oral cavity. Knowledge of common congenital, developmental, infectious, and neoplastic conditions that affect the mouth and its structures can help physicians recognize and manage these lesions appropriately. Although many lesions are benign and regress spontaneously, others may require drainage, administration of medications, or surgical excision. Evaluation and management of some oral conditions may necessitate interaction among the pediatrician, dentist, and oral surgeon.

EPIDEMIOLOGY

Oral pathology is common. Benign oral lesions, such as gingival cysts, occur in about 75% of newborns. The reported incidence of natal teeth (teeth present at birth) is about 1 in every 3000 live births; the incidence increases in infants with cleft lip or palate. Developmental abnormalities such as geographic tongue and hyper- or hypodontia are evident in 1 to 2% and 4 to 7% of individuals, respectively. The incidence of hypodontia in the permanent dentition is about 7% (less than 1% in the primary dentition). The teeth most commonly missing are the third molars, maxillary lateral incisors, and mandibular second premolars. The incidence of supernumerary permanent teeth is 3 to 4%, occurring most often in the area of the maxillary central incisors.

Infections of the mouth are even more common. Although the rate of dental caries in the United States has significantly declined in the past 10 to 20 years, largely because of the use of systemic fluoride, approximately 50% of school children either have dental caries or a history of gingivitis.

CLINICAL PRESENTATION

Little or no discomfort is associated with even extensive dental caries. Untreated caries may result in destruction of most of the tooth. When infection extends to the dental pulp (pulpitis), significant pain may occur. Dental abscesses may present with fever, severe facial pain, and swelling. Aphthous ulcers are characteristically extremely painful. Even small lesions can produce a disproportionate amount of discomfort.

Children with gingivitis present with red, swollen mucosa that may bleed with toothbrushing. Children with primary herpetic gingivostomatitis present with fever, often as high as 103–104° F (39.4–40.0° C); irritability; anorexia due to pain on chewing and swallowing; and scattered vesicular lesions on the mucous membranes of the lips, tongue, and gingivae, which may also be erythematous and swollen. Herpangina, like herpetic gingivostomatitis, may be associated with fever (frequently high), irritability, and anorexia. The vesicular lesions are usually confined to the oropharynx (e.g., pharynx, tonsils, soft palate), sparing the gingiva and anterior oral cavity.

Candidiasis, or thrush, typically appears as small, white plaques on the buccal mucosa or tongue. Children are usually asymptomatic.

PATHOPHYSIOLOGY

Neonatal Abnormalities

Gingival cysts in newborns are due to entrapment of tissues during embryologic development. Histologically, **congenital epulis** consists of sheets of granular cells in the connective tissue underlying the epithelium. **Melanotic neuroectodermal tumor of infancy** is characterized by clusters of small, neuroblast-type cells lying within the alveolar spaces lined with endothelial-type, melanin-containing cells.

Developmental Abnormalities

The etiology of **geographic tongue,** or benign migratory glossitis, is unknown, but this chronic, often recurring condition has been associated with stress. **Mucoceles** are usually due to trauma to one of the minor salivary glands. **Enamel abnormalities** may be due to local or systemic infections, excessive fluoride ingestion, or nutritional deficiencies.

Tooth Discoloration

Extrinsic staining is due to material adhering to the surfaces of the teeth. **Intrinsic staining** results from the incorporation of excessive levels of endogenous substances, including normal pigments, such as hemoglobin or bilirubin, or exogenous substances, such as tetracycline or fluoride, into the developing enamel.

Oral Infections

The process of the formation of **dental caries** requires the interaction of dietary carbohydrates, particularly sucrose, and dental plaque. Dental plaque is a dense material composed of salivary products, food debris, and bacteria that forms along the margins of the teeth

and gums. The bacteria in plaque, most commonly *Streptococcus mutans*, produce organic acids that demineralize the outer surfaces of the teeth through the fermentation of carbohydrates. Left untreated, caries can progress, and eventually lead to necrosis of the pulp and cavitation of the tooth. The frequency of carbohydrate consumption and duration of contact with the tooth (relative stickiness of the substance) are more important than the total amount of carbohydrates consumed.

Nursing bottle caries are caused by the pooling of carbohydrate-containing liquids around the teeth. These caries are seen most often in infants who sleep with a bottle in their mouth.

Primary herpetic gingivostomatitis is caused by herpes simplex virus, usually type 1.

The etiology of **aphthous ulcers** is unknown, but stress and local trauma are believed to be predisposing factors.

DIFFERENTIAL DIAGNOSIS

Oral pathology may be divided into several categories: neonatal abnormalities, developmental abnormalities, tooth discoloration, and oral infections (Table 45–1).

TABLE 45–1. Common Oral Lesions in Children

Neonatal Abnormalities
Natal teeth
Benign gingival cysts
   Epstein's pearls
   Bohn's nodules
   Dental lamina cysts
Congenital epulis
Melanotic neuroectodermal tumor of infancy
Developmental Abnormalities
Soft tissues
   Generalized gingival hyperplasia
   Benign migratory glossitis (geographic tongue)
   Mucoceles and ranulas
Hard tissues (teeth)
   Variations in tooth number (hyper- and hypodontia)
   Variations in size and shape of teeth
   Defective enamel formation (hypoplasia or hypocalcification)
Tooth Discoloration
Extrinsic staining
   Poor oral hygiene
   Smoking
   Food or drink
   Medication
Intrinsic staining
   Endogenous (e.g., hemoglobin, bilirubin)
   Exogenous (e.g., tetracycline, fluoride)
Oral Infections
Bacterial
   Dental caries
   Nursing bottle caries
   Dental abscesses
   Gingivitis
Viral
   Primary herpetic gingivostomatitis
   Herpangina
   Aphthous ulcers
Fungal
   Candidiasis (thrush)

Neonatal Abnormalities

Natal teeth are present in the oral cavity at the time of birth, whereas **neonatal teeth** erupt during the first month of life. Most natal teeth are primary teeth that have erupted early, not supernumerary teeth. The most commonly affected teeth are the mandibular central incisors. These teeth are often loose due to immature root development. The two most common associated problems involve difficulty with breast-feeding (biting the mother) and potential aspiration of teeth.

Benign gingival cysts are commonly seen in newborns. **Epstein's pearls** are most common. They are small, white, keratin-filled lesions located along the midline of the palate. **Bohn's nodules** appear as multiple, firm, grayish-white lesions located along the gums and only occasionally on the palate. Unlike Epstein's pearls, these contain remnants of mucous gland structures as well as keratin. **Dental lamina cysts** are remnants of dental lamina epithelium that appear as small, cystic lesions along the crests of the mandibular and maxillary mucosa.

Two benign tumors that are seen during infancy are congenital epulis and melanotic neuroectodermal tumor of infancy. **Congenital epulis** is a rare, benign soft tissue tumor usually located on the anterior portion of the maxillary (most likely) or mandibular mucosa at birth. Over 90% of cases occur in girls. Solitary lesions are most common, but about 10% are multiple. **Melanotic neuroectodermal tumor of infancy** is a benign but locally aggressive tumor that presents during the first year of life. It usually appears as a grayish-blue, firm mass along the anterior aspect of the maxillary mucosa.

Developmental Abnormalities

Common soft tissue abnormalities include generalized gingival hyperplasia, geographic tongue, mucoceles, and ranulas. **Generalized gingival hyperplasia** may be idiopathic, secondary to drugs such as phenytoin and cyclosporine, genetically transmitted (fibromatosis gingivae), or transiently associated with tooth eruption. A nonspecific pathologic entity, it is characterized by gingival overgrowth that may secondarily become inflamed or edematous. **Geographic tongue** is characterized by painless, irregularly shaped, red patches with white borders located on the dorsum and lateral borders of the tongue. Affected areas are devoid of filiform papillae. Lesions regress and reappear spontaneously over a period of weeks to months, producing a migratory appearance.

Mucoceles and ranulas are benign soft tissue tumors of the oral cavity. **Mucoceles** are painless, smooth, fluid-filled translucent or bluish lesions that are most often found on the mucosa of the lower lip. They may increase and decrease in size. Ranulas are mucoceles located in the floor of the mouth.

Hard tissue abnormalities include variations in tooth number (hyperdontia and hypodontia), size and shape, and hypoplasia or hypocalcification of teeth. **Hypodontia** occurs when tooth buds fail to form. Hypodontia may be associated with ectodermal dysplasia syndromes.

Hyperdontia is the occurrence of supernumerary teeth. **Variations in size and shape of teeth** result from disturbances during tooth development. These changes are clinically significant only if they cause problems with crowding or alignment of the other teeth. Defective enamel formation may present as **hypoplasia** (pitting or thinning of the enamel) or **hypocalcification** (chalky or white lesions on the surfaces of the teeth).

Tooth Discoloration

Discoloration may be extrinsic or intrinsic. **Extrinsic stains** are usually due to poor oral hygiene, smoking, foods or drinks and medications (e.g., children taking liquid iron supplements may develop brownish-black stains on their teeth). **Intrinsic stains** may be secondary to endogenous or exogenous substances. Infants with erythroblastosis fetalis or severe neonatal jaundice are at risk for staining secondary to high plasma levels of hemoglobin or bilirubin. Tetracycline is incorporated into calcifying teeth and produces a yellow to brown to dark gray discoloration.

Oral Infections

Bacterial Infections

Dental caries, a multifactorial disease, causes progressive destruction of teeth. Lesions initially appear as opaque or yellowish-brown defects on the surface of the enamel. Severe involvement can present as complete destruction of the involved teeth. Caries may affect the smooth surfaces of the teeth, especially those between adjacent teeth, but they occur more commonly in the pits and fissures of the chewing surfaces of the teeth.

Nursing bottle caries, or baby bottle tooth decay, is a specific form of caries that occurs typically in children 12 to 24 months of age. The most commonly affected teeth are the maxillary incisors, followed by the cuspids and the first molars. The lower incisors are usually spared because of the protective barrier provided by the tongue. Opaque or chalky discolorations of the teeth are the earliest sign of decay. These areas become darkly eroded, and eventually tooth loss results.

Dental abscesses are most often the result of untreated dental caries. Once tooth necrosis occurs, bacteria may invade the alveolar bone and produce dental abscesses. Associated complications include sepsis and facial cellulitis.

Gingivitis is an infection of the gingiva that produces inflammatory changes. It is usually secondary to poor oral hygiene, resulting in accumulation of dental plaque around the apices of the teeth at the gingival margin (gum line). This condition may also be seen in children with diabetes mellitus, neutropenia, thrombocytopenia, and leukemia.

Viral Infections

Viral infections of the mouth are quite common in children. Gingivostomatitis is an infection of the gingiva and other parts of the oral mucosa. **Primary herpetic**

gingivostomatitis primarily affects children one to three years of age. The associated vesicles are painful, and when these vesicles rupture, shallow ulcers form. **Herpangina**, a form of stomatitis, is an infection of the oral mucosa that spares the gingiva. Caused by the coxsackie A group of viruses, it is usually characterized by painful vesicles on the mucosa of the soft palate and posterior pharynx. Although herpangina most commonly affects children under five years of age, older children may also be afflicted. **Aphthous ulcers**, or canker sores, are of unclear etiology, but may be related to trauma or viruses. These shallow, 3–4-mm ulcers, with an erythematous ring, occur singly or multiply, most often on the floor of the mouth or the mucous membranes of the lips. The painful lesions usually begin during adolescence or young adulthood and often recur.

Fungal Infections

Candidiasis, or thrush, is caused by *Candida albicans*. This condition is seen mostly in infants, but it also occurs in children who are receiving antibiotic therapy or who are immunosuppressed. Creamy white plaques on the buccal mucosa or tongue that are difficult to remove and may cause bleeding when scraped are characteristic of candidiasis. Candidal diaper rash may be associated with oral thrush.

EVALUATION

History

Any parental concerns regarding disruptions in the child's daily activities (e.g., decreased appetite, irritability) due to the lesion in question should be noted. The length of time the lesion has been present, whether it is painful, and whether the child has recently taken or is currently taking any medications are important to determine (Questions Box).

Physical Examination

Physical examination begins with an inspection of all structures in the mouth (e.g., lips, gums, teeth, mucosal surfaces) and an assessment of oral hygiene. Gingival swelling, erythema, and friability should be noted. The number of teeth should be counted, and any unusual shapes or stains should be described. Any obvious le-

sions within the oral cavity should be assessed in terms of location, color, size, shape, and tenderness.

Laboratory Tests

A CBC and blood culture may be obtained if systemic symptoms (e.g., fever) are associated with a dental abscess. Ulcers can be scraped for viral isolation or microscopic examination (Tzanck smear), looking for the multinuclear giant cells characteristic of herpetic infection. The diagnosis of thrush can be made by scraping the lesion, mixing the material with KOH, and viewing the characteristic hyphae on microscopic examination. This is rarely necessary, however, because the diagnosis can usually be made on clinical appearance.

Imaging Studies

Dental x-rays may be required in the evaluation of natal teeth, dental caries, or dental abscesses. Such x-rays may also be used to differentiate supernumerary teeth from natal teeth that are prematurely erupted primary teeth. Early radiographic identification of supernumerary teeth is important because they may interfere with eruption and alignment of future teeth.

MANAGEMENT

Neonatal Abnormalities

The vast majority of natal teeth are true primary teeth. Premature extraction may lead to overcrowding of the permanent teeth because the space once occupied by the extracted tooth may become occupied by the adjacent primary teeth. Only loose teeth that pose a danger of aspiration, are supernumerary, or cause discomfort to the mother or child should be removed. All gingival cysts are benign and resolve within a few weeks. Both congenital epulis and melanotic neuroectodermal tumors respond to surgical excision with infrequent recurrence.

Developmental Abnormalities

Meticulous oral hygiene should be stressed for children on phenytoin therapy. Phenytoin-induced gingival hyperplasia may require surgical excision of the excessive tissue. However, recurrence is common. Both mucoceles and ranulas require surgical excision of the lesion and the associated minor salivary gland to prevent recurrence. Children with hard tissue abnormalities should be referred to a pediatric dentist for further evaluation.

Tooth Discoloration

Tetracycline should not be given to pregnant women or children under the age of 8 to 10 years because it produces intrinsic staining of the teeth. Because tetracycline crosses the placenta and affects developing teeth in the fetus, it should not be prescribed to

---

Questions: Common Oral Lesions

- How long has the child had the lesion?
- Is the lesion painful?
- Did the child recently injure the affected area?
- Has the child had any fever?
- Is the child eating as usual?
- Does the child have any other lesions?
- Is the child currently taking any medications? Has the child recently taken any medications?

pregnant women. Green staining may result from algal growth on the teeth. Such extrinsic stains can be removed with cleaning.

Oral Infections

Most dental caries can be prevented through **good oral hygiene, proper diet,** and **preventive dental care.** The best method for prevention of smooth surface caries involves the **regular use of systemic fluorides.** Initiation of caries on chewing surfaces may be prevented by the application of **dental sealants** to these surfaces. **Prevention** is the best treatment for nursing bottle caries. Parents should be counseled never to nurse their children to sleep or put them to bed with a bottle containing anything but water.

Gingivitis in its early forms responds to improved oral hygiene and daily plaque removal with toothbrushing. Professional dental care may be required for more extensive disease. In both primary herpetic gingivostomatitis and herpangina, lesions heal spontaneously in one to two weeks. Treatment is supportive. Acetaminophen may be used for fever and pain control, and fluids, including cold liquids and Popsicles, should be encouraged because they may be soothing to inflamed tissues. Application of topical anesthetics such as viscous lidocaine should be discouraged because of the risk of absorption and seizures.

Aphthous ulcers (canker sores) heal spontaneously. Treatment is supportive and aimed at minimizing pain and shortening the duration of the lesions. Rinsing the mouth with a **topical antibiotic** (e.g., 250-mg capsule of tetracycline dissolved in 15 mL of water) may help reduce pain and prevent the overgrowth of opportunistic microorganisms. Mouthwashes containing hydrogen peroxide promote oral hygiene as well and should be used frequently. Topical steroid ointment (e.g., 0.1% triamcinolone dental paste) and systemic steroid therapy (in adults with extensive lesions) are other therapeutic options. Omeprazole has also been used for extensive, chronic aphthous ulcers, particularly in immunodeficient patients.

Treatment of candidiasis involves administration of **nystatin** suspension four times a day until the lesions resolve (generally one to two weeks). An alternative treatment is direct application to the lesions of a 1% gentian violet solution several times a day. Because it stains the skin and mucous membranes a bluish-purple color, it may not be well-accepted. Recurrent or refractory infection may warrant evaluation of the immune system.

Case Resolution

The child described in the case history at the beginning of this chapter appears to have a mucocele. She should be referred to either an oral or head and neck surgeon for surgical excision of the lesion.

Selected Readings

Dilley, D. C., M. A. Siegel, and S. Budnick. Diagnosing and treating common oral pathologies. Pediatr. Clin. North Am. 38:1227–1264, 1991.

Dunlap, C. L., B. F. Barker, and J. W. Lowe. Ten oral lesions you should know. Contemp. Pediatr. 8:16–28, 1991.

Mueller, W. A. When baby teeth decay. Contemp. Pediatr. 10:75–83, 1993.

Nazif, M. M., et al. Oral disorders. *In* Zitelli, B. J., and H. W. Davis. Atlas of Pediatric Physical Diagnosis, 2nd ed. Philadelphia, J.B. Lippincott, 1992.

CHAPTER 46

OTITIS MEDIA

Monica Sifuentes, M.D.

H$_x$ An 18-month-old male infant is brought to your office with a two-day history of fever and decreased intake of feedings. He has had symptoms of an upper respiratory infection (URI) for the past four days but no vomiting or diarrhea. Otherwise he is healthy.

The infant appears tired but not toxic. On physical examination the vital signs are normal except for a temperature of 38.8° C. The left tympanic membrane (TM) is erythematous and injected, with yellow pus behind the membrane. The light reflex is splayed, and mobility is decreased. The right tympanic membrane is gray and mobile, with a sharp light reflex. The neck is supple with shotty anterior cervical adenopathy, and the lungs are clear.

This is the infant's fourth documented ear infection in six months. He has a 10- to 15-word vocabulary, and no one smokes in the household.

Otitis media (OM) is the second most common reason after well child care for a visit to the pediatrician. It is estimated that approximately 30 million office visits per year involve the evaluation and treatment of OM and that billions of dollars are spent annually for OM care. Moreover, more than a quarter of all prescriptions written each year for oral antibiotics are for the treatment of middle ear infections. In addition, many surgical procedures such as myringotomy with tympanostomy tube placement or tonsillectomy and adenoidectomy are performed on children for treatment of recurrent disease. Therefore, the primary care physician must have a good understanding of this pediatric condition.

OM can be classified into the following four categories: acute OM with or without effusion, persistent middle ear effusion, recurrent acute OM, and chronic OM with effusion. It is important to distinguish between each of these entities because their presentation and management differ.

Acute OM (acute suppurative or purulent OM) is the sudden onset of inflammation of the middle ear, which is often accompanied by fever and ear pain. **Persistent middle ear effusion,** or subacute OM, is the presence of middle ear fluid after antimicrobial treatment. Resolution of acute inflammatory signs has occurred, with persistence of a more serous, less purulent effusion. Although the fluid may persist for two to three months, it resolves within three to four weeks in 50% of cases. **Recurrent OM** is defined as frequent episodes of acute OM with complete clearing between each case. This condition affects approximately 20% of children who are "otitis prone"; such children are usually infants who have their first infection at less than a year of age. **Chronic OM with effusion** (serous OM, secretory OM, or nonsuppurative OM) is a chronic condition characterized by persistence of fluid in the middle ear for three months or longer. The TM is retracted or concave with impaired mobility and shows no signs of acute inflammation, and affected children may be asymptomatic. These individuals are at greatest risk for developing hearing deficits and speech delay.

EPIDEMIOLOGY

The overall prevalence of OM is 15 to 20%, with the highest peak at 6 to 36 months of age. An additional smaller peak occurs at about four to six years. OM is relatively uncommon in older children and adolescents. The condition is more common in boys than girls, and the prevalence is greater in Alaskan natives and Native Americans than in Caucasians.

Several epidemiologic risk factors for OM have been identified, including familial predisposition; low socioeconomic status; altered host defenses (acquired or congenital immunodeficiencies); environmental factors, such as day care attendance and passive smoke exposure; and the presence of an underlying condition such as a cleft palate or other craniofacial anomaly. Children with Down, Goldenhar's, and Treacher Collins syndromes also have an increased risk of OM as well. As one might expect, the highest rate of OM occurs during the winter months and in early spring, coinciding with peaks in the incidence of URIs.

Breast-feeding, which provides infants with immunologic protection against URIs, other viral and bacterial infections, and allergies, is thought to have a preventive effect. It has also been hypothesized that facial musculature develops differently in breast-fed infants, thus influencing eustachian tube function and preventing aspiration of fluid into the middle ear. Positioning during breast-feeding also has been hypothesized to have some protective effect, although this may not be as important as the role of an immune factor in breast milk.

CLINICAL PRESENTATION

Children with OM have a history of fever and ear pain. Associated symptoms include URI, cough, diarrhea, and nonspecific complaints such as decreased appetite or irritability. Purulent otorrhea with minimal ear pain and hearing loss may also occur (D_x Box).

PATHOPHYSIOLOGY

The most important factor in the pathogenesis of OM is abnormal function of the eustachian tube (Fig. 46–1). Reflux, aspiration, or insufflation of nasopharyngeal bacteria into the middle ear via the dysfunctional eustachian tube may lead to infection. Hematogenous spread of microorganisms is another cause of infection. Less often, primary mucosal disease of the middle ear from allergies or abnormal cilia may lead to OM.

The causative microorganisms for OM are *Streptococcus pneumoniae, Haemophilus influenzae,* and *Moraxella*

D_x Otitis Media

- Ear pain or otorrhea
- Possibly fever
- Abnormal TM
- Erythema or injection of TM
- Pus behind TM
- Bulging appearance
- Distorted or absent light reflex
- Decreased mobility via pneumatic otoscopy

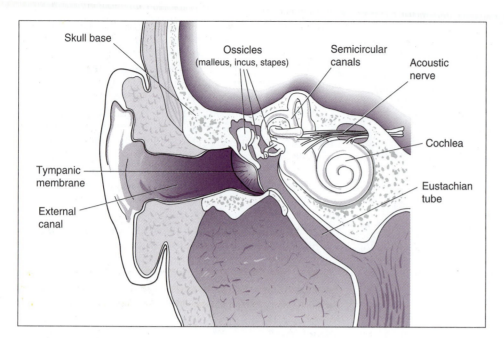

FIGURE 46–1. *Relationship of middle ear to external and inner ears.*

catarrhalis. Group A streptococcus, *Staphylococcus aureus*, and anaerobic bacteria are other less common causes. Respiratory viruses such as RSV, adenovirus, rhinovirus, and influenza A also play a role.

Eustachian tube dysfunction occurs primarily for two reasons: abnormal patency and obstruction. Obstruction is either functional (secondary to collapse of the eustachian tube), mechanical (from intrinsic or extrinsic causes), or both. Functional obstruction or collapse of the eustachian tube occurs commonly in infants and young children because the tube is less cartilaginous and therefore less stiff than in adults. In addition, the tensor veli palatini muscle is less efficient in this age group. Intrinsic mechanical obstruction of the eustachian tube occurs as the result of inflammation secondary to a URI or allergy. Extrinsic causes of mechanical obstruction include masses such as tumors or adenoidal enlargement.

DIFFERENTIAL DIAGNOSIS

The most common cause of otalgia, or ear pain, is acute OM. Other causes include mastoiditis, which is almost always accompanied by OM; otitis externa; and referred pain from the oropharynx, teeth, adenoids, or posterior auricular lymph nodes. A foreign body in the canal can produce similiar symptoms. In children with ear pain, a search for any of these other conditions must be undertaken if the TM appears completely normal.

EVALUATION

History

It is important in the history to differentiate nonspecific symptoms of otitis from those indicating a more serious condition such as meningitis (Questions Box).

For infants or children with a history of persistent or recurrent OM, it is important to find out when they had their last documented infection and what treatment they received.

Physical Examination

To diagnose OM, the TM must be visualized. Occasionally this may be difficult because of otorrhea, and the diagnosis is then made clinically. In all other cases, the position, color, degree of translucency, and mobility of the TM must be evaluated. Classically, in acute OM the TM is full or bulging, hyperemic, opaque, and has limited or no mobility. In addition, the light reflex is usually distorted or absent. In the case of a persistent or chronic OM, signs of inflammation are usually absent and the TM may be retracted, with limited or no mobility.

Associated physical findings with an uncomplicated middle ear infection may include posterior auricular and cervical adenopathy. Other significant findings on physical examination are pain on movement of the

---

Questions: Otitis Media

- Does the infant or child have fever, ear pain, hearing loss, or otorrhea?
- Is the infant or child inconsolable or lethargic?
- Has the infant or child had a previous ear infection? If so, when?
- Did the child complete the course of prescribed antibiotics?
- How many ear infections has the child had in the past year?
- Is the child taking any medication to prevent recurrent OM?
- Does the child appear to hear?
- Is the child's speech development normal?
- Does the child attend day care?
- Is the child exposed to passive smoke?

FIGURE 46–2. *Three ways to position the infant or child for examination of the ear.*

pinna, anterior ear displacement, posterior auricular pain, and evidence of peripheral facial nerve (cranial nerve VII) paralysis. The presence of these findings suggests other diagnoses such as an associated otitis externa or mastoiditis.

Positioning of infants or young children for examination of the ear can be difficult. Several methods have been described, including allowing parents to hold the child in their arms or on their laps or restraining the child on the examination table with or without a papoose board (Fig. 46–2). In addition, it may be difficult to visualize the TM in infants because the external auditory canal is slightly angulated. Lateral retraction of the pinna may help correct this problem.

Laboratory Tests

Although the diagnosis of OM is suspected on the basis of the history and then verified on physical examination, tympanometry may be helpful in distinguishing the normal ear from one with an effusion. In acute cases audiometry is of limited diagnostic value, but it is helpful in evaluating the effects of a persistent, recurrent, or chronic middle ear effusion on hearing.

Tympanocentesis is the most definitive method of verifying the presence of middle ear fluid and of recovering the organism responsible for the infection. Indications for tympanocentesis or myringotomy are listed in Table 46–1. Nasopharyngeal cultures are not helpful because they do not seem to correlate highly with middle ear fluid cultures.

MANAGEMENT

Oral antibiotics are the mainstay of medical treatment for acute OM (Table 46–2). Several studies have been conducted to evaluate second- and third-generation cephalosporins as well as other newer antibiotics. Amoxicillin remains the first-line drug of choice. It is effective in treating 80 to 85% of cases of acute OM, is well tolerated by children, has few adverse side effects, and is inexpensive. More important, amoxicillin is active both in vitro and in vivo against *S. pneumoniae* and nontypable *H. influenzae,* the most common organisms that cause acute OM.

Trimethoprim-sulfamethoxazole (TMP-SMZ, Bactrim, Septra) and erythromycin-sulfisoxazole (Pediazole) are usually considered second-line therapy. They are both effective against β-lactamase-producing bacteria (10–30% of *H. influenzae* and most *M. catarrhalis*). TMP-SMZ,

---

TABLE 46–1. Indications for Tympanocentesis or Myringotomy in Children with Otitis Media

Otitis media (OM) in patients with severe ear pain, serious illness or appearance of toxicity

Unsatisfactory response to antimicrobial therapy

Onset of OM in children receiving appropriate and adequate antimicrobial therapy

OM associated with confirmed or potential suppurative complications, such as mastoiditis or meningitis

OM in newborns, sick neonates, or immunodeficient patients, in each of whom an unusual organism may be present

---

TABLE 46–2. Considerations in Antimicrobial Drug Selection

Age

Associated illnesses

History of otitis media

Drug hypersensitivity

Cost and coverage

Compliance issues

however, is not effective against group A streptococcus. Factors to consider when prescribing these drugs are dosing intervals and side effects. Compliance may be an issue with Pediazole because it is taken four times a day. TMP-SMZ is taken twice daily. The erythromycin in Pediazole may also cause undesirable vomiting and abdominal pain. In addition, both of these medications contain a sulfonamide, so the risk of serious reactions such as Stevens-Johnson syndrome is not negligible.

Amoxicillin-clavulanic acid (Augmentin) and cefixime (Suprax) are used in cases of resistant organisms. The main disadvantage of these medications is cost; in the case of Augmentin, side effects such as diarrhea, which occurs in 30 to 50% of patients, may also be a problem. An attractive advantage of Suprax is the once-a-day dosing. Some clinicians have advocated cefaclor (Ceclor) as another treatment option; cost, inadequate antimicrobial coverage, and adverse reactions such as serum sickness make it less popular, however.

Although most practitioners prescribe these antibiotics for 10 days, they may be given for up to 14 days. After beginning correct medical therapy, children should be afebrile and subjectively feeling better in 48 to 72 hours. They should remain afebrile throughout the remainder of the antibiotic course.

Adjunctive medications such as topical analgesics and antipyretics are important therapeutic options and should be prescribed for children with significant pain or fever. Antihistamines, decongestants, or steroids play no documented role in the treatment of OM with effusion.

Most resolving middle ear effusions seen after an OM in otherwise healthy children do not need to be treated, and the "wait-and-watch" approach can be taken. In the symptomatic patient (recurrent fever, pain, or hearing loss), second-line antibiotic treatment is in order. Children should then be reexamined in three to four weeks.

Chemoprophylaxis is indicated in "otitis prone" children as a means of protecting them from the serious consequences of recurrent OM such as permanent hearing loss. Children who have three or more documented ear infections in six months or four episodes in 12 months and those with a positive family history of otitis are candidates for prophylaxis. In addition, infants who are plagued with ear infections beginning at less than 1 year of age should be considered for preventive therapy. Before the initiation of chemoprophylaxis, however, children must be free of all signs and symptoms of an acute infection.

Amoxicillin and sulfisoxazole are safe and effective drugs for daily prophylaxis. Half the therapeutic dose given once daily is appropriate. To increase compliance, the dosage should probably be given at the same time each day. Dosages are: Amoxicillin, 20 mg/kg/d, and sulfisoxazole, 50 mg/kg/d. Although TMP-SMZ is also effective and is used by some clinicians, it is currently not recommended for prophylaxis.

Current recommendations are to continue the chemoprophylaxis for three to six months or during the winter and spring seasons when the incidence of respiratory illnesses is highest. Children should then be reexam-

ined at 1–2-month intervals to ensure the resolution of any residual effusions. Any acute infections should be treated accordingly with full dosages of an alternative regimen.

Frequent bouts of OM also require a further search for respiratory allergies, sinusitis, immunologic deficiencies, and anatomic abnormalities such as a submucosal cleft palate or nasopharyngeal tumor. Any suspicion of a hearing deficit requires that a BAER or audiogram be performed, depending on the age of the child.

Failure of prophylactic medication and chronic effusions warrants a referral to an otolaryngologist for further evaluation for pressure equalization tubes or tonsillectomy and adenoidectomy. Other reasons for consultation include any evidence of hearing loss; the presence of any anatomic abnormality, such as a defect of the TM (perforations, cholesteatomas) or intranasal problems (deviated septum, polyp); signs and symptoms of an OM but normal physical examination; and a predisposition to chronic-recurrent OM (i.e., children with a cleft palate or Down syndrome).

PROGNOSIS

Complications associated with OM are much less common with early antibiotic therapy but occasionally occur. They can be divided into two categories: extracranial and intracranial. Extracranial complications include perforation of the TM, conductive and sensorineural hearing loss, cholesteatoma, mastoiditis, facial nerve (cranial nerve VII) paralysis, osteomyelitis of the temporal bone, and Bezold's abscess. Intracranial complications are meningitis, extradural as well as subdural abscesses, lateral venous sinus thrombosis, brain abscess, and hydrocephalus.

Case Resolution

In the case presented at the beginning of the chapter, the child displays the classic signs and symptoms of acute OM: fever, URI, decreased appetite, and an abnormal TM. He should be treated for 10 to 14 days with oral antibiotics and then placed on prophylaxis to prevent further infections. The prognosis is good, given his normal speech development.

Selected Readings

Bluestone, C. D. Modern management of otitis media. Pediatr. Clin. North Am. 36:1371–1387, 1989.

Bluestone, C. D., and J. O. Klein. Otitis Media in Infants and Children. Philadelphia, W. B. Saunders, 1988.

Bluestone, C. D., J. S. Stephenson, and L. M. Martin. Ten-year review of otitis media pathogens. Pediatr. Infect. Dis. J. 11:S7–S11, 1992.

Duncan, B., et al. Exclusive breast-feeding for at least four months protects against otitis media. Pediatrics 93:867–872, 1993.

Giebink, G. S., D. M. Canafax, and J. Kempthorne. Antimicrobial treatment of acute otitis media. J. Pediatr. 119:495–500, 1991.

Howie, V. M. Otitis media. Pediatr. Rev. 14:320–323, 1993.

Klein, J. O. Preventing recurrent otitis: what role for antibiotics? Contemp. Pediatr. 11:44–60, 1994.

The Otitis Media Guidelines Panel. Managing otitis media with effusion in young children. Pediatrics 94:766–773, 1994.

Paradise, J. L. Antimicrobial drugs and surgical procedures in the prevention of otitis media. Pediatr. Infect. Dis. J. 8:S35–S37, 1989.

Pichichero, M. E., and C. L. Pichichero. Persistent otitis media. I. Causative organisms. Pediatr. Infect. Dis. J. 14:178–183, 1995.

Pichichero, M. E., and C. L. Pichichero. Persistent otitis media. II. Antimicrobial treatment. Pediatr. Infect. Dis. J. 14:183–188, 1995.

Ruuskanen, O., and T. Heikkinen. Otitis media: etiology and diagnosis. Pediatr. Infect. Dis. J. 13:523–526, 1994.

Teele, D. W. Strategies to control recurrent acute otitis media in infants and children. Pediatr. Ann. 20:609–616, 1991.

Wright, P. F., J. Thompson, and F.H. Bess. Hearing, speech, and language sequelae of otitis media with effusion. Pediatr. Ann. 20:617–621, 1991.

CHAPTER 47

HEARING IMPAIRMENTS

Monica Sifuentes, M.D.

H$_x$ A 15-month-old girl is brought to the office because she has not yet begun to speak. The child was the full-term product of an uncomplicated pregnancy. Her 25-year-old mother, who began to receive regular prenatal care during the second month of gestation, had no documented infections during the pregnancy, took no medications, and has denied using illicit drugs or alcohol. The 27-year-old father is reportedly healthy. There is no family history of deafness, mental retardation, or consanguinity.

The girl, who is otherwise healthy, has never been hospitalized, but she has had three documented ear infections. She rolled over at four to five months of age, sat at seven months, and walked at 13 months. She is able to scribble. The parents report that their daughter smiles appropriately, laughs occasionally, and plays well with other children. As an infant, the girl cooed and babbled, but she now points and grunts to indicate her needs. She does not respond to loud noises by turning her head.

The child's growth parameters, including head circumference, are normal for age. The rest of the physical examination is unremarkable.

Questions

1. When should deafness be suspected in infants or children?
2. What is the relationship between hearing loss and language development?
3. What are the major causes of deafness in children?
4. What neonates are at risk for the development of hearing deficits?
5. What methods are currently available to evaluate hearing in infants and children?
6. What are the important issues to address with families who have infants or children with suspected hearing impairments?

Children may either be born deaf or may develop the condition during childhood. A mild hearing deficit occurs with a 30–40 decibel (dB) loss. Severe hearing loss, on the other hand, is defined as 60–80 dB, and profound loss is 85 dB and above. The most important period for language and speech development is generally the first three to four years of life, and reduced hearing acuity during this time can greatly interfere with this important process. When these crucial years for language and speech development are lost, children's social, emotional, cognitive, and academic development can be affected (see Chapter 15, Language Development). Their potential financial and vocational status may also be influenced. Therefore, primary care physicians must have a clear understanding of when to suspect deafness in infancy and early childhood and must be familiar with its evaluation.

EPIDEMIOLOGY

The prevalence of deafness in children is approximately 0.1% at birth; approximately 1 of every 1000 children is born severely to profoundly deaf. The average age at diagnosis of most children who are born deaf is now two to three years. Current methods of screening miss approximately 50% of infants who are born with hearing impairments, and lesser degrees of deafness may go undetected for several years. A careful assessment of language development is therefore essential at each patient encounter.

An estimated 20 to 30% of children who are hearing impaired developed the condition during childhood. In addition, 70% of children with acquired hearing loss are initially identified by the parents rather than physicians.

Graduates of the neonatal intensive care unit have a significant risk of bilateral sensorineural hearing loss (1–3%); associated factors such as prematurity (birth weight <1500 grams) and neonatal sepsis increase this risk. Other factors associated with deafness in infancy include meningitis, parental consanguinity, craniofacial malformations, congenital viral infections, hyperbilirubinemia, perinatal asphyxia, and a family history of deafness.

CLINICAL PRESENTATION

Children with hearing impairments appear to physicians most commonly with delayed speech. Parents may be concerned that the toddler is indicating his needs by grunting and pointing rather than by using words. Children also may be displaying behavioral problems, such as temper tantrums or aggressive play with other children. In addition, they can present with no intelligible speech (D$_x$ Box).

PATHOPHYSIOLOGY

Mechanism of Hearing

Sounds in the form of pressure waves are carried from the external environment through the external auditory canal to the tympanic membrane (TM). These waves are then converted to mechanical vibrations by the ossicles, and the mechanical vibrations are then transmitted from the TM to the inner ear, where they are

transformed to fluid vibrations. Finally, these fluid vibrations are converted into nerve impulses by nerve endings located in the cochlea in the inner ear. These impulses are conducted via the auditory nerve to higher levels (Figure 47–1).

Hearing impairments can be classified either according to the part of the auditory system affected or as the cause of the hearing loss.

Types of Hearing Loss

The tympanic membrane, the ossicles, or both, are affected in **conductive hearing loss.** Various conditions, infections, or anomalies that affect the middle ear such as otitis media or ossicular discontinuity result in this type of hearing loss. Middle ear effusions rarely cause more than a 20–30 dB loss. The cochlea or inner ear is affected in **sensorineural hearing loss.** Congenital infections, anomalies, and genetic disorders lead to this type of loss. A **mixed disorder** has characteristics of both conductive and sensorineural losses. In a **retro-cochlear hearing loss,** the auditory nerve, brain stem, or cortex is affected.

ETIOLOGY OF HEARING IMPAIRMENT (TABLE 47–1)

Severe to profound hearing loss has three main causes: genetic, acquired, and malformative. Genetic causes account for at least 50% of cases; primarily these are isolated, sporadic cases without ready explanation. These genetic mutations may result in different types of deafness with various presentations and outcomes: that is, the hearing loss may be conductive, sensorineural, or mixed, and may be static or progressive with the initial presentation either in infancy or later childhood. Most instances of congenital sensorineural hearing loss are autosomal recessive (75%). The estimated recurrence

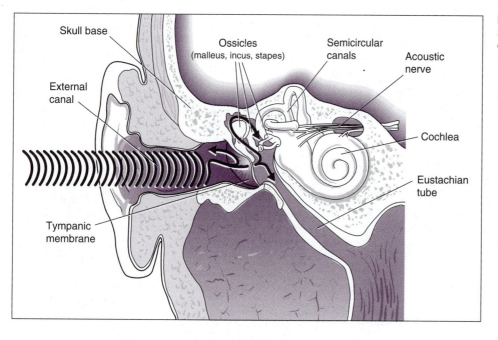

FIGURE 47-1. *Sound waves passing through the external ear into the middle ear.*

Skull base

Ossicles
(malleus, incus, stapes)

Semicircular
canals

Acoustic
nerve

External
canal

Cochlea

Eustachian
tube

Tympanic
membrane

TABLE 47–1. Major Causes of Childhood Deafness

Genetic
Acquired
  Infections
    Congenital—CMV, rubella, toxoplasmosis, HSV, syphilis
    Acquired—bacterial meningitis, mastoiditis, otitis media, mumps
  Complications associated with prematurity
  Ototoxic medications
  Hyperbilirubinemia
  Head trauma
  Acoustic trauma
Malformations
Unknown

Modified, with permission, from Rapin, I. Hearing disorders. Pediatr. Rev. 14:44, 1989.

rate in siblings is 10% if the cause of hearing loss in the initial case is unknown.

Acquired causes include congenital infections, bacterial meningitis, hyperbilirubinemia, complications of prematurity, and exposure to ototoxic medications. Cytomegalovirus is probably the most frequently unrecognized congenital infection causing deafness; however, toxoplasmosis, rubella, herpes simplex, and syphilis can also be implicated. With bacterial meningitis, where the incidence of hearing loss can be as high as 20%, *Streptococcus pneumoniae* is likely to become the most prevalent cause; the incidence of *Haemophilus influenzae* infection has decreased tremendously in young children with the advent of vaccine administration. The role of steroids in the treatment of bacterial meningitis has also contributed greatly to the decrease in sensorineural hearing loss in survivors. The problem of untreated significant hyperbilirubinemia in term newborns is rare in the United States and other developed countries. Prematurity, however, is not uncommon, but it is still unclear which of the associated complications are responsible for the higher rates of severe hearing loss in this group compared to full term infants. Some antibiotics, such as the aminoglycosides, and other medications like furosemide can be irreversibly ototoxic; other drugs cause only transient effects.

Any head injury causing significant middle ear trauma may also lead to deafness in children. Repeated acoustic trauma such as that associated with continuous or significant exposure to loud noise can also cause irreversible hearing loss.

Malformations are the least common cause for severe to profound hearing loss in infants and children. These include ear malformations in neonates and children with midfacial anomalies, such as a cleft lip or palate. In contrast, profound malformations of the external and middle ears, such as microtia or absence of the external canal and tympanic membrane and fusion of the ossicles, can cause a maximum loss of about 60 dB if the cochlea is normal. Specific syndromes like Down's syndrome and Goldenhar's syndrome frequently are associated with hearing impairment. In addition, multiple syndromes with and without anomalies of the head and neck may lead to hearing impairment, and affected children must be evaluated on an individual basis.

DIFFERENTIAL DIAGNOSIS

In addition to hearing loss, communication disorders should be considered in infants or children with delayed speech and language development. These include problems with speech perception, language comprehension, formulation of language output, and speech production. Unrecognized conditions such as mental retardation can be responsible for some of these disorders. Other etiologies include specific central nervous system deficits as well as impairments of fine motor control of the oropharynx.

EVALUATION

History

Because the primary symptom of deafness is failure to learn to speak at the appropriate age, the most important aspect of the history in children with possible hearing loss is determining whether speech is developing normally. Even deaf infants may begin cooing and babbling in infancy, and these early attempts at verbalization are not useful milestones for assessment of hearing loss. It helps to ask parents whether they are at all suspicious or concerned about their children's speech or hearing. Guidelines to assess language development are found in Table 47–2. (See Chapter 15, Language Development.) An assessment of risk factors for deafness, such as history of prematurity, hyperbilirubinemia, neonatal sepsis, and asphyxia is also important (Questions Box).

TABLE 47–2. SNHL Guidelines for Quick Clinical Screening*

4 months
Coos or "sings" a vowel sound
Takes turns listening, and vocalizes when you're quiet
Recognizes the sound of a parent's voice
7 months
Laughs out loud
Looks toward the sound when he hears it
Coos independently, mainly using vowels
10 months
Makes a raspberry (or Bronx cheer) or bubbles
Says "mama" or "dada" (not necessarily to the correct person)
Understands "no"
14 months
Uses the words "mama" and "dada" for the correct person
Obeys a command (like "stop," "come here," or "give me") and understands words like "up" and "milk"
16 months
First words, in addition to "mama" and "dada" (e.g., shoe)
18 months
Able to identify objects in pictures (e.g., doggie, cup, baby)
Multiple-word (4–5) vocabulary
2 years
Several two-word sentences
30–60 words of vocabulary
2½ years
Uses "me" and "you" (but may reverse the meaning)
Vocabulary can increase to 500–1000 words

*SNHL: sensorineural hearing loss.
Reproduced, with permission, from Epstein, S., et al. Sensorineural hearing loss. Pediatr. Clin. North Am. 36:1517, 1989.

Physical Examination

A brief but complete physical examination should be performed on all children. In particular, any dysmorphic facial features that may suggest the presence of a syndrome with an associated hearing deficit should be noted. Other anomalies of the head and neck should be noted as well. The pinna and external ear canals should be carefully inspected for abnormalities and patency, respectively. In addition, the tympanic membranes should also be visualized and assessed for the presence of a middle ear effusion that may influence subsequent audiologic tests. The oropharynx should be examined for a cleft palate or a bifid uvular, which may be associated with a submucous cleft. The manner in which children communicate with parents should be noted, if possible.

Laboratory Tests

Although tympanometry is not a hearing test, it can be useful to assess the presence of fluid in the middle ear as well as the mobility of the tympanic membrane. Tympanometry can be particularly helpful with uncooperative, crying children in whom the detection of any problems based solely on the appearance of the TM and insufflation is difficult. Different types of hearing tests for evaluating infants and children for possible hearing deficits are available to general pediatricians (Table 47–3). These tests should be used in conjunction with audiologic and otolaryngologic consultations. In the case of high-risk infants, testing should be repeated several times during the first two years of life and should be considered normal only after at least two tests are performed.

TABLE 47–3. Tests to Evaluate Hearing

Acoustic reflexes
Behavioral audiometry
Brain stem auditory-evoked response (BAER)
Evoked otoacoustic emissions: newer type of newborn screening
Standard audiometric testing

Other diagnostic tests to consider in infants include titers for congenital infections and fluorescent treponemal antibody absorption (FTA-ABS) tests for syphilis. Thyroid function tests are used to rule out Pendred's syndrome in school-age children with goiters. One-third of affected children have an associated sensorineural hearing defect. Proteinuria and hematuria should also be ruled out by urine dip stick, especially in boys with a positive family history of deafness and renal failure, which is suggestive for Alport's syndrome.

Imaging Studies

A renal ultrasound should be obtained in infants with pinna abnormalities. Occasionally, a CT or MRI scan of the temporal bone may be used to view the anatomy of the middle and inner ear, particularly in cases of a suspected cochlear/vestibular malformation or fistula.

MANAGEMENT

Once infants or children are found to have a hearing impairment, careful follow-up is necessary so that no further hearing loss occurs. The role of primary care providers thus becomes even more crucial. Both parents and other family members may initially be devastated by the diagnosis of a hearing impairment, especially if the loss is severe to profound, and they probably will have multiple questions about children's medical prognosis and educational future. The possibility of further speech and language development may also be a foremost concern in their minds. In addition to providing patients with comprehensive care, all of the parents' questions and concerns must be addressed and anticipated.

Future Audiologic Evaluations

In newly diagnosed patients with sensorineural hearing loss, **audiograms** should be repeated every three months in the first year and then every six months when children are in preschool. The test should be repeated at least annually after children have begun school. Continued monitoring is essential to detect any progression of hearing loss, especially in the less affected ear.

Assistive Devices

Although **hearing aids** do not restore hearing, all children with conductive as well as sensorineural hearing loss benefit from amplification. Several different types of hearing aids are available for children; these devices should be fitted appropriately and adjusted regularly. In addition, it is also recommended that all patients receive bilateral hearing aids to improve auditory localization and training, particularly in the context of different learning situations. In reality, unfortunately, many children do not use bilateral hearing aids, either because their families do not have the necessary financial resources or because one is lost, damaged, or malfunctioning. **Closed-caption television** (signed or subtitled) is another method of auditory training. In addition, **teletype telephone systems** are available for children who can read or wish to learn how to read.

At one time, **cochlear implants** were considered purely experimental and perhaps even dangerous because of a significant risk of permanent damage at implantation. However, they are currently being used in children with profound sensorineural hearing loss, particularly those who have acquired postlingual deafness. A majority of patients with implants show significant improvement in communication skills.

Education and Communication

Much controversy exists regarding the optimal method of communication for deaf children. **Oral communication (lip reading)** and **sign language** each have their advantages as well as disadvantages depending on children's age, the type of deafness, and whether the deficit is congenital or acquired. Whether the children already know a language is also important to consider. The preferred methods seem to vary from region to region; therefore schools, other institutions, and resource groups often use the most popular communication method in a particular area.

Whether to "mainstream" children with severe hearing loss in a regular classroom with an interpreter or place them in a school for deaf children is another controversial issue. Parents should be encouraged to explore the possibilities of each option and to make a decision based on the individual needs of their children and not current trends. The expertise of an educator who is knowledgeable in this field can also be helpful when making this decision.

Outside Resources and Referrals

Newly diagnosed children should be evaluated by **ophthalmologists** and medical **geneticists**. Any refractory error should be treated and followed closely, because children with severe hearing difficulties are so dependent on vision. A complete eye examination may also reveal retinal lesions that contribute to diagnosing the etiology of the hearing loss. A genetics evaluation is important for diagnostic reasons as well as for providing families with information and counseling about recurrence.

Support groups and referrals to national organizations for hearing impaired individuals can be valuable resources for parents and families. Resources for financial support should also be explored. Agencies with multidisciplinary teams are particularly important in infants or children with other associated handicaps.

PROGNOSIS

The goal of early recognition and treatment of hearing loss is to minimize the possible long-term sequelae of persistent speech and language problems. An additional goal is to prevent the development of learning disabilities. Most children, however, do well with early recognition and intervention, and learn to communicate using sign language, lip reading, or a combination of both methods.

Case Resolution

In the case presented at the beginning of the chapter, the child clearly has a hearing deficit. She does not turn to loud noises, she has not developed any specific words, and she indicates her needs nonverbally. Although there are no obvious historical risk factors for hearing loss, a behavioral audiogram should be performed. The physician's suspicion should be discussed with the family, and a follow-up visit should be arranged to review the hearing test results as soon as possible.

Selected Readings

Epstein, S. and J. S. Reilly. Sensorineural hearing loss. Pediatr. Clin. North Am. 36:1501–1520, 1989.

Gerhardt, K. J. Prenatal and perinatal risks of hearing loss. Semin. Perinatol. 14:299–304, 1990.

Rapin, I. Hearing disorders. Pediatr. Rev. 14:43–49, 1993.

Ruben, R. J. Diagnosis of deafness in infancy. Pediatr. Rev. 9:163–166, 1987.

Tharpe, A. M. and F. H. Bess. Identification and management of children with minimal hearing loss. Int. J. Pediat. Otorhinolaryngol. 21:41–50, 1991.

U.S. Department of Health and Human Services. Early identification of hearing impairment in infants and young children. NIH Consensus Statement 11:1–20, 1993.

Wright, P. F., J. Thompson, and F. Bess. Hearing, speech, and language sequelae of otitis media with effusion. Pediatr. Ann. 20:617–621, 1991.

SORE THROAT

Stanley H. Inkelis, M.D.

Hx
    An eight-year-old girl has had a sore throat and fever for two days. She also has pain on swallowing, a headache, and a feeling of general malaise but no stridor, drooling, breathing difficulty, or rash. Other than the current illness, the girl is in good health. Although she has had sore throats in the past, she has never had one this severe. One week ago both her mother and father had a sore throat and fever that resolved after five days with no medication.
    The child has a temperature of 102.2° F (39.0° C). The physical examination is normal except for red tonsils with exudate bilaterally, palatal petechiae, and tender cervical lymphadenopathy.

Questions

1. What are the causes of sore throat in children?
2. What is the appropriate evaluation of children with sore throat? What laboratory tests are necessary?
3. What is the appropriate management for children with sore throat?
4. When should otolaryngologic consultation be obtained?

Sore throat, one of the most common illnesses seen by the primary care physician, is a painful inflammation of the pharynx, tonsils, or surrounding areas. In most cases, children with sore throat have mild symptoms that require little or no treatment. Sore throat may be the presenting complaint of a severe illness such as epiglottitis or retropharyngeal abscess, however. Small children are not able to define their complaints very well, which makes a careful history from parents or other care givers and a good physical examination essential for correct diagnosis. Optimal management of sore throat, especially if group A beta-hemolytic streptococcus is suspected, is still very controversial.

EPIDEMIOLOGY

Five percent of all pediatric visits are for pharyngitis. Sore throats are most common in children five to eight years of age, and they continue to occur during later childhood. They are uncommon in children under one year of age. Like other respiratory infections, sore throats occur most often in the late fall and winter months. Approximately 11% of all school-age children receive medical care for pharyngitis. Fifteen to 40% of cases of pharyngitis in these children are caused by group A beta-hemolytic streptococcus.

The organisms that cause bacterial and viral pharyngitis, are present in saliva and nasal secretions and are almost always transmitted by close contact. Spread from child to child in school is the common mode of transmission.

CLINICAL PRESENTATION

The clinical presentation of sore throat is variable and often depends on etiology (D_x Box and see Differential Diagnosis). Most children with sore throat present with sudden onset of pain and fever. The height of the fever is variable and is typically higher in younger children. In older children, especially if the sore throat is associated with a common cold, fever is minimal or absent. The throat or tonsils are red, and the breath may be malodorous. Headache, nausea, vomiting, and abdominal pain may occur, especially if children are febrile. The appetite may be decreased. Children may be less active than usual.

In children with the common cold, rhinorrhea and postnasal discharge are present. A pharyngeal and tonsillar exudate is not typical. Although the cervical lymph nodes may be enlarged, they are usually not very tender. In contrast, children with streptococcal pharyngitis typically have high fever, pharyngeal and tonsillar exudate, and tender cervical lymph nodes.

PATHOPHYSIOLOGY

Various bacterial and viral organisms lead to sore throat by causing inflammation in the ring of posterior

---

Dx | **Sore Throat**

VIRAL
- Pain in throat
- Fever (variable)*
- Rhinorrhea (common)
- Cough (common)
- Erythema of pharynx or tonsils
- Follicular, ulcerative, exudative lesions of pharynx or tonsils*

BACTERIAL
- Pain in throat
- Fever
- Marked erythema of pharynx or tonsils
- Tonsillar and posterior pharyngeal wall exudate
- Tender, swollen cervical lymphadenopathy
- Positive rapid antigen test or throat culture

*Dependent on etiology (see Differential Diagnosis).

pharyngeal lymphoid tissue that consists of the tonsils, adenoids, and surrounding lymphoid tissue. This ring of tissue, called Waldeyer's ring, drains the oral and pharyngeal cavity and defends against infection of the mouth and throat. Other host defenses that protect against infection include the sneeze, gag and cough reflexes, secretory IgA, and a rich blood supply.

Viral sore throats may be acquired by inhalation or self-inoculation from the nasal mucosa or conjunctiva. The local respiratory epithelium becomes infected with the virus, and inflammation occurs. In some instances, inflammatory mediators may be responsible for the pain of sore throat. Group A streptococcus and other bacterial organisms directly invade the mucous membranes. Enzymes produced by this organism, streptolysin O and hyaluronidase, aid in the spread of infection.

DIFFERENTIAL DIAGNOSIS

Although most children who present with sore throat have common viral or bacterial pharyngitis, other less common disorders such as infectious mononucleosis, epiglottitis, retropharyngeal abscess, or peritonsillar abscess should be considered.

Viral Infection

Viral infection, the most common cause of sore throat in children, is most often associated with a URI caused by a rhinovirus. Cough and rhinorrhea associated with a sore throat suggest this etiology.

Adenovirus often leads to exudative pharyngitis, frequently in children less than three years old. Pharyngoconjunctival fever, caused by adenovirus 3, is characterized by a high fever (temperature: >102.2° F [39.0° C]) for several days, conjunctivitis, and exudative tonsillitis.

Coxsackie virus and **echovirus** (enteroviruses) are the usual cause of herpangina. Vesicles and ulcers are generally apparent on the anterior tonsillar pillars and soft palate. They may also be found on the tonsils, pharynx, or posterior buccal mucosa. Children may have a high fever (temperature: >102.2° F [39.0° C]), irritability, and refuse to eat or drink; dehydration may result. Coxsackie virus A16 causes hand-foot-and-mouth disease, which is characterized by ulcerative oral lesions on the tongue and buccal mucosa and, less frequently, on the palate and anterior tonsillar pillars. Vesicular and papulovesicular lesions are evident on the hands and feet and occasionally on other parts of the body. Enteroviral infections typically occur in the late spring, summer, and early fall.

Herpes simplex virus may lead to pharyngotonsillitis but may be distinguished from most of the enteroviral infections for two reasons. One, it almost always involves the anterior portion of the mouth and lips, and two, it is associated with a gingivitis (herpes gingivostomatitis). The lesions often appear as whitish-yellow plaques with an erythematous base, and they are sometimes ulcerative. This illness is characterized by a high fever (temperature: 102.2° F [39.0° C]) for up to

7 to 10 days and frequent refusal to eat or drink because of the painful lesions. Dehydration may occur.

EBV may cause exudative pharyngotonsillitis either alone or as part of the infectious mononucleosis syndrome that includes fever, malaise, lymphadenopathy, and hepatosplenomegaly.

Bacterial Infection

Group A beta-hemolytic streptococcus is the most common cause of bacterial sore throat in children over three years of age. The pharynx is typically very red and sometimes edematous, and the tonsils are red, enlarged, and covered with exudate. Children may also have dysphagia, fever, vomiting, headache, malaise, and abdominal pain. Swollen anterior cervical lymphadenopathy and petechiae on the soft palate and uvula are usually apparent. In addition, the occurrence of a scarlatiniform rash, "strawberry tongue," and Pastia's lines (petechiae in the flexor skin creases of joints) indicates scarlet fever, which is diagnostic of Group A streptococcal infection (see Chapter 93, Maculopapular Rashes). Sore throat from group A beta-hemolytic streptococcus typically occurs in the winter and spring. Rheumatic fever and glomerulonephritis are nonsuppurative complications of group A streptococcal infection.

Group B, C, and G beta-hemolytic streptococci (non-group A beta-hemolytic streptococci) have all been isolated from children with pharyngitis. *Streptococcus pneumoniae* and *Staphylococcus aureus* infrequently cause pharyngitis in children. Although *Corynebacterium diphtheriae* (diphtheria) rarely causes sore throat in immunized children, this organism should be considered in nonimmunized children who have exudative pharyngotonsillitis and a grayish pseudomembrane that bleeds when removal is attempted.

Chlamydia trachomatis can lead to pharyngitis in young adults, but its role as the cause of sore throat in children remains unclear. *Mycoplasma pneumoniae* does not usually produce sore throat in children unless they have lower respiratory tract disease. *Neisseria gonorrhoeae* may lead to sore throat in sexually active adolescents. Its occurrence in prepubertal children is often secondary to sexual abuse. The appearance of the throat is not characteristic, and diagnosis is made by cultures when the degree of suspicion is high. **Tularemia** is a rare cause of exudative pharyngitis in children but should be suspected if contact with wild animals has occurred.

Other Causes

Candida albicans may be responsible for sore throat in infants and in children who are immunocompromised or taking antibiotics. Children with oral candidiasis usually present with whitish plaques on the labial or buccal mucosa that do not wipe off easily. When the pharynx and tonsils are involved, some discomfort or dysphagia, but usually not significant pain, may occur.

Retropharyngeal abscess typically occurs in children less than four years of age. Sore throat is associated with this condition, but it is usually more evident only when swallowing. Fever, refusal to swallow, drooling, stridor, and meningismus in toxic-appearing children suggest this diagnosis.

Epiglottitis (supraglottitis), almost always secondary to infection with *Haemophilus influenzae type b*, may present as sore throat. This condition typically affects children two to seven years of age who present with signs of toxicity, stridor, difficulty swallowing, and drooling. In relatively well-appearing children with sore throat but no stridor, neither epiglottitis nor retropharyngeal abscess is a likely cause of sore throat.

Children with croup may have sore throat and stridor, but they do not usually appear toxic and do not have difficulty swallowing. Affected children are usually between six months and three years of age (see Chapter 37, Stridor and Croup).

Trauma from penetrating objects, burns, or exposure to caustic materials may cause sore throat in children. Household smoking may also lead to pharyngeal irritation. In addition, allergic rhinitis with postnasal drip may result in sore throat. Tumor rarely causes sore throat in children but should be considered if a mass is present or pharyngeal inflammation persists. Persistent sore throat may also be a symptom of Kawasaki syndrome.

EVALUATION

History

A thorough history often reveals the etiology of the sore throat (Questions Box). Questions regarding duration, fever, headache, vomiting, pain on swallowing, rash, oral lesions, abdominal pain, and history of contact with other family members or classmates with similar symptoms suggest the most common causes of sore throat (infections with viruses and group A beta-hemolytic streptococcus). A history of rapid onset of fever, toxicity, difficulty swallowing, drooling, and respiratory distress suggest epiglottitis and retropharyngeal abscess. Voice changes suggest peritonsillar abscess or tonsillar hypertrophy associated with infectious mono-

---

Questions: Sore Throat

- How long has the child had a sore throat?
- Does the child have fever, headache, or vomiting?
- How rapid was the onset of fever?
- Does the child have pain on swallowing?
- Are there any voice changes?
- Does the child have a rash or oral lesions?
- Does the child have abdominal pain?
- Does the child have any ill contacts?
- Are the child's immunizations up-to-date?
- Is the child having any difficulty breathing?
- Does the child have a history of allergies?
- Has the child suffered any trauma to the throat or neck?
- Has the child been exposed to environmental smoke?
- (For sexually active adolescents or children with a history of sexual abuse with nonresponding sore throats) Has there been any oral sexual activity?

---

nucleosis (EBV). Immunization history or history of immigration from a developing country helps assess the risk of diphtheria. Oral sexual activity suggests the possibility of an STD. A history of allergies, trauma, and environmental smoke may help diagnose other causes of sore throat. Red or pink eye with a rash, persistent fever (> 5 days), and sore throat suggest Kawasaki syndrome.

Physical Examination

A general physical examination should be performed. It is important to note whether children appear toxic. The skin should be examined for a scarlatiniform, sandpaper-like rash, a vesicular rash involving the hands and feet, or a generalized maculopapular rash. The eyes should be evaluated for conjunctivitis and the nose for rhinorrhea (serous or purulent). The mouth, pharynx, and tonsils should be examined for vesicular lesions, ulcers, and gingivitis. The pharynx should be checked for redness, exudate, vesicles, edema, and foreign bodies. The tonsils and uvula should be examined for these same findings as well as asymmetry, and the neck should be checked for nuchal rigidity. The lymph nodes should be evaluated for enlargement (adenopathy) and inflammation (adenitis). The abdomen should be examined for hepatosplenomegaly.

Laboratory Tests

Although many signs and symptoms may suggest streptococcal pharyngitis, diagnosis can be confirmed only with laboratory tests. The **throat culture** is the "gold standard" for diagnosis. However, it has a false-negative rate of 10% and a false-positive rate of up to 50%, because streptococcal carriers are not infected with the organism at the time they present with sore throat. Nevertheless, throat culture is the most reliable way to confirm streptococcal infection.

Rapid streptococcal antigen tests are available for "on-the-spot" diagnosis. False-positive results are uncommon (specificity: 88–100%), but false-negative tests are common (sensitivity: 72–95%). Because a negative test does not exclude a streptococcal infection, it should be confirmed by throat culture. An antistreptolysin-O titer and an anti-DNAase-B titer may help diagnose a recent streptococcal infection if the throat culture is negative.

Differentiating between viral and bacterial pharyngitis is often difficult, and the rapid streptococcal antigen tests and throat cultures should be reserved for patients who have signs and symptoms common for both illnesses. For example, afebrile children with a sore throat, runny nose, and cough who have slight pharyngeal erythema almost certainly have viral pharyngitis and do not need further workup. On the other hand, children with fever, exudative tonsillitis, red pharynx and tonsils, or exposure to an individual with streptococcal pharyngitis may need further confirmation by throat culture to determine if the pharyngitis is bacterial.

Viral throat cultures and acute and convalescent titers to determine viral pharyngitis are rarely indicated unless systemic infection occurs (e.g., herpes encephalitis). EBV infection can be determined by specific serologic assays, but a heterophil agglutination test is the test of choice for diagnosing infectious mononucleosis. However, it may be negative in children younger than four years of age or early in the course of the infection. Only 75% of infected children between two and four years of age are identified by this test, and less than 30% of children under two years of age are identified. The monospot test, a rapid slide test for heterophil antibodies, may remain positive for months after the infection and may suggest the diagnosis of infectious mononucleosis in children who do not have this disorder. A CBC with more than 50 to 60% lymphocytes or more than 10% atypical lymphocytes is suggestive of mononucleosis.

Culture or fluorescent antibody evaluation of the pseudomembrane may be used to diagnose diphtheria. Culture or presence of serum agglutinins confirms tularemia. Thayer-Martin culture plates should be used to diagnose suspected gonorrheal sore throat.

Imaging Studies

If epiglottitis or retropharyngeal abscess is suspected but is not clinically apparent, a lateral neck x-ray may be obtained. The x-ray should be performed with a physician in attendance who is capable of performing endotracheal intubation in case the child has respiratory difficulties (see Chapter 37, Stridor and Croup).

MANAGEMENT

The management of children with sore throat is based on the etiology of the condition. The early recognition of potentially serious conditions based on history and physical examination is essential to providing optimal care. **Otolaryngologic consultation** should be obtained in children with peritonsillar abscess, retropharyngeal abscess, epiglottitis, significant pharyngeal trauma, or pharyngeal tumor. Recurrent tonsillitis, especially in children who miss school, may be a reason for referral to an otolaryngologist.

Outpatient Treatment

In most cases of children with sore throat, the physician must differentiate between viral and streptococcal pharyngitis. Viral sore throat can be managed symptomatically. Treatment of pain and discomfort with **analgesics** and maintenance of **hydration** are the mainstays of therapy for young children with viral sore throat. Gargling with warm water and sucking on hard candy may provide additional symptomatic relief for older children.

The pain from lesions of herpes stomatitis sometimes responds to acetaminophen. For those children with persistent pain, acetaminophen with codeine may be helpful. **Anesthetics** such as lidocaine may also de-

crease the pain. Lidocaine can be placed on a gloved finger and applied directly on the oral lesions of the tongue, labial, and buccal mucosa. It is best used about 30 minutes before feeding or drinking, especially in children who refuse to drink. Lidocaine should be used cautiously because it can suppress the gag reflex. The dose should never exceed 3 mg/kg/dose. Too much lidocaine may result in seizures. Antacids to coat the mucosa or a mixture (1 part each) of lidocaine, diphenhydramine (Benadryl), and kaolin-pectin (Kaopectate), either gargled or applied are alternative analgesics.

In children without clear-cut evidence of streptococcal pharyngitis, a positive rapid streptococcal antigen test helps direct antibiotic treatment. A negative test in the presence of positive symptoms should be accompanied by a throat culture. Patients can await the results of culture before beginning antibiotic therapy. **Antibiotics** are indicated in children without confirmation from rapid streptococcal tests or cultures, who appear toxic, who have scarlet fever or peritonsillar cellulitis/abscess, or who have a past history of rheumatic fever. Most evidence suggests that early treatment results in more rapid clinical improvement, although this is controversial. The experienced physician may treat children with antibiotics on clinical grounds alone. Rheumatic fever can be prevented if treatment is started within nine days of sore throat symptom development. Glomerulonephritis probably is not affected by antibiotic therapy.

Children with streptococcal pharyngitis should be treated with antibiotics to relieve symptoms; shorten the course of their illness; and prevent disease dissemination, suppurative complications, and rheumatic fever. Penicillin is the antibiotic of choice. It may be administered orally as phenoxymethyl penicillin, 50 mg/kg/day every six hours for 10 days (maximum: 250 mg qid for children; 500 mg qid for adults), or intramuscular benzathine penicillin. (See Table 48–1 for dosage information.)

If the risk of noncompliance is high or if the risk of complication is great (e.g., children have a history of rheumatic fever), the penicillin should be administered intramuscularly. Intramuscular penicillin has two disadvantages: (1) pain associated with the injection and (2) increased incidence of a potentially more severe allergic reaction. Bicillin C-R, which contains benzathine peni-

TABLE 48–1.   Antibiotics Used in the Management of Sore Throat in Children

Drug	Dosage
Phenoxymethyl penicillin	50 mg/kg/day (up to 250 mg qid) PO q6h for 10 days
Benzathine penicillin	600,000 units (<60 lb); 1.2 million units (> 60 lb)
Erythromycin	30–50 mg/kg/day in 3–4 divided doses
Rifampin	10 mg/kg/dose PO q12h for 4 days
Clindamycin	20 mg/kg/day (maximum of 450 mg/day) PO q8h for 10 days
Ceftriaxone	125 mg (< 100 lb) IM; 250 mg (> 100 lb) IM
Doxycycline	100 mg PO two times a day for 7 days (≥ 9 years)

cillin and procaine penicillin, is the preferable form of delivering penicillin intramuscularly because it causes less pain and less severe local reaction. It may be given in a 600,000:200,000 unit ratio in children less than 60 pounds. Erythromycin may be substituted in children who are allergic to penicillin.

Many children are asymptomatic carriers of group A streptococci. In general, these children do well, and eradication of the bacteria is not necessary. Cultures after treatment are generally not recommended, except for children with recurring or persistent symptoms or those with a previous history of rheumatic fever. If cultures remain positive, these children may be treated with benzathine penicillin and oral rifampin in an attempt to eradicate the organism (see Table 48–1 for dosages). Clindamycin may be more effective in eradication of the organism from symptom-free carriers (see Table 48–1 for dosages).

M. pneumoniae pharyngitis is usually associated with a generalized infection. Because it is often a self-limited illness, it does not require antibiotic therapy unless symptoms persist. Erythromycin (30–50 mg/kg/day) is the drug of choice.

Diphtheria is a life-threatening infection that requires prompt diagnosis and treatment. Penicillin G or erythromycin must be given to kill *C. diphtheriae* and, in addition, equine antitoxin must be administered to neutralize the exotoxin. Tularemia is treated with streptomycin or gentamicin.

For gonococcal pharyngitis caused by *N. gonorrhoeae*, intramuscular ceftriaxone is the drug of choice (see Table 48–1 for dosages). Oral doxycycline should also be given to children nine years of age or older to cover associated *C. trachomatis* infection (see Table 48–1 for dosages). Erythromycin may be used for younger children. Children should be examined and cultured for STDs in other sites and should have a serologic test for syphilis. Sexual abuse should be considered in all cases of gonococcal pharyngitis, particularly in prepubertal children.

Children with croup usually respond to cool mist. Oral nystatin can be used in children with oral candidiasis.

Inpatient Treatment

Children with sore throat should be admitted to the hospital if they have airway obstruction or need intravenous hydration or antibiotics. Children with retropharyngeal abscess, peritonsillar abscess, and epiglottitis require intravenous antibiotics. Intravenous hydration is occasionally needed for patients with severe herpes stomatitis who will not drink because of pain and become dehydrated.

The role of tonsillectomy in recurrent sore throat is still controversial. Indications are not clearly defined, and in many cases, surgery is not indicated.

Education

Both patients and families should receive general education about sore throats. Medication for pain with drugs such as acetaminophen or ibuprofen is useful, especially if children are having difficulty swallowing. Gargling with warm salt water or sucking on hard candy may soothe the pain of sore throat. Children with bacterial pharyngitis may return to school after 24 hours of antibiotic therapy and the disappearance of fever. The practitioner should recommend that symptomatic family members see a physician. Parents should call or return to the physician if their children have respiratory or swallowing difficulties, drooling, severe pain, or fever (temperature: > 101.0° F [38.3° C]) for more than 48 hours after the initiation of appropriate antibiotics.

PROGNOSIS

The prognosis for children with viral sore throat is excellent because of its self-limited nature. The outlook for children with streptococcal sore throat is also excellent. If the infection is not diagnosed and treated appropriately, however, suppurative and nonsuppurative complications (e.g., rheumatic fever, acute glomerulonephritis) may occur. With early diagnosis and prompt treatment, the prognosis for unusual, life-threatening causes of sore throat is also very good.

Case Resolution

In the case presented, the child has palatal petechiae and tonsillar exudate, which are signs and symptoms consistent with streptococcal pharyngitis. A rapid streptococcal antigen test or throat culture should be performed, and if positive, the child should be treated accordingly. If the test is negative and the child is ill-appearing, treatment may be started and either continued or stopped, depending on the results of the throat culture. If a positive rapid streptococcal test or throat culture indicates that the parents had strep throat, they should be empirically treated with antibiotics to prevent rheumatic fever.

EBV infection can present in a similar manner. If the child continues to be ill after a negative throat culture, workup for EBV should be considered.

Selected Readings

Barkin, R. M., and P. Rosen. Pharyngotonsillitis (sore throat). *In* Barkin, R. M., and P. Rosen (eds.). Emergency Pediatrics, 4th ed. St. Louis, C.V. Mosby, 1994, pp. 552–555.

Berkowitz, C. D., et al. Cooperative study of latex agglutination to identify group A streptococcal antigen on throat swabs in patients with acute pharyngitis. J. Pediatr. 107:89–92, 1985.

Denny, F. W. Current problems in managing streptococcal pharyngitis. J. Pediatr. 111:797–806, 1987.

Fleisher, G. R. Sore throat. *In* Fleisher, G. R., and S. Ludwig (eds.). Textbook of Pediatric Emergency Medicine, 3rd ed. Baltimore, Williams & Wilkins, 1993, pp. 469–473.

Gerber, M. A., et al. Lack of impact of early antibiotic therapy for streptococcal pharyngitis on recurrence rates. J. Pediatr. 117:853–858, 1990.

Gooch, W. M. III. Alternatives to penicillin in the management of group A streptococcal pharyngitis. Pediatr. Ann. 810–815, 1992.

Koomson, B., and D. M. Jaffe. Pharyngeal disease. *In* Reisdorff, E. J., M. R. Roberts, and J. G. Wiegenstein. Pediatric Emergency Medicine. Philadelphia, W. B. Saunders, 1993, pp. 623–628.

Niederman, L. G., and J. F. Marcinak. Sore throat. *In* Dershewitz, R. A. Ambulatory Pediatric Care, 2nd ed. Philadelphia, J.B. Lippincott, 1993, pp. 315–319.

Paradise, J. L. Etiology and management of pharyngitis and pharyngotonsillitis in children: a current review. Ann. Otol. Rhinol. Laryngol. 101:51–57, 1992.

Pichichero, M. E., et al. Adverse and beneficial effects of immediate treatment of group A beta-hemolytic streptococcal pharyngitis with penicillin. Pediatr. Infect. Dis. J. 6:635–643, 1987.

Pichichero, M. E., et al. Comparative reliability of clinical, culture, and antigen detection methods for the diagnosis of group A beta-hemolytic streptococcal tonsillopharyngitis. Pediatr. Ann. 21:798–805, 1992.

Putto, A. Febrile exudative tonsillitis: viral or streptococcal? Pediatrics 80:6–12, 1987.

CHAPTER 49

NOSEBLEEDS

Stanley H. Inkelis, M.D.

H$_x$ A three-year-old boy is brought to the office one winter day. He has had four nosebleeds in the past week as well as a cold with a runny nose and cough, which began the day before the first nosebleed. The nosebleeds occurred either at night or during sleep and stopped spontaneously or with gentle pressure. Other than the cold and nosebleeds, the boy is in good health. He is active, with bruises over both tibias but none elsewhere. The many cuts and scrapes he has had in the past resulted in minimal bleeding. His family has no history of a bleeding disorder or easy bruisability.

The child's physical examination is entirely normal, except for a small amount of blood in the left anterior naris.

Questions

1. What are the common causes of nosebleeds in children?
2. What systemic diseases are associated with nosebleeds?
3. How should nosebleeds be evaluated in children?
4. How should minor and severe nosebleeds be managed in children?

Nosebleed, or epistaxis, occurs commonly in children, especially in those between the ages of 2 and 10 years. In most cases, nosebleeds are secondary to local trauma and can be cared for by primary care physicians. In rare instances, however, a nosebleed may be difficult to control or may be a manifestation of a serious systemic illness. Referral to an otolaryngologist or a hematologist/oncologist is usually not required except in these situations, and hospitalization is generally unnecessary. Parents and children, who are often frightened by nosebleeds, frequently overestimate the amount of blood lost. Understanding and reassurance are important in allaying anxiety.

EPIDEMIOLOGY

Thirty percent of children have one nosebleed by the time they are 5 years of age. In children between the ages of 6 and 10, the frequency increases to 56%. Nosebleeds are rare in infancy and infrequent after puberty. They occur much more frequently in the late fall and winter months, when URIs are common, environmental humidity is relatively low, and the use of heating systems results in dryness. Nosebleeds are also more common in children who live in dry climates, especially if they have a URI or allergic rhinitis.

CLINICAL PRESENTATION

Most children with nosebleeds have a history of bleeding at home and have minimal or no bleeding at the time of presentation (D$_x$ Box). With anterior nosebleeds, blood exits almost entirely from the anterior portion of the nose. With posterior nosebleeds, most of the bleeding occurs in the nasopharynx and mouth, although some blood exits through the nose as well. Posterior nosebleeds are heavier and more difficult to control, and children may present in a hemodynamically unstable condition.

Children with bleeding disorders may have recurrent nosebleeds and a history of prolonged bleeding, easy bruisability, or multiple bruises in unlikely locations. In unusual situations, children with GI or respiratory tract bleeding may present with blood exiting through the nose. Alternatively, some children who present with hematemesis have vomited swallowed nasal blood.

PATHOPHYSIOLOGY

Nosebleeds may be either anterior or posterior in origin. The large majority of nosebleeds in children

Dx Nosebleeds

- Blood in anterior nares, nasopharynx, or mouth
- History of any of the following:
  - Frequent digital manipulation (nose picking)
  - URI (recent)
  - Allergic rhinitis
  - Dry climate
  - Foreign body in nose
  - Trauma to nose
  - Prolonged or difficult to stop bleeding or easy bruisability
- Physical examination consistent with any of the following:
  - Rhinorrhea
  - Dry, cracked nasal mucosa
  - Foreign body in nose
  - Trauma to nose
  - Multiple bruises

(90%) are anterior and are more easily controlled than posterior nosebleeds. The anteroinferior portion of the nasal septum, about 0.5 cm from the tip of the nose, known as Kiesselbach's plexus or Little's area, is the most common part of the nose involved in anterior nosebleeds. This area is supplied by the anterior and posterior ethmoidal arteries, the sphenopalatine artery, and the septal branches of the superior labial artery (Fig. 49–1). The mucosa covering the area is thin and friable, and the small vessels supplying the nasal mucous membrane have little structural support. Congestion of the vessels caused by conditions such as a URI or drying of the mucosa from low environmental humidity makes this area susceptible to bleeding.

Posterior nosebleeds generally arise from the turbinate or nasal wall. Significant bleeding, usually from a branch of the sphenopalatine artery, may occur.

DIFFERENTIAL DIAGNOSIS

Trauma from nose picking and **inflammation** of the nasal mucosa from a URI are by far the most common causes of nosebleeds in children. Repetitive, habitual nose picking results in the formation of friable granulation tissue that bleeds when traumatized (epistaxis digitorum). Mucosal inflammation predisposes children to bleeding because of erosion of congested blood vessels. As the nasal mucosa dries, it may lead to crust formation and cracking. Bleeding may occur spontaneously, but more often it results from forceful nose blowing and sneezing that increases venous pressure in the more vascularized nasal septum.

Viral respiratory infections, such as measles, infectious mononucleosis, and influenza, may also predis-

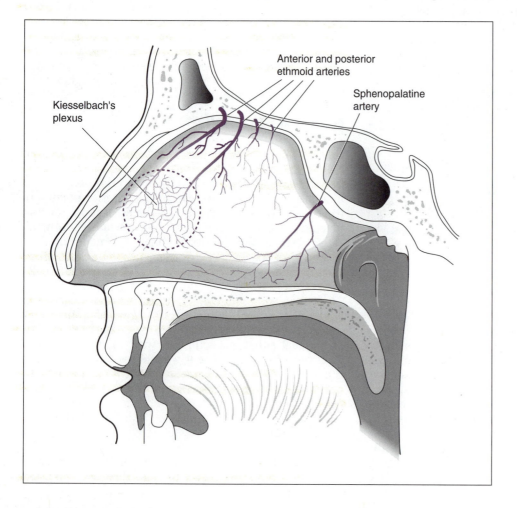

Kiesselbach's plexus

Anterior and posterior ethmoid arteries

Sphenopalatine artery

FIGURE 49–1. *Vascular supply of nasal septum. Note the confluence of vessels that forms Kiesselbach's plexus.*

pose children to nosebleeds because of their local inflammatory effect. Nosebleeds in children with these infections are more common in areas of low environmental humidity. Many children with no URI-like symptoms also suffer from nosebleeds in such environments, usually in winter, when inhaling dry hot air from heating systems causes desiccation of the nasal mucosa (rhinitis sicca). **Allergic rhinitis** with inflammation and subsequent drying may also lead to nosebleeds. Children with allergic rhinitis who take decongestants may be more likely to suffer from nosebleeds.

Foreign bodies may cause direct trauma or pressure necrosis to the vessels of the nasal mucosa. **External trauma** can cause either tears to the nasal mucosa or nasal fractures. If bleeding from mucosal vessels occurs but the mucosa remains intact, a septal hematoma may develop. Abscess formation or septal perforation may occur if the septal hematoma is not drained.

Although nosebleeds are usually benign conditions, they may be the first sign of serious illness. Persistent or recurrent nosebleeds with no obvious cause should raise the suspicion of **bleeding disorders**. Thrombocytopenia is the most common coagulation defect causing nosebleeds. Idiopathic thrombocytopenic purpura is the most frequent thrombocytopenic disorder associated with nosebleeds. Leukemia and HIV must be strongly considered and ruled out in children with nosebleeds and thrombocytopenia.

The most commonly inherited bleeding disorder associated with nosebleeds is von Willebrand's disease, an autosomal dominant bleeding disorder characterized by varying degrees of factor VIII deficiency and platelet dysfunction (decreased platelet adhesiveness). Hemophilia (factor VIII, IX, or XI deficiency) and Glanzmann's thrombasthenia are other inherited bleeding disorders that may lead to nosebleeds. Hepatic disease, severe vitamin K deficiency, or malabsorption syndrome is associated with an acquired coagulopathy, which may present with nosebleed.

Nosebleeds may be a manifestation of **blood vessel disorders,** either hereditary or acquired. Osler-Weber-Rendu syndrome (hereditary hemorrhagic telangiectasia) is an inherited autosomal dominant disease with multiple mucosal telangiectasias, especially in the nose. Because telangiectasias are deficient in muscular and connective tissue, these telangiectasias may rupture spontaneously and bleed profusely. Vitamin C deficiency, an acquired blood vessel disorder, is associated with nosebleeds.

Neoplasms, particularly malignancies, are uncommon causes of nosebleeds in children. Polyps are usually present in association with cystic fibrosis or allergies. Capillary, cavernous, and mixed hemangiomas may occur in the nose. Juvenile nasopharyngeal angiofibroma occurs almost exclusively in adolescent males, who present with nasal obstruction and bleeding. Rhabdomyosarcomas, lymphomas, and squamous cell carcinomas of the nose, sinuses, or nasopharynx are rare causes of nosebleeds.

Drugs such as aspirin and NSAIDs, which interfere with platelet function, and warfarin and heparin, which inhibit clotting factors, increase the risk of nasal hemorrhage with minor trauma, infection, or inflammation. Cocaine snorting may cause nasal septal perforation and nosebleeds.

Hypertension is rarely associated with nosebleeds in children. Wegener's granulomatosis and lethal midline granuloma are rare, idiopathic, inflammatory diseases in children that lead to nasal tissue destruction and bleeding. Nosebleeds during menstruation may be secondary to endometriosis with ectopic endometrial tissue implants in the nasal cavity.

EVALUATION

History

A thorough history often reveals the etiology of the nosebleed (Questions Box). In addition, information concerning the side of the nose from which the bleeding occurred, the amount of bleeding, the measures used to stop the bleeding, and the time required to stop the bleeding may be helpful.

Physical Examination

A general physical examination should be performed. In children with significant blood loss, particular attention should be directed toward the mental status and vital signs to determine children's hemodynamic stability. If vital signs are normal, these children should also be evaluated for orthostatic changes.

In addition, the skin and mucous membranes should be checked carefully for petechiae, purpura, and ecchymosis, which are signs of easy bruisability. The abdomen should be examined for hepatosplenomegaly. Telangiectasias in the oropharynx or mucous membranes suggest Osler-Weber-Rendu syndrome. The oropharynx and nasopharynx should be examined for masses and blood dripping downward from a posterior bleed. The nose should then be inspected for the site of bleeding.

Questions: Nosebleeds

- Does the child pick his or her nose?
- Has the child suffered any trauma recently?
- Has the child recently had a URI?
- Has the child recently had any systemic viral or bacterial illness?
- Does the child have any allergies?
- Is the child exposed to dry conditions (e.g., dry climate, dry heat, dehumidified air)?
- Has the child put or tried to put foreign objects in his or her nose?
- Is there a history of easy bruisability or prolonged, difficult-to-stop bleeding in the child or family?
- Does the child use any aspirin or aspirin-containing medications?
- Which side of the nose was bleeding?
- How extensive was the bleeding?
- Did the child spit out or swallow blood? Was there blood in the mouth?
- What measures were used to stop the bleeding? How long did it take to stop the bleeding?
- Was this the first nosebleed? If the nosebleeds are recurrent, how often do they occur and how long do they last?

Diagnostic Studies

Laboratory tests are rarely indicated in most children with nosebleeds. A hematocrit/hemoglobin should be obtained if the nosebleeds are severe or recur frequently. Blood for type and cross-match should be sent in children who have signs or symptoms of hypovolemia (increased pulse; cool, clammy skin; increased capillary refill; decreased blood pressure; etc.) or a marked drop in hematocrit. If the history or physical examination suggests that a coagulopathy may be present, a CBC with platelet count, PT, and PTT should be obtained.

X-rays and other imaging studies are rarely necessary in children with nosebleeds.

MANAGEMENT

Children who present to primary care physicians with a history of a nosebleed or nosebleeds that have resolved spontaneously or with application of pressure to the nose need no further treatment in the office setting, provided that the history and physical examination are consistent with a benign cause of the nosebleed. These children or their parents should be instructed to apply **petroleum jelly** (Vaseline) or an antibiotic ointment inside the septal portion of the involved naris twice a day for three to five days with a cotton-tipped swab (Q-tip) or with the little finger. Often the child's little finger is used because it is nonthreatening and it "knows where to go." Further nose picking should be discouraged, and fingernails should be trimmed to minimize trauma. In addition, a bedside **humidifier** helps to moisturize the air, especially in dry climates or during the winter when forced hot air heat is used. Children whose noses moisten from rhinorrhea and then dry and crack also benefit from humidified air. Buffered saline nasal spray may also be helpful.

Children or parents should be given advice about how to care for nosebleeds at home. These instructions can also be given to parents who seek advice over the telephone about how to stop children's nosebleeds. Practitioners should reassure parents and children that most nosebleeds are easily controlled. Children should sit upright and lean forward slightly while **direct pressure** is applied to the naris. External compression of the nares between two fingers for 5 to 10 minutes should be sufficient. Pressure applied on the anterior and midportion of the nose rather than at the base is more effective in stopping the bleeding because most nosebleeds occur in these parts of the nose.

Children who are actively bleeding through the nose when seen by primary care physicians should be positioned sitting upright and leaning forward slightly, and they should be given a basin and facial tissue. Direct pressure should be applied by a nurse or physician. A cotton dental roll may be placed under the upper lip to compress the labial artery in older children in whom concern about displacement and possible aspiration of the cotton is minimal. If the bleeding continues after external compression, children should be instructed to blow their noses to remove as much clot as possible. Fresh blood should be removed with suction. Cotton pledgets moistened with a few drops of a topical vasoconstrictor, such as 0.25% phenylephrine (Neo-Synephrine) or epinephrine (1:1000) or topical thrombin, should be inserted into the side of the nose involved. Pressure should then be applied for an additional 10 minutes.

If the bleeding persists, **cauterization** of the bleeding site with a silver nitrate stick for no more than three seconds is indicated. Continued bleeding is slowed by cauterizing the four quadrants surrounding the bleeding point to interrupt flow from surrounding vessels. Cauterization is often difficult in children, and consultation with an otolaryngologist is advisable. Cauterization should not be performed in children with a bleeding diathesis.

If the bleeding continues, an absorbable **nasal pad** with Oxicel, Surgicel, or Gelfoam may be directly applied to the bleeding site to form an artificial clot. Avitene, a microfibrillar collagen material, provides for platelet aggregation and clot formation when applied to the bleeding site. Continued uncontrolled bleeding requires anterior **nasal packing** with antibiotic-impregnated, one-inch petrolatum gauze strips, which should remain in place for approximately two to three days. Prophylactic **antibiotics** should be started because sinusitis is a complication of anterior nasal packing.

Posterior nosebleeds, which are more difficult to control, should be suspected if (1) the measures described previously are ineffective, (2) bleeding is vigorous and the cause cannot be identified, or (3) most of the bleeding is into the nasopharynx and mouth. A posterior nasal pack using a Foley catheter or an intranasal balloon is indicated to control posterior nosebleeds. This pack is left in place for two to five days, and children should be started on antibiotics to prevent sinusitis.

The need for **otolaryngologic consultation** depends on the experience of the individual physician and the availability of consultation. Prompt consultation, if available, should be obtained for children with severe nosebleeds who need volume replacement, for children with nosebleeds that do not stop or recur after the above measures have been taken, for children who may need anterior or posterior nasal packing, and for children with recurrent, difficult-to-stop nosebleeds. In some cases, obtaining consultation before cauterization with silver nitrate is advisable. Children with septal hematomas, tumors, polyps, and telangiectasias should be referred to an otolaryngologist for further care. Children with a documented or suspected bleeding disorder should be referred to a hematologist.

Children with severe nosebleeds should have an intravenous line started early; blood sent for type and cross-match; and fluids replaced, depending on the amount of blood loss and physical evidence of hypovolemia. In children who are frightened or in whom certain procedures (e.g., cauterization of bleeding site, drainage of septal hematoma) are performed, sedation should be strongly considered. Pain medication should be used in children who need anterior or posterior packing. If procedures that cause undue pain or discomfort are necessary, general anesthesia in an operating room setting may be indicated.

Hospitalization is not often necessary for children with nosebleeds. However, children who are hemodynamically unstable on presentation or who need placement of a posterior nasal pack usually require inpatient treatment. Hospitalization may be necessary for children with difficult-to-stop bleeds who need an anterior nasal pack or who have a bleeding disorder or underlying chronic illness such as leukemia or HIV infection.

PROGNOSIS

The prognosis for nosebleeds in children is excellent. Almost all nosebleeds are easily controlled with a minimal amount of home care or medical management. Surgery is rarely indicated. Complications associated with significant nosebleeds include hypovolemia from blood loss and sinusitis from anterior or posterior nasal packs. Even for rare causes of nosebleeds, the prognosis is very good with prompt diagnosis and treatment.

Case Resolution

In the case presented, the boy has experienced several nosebleeds of short duration associated with a URI and winter dryness. His history and physical examination are unremarkable for a bleeding disorder or chronic illness. The small amount of blood in his nose is consistent with an anterior nosebleed originating from Kiesselbach's plexus with inflammation and drying of the nasal mucosa. Laboratory tests are not indicated. The parents should be instructed to apply petroleum jelly to the septal portion of the left side of the child's nose twice a day for three to five days and to humidify the child's bedroom. They should also be reassured that their child has a common condition that he will outgrow.

Selected Readings

Friedman, E. M. Epistaxis. *In* Dershowitz, R. A. (ed.). Ambulatory Pediatric Care, 2nd ed. Philadelphia, J. B. Lippincott, 1993, pp. 308–310.

Guarisco, J. L., and H. D. Graham, III. Epistaxis in children: causes, diagnosis, and treatment. Ear Nose Throat J. 68:522–538, 1989.

Henretig, F. M. Epistaxis. *In* Fleisher, G. R., and S. Ludwig (eds.). Textbook of Pediatric Emergency Medicine, 3rd ed. Baltimore, Williams & Wilkins, 1993, pp. 175–177.

Josephson, G. D., F. A. Godley, and P. Stierna. Practical management of epistaxis. Med. Clin. North Am. 75:1311–1320, 1991.

Katsanis, E., et al. Prevalence and significance of mild bleeding disorders in children with recurrent epistaxis. J. Pediatr. 113:73–76, 1988.

Mulbury, P. E. Recurrent epistaxis. Pediatr. Rev. 12:213–217, 1991.

Perretta, L. J., B. L. Denslow, and C. G. Brown. Emergency evaluation and management of epistaxis. Emerg. Med. Clin. North Am. 5:265–277, 1987.

Potsic, W. P., and S. D. Handler. Otolaryngology emergencies (epistaxis). *In* Fleisher, G. R., and S. Ludwig (eds.). Textbook of Pediatric Emergency Medicine, 3rd ed. Baltimore, Williams & Wilkins, 1993, pp. 1377–1379.

Santamaria, J. P., and T. J. Abrunzo. Ear, nose, and throat (epistaxis). *In* Barkin, R. M. (ed.). Pediatric Emergency Medicine. St. Louis, C.V. Mosby, 1992, pp. 646–650.

Wallace, L., and M. R. Clark. Epistaxis. *In* Reisdorff, E. J., M. R. Roberts, and J. G. Wiegenstein (eds.). Pediatric Emergency Medicine. Philadelphia, W. B. Saunders, 1993, pp. 629–634.

Werner, E. J., et al. Prevalence of von Willebrand disease in children: a multiethnic study. J. Pediatr. 123:893–898, 1993.

C H A P T E R   5 0

STRABISMUS

Geeta Grover, M.D.

Hₓ   The mother of an eight-month-old infant complains that every time her son looks to either side his eyes seem "crossed." Otherwise he is growing and developing normally. A symmetric pupillary light reflex, bilateral red reflex, and normal extraocular eye movements in all directions are noted on physical examination of the eyes.

Questions

1. What is strabismus?
2. What conditions make infants' eyes appear "crossed"? What is the differential diagnosis?
3. What tests are used in the office evaluation of children suspected of having strabismus?

4. Which infants with "crossed" eyes require referral for further evaluation and treatment?

Strabismus refers to any abnormality in ocular alignment. It is one of the most common eye problems observed in infants and children. The pediatrician plays an important role in the early detection and prompt referral of children with suspected ocular alignment abnormalities.

EPIDEMIOLOGY

Strabismus affects approximately 3% of the population, and the condition is seen most commonly in children under six years of age. About 50% of all affected children have a positive family history of strabismus, although the exact genetic mode of inheritance is unclear. Up to 75% of normal infants have transient intermittent strabismus during the first three months of life.

CLINICAL PRESENTATION

Children with ocular misalignment have an asymmetric corneal light reflex test. Eye movement is noted with cover testing. Children with paralytic strabismus may present with torticollis or head tilting in an effort to avoid diplopia (D_x Box).

PATHOPHYSIOLOGY

Normal binocular vision is the result of the fusion of images from both eyes working synchronously across the visual field. Six extraocular muscles control all eye movements. Orthophoria is proper alignment of the eyes, and strabismus results from an imbalance in muscle movements.

Strabismus

The classification of strabismus is complex. Based on etiology, it may be considered nonparalytic (comitant) or paralytic (noncomitant). Strabismus may also be classified as congenital or acquired, intermittent or constant, alternating or unilateral, or convergent or divergent.

In **nonparalytic strabismus,** the extraocular muscles and the nerves that control them are normal. The degree of deviation is constant or nearly constant in all directions of gaze. Nonparalytic strabismus is the most common type of strabismus seen in children, and congenital or infantile esotropia is usually of this kind. Ocular or visual defects such as cataracts or high refractive errors occasionally cause nonparalytic strabismus.

In **paralytic strabismus,** paralysis or paresis of one or more of the extraocular muscles produces a muscle imbalance. The deviation is asymmetric, and characteristically the degree of deviation is worse in the direction of gaze of the affected muscle.

Paralytic strabismus may be congenital or acquired. **Congenital strabismus** may result from birth trauma, muscle anomalies, abnormal development of the cranial nerve nuclei, or congenital infections affecting the eyes. **Acquired strabismus** due to extraocular muscle palsies usually indicates the presence of a serious underlying condition, such as an intracranial tumor, a demyelinating or neurodegenerative disease, myasthenia gravis, a progressive myopathy, or a CNS infection. Children may present with a complaint of double vision or a compensatory torticollis (head tilt) to avoid double vision (diplopia).

Intermittent (latent) misalignment of the eyes is referred to as **heterophoria.** Under normal conditions, the fusional mechanisms of the CNS maintain eye alignment. Eye deviation is appreciated only under certain conditions, such as illness, fatigue, stress, or when fusion is interrupted by occluding one eye (e.g., during cover testing). Some degree of heterophoria may be found in almost all individuals and it is usually asymptomatic. Larger degrees of heterophoria may give rise to troublesome symptoms such as headaches, transient diplopia, or asthenopia (eye strain).

Constant misalignment of the eyes is referred to as **heterotropia.** This condition occurs because normal fusional mechanisms are unable to control eye deviation; children are unable to use both eyes together to fixate on an object. Heterotropias may be alternating and involve either one or both eyes. In alternating tropias, both eyes appear to deviate equally, and vision generally develops normally in each eye because children have no preference for fixation. If strabismus affects one eye, the other eye is always used for fixation, and there is danger of amblyopia or loss of vision in the deviating eye.

Convergent deviation, a "turning in" or "crossing" of the eyes, is called an esodeviation (e.g., esotropia or esophoria). Divergent deviation, a "turning out" of the eyes, is an exodeviation. The prefixes hyper- and hypo- are used for upward and downward vertical deviations, respectively. Esodeviations are the most common type of ocular misalignment, accounting for 50 to 75% of all cases of strabismus. Vertical deviations represent less than 5% of all cases of strabismus.

Amblyopia

Amblyopia, a potential complication if strabismus is not corrected in a timely manner, refers to poor vision in one eye, or rarely both, despite correction of any

---

D_x	**Strabismus**

- Head tilt
- Blurred vision
- Double vision (diplopia)
- Squint
- Asymmetric corneal light reflex
- Eye movement with cover testing

refractive errors. If children have no significant refractive error and the visual acuity of one eye is worse than the other, they probably have amblyopia. Amblyopia is most commonly associated with strabismus that develops in children who are younger than four years of age. Early diagnosis of strabismic amblyopia is essential because restoration of normal vision after six to seven years of age may be difficult.

Amblyopia may be classified as organic or functional. **Organic amblyopia** results from a lesion or developmental defect in one of the structures of the eye or its visual pathways. **Functional amblyopia,** which includes strabismic, deprivation, and refractive amblyopia, leads to poor vision in one eye with no recognized organic cause. Refractive amblyopia refers to a blurring of the retinal image due to bilateral large or asymmetric refractive errors. Deprivation amblyopia is the lack of formation of a retinal image, usually in one eye (e.g., due to a congenital cataract, corneal opacity, total ptosis). In strabismic amblyopia, the immature or developing brain suppresses images from the deviating eye to prevent diplopia. If the strabismus is not corrected while the brain's visual pathways are still malleable (i.e., before approximately 6–7 years of age), children may have some degree of permanent visual loss in the deviating eye.

DIFFERENTIAL DIAGNOSIS

The differential diagnosis of strabismus may be divided into three categories: transient neonatal strabismus, congenital or infantile strabismus, and acquired strabismus. True strabismus must be differentiated from the illusion of deviation created by facial asymmetry or anatomic variations.

Transient Neonatal Strabismus

Eye alignment in normal infants during the first two to three months of life may vary from normal to intermittent esotropia or exotropia. These deviations are believed to result from CNS immaturity and resolve spontaneously in the vast majority of children by four months of age. If such deviations are constant or persist beyond this age, children should be referred to an ophthalmologist for further evaluation.

Congenital or Infantile Strabismus

This type of strabismus is defined as a deviation that occurs during the first six months of life. Because the deviation may not always be present at birth, the term "infantile" may be more accurate. The differential diagnosis of infantile strabismus is presented in Table 50–1. **Pseudoesotropia** is an illusion or apparent deviation and not a true deviation. In many infants, the broad, flat nasal bridge and prominent epicanthal folds may obscure a portion of the sclera near the nose and create the appearance of esotropia (Fig. 50–1). This illusion resolves as children mature. Symmetric corneal light reflexes or normal cover tests differentiate pseudoesotropia from true esotropia.

TABLE 50–1. Differential Diagnosis of Strabismus
Congenital or Infantile Strabismus
Esodeviations
Infantile esotropia
Pseudoesotropia
Möbius syndrome
Exodeviations
Congenital exotropia
Congenital third nerve paralysis
Abnormalities of the bony orbit (Crouzon's syndrome)
Both Esodeviations and Exodeviations
Duane's syndrome (esotropia more common than exotropia)
Acquired Strabismus
Esodeviations
Accommodative esotropia
Benign sixth cranial nerve palsy
Exodeviations
Intermittent exotropia
Overcorrection after surgery for esotropia
Both Esodeviations and Exodeviations
Poor vision
Orbital trauma causing entrapment of extraocular muscles
Intracranial tumors or tumors involving the orbit (e.g., retinoblastoma)
Myasthenia gravis
Central nervous system (CNS) infection (e.g., meningitis)
CNS tumor
Orbital cellulitis

Esotropia is one of the more common types of childhood strabismus. The constant deviation of infantile esotropia is usually readily apparent because of the large angle of deviation. Affected children usually have good bilateral vision because of the alternation of fixation from one eye to the other. Cross-fixation, in which children look to the left with the adducted right eye and to the right with the adducted left eye, may be evident because of the large angle of deviation.

Infantile exotropia is less common than esotropia. Like esotropia, exotropia develops within the first six months of life and is characterized by a large angle of deviation. Other causes of infantile exotropia include congenital third nerve palsy (paralytic strabismus) and abnormalities of the bones of the orbit (e.g., Crouzon's syndrome).

FIGURE 50–1. *Child with pseudoesotropia.* Note the wide nasal bridge and prominent epicanthal folds.

Acquired Strabismus

Acquired strabismus may result from a variety of causes (see Table 50–1). Accommodative esotropia and intermittent exotropia are two common types of acquired strabismus. **Accommodative esotropia** typically develops in children between two and three years of age but may appear as early as six months or as late as eight years. Children with hyperopia use accommodation (alteration in the shape of the lens) to see clearly. The accommodative reflex is closely linked to convergence; when accommodation occurs, so does convergence. If children have severe hyperopia (farsightedness), the amount of convergence that occurs with accommodation may be severe and lead to the development of esotropia. Such esotropia is usually intermittent initially and only gradually becomes constant.

Intermittent exotropia, the most common form of exodeviation seen in children, develops between birth and four years of age. Although it begins as an intermittent condition in which children's eyes appear to deviate outward, especially when they are tired, ill, or fixating at a distance, the exotropia can become constant with time. Children may also close one eye in bright sunlight, presumably in an effort to prevent diplopia.

EVALUATION

History

The evaluation of infants or children suspected of having strabismus should begin with a thorough family history; strabismus often runs in families (Questions Box). Parental description of the ocular deviation is useful, because misalignments, especially intermittent deviations that may only become manifest when children are tired, may not always be evident during the office visit. A history of head or orbital trauma may help in the evaluation of acquired strabismus.

Physical Examination

On physical examination, the presence of any dysmorphic features and structural abnormalities of the face or neck (e.g., torticollis) should be noted. Children with paralytic strabismus may compensate for their paretic lesion by tilting their head to avoid diplopia.

It is important that visual screening of children begin during the neonatal period. Newborn screening should emphasize the presence of a bilateral red reflex. An abnormal red reflex or a white reflex may indicate the presence of a cataract or retinoblastoma. Evaluation

for ocular alignment should begin at the four-month health maintenance visit. Intermittent misalignment of the eyes is often seen in normal infants who are younger than four months of age. However, constant misalignment requires immediate attention at any age.

Vision Testing

Testing of visual acuity is essential in the evaluation of children with suspected strabismus. Such testing may be performed as early as three years of age, if children are cooperative. Charts with symbols, figures, or letters can be used. The traditional Snellen eye chart with letters can generally be used in children who are four years of age. Decreased vision in one eye may be indicative of ocular abnormalities, including ocular deviations.

Tests for Strabismus

The two basic tests for strabismus that can be easily performed in the office are the corneal light reflex test, or Hirschberg test, and the cover tests. The pediatrician should be comfortable performing both tests.

The **corneal light reflex test** is the simplest and quickest test for the evaluation of strabismus. In this test, a penlight is projected simultaneously onto the corneas of both eyes as the child looks straight ahead. The examiner compares the placement of the corneal light reflex in each eye with respect to the center of the pupil. If the eyes are straight, the reflection appears symmetrically in the center of both pupils or on the same point on each cornea. If the light reflex appears off center in one eye as compared to the other, an ocular deviation or tropia is present. Nasal deviation of the light reflex on the cornea indicates exotropia on that side; temporal deviation signifies esotropia; and superior or inferior deviation indicates hypo- and hypertropia, respectively.

Unlike the corneal light reflex test, which may be performed even in uncooperative children, the **cover tests** require children's cooperation and ability to fixate on a specified object. These tests are used to detect heterophorias. Two types of cover tests, alternate-cover and cover-uncover, are used. Only the alternate-cover test detects both heterophorias and heterotropias. This test may be preferred by the primary care physician as a screening tool; the cover-uncover test detects only manifest deviations or heterotropias. In the alternate-cover test, one eye and then the other is covered as the child fixates on an object at a distance. If neither eye moves as the cover is moved rapidly between the eyes, the eyes are in alignment or orthophoric. With heterotropia, the deviating eye moves when the fixating eye is occluded; in heterophoria, the deviating eye moves when it is uncovered (Fig. 50–2).

The alternate-cover test may be illustrated with the following example. A child presents with constant esotropia of the left eye. When the right or fixating eye is occluded, the left eye is forced to fixate so that the child can see, and the left eye moves outward as the

---

Questions: Strabismus

- Does the child have a family history of strabismus?
- Does the child constantly tilt the head toward one side?
- Does the child squint?
- Has the child complained of blurred or double vision?
- Does the child close one eye in bright sunlight?
- Has the child had any recent trauma to the eyes or head?

FIGURE 50-2. *Alternate-cover test in the detection of strabismus.* Normally, both eyes appear to be aligned and centrally fixed.
A. *Detection of esotropia. The right eye is fixating and a left esotropia is present. When the right or fixating eye is covered, the left eye moves outward (toward the center).*
B. *Detection of esophoria. The eyes are aligned with a left esophoria. When the left eye is covered, it deviates inward. As the occluder is moved from the left eye to the right eye, the left eye moves outward to a position of fixation.*

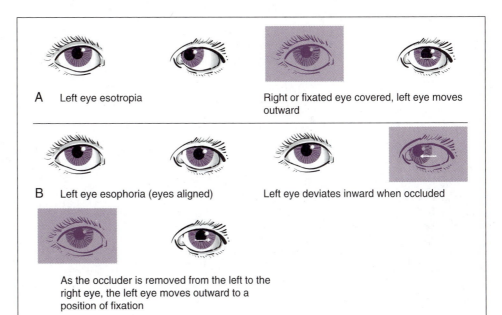

A Left eye esotropia

Right or fixated eye covered, left eye moves outward

B Left eye esophoria (eyes aligned)

Left eye deviates inward when occluded

As the occluder is removed from the left to the right eye, the left eye moves outward to a position of fixation

right eye is occluded. In the case of a child with an esophoria or latent deviation of the left eye, the eye deviates inward when it is occluded, because it is not being forced to fixate. As the occluder is removed from the left eye to the right, the left eye moves outward and returns to a position of fixation.

The alternate-cover test may be more difficult to interpret in children with bilateral or alternating strabismus who use both eyes in turn for fixation. It is not necessary for the pediatrician to identify exactly what type of strabismus is present; abnormal movement should be noted and children should be referred for further evaluation. An ophthalmologist is able to perform a more detailed examination.

MANAGEMENT

The goal of management is the attainment of the best possible vision in each eye. The sooner deviations are corrected, the better are children's chances for equal bilateral vision. Treatment includes correction of any underlying refractive error with **corrective lenses.** Such lenses, which remedy the refractive error and minimize the need for accommodation, are used to treat accommodative esotropia.

Children who do not see equally well from both eyes may be at risk for amblyopia if they preferentially fixate with only one eye. If detected, amblyopia should be corrected with occlusion therapy of the fixating "good" eye. **Occlusion therapy** forces children to use the amblyopic eye. This treatment is best accomplished by constantly patching the eye with better vision during waking hours. Children require repeat evaluations and close monitoring during this therapy.

If nonsurgical methods fail to align the eyes, surgical correction may be necessary. **Surgery** may be used to achieve the best possible ocular alignment and is usually required for treatment of infantile esotropia. It is

generally performed in children between six months and two years of age, while the visual system is still pliable enough to allow for development of postsurgical binocular vision. Surgery also may be needed in children with intermittent exotropia if the frequency or deviation is increasing.

PROGNOSIS

Certain conditions, such as pseudoesotropia or infrequent intermittent exotropia, may resolve as children mature. Others, such as infantile esotropia, require early detection and treatment to achieve the best binocular vision. Amblyopia and permanent vision loss may result if correction of strabismus is delayed.

Case Resolution

The infant in the case history has pseudoesotropia. Although the boy's eyes appear to deviate, the corneal light reflex and cover tests are normal. Physical examination reveals prominent epicanthal folds and a broad, flat nasal bridge.

Selected Readings

Catalano, J. D. Strabismus. Pediatr. Ann. 19:289–297, 1990.

Cheng, K. P., A. W. Biglan, and D. A. Hiles. Pediatric ophthalmology. *In* Zitelli, B. J., and H. W. Davis. Pediatric Physical Diagnosis, 2nd ed. Philadelphia, J. B. Lippincott, 1992, pp. 19.1–19.39.

Crouch, E. R., and E. R. Crouch. Pediatric vision screening: why? when? what? how? Contemp. Pediatr. 8:9–30, September 1991. (Special issue.)

Frankel, C. A. Strabismus. *In* Hoekelman, R. A. (ed.). Primary Pediatric Care, 2nd ed. St Louis, Mosby-Year Book, 1992, pp. 1068–1073.

Lavrich, J. B., and L. B. Nelson. Diagnosis and treatment of strabismus disorders. Pediatr. Clin. North Am. 40:737–752, 1993.

INFECTIONS OF THE EYE

Geeta Grover, M.D.

H$_x$ A 10-day-old infant has a one-day history of red, watery eyes and nonproductive cough with no fever. The girl is breast-fed and continues to eat well. She was the 7 lb, 2 oz (3238 g) product of a term gestation, born via normal spontaneous vaginal delivery without complications to a 26-year-old woman. The pregnancy was also uncomplicated. No one at home is ill.

On examination, the infant is afebrile with normal vital signs. Examination of the eyes reveals bilateral conjunctival injection with only a mild amount of purulent discharge. Bilateral red reflexes are present. The rest of the physical examination is within normal limits.

Questions

1. What is the differential diagnosis of conjunctivitis both during and following the neonatal period?
2. What laboratory tests, if any, should be performed?
3. When is a chest x-ray indicated in the evaluation of neonates with conjunctivitis?
4. What are management strategies for eye infections?

Infections of the eye and surrounding structures are commonly seen by pediatricians. Such infections range in severity from more common problems such as blepharitis and conjunctivitis, which lack serious sequelae, to more severe and less common infections such as periorbital and orbital cellulitis. The presenting complaint in many children with eye infections is a red-appearing eye. Familiarity with the common causes of a red eye makes prompt diagnosis and treatment possible.

EPIDEMIOLOGY

Conjunctivitis, which affects children of all ages, is perhaps the most common eye infection of childhood. The incidence of conjunctivitis in the newborn period is estimated to range from 1.6 to 12%. The incidence of chlamydial conjunctivitis is about 8 per 1000 live births. About two thirds of acute childhood conjunctivitis has a bacterial etiology, and one third is viral. *Haemophilus influenzae* and *Streptococcus pneumoniae* are the most common bacterial agents and account for about 40% and 10% of culture-proven cases, respectively. *Staphylococcus aureus* is isolated from the conjunctivae of children with acute conjunctivitis, but it is found with about the same frequency in the eyes of children without conjunctivitis. Adenovirus is the most common viral isolate. Most cases of acute conjunctivitis in young adults have a viral etiology. Serious eye infections such as periorbital and orbital cellulitis occur far less often.

CLINICAL PRESENTATION

Red eyes are a common presenting sign of infections of the eyelids and conjunctivae. Eyelid edema and erythema surrounding the eye characterize periorbital and orbital cellulitis. Proptosis, abnormal extraocular movement, or loss of visual acuity may signal spread of the infection beyond the orbital septum (orbital cellulitis) (D$_x$ Box).

PATHOPHYSIOLOGY

Eye infections may be divided into two types: those affecting the structures surrounding the orbit and those involving the orbital contents themselves (Fig. 51–1). Although all structures surrounding the eye may potentially become inflamed or infected, the eyelids, nasolac-

---

D$_x$ Eye Infections

EYELID INFECTIONS
- Redness
- Itching (blepharitis)
- Burning (blepharitis)
- Scales at the base of the lashes (seborrheic blepharitis)
- Swelling (external hordeolum and chalazion)
- Pain (external hordeolum)

CONJUNCTIVITIS
- Conjunctival injection and edema
- Excessive tearing
- Discharge or crusting
- Itching (allergic conjunctivitis)

PERIORBITAL CELLULITIS
- Unilateral eyelid edema
- Erythema surrounding the eye
- Pain
- Fever

ORBITAL CELLULITIS
- Eyelid edema
- Proptosis
- Decreased extraocular movements
- Loss of visual acuity
- Fever
- Ill appearance
- Associated sinusitis

FIGURE 51–1. *The eye and surrounding structures.*

rimal drainage system (dacryocystitis; see Chapter 52, Excessive Tearing), conjunctiva, and cornea are most commonly involved. Orbital cellulitis is defined as an infection of the orbital structures posterior to the orbital septum. The orbital septum, an extension of the periosteum of the bones of the orbit, extends to the margins of both the upper and lower eyelids, and provides an anatomic barrier to the spread of most infectious and inflammatory processes. Preseptal, or periorbital, cellulitis is localized to structures superficial to the orbital septum, whereas septal, or orbital, cellulitis implies that the disease process involves orbital structures extending beyond the septum.

DIFFERENTIAL DIAGNOSIS

Infections of the eye are included in the differential diagnosis of conditions presenting with red eye (Table 51–1). Also included in the differential diagnosis are congenital, inflammatory, traumatic, and systemic processes. Although infection and irritation are by far the most common causes of an acute onset of red eye, other possibilities, especially trauma, glaucoma, or underlying systemic disease, must be considered.

Eyelid Infections

Common conditions of the eyelid and its related structures are blepharitis, hordeolum, and chalazion.
Blepharitis is an inflammation of the lid margins. This condition, which is often bilateral, may be chronic or recurrent. The two most common causes of blepharitis are staphylococcal infection and seborrheic dermatitis. Children with staphylococcal blepharitis often present with scales at the base of the lashes, ulceration of the lid margin, and loss of lashes. The infection may spread to the conjunctiva or cornea, producing conjunctivitis or keratitis. In contrast, seborrheic bleph-

aritis is characterized by greasy, yellow scales attached to the base of the lashes. In addition, associated seborrhea of the scalp or eyebrows may be present. Mixed staphylococcal-seborrheic infections, which occur as staphylococcal superinfection, may complicate seborrheic blepharitis. Less commonly seen forms of blepharitis are parasitic blepharitis, which results from infestation of the lids by the head louse, *Pediculus capitis,* or crab louse, *P. pubis,* and primary or recurrent herpes virus type 1 infections that may manifest as clusters of vesicles on the eyelids.

The glands of the eyelid can also be infected. *S. aureus*

TABLE 51–1.   Differential Diagnosis of Red Eye

Congenital Anomalies
Nasolacrimal duct obstruction
Congenital glaucoma
Infection
Keratitis
Conjunctivitis
Dacryocystitis
Periorbital and orbital cellulitis
Inflammation
Blepharitis
Hordeolum
Chalazion
Trauma
Corneal abrasion
Foreign body
Blunt trauma: hyphema, perforating injuries
Exposure to chemicals or other noxious substances
Systemic Illnesses
Kawasaki's disease
Varicella
Measles
Lyme disease
Stevens-Johnson syndrome
Ataxia-telangiectasia
Juvenile rheumatoid arthritis

is the most common organism. An external **hordeolum,** or common stye, results from an infection of the glands of Moll or Zeis located along the lid margins. Affected children present with a well-circumscribed, painful swelling along the lid margin that generally ruptures spontaneously and resolves without complications. An internal hordeolum, on the other hand, is an acute infection of the meibomian glands that tends to be larger and ruptures through either the skin or the conjunctival surface.

A **chalazion** is a chronic granulomatous inflammation of the meibomian glands that is caused by retention of secretions. The resulting firm, nontender, slow-growing mass within the upper or lower eyelid may be painful if secondary infection is present.

Infections of the Conjunctiva

Conjunctivitis refers to any inflammation of the conjunctiva. The condition may be allergic, chemical, viral, or bacterial in etiology. In addition, it may be a sign of systemic disease such as Kawasaki's disease or Stevens-Johnson syndrome.

Acute conjunctivitis, or pink eye, is common during childhood and can be extremely contagious. The usual signs are conjunctival injection, tearing, discharge, crusting of the lashes, and conjunctival edema (chemosis). Pain and decreased vision are uncommon symptoms and may signal corneal involvement.

In general, it is difficult to distinguish bacterial conjunctivitis from viral conjunctivitis on clinical features alone. Certain clinical characteristics may guide the diagnosis. The average age of children affected with **bacterial conjunctivitis** tends to be younger than for viral conjunctivitis, which is more frequent in adolescents; however, considerable overlap occurs. Children with bacterial conjunctivitis typically present with an acute onset of unilateral or bilateral injection and edema of both the palpebral and bulbar conjunctiva, minimal to copious purulent discharge, and crusting of the eyelashes. Children may have difficulty opening their eyes on awakening in the morning because of the crusting of the exudate. An association between conjunctivitis and concomitant otitis media has been well described. *H. influenzae,* which is often resistant to ampicillin, is the pathogen most commonly isolated from affected children.

The diagnosis of **viral conjunctivitis** is considered if signs of viral URI (e.g., low-grade fever, cough, rhinorrhea) are evident. Viral infection is associated with unilateral rather than bilateral mild conjunctival injection, watery or thin mucoid discharge, and only mild lid edema and erythema. Adenoviral infection is usually bilateral, with significant conjunctival injection and chemosis of the lids, and is often accompanied by a tender preauricular lymph node. Epidemic keratoconjunctivitis is a highly contagious form of adenoviral conjunctivitis. Affected children often complain of foreign body sensation beneath the lids or photophobia due to corneal involvement. Pharyngeal conjunctival fever, another presentation of adenoviral conjunctivitis,

usually manifests as conjunctivitis in association with pharyngitis and fever.

Infants who suffer from **chronic or recurrent conjunctivitis** may have an obstruction of the nasolacrimal duct, whereas older children with chronic conjunctivitis may have allergic diseases, recurrent blepharitis, or chlamydial infections. Blepharitis is the most common cause of chronic conjunctivitis in older children. *S. aureus* is frequently implicated in these infections.

Itching, tearing, and conjunctival edema are the hallmarks of **allergic conjunctivitis,** a noninfectious form of conjunctival inflammation often seen in children with other allergic disorders such as asthma or hay fever. Conjunctival injection tends to be mild, bilateral, and seasonal. The etiology is most often a hypersensitivity to pollens, dust, or animal hair. Vernal conjunctivitis is a particularly severe form of allergic conjunctivitis seen primarily during childhood. Usually bilateral, it occurs more frequently in boys. The majority of cases occur during the spring and summer. Severe itching and tearing are the most frequent complaints. The conjunctivae of the upper eyelid may have a cobblestone appearance due to the accumulation of inflammatory cells, or there may be small, elevated lesions of the bulbar conjunctiva at the corneal limbus. The pathogenesis is unclear, but atopy appears to play a role.

Chlamydial conjunctivitis frequently affects both neonates and adolescents. Inclusion conjunctivitis is an acute infection of the eyes caused by sexually transmitted *Chlamydia trachomatis* (usually serotypes D through K). This condition may be seen in neonates or sexually active adolescents. Trachoma, the most common cause of impaired vision and preventable blindness worldwide, is a chronic conjunctivitis usually caused by *C. trachomatis* serotypes A, B, and C. Although this disease is rarely seen in North America, it is endemic among certain populations, especially Native American. Inclusion conjunctivitis and endemic trachoma are both characterized initially by conjunctivitis with small lymphoid follicles in the conjunctiva.

Neonatal conjunctivitis, or ophthalmia neonatorum, occurs during the first month of life. The major causes of neonatal conjunctivitis are chemical, chlamydial, and bacterial (in decreasing order of frequency). Ophthalmia neonatorum may be produced by the same bacteria that cause childhood conjunctivitis but also results from organisms such as *C. trachomatis* or *Neisseria gonorrhoeae*. Newborns may acquire these latter pathogens following premature rupture of membranes or passage through an infected or colonized birth canal. *C. trachomatis* is the organism most commonly identified. It has been isolated from 17 to 40% of neonates with conjunctivitis. Infants born to mothers with active cervical chlamydial infection have a 20 to 50% chance of developing chlamydial conjunctivitis. Viruses are uncommon causes of neonatal ocular infections. Herpes simplex virus (HSV) is the primary viral agent involved in neonatal conjunctivitis. The presence of characteristic vesicular skin lesions or corneal dendritic lesions helps in the diagnosis.

The time of onset of symptoms is related to the etiologic agent. Inflammation secondary to the silver nitrate drops instilled at birth to prevent gonococcal infection presents as mild conjunctivitis 12 to 24 hours after birth in 10 to 100% of treated newborns. This condition usually resolves spontaneously in 24 to 48 hours. Conjunctivitis due to *N. gonorrhoeae* appears two to five days after birth and is associated with copious purulent discharge. Conjunctivitis due to *C. trachomatis* occurs at 5 to 14 days, a result of a longer incubation period. The time of onset and the severity of symptoms of these two conditions may overlap, however. The presentation of gonococcal infection may be delayed for five days or more because of the partial suppression of the infection by the prophylactic drops instilled at birth. Chlamydial infection can vary in severity from mild erythema of the eyelids to severe inflammation and copious purulent discharge. Gonococcal conjunctivitis is considered a medical emergency because the gonococcus can penetrate the cornea, resulting in corneal ulceration and perforation of the globe within 24 hours if untreated. Chlamydial infection is primarily localized to the palpebral conjunctiva and only rarely affects the cornea.

Concomitant nasopharyngeal chlamydial infection is commonly seen. Spread of the organism from the nasopharynx to the lungs is a sequela of colonization. Ten to 20% of infants with conjunctivitis have chlamydial pneumonia. It may occur either simultaneously with the conjunctivitis or up to four to six weeks later. Affected infants are usually afebrile and present with symptoms of increasing tachypnea and cough.

Infections of the Eye and Surrounding Tissues

Preseptal cellulitis and **orbital cellulitis** are two serious infections of the eye and surrounding structures. Although these infections are not as frequent as those that are limited to the eye, they have serious sequelae. The preseptal space is defined by the skin of the eyelid on one side and the orbital septum on the other. Children with preseptal, or periorbital, cellulitis usually present with acute onset, and unilateral upper and lower eyelid edema, erythema, and pain. The condition is often associated with systemic signs and symptoms such as ill appearance, fever, and leukocytosis. The eye itself usually appears normal. Infection may follow hematogenous seeding of the preseptal space, most often with *H. influenzae* type b or *S. pneumoniae*, or traumatic breaks in the skin that usually lead to *S. aureus* infection.

Orbital cellulitis is an infection of the contents of the orbit posterior to the orbital septum. Usually an insidious onset of eyelid edema, proptosis, decreased extraocular movements, and loss of visual acuity occurs. As with periorbital cellulitis, children are often febrile and ill-appearing. Contiguous spread of infection from adjacent sinusitis (most often ethmoid) is the most common cause. The organisms most often involved are the same as those in acute sinusitis (*S. aureus, S. pneumoniae,* nontypeable *H. influenzae,* and *Staphylococcus pyogenes*). Untreated, the infection may progress to orbital abscess formation.

Primary herpes simplex infection can affect the skin surrounding the eyes as well as the eye itself. Most such infections are caused by HSV type 1, although type 2 infections may be seen in newborns. Children with **herpetic infections of the eye** usually present with unilateral skin vesicles and a mild conjunctivitis or keratitis. Herpetic keratoconjunctivitis can recur following fever, exposure to sunlight, or mild trauma. The characteristic corneal lesion of herpes keratitis is the dendritic corneal ulcer, which appears as a tree-branch pattern on fluorescein staining of the cornea. Although this lesion may be seen with primary infection, it is more common in recurrent infections. Skin vesicles may not appear with recurrences, which makes it difficult to distinguish herpetic infection from other causes of conjunctivitis. Empiric topical steroid treatment for presumed viral conjunctivitis should be avoided for this reason; steroids may lead to progression of the herpetic infection and permanent corneal scarring.

Neonatal herpetic infections of the eye primarily result from HSV 2. Infections may be isolated to the eye or the eye may be infected secondarily due to CNS or disseminated disease. Proper diagnosis is important, because disseminated herpetic disease has a mortality of about 85%, and CNS disease has a mortality of 50%. Isolated herpetic eye disease is actually quite rare in neonates.

EVALUATION

History

A careful history taken from the parent or primary caregiver as well as the child can guide the diagnosis (Questions Box). It is important to exclude the possibility of ocular trauma or exposure to noxious chemicals when evaluating children with red, irritated eyes.

Physical Examination

A thorough examination of the eyes should be performed. The eyelids, conjunctiva, and cornea should be inspected for evidence of inflammation or foreign bodies. The presence of any discharge or crusting of the eyelids as well as light sensitivity or pain should be

---

Questions: Eye Infections

- How long has the child had symptoms?
- Is the child having any difficulty seeing clearly? Is he or she complaining of light sensitivity?
- Has the child had fever, cold symptoms, or purulent nasal discharge (e.g., green or yellow)?
- Are the eyes pruritic (itchy) or painful?
- Does the child have difficulty opening the affected eye on awakening in the morning or after naps?
- Have the parents noticed any discharge from the eyes or crusting around the eyelids?
- Is the child complaining of earache or sore throat?
- Does the child have allergies, asthma, or hay fever?

noted. Extraocular movements should be checked, and their symmetry should be noted. Visual acuity should be determined, and an ophthalmoscopic examination of the retina should be performed whenever possible. In addition, it is important to perform a thorough head and neck examination, noting the presence of associated sinusitis, otitis media, or pharyngitis.

Laboratory Tests

Laboratory assessment is guided by the history and physical examination. Although clinical differentiation between a bacterial and viral etiology is difficult, cultures are usually not required, because acute conjunctivitis in children is a self-limited disease. In neonatal conjunctivitis, however, the time of onset of illness and the clinical findings overlap, and Gram's stain and cultures are essential. Gonococcal infection is assessed by both Gram's stain and culture. Treatment may be initiated on the basis of Gram's stain alone because of the serious potential for corneal involvement and subsequent loss of visual acuity.

If HSV is suspected, viral cultures should be obtained. If chlamydial infection is suspected, a nasopharyngeal culture should be sent in addition to conjunctival scraping. Purulent material may be examined for gonococci, but conjunctival scrapings are required for chlamydia, because chlamydia is an obligate intracellular parasite.

Laboratory assessment of periorbital cellulitis includes a CBC, blood culture, and a lumbar puncture in young infants or in children with signs of meningeal irritation. The reported prevalence of meningitis is 1% in children with periorbital cellulitis, and it is 10% in children with bacteremia and periorbital cellulitis. As with periorbital cellulitis, laboratory assessment of orbital cellulitis includes a CBC and blood culture.

Imaging Studies

Imaging studies are required infrequently in the assessment of eye infections. A chest x-ray to detect pneumonia should be taken if infants with neonatal conjunctivitis have respiratory symptoms. Characteristic features on chest x-ray include hyperinflation and diffuse or patchy interstitial infiltrates. In orbital cellulitis, a CT scan of the orbit and sinuses may be useful for assessing the degree of involvement.

MANAGEMENT

The majority of common eye infections either resolve spontaneously or respond readily to **hygiene** and **topical antibiotics.** Treatment of both staphylococcal and seborrheic blepharitis consists of daily lid hygiene (usually at bedtime), including application of a warm compress and removal of the scales and crusts with a moistened, warm washcloth. The eyelashes and lid margins may also be scrubbed with a cotton-tipped applicator soaked in a 50:50 mixture of baby shampoo and water. When staphylococcal blepharitis is present,

an ointment containing an antistaphylococcal antibiotic agent such as erythromycin may be applied to the eyelids after cleansing. Treatment of parasitic blepharitis consists of application of petrolatum ophthalmic ointment several times a day for one week, followed by removal of the remaining parasites and their ova with tweezers or forceps.

Treatment for both external and internal hordeolum consists of application of warm compresses several times a day and local application of an antistaphylococcal ointment. Once the infection comes to a head or point, the hair at the center of the external hordeolum can sometimes be removed with tweezers, thereby creating an opening and allowing the infection to drain. Occasionally, surgical excision and drainage may be required if the abscess does not resolve (more common for internal hordeolum than external hordeolum). Unlike the hordeolum, a chalazion generally requires surgical excision, because spontaneous resolution is uncommon.

The vast majority of cases of acute childhood conjunctivitis can be managed successfully by primary care physicians. Appropriate treatment depends on making the correct diagnosis. Empiric treatment with topical antibiotic preparations is usually initiated. Polymyxin-bacitracin, trimethoprim-polymyxin, and sodium sulfacetamide are some of the more commonly prescribed antibiotics. Antibiotic ointments may be easier to instill in infants and young children. Antibiotic drops should be used in older children during the day because these preparations do not interfere with vision. Ointments may be used at bedtime. Systemic therapy can be considered for concomitant conjunctivitis and otitis media. If symptoms persist for more than 7 to 10 days or if the diagnosis is in question, appropriate cultures should be taken. Complicated cases such as suspected herpetic or gonococcal infection, foreign bodies that cannot be removed easily, loss of visual acuity, presence of significant pain, those involving children with a history of recent penetrating ocular trauma or surgery, and those involving children who use contact lenses should be referred to an ophthalmologist immediately.

Chronic conjunctivitis can be managed with cool compresses. Topical decongestant drops may provide symptomatic relief if treatment is indicated. Vernal conjunctivitis may be treated with topical cromolyn sodium drops. Corticosteroid therapy may be considered. Caution should be used when prescribing corticosteroid preparations for the eye, however, because they may lead to progression of an undiagnosed herpetic eye infection.

Treatment of neonatal conjunctivitis depends on the diagnosis. If gonococcal infection is suspected and Gram's stain is positive for gram-negative diplococci, immediate parenteral therapy with ceftriaxone should be initiated. Chlamydial conjunctivitis should be managed with systemic rather than topical treatment to prevent systemic disease. Oral erythromycin is the drug of choice. Although oral treatment provides adequate local antibiotic levels, topical erythromycin ointment may be used in conjunction with systemic therapy to provide more prompt relief of ophthalmic symptoms.

Empiric parenteral antibiotic therapy (e.g., cefuroxime) should be initiated for periorbital cellulitis. Repeat evaluations for signs of progression should be performed frequently during the initial 24 to 48 hours. If orbital cellulitis is suspected, an ophthalmologist should be consulted, and hospitalization and systemic antibiotics should be instituted. Surgical drainage of the sinuses or of an orbital abscess is sometimes necessary.

Children with suspected herpetic infection should be referred to an ophthalmologist. Intravenous acyclovir is often recommended for the treatment of isolated herpetic eye infections in neonates.

PROGNOSIS

The majority of common eye infections such as blepharitis, hordeolum, and acute childhood conjunctivitis resolve without sequelae. Recurrence is common for hordeolums, and periorbital cellulitis may be a potential complication in rare or untreated cases. Unlike acute conjunctivitis, chronic conjunctivitis may not be self-limited. Appropriate diagnosis and management are extremely important to prevent serious sequelae in some children. For example, endemic trachoma may progress to produce conjunctival scarring, pannus formation, and even blindness if not appropriately treated with systemic erythromycin or tetracycline.

Periorbital cellulitis generally resolves without sequelae if treated promptly with systemic antibiotics. Orbital cellulitis should be considered a true ophthalmologic emergency because the potential for complications is high. The optic nerve may become involved, resulting in loss of vision or spread of the infection into the cranial cavity. This spreading may lead to meningitis, cavernous sinus thrombosis, or brain abscess.

Case Resolution

The infant presented in the case history has neonatal conjunctivitis. A Gram's stain of the purulent discharge should be examined, and cultures should be taken from the eye and nasopharynx. If the Gram stain is negative for gonococci, empiric treatment may begin with oral erythromycin.

Selected Readings

Gigliotti, F. Acute conjunctivitis of childhood. Pediatr. Ann. 22:353–356, 1993.

King, R. A. Common ocular signs and symptoms in childhood. Pediatr. Clin. North Am. 40:753–766, 1993.

Malinow, I., and K. R. Powell. Periorbital cellulitis. Pediatr. Ann. 22:241–246, 1993.

O'Hara, M. A. Ophthalmia neonatorum. Pediatr. Clin. North Am. 40:715–725, 1993.

Persaud, D., W. J. Moss, and J. L. Munoz. Serious eye infections in children. Pediatr. Ann. 22:379–383, 1993.

Wagner, R. S. The differential diagnosis of the red eye. Contemp. Pediatr. 8:26–48, 1991.

Weiss, A. H. Chronic conjunctivitis in infants and children. Pediatr. Ann. 22:366–374, 1993.

CHAPTER 52

EXCESSIVE TEARING

Geeta Grover, M.D.

H$_x$ A four-week-old infant girl has had a persistent watery discharge from the left eye since birth. Her mother has noticed white, crusty material on her daughter's eyelids for the past few days. The infant's birth and medical history are unremarkable. Examination of the eyes, including bilateral red reflexes and symmetric extraocular movements, is normal, except that the left eye appears "wetter" than the right.

Questions

1. What is the differential diagnosis of excessive tearing in infancy?

2. How do physical findings such as corneal enlargement and haziness influence the differential diagnosis?

3. How should infants with excessive tearing be managed?

Infants or young children with excessive tearing or epiphora in one or both eyes are a common pediatric ophthalmologic concern. The pediatrician must be capable of differentiating benign causes of this common childhood condition from other more serious illnesses, such as glaucoma, that potentially threaten vision.

EPIDEMIOLOGY

Congenital obstruction of the nasolacrimal duct or dacryostenosis, which occurs in 1 to 6% of newborn infants, is the most common cause of excessive tearing in infancy. Spontaneous resolution of this obstruction before six months of age is common.

In contrast, congenital or infantile glaucoma, a serious cause of excessive tearing, is quite rare; the incidence is about 1 in 10,000 live births. Although glaucoma may be present at birth, onset during the first few weeks to months of life is more common. Approximately 25% of cases are diagnosed at birth and 80% by one year of age. The majority of affected infants are male; the male: female ratio in older infants is 2:1. Infantile glaucoma appears to have a multifactorial inheritance pattern, but the majority of cases are sporadic. In families with one affected child or a parental history of infantile glaucoma, the chance of having a child with glaucoma is about 5%. Although glaucoma may be unilateral or bilateral, the vast majority of children (75–90%) who present before three months of age have bilateral glaucoma.

CLINICAL PRESENTATION

Infants with dacryostenosis usually present with a history of a mucoid eye discharge and crusting along the eyelid margins. The affected eye appears "wetter" than the normal eye, and a small pool of tears may be noted along the lower eyelid. Infants with glaucoma characteristically present with excessive tearing, rhinorrhea, photophobia, and corneal haziness (D$_x$ Box).

PATHOPHYSIOLOGY

Tears serve many important functions within the visual system. As well as lubricating the eyes, they provide them with oxygen and antibacterial substances. The tear film is composed of three layers: oily, mucoid, and aqueous. The lacrimal system (Fig. 52–1) produces and drains tears away from the eyes and into the nose. The accessory lacrimal glands of Krause and Wolfring, located behind the upper and lower eyelids in the conjunctival cul-de-sac, are responsible for the basal secretion of tears necessary to keep the eyes moist and lubricated, and the lacrimal gland itself produces reflex tears or tears due to emotions. Reflex tearing is usually present shortly after birth but may be delayed for

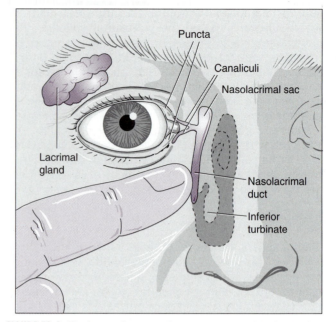

FIGURE 52-1. *The lacrimal system, showing massage of the lacrimal sac.*

several weeks to months until the lacrimal gland begins to function. Tears drain away from the eyes through the superior and inferior puncta into the superior and inferior canalicula and finally into the nasolacrimal duct, which drains beneath the inferior turbinate in the nose.

Excessive tearing during infancy may result from either increased production of tears or obstruction of drainage. Outflow obstruction, most often due to obstruction of the nasolacrimal duct or dacryostenosis, is the most common cause of excessive tearing in infancy. The obstruction is usually unilateral and occurs during fetal development. Most commonly, a congenital narrowing of the duct or a persistent, thin membrane obstructs it. The membrane is usually located in the distal or nasal segment of the duct rather than in the proximal portion. The term "dacryocystitis" is used if acute infection or inflammation is associated with the obstruction. If both the canaliculi and the nasolacrimal duct are obstructed, a mucocele over the nasolacrimal sac may be noted at birth. This sac appears as a bluish, firm mass located below the medial canthus. Atresia of some portion of the drainage system may also occur, but this is extremely rare.

The most common reason for excessive production of tears is **eye irritation** (e.g., due to a foreign body in the eyelid or corneal abrasion). The congenital paradoxical gustolacrimal reflex, or **crocodile tears,** is a rare disorder that may also produce epiphora. In this disorder, an abnormal connection between the salivary and lacrimal glands produces unilateral and sometimes bilateral tearing with salivation. This condition may also be acquired secondary to facial trauma.

Glaucoma is the most serious and potentially sight-threatening etiology for excessive production of tears. Glaucoma refers to an increase in intraocular pressure that is severe enough to damage the eye and alter

---

D$_x$ Excessive Tearing

- Conjunctival injection or edema
- Crusting of the eyelids
- Rhinorrhea
- Photophobia
- Corneal haziness
- Reflux of tears with gentle pressure on medial canthus
- Wetness of eye

vision. In infants and children, glaucoma is usually a result of a developmental abnormality of the iridocorneal angle interfering with drainage of aqueous humor from the anterior chamber. Young infants differ from adults in that the globe in infants' eyes is distensible; the increased intraocular pressure not only produces corneal enlargement and edema but also expands the globe itself. Breakdown of the corneal epithelium and resultant irritation of the eyes produce reflex tearing. Untreated glaucoma may lead to optic nerve damage with resultant loss of visual acuity and even blindness.

Glaucoma in children younger than three years of age is referred to broadly as infantile glaucoma, and glaucoma that occurs in children between three and 20 years of age is called juvenile glaucoma. Infantile glaucoma is further classified as being primary or secondary. Primary glaucoma refers to isolated abnormalities of the iridocorneal angle, whereas secondary glaucoma may be associated with other ocular or systemic diseases. Juvenile glaucoma is a form of open-angle glaucoma.

DIFFERENTIAL DIAGNOSIS

Table 52–1 outlines the differential diagnosis of excessive tearing in infancy. Although obstruction of the nasolacrimal duct is the most common cause of excessive tearing in infants, it is important to consider and rule out glaucoma when evaluating infants with this complaint. The presence of rhinorrhea in association with epiphora distinguishes infantile glaucoma from dacryostenosis. Rhinorrhea is not associated with dacryostenosis because the nasolacrimal duct is obstructed, and no tears drain out of the nose. Unlike dacryostenosis, which is usually unilateral, infantile glaucoma is very commonly bilateral.

Acute onset of excessive tearing in older children is usually due to ocular irritation. Any irritation of the conjunctiva, cornea, or eyelids may produce tearing. Conjunctivitis and corneal abrasion, usually secondary to a retained foreign body or herpes simplex keratoconjunctivitis, are the two most common causes. Eye infections are discussed in Chapter 51.

TABLE 52–1. Differential Diagnosis of Excessive Tearing in Infants

Increased Production

Infantile glaucoma
Irritation
  Conjunctivitis
  Corneal abrasion
  Foreign body under the eyelid
Congenital paradoxical gustolacrimal reflex (crocodile tears)

Outflow Obstruction

Nasolacrimal duct obstruction (dacryostenosis)
Anomalies of the lacrimal drainage system
  Mucocele of the lacrimal sac
  Atresia of the lacrimal punctum or canaliculus
Nasal congestion
Craniofacial anomalies involving the midface

Questions: Excessive Tearing

- How old was the child when the excessive tearing appeared?
- Are one or both eyes affected?
- Is there a family history of infantile glaucoma?
- Is the child photophobic or light-sensitive (e.g., closes the eyes in bright sunlight)?
- Has the child had any persistent, watery discharge?
- Does the child have difficulty opening the affected eye on awakening in the morning or after a nap?

EVALUATION

History

Evaluation of excessive tearing should begin with a thorough history. The nature of the discharge (i.e., watery, mucoid, or purulent) should be noted. Parents or other care givers should be questioned about the appearance of the child's eyes (Questions Box). The excessive mucoid discharge in the medial canthal region and on the eyelashes is usually more noticeable to the family than the increased tearing. Crusting along the eyelashes caused by drying of the mucoid material is usually noted when children awaken in the morning or after a nap. Mucopurulent discharge may be noted if an associated acute infection is present (dacryocystitis).

Physical Examination

A careful examination of the eyes in infants includes inspection, evaluation of extraocular movements, and funduscopic examination. Funduscopic examination may be difficult in this age group, but bilateral red reflexes should at least be elicited. Signs of **dacryostenosis**, which usually appear days to weeks after birth, include tearing, mucoid discharge, and crusting of the eyelids. Tearing may be as mild as an increased wetness of the affected eye; this is best evaluated prior to disturbing children. Visible overflow of tears from the affected eye is unusual, and is typically seen only when the eye is irritated (e.g., due to cold or wind). If dacryostenosis is present, associated conjunctival injection, erythema, and edema of the eyelids or systemic signs of infection such as fever may be noted. Dacryocystitis may also spread to the surrounding tissues, producing a periorbital cellulitis. Gentle pressure along the medial canthal region over the lacrimal sac may produce a reflux of tears or mucoid discharge onto the surface of the eye, thus confirming the diagnosis of obstruction. If the diagnosis is uncertain, fluorescein dye should be placed in the eye and observed for a few minutes. If an obstruction of the duct is present, the fluorescein will not disappear as expected, and no dye will exit through the nose. The cornea may be examined after instillation of fluorescein dye if an ocular foreign body or corneal abrasion is the suspected cause of the excessive tearing.

In addition to excessive tearing, other clinical signs of infantile glaucoma include blepharospasm (spasmodic winking of the eyelids), photophobia, corneal enlargement and corneal haziness due to corneal edema, progressive enlargement of the eye (buphthalmos), and cupping and atrophy of the optic nerve. A corneal diameter greater than 12 mm in infants is suggestive of infantile glaucoma. Corneal edema is more common in younger infants (< 3 months of age) and may cause the red reflex to appear dull in the affected eye. The optic cup may be enlarged. A cup-to-disk ratio greater than 0.3 or an asymmetry of the ratio between the eyes may indicate glaucoma.

As in adults, loss of visual fields occurs in children with glaucoma. Visual fields are difficult to evaluate in young children because of their inability to cooperate with the examination. Suspected cases of glaucoma should be referred to an ophthalmologist for further evaluation, including measurement of intraocular pressure. Pressures greater than 20 mm Hg are suggestive of glaucoma (normal pressures are 10 to 20 mm Hg in infants and young children as well as in adults).

Laboratory Tests

Routine laboratory assessment is generally not necessary.

MANAGEMENT

Spontaneous resolution of dacryostenosis is common by six to eight months of age. The primary medical treatment of uncomplicated nasolacrimal duct obstruction consists of **local massage** and **cleansing** beginning when the symptoms are noted. Parents are instructed to massage the nasolacrimal duct several times a day by applying firm, downward pressure over the medial canthal region with their finger and then sliding the finger down towards the mouth (Creiger maneuver) (see Fig. 52–1). This maneuver attempts to move fluid trapped within the nasolacrimal sac down through the duct in an attempt to break the obstruction with hydrostatic pressure. Parents may be asked to cleanse the eyes with warm water before performing this maneuver. Antibiotic ointments and drops should be prescribed only if the discharge is purulent or associated conjunctivitis is evident.

Controversy exists regarding when probing of the nasolacrimal duct should be performed. Many ophthalmologists prefer probing the duct before children are six months of age, because prior to this time the procedure may be performed in the office without general anesthesia. Others state that over 90% of obstructions resolve with conservative medical management by 12 months of age and prefer to delay probing until the age of 12 to 15 months. At this age the procedure needs to be performed under general anesthesia. Deciding when to proceed with the probing depends on the standard of practice within the community, the severity of symptoms, the response to medical management, and the level of parental concern.

Ophthalmologic referral is necessary for affected infants by six months of age if the obstruction has not resolved. Referral should be made sooner if symptoms are severe or infections recur. Suspected cases of infantile glaucoma should be immediately referred to an ophthalmologist because if the condition is left untreated, it may progress to blindness. **Surgery** is the primary treatment. The goal is to normalize intraocular pressure and minimize irreversible corneal and optic nerve damage.

PROGNOSIS

The majority of cases of dacryostenosis resolve spontaneously during the first year of life without further sequelae. Infantile glaucoma, if left untreated, may progress to blindness. The visual prognosis depends on several factors, including the age at onset of glaucoma (the earlier the onset, the worse the prognosis) and the degree of myopia caused by the enlargement of the eye. In addition, amblyopia, secondary to either deprivation due to corneal opacities or unequal refractive errors, is often seen (see Chapter 50, Strabismus).

Case Resolution

The infant presented in the case history at the beginning of the chapter has dacryostenosis. She can be managed with medical treatment such as local massage and cleansing at this stage. If her symptoms persist beyond the age of six months, consultation with an ophthalmologist is recommended.

Selected Readings

Calhoun, J. H. Disorders of the lacrimal apparatus in infancy and childhood. *In* Nelson, L. B., J. H. Calhoun, and R. D. Harley. Pediatric Ophthalmology, 3rd ed. Philadelphia, W. B. Saunders, 1991.

Howard, C. W. The baby with too many tears: what to do and how to do it. Int. Pediatr. 5:239–242, 1990.

Lavrich, J. B., and L. B. Nelson. Disorders of the lacrimal system apparatus. Pediatr. Clin. North Am. 40:767–776, 1993.

Wagner, R. S. Glaucoma in children. Pediatr. Clin. North Am. 40: 855–867, 1993.

NECK MASSES

Stanley H. Inkelis, M.D.

Hₓ A 2-year-old boy is brought to the office with a one-day history of an enlarging red, tender "bump" beneath his right mandible. He has a fever of 101.6° F (38.5° C) and sores around his nose, upper lip, and cheek. These sores have been present for three days and have not responded to an over-the-counter antibiotic ointment. He had a URI one week ago, which has almost entirely resolved. He is otherwise in good health. The family has no history of tuberculosis or recent travel, and the child has not been playing with cats or other animals.

The physical examination is completely normal except for fever, mild rhinorrhea, honey-crusted lesions on the nares and upper lip, and a 4 x 5-cm, right submandibular neck mass that is erythematous, warm, and tender to palpation.

Questions

1. What are the common causes of neck masses in children?
2. What steps are involved in the evaluation of children with neck masses?
3. What clinical findings suggest that neck masses are neoplasms? When should neck masses be biopsied or removed?
4. What is involved in the treatment of the different types of neck masses in children?
5. When should children with neck masses be referred for further consultation?

Neck masses are any swellings or enlargements of the structures in the area between the inferior mandible and the clavicle. Normal variants, such as the angle of the mandible or tip of the mastoid, may occasionally appear as swellings, and parents sometimes confuse these with neck masses. If the swelling is not a normal structure, a well-directed history and physical examination usually determine the etiology.

Lymphadenopathy from viral or bacterial throat infections is the most common cause of neck mass in children. Therefore, neck masses are common because children frequently have sore throats. Most parents know about "swollen lymph glands," and they usually do not seek medical advice unless the glands become very large or do not recede in a few days. Neck masses in children may have many other causes besides lymphadenopathy. Most of these masses may be categorized as inflammatory, neoplastic, traumatic, or congenital in origin.

EPIDEMIOLOGY

Most neck masses are benign. Almost 50% of all 2-year old children have palpable cervical lymph nodes. Although more than 25% of malignant tumors in children are found in the head and neck region (this is the primary site in only 5%), less than 2% of suspicious head and neck masses are malignant.

The epidemiology of neck masses of infectious origin depends on the infectious agent itself, geographic location of the child, and the child's socioeconomic status. Neck masses of viral origin may be related to focal infection of the oropharynx or respiratory tract but are often associated with generalized adenopathy. Neck masses of bacterial origin typically occur from normal bacterial flora of the nose, mouth, pharynx, and skin. These organisms are not usually transmitted from person to person. Pathologic flora such as group A streptococcus and *Mycobacterium tuberculosis* that result in neck masses can spread by human-to-human contact, however.

CLINICAL PRESENTATION

Children with neck masses present in a variety of different ways depending on the etiology of the mass. Typically a swelling or enlargement in the neck, which parents often notice more than children, is evident. Associated signs and symptoms include fever, upper respiratory tract infection, sore throat, ear pain, pain or tenderness over the mass, changes in skin color over the mass, skin lesions of the head or neck, and dental caries or infections (Dₓ Box). Malignant tumors are usually slow-growing, firm, fixed, nontender masses. Congenital neck masses and benign tumors, which have frequently been present since birth or early infancy, are soft, smooth, and cystlike and may be recurrent. Neck masses associated with trauma are often rapidly evolving and may lead to airway obstruction.

PATHOPHYSIOLOGY

The pathophysiology of neck masses in children is dependent on etiology. Most neck masses are related to inflammation or infection of lymph nodes. Enlargement of lymph nodes usually results from proliferation of intrinsic lymphocytes or histiocytes already present in the lymph node (e.g., lymphadenopathy caused by a viral infection) or from infiltration of extrinsic cells (e.g., lymphadenitis, metastatic tumor). Neck masses from trauma occur from leakage of fluid into the neck, and

D$_x$ Neck Masses

INFLAMMATORY/INFECTIOUS
- Swelling or enlargement in the neck
- Fever
- Sore throat, dental infection, skin infection of head or neck
- Pain or tenderness over the mass (usually)

NEOPLASTIC
- Slowly enlarging mass
- Unilateral, discrete
- Firm or rubbery
- Fixed to tissue
- Deep within the fascia
- Nontender (usually)

CONGENITAL
- Enlargement in neck (usually present since birth or soon after)
- Soft, smooth, cyst-like
- Nontender (unless infected)
- Recurrent

scratch disease, toxoplasmosis, fungal infection, and *M. tuberculosis* infections may be associated with lympadenopathy that may later progress to lymphadenitis. Viral illnesses, including EBV (mononucleosis), adenovirus, enterovirus, herpes virus, and CMV, commonly cause lymphadenopathy and lymphadenitis.

Lymphadenitis is infection or inflammation of the lymph node, which occurs because neutrophils infiltrate the node, leading to necrosis and abscess formation. This condition is usually associated with proximal bacterial infection that drains to the affected nodes by connecting afferent lymphatic channels. Lymphadenitis is often a progression of disease, resulting in enlarged nodes that measure 2–6 cm. These nodes, which are typical of bacterial disease, are often termed "hot" nodes, and they are erythematous, warm, tender, and sometimes fluctuant. "Cold" nodes or "cold" lymphadenitis usually represents subacute or chronic inflammation of lymph nodes. Unlike hot nodes, cold nodes are not warm to the touch and are usually not as tender. They are usually not suppurative and may be

congenital anatomic abnormalities become apparent because of fluid collection or infection of the defect. The parotid gland may be enlarged from inflammation (e.g., blocked sialic duct), infection (e.g., mumps), or tumor (e.g., rhabdomyosarcoma), but the swelling primarily involves the face rather than the neck and obscures the angle of the jaw.

DIFFERENTIAL DIAGNOSIS

Neck masses in children are usually the result of inflammation or infection of lymph nodes, tumors of lymph nodes and other neck structures, trauma, and congenital lesions. The location of the mass is often a clue to its etiology (Fig. 53–1).

Lymphadenopathy/Lymphadenitis

Lymphadenopathy is lymph node enlargement or hyperplasia secondary to localized infection or antigenic stimulation proximal to the involved node or nodes. Because lymphoid tissue steadily increases until puberty, palpable lymph nodes, including those in the cervical area, are a common, normal finding in children. Any lymph node in the neck larger than 10 mm qualifies as cervical lymphadenopathy.

The most common cause of cervical lymphadenopathy is a viral infection of the upper respiratory tract. Lymphadenopathy usually begins and resolves with the acute infection. Occasionally the swelling remains for several days or months, however, and children present because of parental concern. Bacterial pharyngitis, usually from infection with group A beta-hemolytic streptococcus, is often associated with cervical lymphadenopathy. Cervical as well as generalized lymphadenopathy may be seen in children with systemic illness (e.g., Kawasaki's syndrome, sarcoid, HIV). Cat-

FIGURE 53–1. *Differential diagnosis of neck mass by location.* *1: Parotid—cystic hygroma, hemangioma, lymphadenitis, parotitis, Sjögren's and Caffey-Silverman syndromes, lymphoma. 2: Postauricular—lymphadenitis, branchial cleft cyst (1st), squamous epithelial cyst. 3: Submental—lymphadenitis, cystic hygroma, thyroglossal duct cyst, dermoid, sialoadenitis. 4: Submandibular—lymphadenitis, cystic hygroma, sialoadenitis, tumor, cystic fibrosis. 5: Jugulodiagastic—lymphadenitis, squamous epithelial cyst, branchial cleft cyst (1st), parotid tumor, normal-transverse process C2, styloid process. 6: Midline neck—lymphadenitis, thyroglossal duct cyst, dermoid, laryngocele, normal-hyoid, thyroid. 7: Sternomastoid (anterior)—lymphadenitis, branchial cleft cyst (2nd, 3rd) pilomatrixoma, rare tumors. 8: Spinal accessory—lymphadenitis, lymphoma, metastasis from nasopharynx. 9: Paratracheal—thyroid, parathyroid, esophageal diverticulum. 10: Supraclavicular—cystic hygroma, lipoma, lymphoma, metastasis, normal-fat pad, pneumatocele of upper lobe. 11: Suprasternal—thyroid, lipoma, dermoid, thymus, mediastinal mass. (Reproduced, with permission, from Fleisher, G.R., and S. Ludwig [eds.]. Textbook of Pediatric Emergency Medicine, 3rd ed. Baltimore, Williams & Wilkins, 1993, p. 321.)*

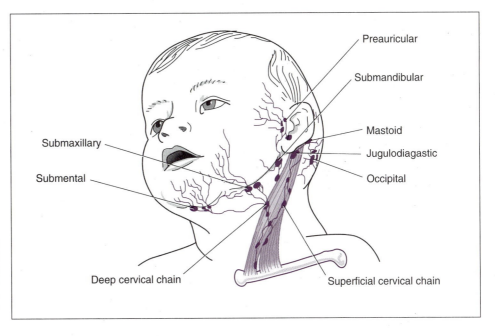

FIGURE 53–2. The lymphatic drainage and lymph nodes involved in infants and children with cervical lymphadenitis. (Reproduced, with permission, from Feigin, R.D., and J.D. Cherry [eds.]. Textbook of Pediatric Infectious Diseases, 3rd ed. Philadelphia, W.B. Saunders, 1992, p. 221.)

difficult to distinguish from nodes that are simply enlarged (Fig. 53–2).

Staphylococcus aureus and group A streptococcus are responsible for 60 to 85% of cases of acute unilateral cervical lymphadenitis. These organisms spread from a primary site to the lymph nodes draining those sites. Common primary sites of infection are the throat; teeth and gums; and skin (lesions), particularly on the scalp or ears. Infections at these sites may result from trauma, such as scratches or scabs, or from primary infection, such as impetigo. *S. aureus* or group B streptococcus usually causes cervical lymphadenitis in neonates or very young infants. Such staphylococcal infections, which are often nosocomially spread from contact in the newborn nursery, present as discrete masses. Group B streptococcus causes the "cellulitis-adenitis" syndrome, which presents as cervical adenitis associated with a facial cellulitis. *Pseudomonas aeruginosa* is an unusual cause of cervical adenitis in newborns.

Mycobacterial disease must always be considered in children of all ages who present with cervical adenitis. Nodes are often multiple, sometimes bilateral, usually nontender, and are not erythematous or warm. In children between 1 and 5 years of age, unilateral rather than bilateral lymph node enlargement usually occurs with atypical mycobacterial infection.

Cat-scratch disease should be considered in children who have cats or kittens or play with them. The infection may result from a cat scratch or from a cat's licking a child's broken skin. If the inoculum is near the head and neck area, cervical adenitis develops. Occasionally, generalized lymphadenopathy is present. An associated papule or papules where the cat scratch or lick occurred may be apparent.

Toxoplasmosis may be accompanied by adenitis, usually in the posterior cervical area. Nodes are painless and may fluctuate in size, and children are often asymptomatic. Multiple lymph nodes are involved in about one third to one half of cases.

Less common bacterial, viral, and fungal causes of cervical adenitis are listed in Table 53–1.

Tumors

Compared to other neck masses, **malignant neck tumors** occur rarely; nevertheless, they should be considered in any children with rapidly enlarging or persistent neck masses. Hodgkin's disease and lymphosarcoma account for approximately two thirds of malignant neoplasms of the head and neck in children. Age is an important factor in determining the likelihood of specific tumors. Neuroblastoma, lymphosarcoma, rhabdomyosarcoma, and Hodgkin's disease are the most frequent tumor types in children under the age of 6 years. Hodgkin's disease and lymphosarcoma occur with almost equal frequency in preadolescent children, followed by thyroid malignancies and rhabdomyosarcoma. Hodgkin's disease is the most common malignancy in adolescents.

Benign neck tumors, with the exception of those mentioned later in the discussion of congenital lesions, are uncommon. They include epidermoid inclusion cysts, lipomas, fibromas, neurofibromas, keloids, goiters, and ranulas (intraoral mucocysts).

Trauma

Trauma to the neck may be associated with bleeding and edema. Large hematomas that affect vital structures are potentially life-threatening. Significant trauma and structural injury usually accompany neck hematomas. In children with mild injuries and neck hematomas, bleeding disorders are a possible cause of neck

TABLE 53–1.   Differential Diagnosis of Neck Masses

Cervical Lymphadenopathy/Lymphadenitis

Bacterial origin
  Staphylococcus aureus
  Group A beta-hemolytic streptococcus
  Mycobacterium tuberculosis
  Atypical mycobacteria
  Cat-scratch disease *(Bartonella henselae)*
  Anaerobes
  Gram-negative enteric bacteria
  Haemophilus influenzae
  Plague
  Actinomycosis
  Diphtheria
  Tularemia
  Brucellosis
  Syphilis
  Group B streptococcus (neonates)
Viral origin
  Epstein-Barr virus (infectious mononucleosis)
  Adenovirus
  Cytomegalovirus
  Herpes virus
  Enterovirus
  Human immunodeficiency virus
  Measles
  Rubella
  Human herpes virus
Fungal origin
  Histoplasmosis
  Coccidioidomycosis
  Aspergillosis
  Candidiasis
  Sporotrichosis
  Cryptococcosis
Parasitic origin
  Toxoplasmosis

Tumor

Malignant
  Hodgkin's disease
  Non-Hodgkin's lymphoma
  Lymphosarcoma
  Rhabdomyosarcoma
  Neuroblastoma
  Leukemia
  Histiocytosis X
  Thyroid tumors
  Nasopharyngeal squamous cell carcinoma
  Salivary gland carcinoma
Benign
  Epidermoid cyst
  Lipoma
  Fibroma
  Neurofibroma
  Keloid
  Goiter
  Osteochondroma
  Teratoma (may be malignant)
  Ranula

Congenital Disorders

Hemangioma
Cystic hygroma (lymphangioma)
Branchial cleft cyst
Thyroglossal duct cyst
Laryngocele
Dermoid cyst
Cervical rib
Sternocleidomastoid tumor

TABLE 53–1.   Differential Diagnosis of Neck Masses
Continued

Trauma

Hematoma (acute or organized)
Subcutaneous emphysema
Foreign body
Arteriovenous malformation

Immunologic Disorders

Local hypersensitivity reaction (sting or bite)
Pseudolymphoma (from phenytoin)
Serum sickness
Sarcoidosis
Caffey-Silverman syndrome
Kawasaki syndrome
Systemic lupus erythematosus
Juvenile rheumatoid arthritis
Kikuchi's disease (necrotizing lymphadenitis)

Miscellaneous

Storage disorders
  Niemann-Pick disease
  Gaucher's disease
Obstructive airway disease (asthma, cystic fibrosis)

masses. Child abuse should also be considered in children who have neck injuries that do not agree with their histories.

A foreign body in the neck may present as a mass because of the foreign body itself (e.g., piece of glass or metal, bullet) or surrounding inflammation. A "crepitant" neck mass following trauma to the neck or chest suggests subcutaneous emphysema from tracheal injury or a pneumomediastinum. Crepitant neck masses may also be seen secondary to pneumomediastinum in children with obstructive lung diseases such as asthma or cystic fibrosis.

Congenital Lesions

Children with congenital neck lesions usually present with a neck mass in early infancy or much later in childhood. Some congenital lesions are not discovered until adulthood. The most common of these benign lesions are thyroglossal duct cysts, branchial cleft cysts, cystic hygromas (lymphangiomas), and hemangiomas (Fig. 53–3).

Thyroglossal duct cysts are almost always midline in the neck and inferior to the hyoid bone. They usually move upward with tongue protrusion or swallowing. Most branchial cleft cysts occur anterior to the middle one third of the sternocleidomastoid muscle. Thyroglossal duct cysts and branchial cleft cysts may also present for the first time as infected neck masses.

Cystic hygromas are usually large, soft, easily compressible masses found in the posterior triangle behind the sternocleidomastoid muscle in the supraclavicular fossa. They transilluminate well. Two thirds of cystic hygromas are present at birth.

Hemangiomas are usually not present at birth but appear in early infancy and may enlarge rapidly. In most cases, they recede spontaneously by 5 to 6 years of age. They are usually much smaller than cystic hygromas, do not transilluminate, and may be recognized by their

FIGURE 53–3. *Head and neck congenital lesions seen in children in frontal and lateral views.* The shaded areas denote the distribution in which a given lesion may be found. A, dermoid cyst; B, thyroglossal duct cyst; C, second branchial cleft appendage; D, second branchial cleft sinus; E, second branchial cleft cyst; F, first branchial pouch defect; G, preauricular sinus or appendage. (Reproduced, with permission, from Fleisher, G.R., and S. Ludwig [eds.]. Textbook of Pediatric Emergency Medicine, 3rd ed. Baltimore, Williams & Wilkins, 1993, p. 1301.)

reddish color (capillary or strawberry hemangioma) or by a bluish hue of the overlying skin (cavernous hemangioma).

Small infants who present with torticollis should be examined for a sternocleidomastoid mass ("tumor"), which represents fibrosis and contracture of that sternocleidomastoid muscle so that the head tilts toward the affected side. Contusion of the sternocleidomastoid muscle from traumatic extraction of head during delivery with subsequent hemorrhage and healing has been implicated as the cause of the fibrotic mass. This mass may have more than one etiology, however. Because the mass occurs following cesarean section and is associated with hip dysplasia and other congenital lesions, some evidence suggests that the condition is sometimes related to abnormal positioning *in utero*. Venous occlusion of the sternocleidomastoid muscle either *in utero* or at the time of delivery has also been proposed as a cause.

EVALUATION

History

A thorough history is important in establishing the etiology of the neck mass (Questions Box).

Physical Examination

A general physical examination should be performed. The neck mass should be examined for anatomic location, color, size, shape, consistency, tenderness, fluctuance, and mobility. The mass should also be measured. The head, neck, and face should be examined for lesions, most often infections, that drain into neck lymph nodes. Lesions can frequently be found on the scalp, neck, face, ears, mouth, teeth, tongue, gums, and throat.

Questions: Neck Masses

- How old is the child?
- How long has the neck mass been present?
- What signs and symptoms are associated with the neck mass?
- Has the child been exposed to tuberculosis?
- Has the child ever drunk any unpasteurized cow's milk?
- Has the child been in contact with any cats or kittens?
- Has the child traveled to areas of endemic diseases such as histoplasmosis or coccidioidomycosis?
- Has the child suffered any trauma recently?
- Does the child have any allergies?
- Does the child have any risk factors for HIV?

Hair styles such as tight braids can sometimes provide ports of entry for bacteria. Occasionally, sinus tracts or fistulas may be the entry point of infection.

In addition, other lymph node groups should be examined to determine if the lymphadenopathy is local or generalized. Particular attention should be paid to the supraclavicular area, because enlarged supraclavicular nodes are more frequently associated with malignant pathology such as Hodgkin's disease.

The chest should be examined for use of accessory muscles, equality of breath sounds, and wheezing. The abdomen should be examined for hepatosplenomegaly.

Laboratory Tests

Laboratory tests are rarely indicated in children with cervical lymphadenopathy or lymphadenitis of acute onset. Although a rapid streptococcal antigen test or throat culture is helpful in children with suspected streptococcal sore throat, it may be unnecessary if antibiotic therapy is empirically prescribed for the lymphadenitis. If the adenitis is fluctuant, aspiration and culture may be helpful in determining the specific bacteriologic diagnosis. A PPD test should be given to all children who present with lymphadenitis.

If the adenitis does not resolve or improve after two to three days of observation or therapy, laboratory tests directed by the history and physical examination should be considered. A CBC with differential and a monospot or heterophil test may be helpful in the diagnosis of infectious mononucleosis. If the mass in the neck is a hematoma and a bleeding disorder is suspected, a CBC with platelet count, PT, and PTT should be obtained. Possible additional tests include an ESR; serologic tests for toxoplasmosis, EBV, CMV, coccidioidomycosis, histoplasmosis, tularemia, and syphilis should be performed if indicated. Skin tests for fungi should be considered in those patients coming from endemic areas. These tests should be placed after serologic tests are performed so that false-positive test results are not obtained.

Similar laboratory tests should be considered for children who present for the first time with enlarged or enlarging lymph nodes of long duration or those who do not respond after two weeks of antibiotic therapy. The physician may choose to do more of these laboratory tests at the initial evaluation or after a therapeutic trial, as the likelihood of viral lymphadenopathy decreases and the possibility of a more unusual etiology increases. HIV testing should also be considered.

Thyroid function tests and thyroid scans should be considered in children with a thyroid mass or suspected thyroglossal duct cyst.

Unless cat-scratch disease is very likely, early lymph node biopsy is indicated for enlarged supraclavicular nodes or lymph nodes in the lower half of the neck, rapidly progressive and enlarging nodes, fixed nodes, nodes deep within the fascia, or firm or hard nodes. Children who have a persistent fever or weight loss despite antibiotic therapy should have a biopsy at one week if a diagnosis has not been established. Asymptomatic children without an established diagnosis should have a biopsy at two weeks if the node increases in size and at six to eight weeks if the node size does not decrease.

Imaging Studies

A chest x-ray should be obtained in all children with suspected tuberculosis or tumor (e.g., enlarged supraclavicular nodes) as well as in children with crepitant neck masses. If a foreign body in the neck is suspected, both anteroposterior and lateral neck x-rays should be obtained.

Ultrasonography is helpful in differentiating cystic from solid masses. MRI may be useful in very select cases where soft tissue detail is necessary for diagnostic purposes.

MANAGEMENT

Neck masses are rarely acutely life-threatening. If neck masses impinge on the airway, children may experience stridor, hoarseness, drooling, increased effort of breathing, unequal breath sounds, or evidence of shock. Resuscitation and stabilization should be initiated immediately. The algorithm in Figure 53–4 outlines the management of cervical lymphadenitis.

Children with lymphadenitis who do not appear toxic and have no evidence of sepsis may be treated empirically with **oral antibiotics** that cover *S. aureus* and group A beta-hemolytic streptococcus. Dicloxacillin (50 mg/kg/day), amoxicillin-clavulanic acid (40 mg/kg/day [amoxicillin]), or a first-generation cephalosporin such as cephalexin (50 mg/kg/day) provides satisfactory coverage. Treatment should be continued for a minimum of 10 days but for no less than five days after resolution of acute signs and symptoms. Lack of clinical improvement after 36 to 48 hours suggests that the diagnosis and proposed therapy need to be reevaluated.

Infants and small children, as well as those older children who do not respond to oral antibiotic therapy, may require admission for **intravenous antibiotics** such as oxacillin or a cephalosporin. Incision and drainage of large, fluctuant nodes should be done, often in consultation with an otolaryngologist, to promote resolution of the lymphadenitis. If *M. tuberculosis* or atypical mycobacterial infection is suspected, incision and drainage should not be done because persistent sinus tracts may result.

Atypical mycobacterial infection is virtually always unresponsive to treatment with antituberculous medications. **Surgical excision** of all visibly affected nodes, deep as well as superficial, is required. Tuberculous mycobacterial adenitis (scrofula) usually responds to short-course medical therapy. Antituberculous medication for six to nine months is recommended.

Lymphadenitis from cat-scratch disease usually resolves on its own. Antibiotic therapy is usually not indicated, but if children are toxic-appearing or admitted for a suppurative adenitis, treatment with trimethoprim-

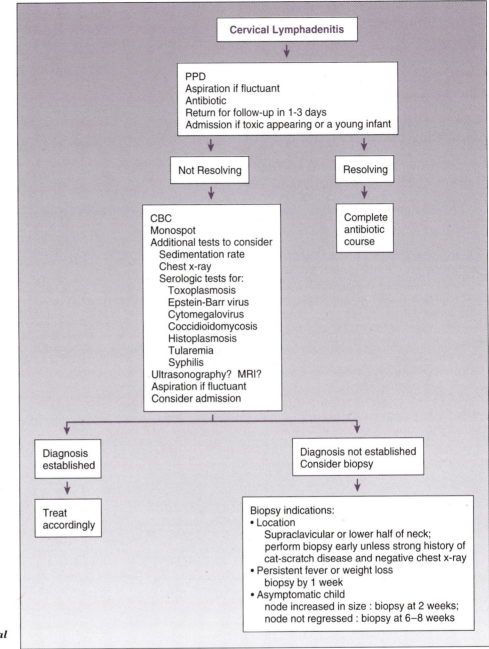

FIGURE 53–4. *Management of cervical lymphadenitis.*

sulfamethoxazole may be beneficial. If the node is fluctuant, **aspiration** is indicated. Total removal of the node is sometimes necessary to effect a cure.

There is no specific therapy for lymphadenitis caused by *Toxoplasma gondii*. Excision of the affected node may be indicated if the diagnosis is questionable.

If a tumor is suspected, consultation with a pediatric oncologist is recommended. The mass should be biopsied for a definitive diagnosis. If it is malignant, a treatment plan should be generated with the appropriate consultants.

Congenital torticollis from fibrosis of the sternocleidomastoid muscle is best treated with nonoperative intervention. Repetitive passive range-of-motion exer-

cises over several weeks usually result in loosening the tight muscle and increasing the range of motion.

Hemangiomas usually resolve by the time children are 5 years of age, and surgical intervention is rarely indicated. Surgical excision is usually indicated for cystic hygromas (lymphangiomas), branchial cleft cysts, and thyroglossal duct cysts. A thyroid scan should be performed before removal of a thyroglossal duct cyst, because the cyst may contain a child's only thyroid tissue. Endocrinologic consultation is recommended in these cases. Thyroid nodules in children may be cancerous, especially in children who have had irradiation to the head and neck region. Consultation with an endocrinologist and surgeon should be obtained. Goiters in children should be evaluated by an endocrinologist.

PROGNOSIS

The prognosis for children with neck masses is generally excellent but differs depending on the cause. Children with an infectious etiology do very well if diagnosed and treated with appropriate antimicrobials. Mycobacterial lymphadenitis may result in sinus tract formation or disseminated disease. Surgical excision usually cures atypical mycobacterial infection. Cat-scratch disease is usually benign and self-limited. Encephalopathy is a rare complication of this disorder.

The prognosis for benign tumors of the neck is excellent. The outlook for children with malignant neck tumors depends on etiology of the tumor and the spread of the malignancy to other organs. Early diagnosis and treatment are clearly important in improving outcome.

Children with neck masses from trauma usually have had significant injury. The outcome often depends on establishment of an airway, provision of ventilatory support, and management of hemodynamic instability. Availability of surgical support is often essential to a good outcome.

Children with congenital lesions of the neck usually have an excellent prognosis. Some lesions resolve spontaneously, while others require simple surgical excision. Cystic hygromas may require multiple operations for complete removal because of their diffuse nature.

Case Resolution

In the case presented, the boy has signs and symptoms consistent with submandibular bacterial cervical lymphadenitis. The location of the neck mass in relation to the honey-crusted lesions (nonbullous impetigo) implicates spread from the primary site of infection to the lymph nodes. Laboratory tests are unnecessary because the child does not appear septic. Culture of the impetigo is of academic interest only because the child will be started empirically on antibiotics directed against *S. aureus* and group A beta-hemolytic streptococcus. If the affected lymph node is fluctuant, aspiration of fluid for culture is indicated, and incision and drainage should be considered. The child should be treated as an outpatient with an oral antibiotic such as cephalexin, amoxicillin-clavulanic acid, or dicloxacillin as well as an analgesic for pain as needed. A PPD skin test should be placed. The child should be followed in one to three days for clinical improvement depending on the severity of the infection.

Selected Readings

Bergman, K. S., and B. H. Harris. Scalp and neck masses. Pediatr. Clin. North Am. 40:1151–1161, 1993.

Bonilla, J. A., and G. B. Healy. Management of malignant head and neck tumors in children. Pediatr. Clin. North Am. 36:1443–1451, 1989.

Burton, D. M., and S. M. Pransky. Practical aspects of managing nonmalignant lumps of the neck. J. Otolaryngol. 21:398–403, 1992.

Butler, K. M., and C. J. Baker. Cervical lymphadenitis. *In* Feigin, R. D., and J. D. Cherry (eds.). Textbook of Pediatric Infectious Diseases, 3rd ed. Philadelphia, W. B. Saunders, 1992, pp. 220–230.

Friedberg, J. Pharyngeal cleft sinuses and cysts, and other benign neck lesions. Pediatr. Clin. North Am. 36:1451–1469, 1989.

Karmody, C. S. Developmental anomalies of the neck. *In* Bluestone, C. D., S. E. Stool, and M. D. Scheetz (eds.). Pediatric Otolaryngology, 2nd ed. Philadelphia, W. B. Saunders, 1990, pp. 1303–1316.

Knight, P. J., A. F. Mulne, and L. E. Vassy. When is lymph node biopsy indicated in children with enlarged peripheral nodes? Pediatrics 69:391–396, 1982.

May, M. Neck masses in children: diagnosis and treatment. Pediatr. Ann. 5:518–539, 1976.

Ruddy, R. M. Neck mass. *In* Fleisher, G. R., and S. Ludwig (eds.). Textbook of Pediatric Emergency Medicine, 3rd ed. Baltimore, Williams & Wilkins, 1992, pp. 318–322.

Smith, K. M., and B. M. Malone. Neck masses. *In* Reisdorff, E. J., M. R. Roberts, and J. G. Wiegenstein (eds.). Pediatric Emergency Medicine. Philadelphia, W. B. Saunders, 1993, pp. 636–639.

Stanievich, J. F. Cervical adenopathy. *In* Bluestone, C. D., S. E. Stool, and M. D. Scheetz (eds.). Pediatric Otolaryngology, 2nd ed. Philadelphia, W. B. Saunders, 1990, pp. 1317–1327.

Zitelli, B. J. Neck masses. *In* Dershewitz, R. A. (ed.). Ambulatory Pediatric Care, 2nd ed. Philadelphia, J. B. Lippincott, 1993, pp. 328–333.

C H A P T E R   5 4

ALLERGIC DISEASE

Julie E. Noble, M.D.

Hx   A 3-year-old girl is rushed to the office by her mother after her daughter develops a pruritic rash, facial swelling, and hoarseness shortly after eating a peanut butter sandwich. Previously she has been well except for recurrent nasal congestion every spring that has responded to antihistamines. She has also had an intermittent skin rash that has been treated with topical steroid creams. She has never had an acute reaction before and has no history of asthma. Her father had asthma as a child, however.

Physical examination reveals a well-developed, 3-year-old girl with marked facial swelling who is in mild respiratory distress. Vital signs, including blood pressure, are normal. Growth parameters are at the 50th percentile. The girl has a diffuse blotchy erythematous rash with central wheals, a hoarse voice, and a mild expiratory wheeze on auscultation of her chest. The remainder of the examination is normal.

Questions

1. What are the various symptoms of allergic disease?
2. What is the appropriate evaluation of children with manifestations of allergic disease?
3. What allergens are common triggers for allergic symptoms?
4. What management is helpful in treatment of children with manifestations of allergic disease?
5. Can allergic disease be prevented?

Allergic disease, which occurs frequently in the general population, is manifested in many ways. Asthma, atopic dermatitis, allergic rhinitis, allergic conjunctivitis, urticaria, angioedema, anaphylaxis, and vomiting and diarrhea (with food allergies) are all types of allergic diseases. These reactions generally result from the production of immunoglobulin E (IgE) on exposure to a foreign antigen. Similar non–IgE-mediated symptoms may occur, but these are not true allergic reactions. The reader should refer to Chapter 55, Wheezing and Asthma, for details concerning asthma, and Chapter 92, Papulosquamous Eruptions, for a review of atopic dermatitis. This chapter focuses on the remaining manifestations of allergies, including food allergies.

EPIDEMIOLOGY

Allergic disease or some form of allergic symptoms is found in 12 to 20% of the general population. The prevalence of symptoms varies depending on the population being investigated. Factors such as age, genetic background, and place of residence are significant. Allergic rhinitis occurs in 10% of children, as does asthma. Up to 8% of children under 3 years of age develop food allergies.

It is generally accepted that if neither parent is atopic (has the allergic tendency to manufacture IgE on antigen exposure), then the chance that children will develop allergic symptoms is less than one in five. If one parent is atopic, the risk doubles. If both parents are atopic, the chance is greater than three in five.

CLINICAL PRESENTATION

Children with allergic disease frequently present with persistent, clear rhinorrhea, sneezing, postnasal drip, or injected pruritic conjunctiva. Skin manifestations in-clude dry, scaling, erythematous rashes, wheals, or subcutaneous swelling (D$_x$ Box). A recurrent cough or wheezing on chest examination is further evidence of allergic disease.

PATHOPHYSIOLOGY

Allergic rhinitis, like all allergic manifestations, is caused primarily by an antigen-antibody reaction involving IgE. Antigen-specific IgE is produced by the B lymphocytes of allergic patients on exposure to a particular antigen. The IgE attaches to mast cells in the conjunctiva and mucous membranes of the respiratory tract. On reexposure, the antigen reacts with this specific IgE on the mast cells, releasing vasoactive mediators including histamine, leukotrienes, kinins, and prostaglandins. These mediators produce vasodilatation and edema, and they also stimulate neural reflexes to produce mucous hypersecretion and sneezing. Eosinophils, induced by chemotactic factors, pour into nasal secretions and release proteins that worsen the edema. Other immunologic mechanisms can also be involved.

Urticaria, the clinical rash produced by vasodilatation and edema of the skin, is the allergic condition that occurs when histamine is released from the dermal mast cells. The antigen-specific IgE is located on these mast cells. Otherwise, the pathophysiology is similar to that of allergic rhinitis. Exposure to that antigen causes release of chemical mediators from the mast cells. Other mechanisms, including physical stimuli, can produce nonallergic urticaria.

Angioedema is the extension of the urticarial process deeper into the dermis of the skin, producing circumscribed swelling. The mucous membranes may be affected. The pathophysiology is the same as for urticaria. A hereditary type of angioedema, which is not allergy-related, is caused by the inherited deficiency of C1 esterase inhibitor.

Anaphylaxis is an acute, systemic allergic reaction resulting from antigen-specific IgE on mast cells and basophils. The pathophysiology is similar to allergic rhinitis but it occurs in mast cells in many locations simultaneously, and prior sensitization to an allergen is essential. Anaphylactic reactions may be life-threatening. Vasodilatation may be so severe that

---

D$_x$ Allergic Disease

- Chronic, clear rhinorrhea
- Conjunctival tearing and pruritus
- Skin findings of atopic dermatitis or urticaria
- Seasonal variability
- Occurrence of symptoms after exposure to an antigen
- Family history of allergic disease
- Conjunctival injection
- Wheezing
- Chronic cough
- Postnasal drip

TABLE 54–1.   Highly Allergenic Foods
Egg white
Cow's milk
Nuts
Fruits (citrus)
Fish and shellfish
Wheat
Soy
Corn

decreased venous return can lead to acute myocardial infarctions and arrhythmias. Reactions can occur in seconds or as late as one hour after exposure. Common antigens that precipitate anaphylactic reactions include injections of foreign serum, drugs, and venous contrast material, and foods or food additives. The drug most frequently implicated is penicillin. Patients initially experience tightness and intense itching of the skin. Nausea, vomiting, and abdominal pain may ensue. Subsequently, the full spectrum of anaphylaxis appears.

A **food allergy** may produce any of the previously described allergic manifestations, including atopic dermatitis and asthma, as well as vomiting, diarrhea, and FTT. Food intolerance, which has a nonimmunologic pathogenesis, should be differentiated from food allergy, which is an IgE-mediated, allergic reaction. The localization of the IgE-sensitized mast cells to that specific antigen determines the symptoms produced by the allergy. The antigen enters through the GI mucosal barrier. Intact food proteins may enter circulation, stimulating the production of antigen-specific IgE.

Major food allergens are usually glycoproteins (Table 54–1), but any food can be sensitizing. Sensitized GI mast cells release mediators, causing vomiting and diarrhea. As a result of the edema and vasodilation, the mucosa becomes more permeable to enteric antigens, resulting in more hypersensitivity and inflammation.

DIFFERENTIAL DIAGNOSIS

In evaluating children with possible allergic disease, other etiologies for the symptoms should be considered and explored. Allergic rhinitis is most often confused with a URI but may also resemble vasomotor rhinitis, sinusitis, or a nasal foreign body. Unlike allergic rhinitis, infectious etiologies of rhinitis result in inflammatory nasal mucosa and possible fever. Foreign bodies elicit a unilateral, purulent, often foul-smelling discharge. Vasomotor rhinitis is usually transient.

Urticaria can resemble insect bites, erythema multiforme, papular urticaria, mastocytosis, or contact dermatitis. Unlike these other rashes, urticaria is very pruritic and transient, without any epidermal break. It may result from an allergic reaction or may occur secondary to an infections etiology. Parasitic, bacterial, fungal, and viral infections can all cause urticaria. Physical stimuli (e.g., sun, cold), exercise, or anxiety can also produce the reaction. In addition, a deficiency in factor H in the complement system may cause a genetic form of urticaria.

Anaphylaxis is usually associated with edema, wheezing, and fever, although it presents like other forms of shock. A history of an acute exposure is more likely to be seen with anaphylaxis.

Food allergies may resemble food intolerances, which are nonallergenic, with regard to clinical presentation. Food intolerances include toxic contamination, metabolic disorders (e.g., lactose intolerance), and reactions to pharmacologic properties of the ingested food. Associated allergic findings (e.g., asthma, atopic dermatitis) may be seen with true allergies. Specific testing of the food, stool, or patient may be necessary to differentiate allergic reactions from food intolerance.

EVALUATION: HISTORY AND PHYSICAL EXAMINATION

Allergic Rhinitis and Conjunctivitis

Practitioners should determine if children with possible allergic rhinitis have a history of symptoms of sneezing, itching, and nasal discharge. The eyes, ears, palate, and throat may itch. Children may also have a history of mouth breathing and snoring at night from nasal obstruction. These symptoms may be seasonal or associated with a specific stimulus. In addition, systemic symptoms of fatigue, headache, anorexia, and irritability may be present.

The history should also include a search for other manifestations of allergies (e.g., wheezing, atopic dermatitis) as well as a family history of atopy. An environmental history of allergen exposure, including pets, is also important to obtain.

The physical examination should be thorough. The skin should be inspected for atopic dermatitis and the lungs for evidence of asthma. The nasal mucosa should be examined with an otoscope. In children with allergic rhinitis, the nasal mucosa is swollen, pale, and sometimes cyanotic with copious clear discharge. Nasal polyps, if present, should be noted. Although polyps are most often present on an allergic basis, they may occur with cystic fibrosis. A transverse crease across the nose ("an allergic salute") can occur from repeated rubbing of the nose. Dark circles under the eyes, termed "allergic shiners," may be present from venous stasis. If affected, the conjunctivae are erythematous with a clear discharge and may have a follicular appearance. The mouth may reveal a high arched palate from chronic mouth breathing, and the pharyngeal follicular lymphoid tissue may be increased (Fig. 54–1).

Complications of chronic allergic rhinitis may be evident on examination. If children have one of these conditions, such as chronic serous otitis, recurrent otitis media, hearing loss secondary to otitis, sinusitis, sleep apnea, or dental malocclusion, the possibility of allergic disease as a cause should be explored.

Urticaria and Angioedema

When children present with an acute rash, questions should include recent exposures, including drugs, dietary changes, new soaps or detergents, and environmental agents. An urticarial rash is acute in onset,

| A | Allergic shiner | B | Nasal crease | C | Open-mouth facies |

FIGURE 54–1. *Characteristic facial features in children with allergic diseases.*
A. *Allergic shiner.*
B. *Nasal crease.*
C. *Open-mouth facies.*

extremely pruritic, and typically evanescent. Evidence of infection and a history of chronic disease or any other allergic disease should be explored.

The rash should be evaluated carefully. An urticarial rash appears as erythematous lesions of various sizes with pale, papular centers. Lesions may coalesce, the rash blanches on pressure, and the skin is intact.

The physical examination should also assess whether other contributing problems, such as infection, are present.

Anaphylaxis

An acute exposure to a foreign antigen (e.g., medication, food, venom) should be elicited in the history of any patient who presents with anaphylaxis.

On physical examination, vital signs indicate hypotension and tachycardia. The skin is erythematous with diffuse edema. Airway edema may produce hoarseness with stridor and wheezing noted on auscultation of the chest. Patients may have severe difficulty breathing. Cardiac examination may reveal arrhythmias.

Food Allergies

An accurate diet diary is essential in diagnosing a food allergy. The timing of symptoms associated with a specific food must be obtained. Personal as well as family history of atopy is important. An elimination diet followed by a challenge helps the diagnostic evaluation. The double-blind, placebo-controlled food challenge is the most accurate assessment for diagnosis.

EVALUATION: LABORATORY TESTS

With allergic rhinitis, as with any allergic disease, the diagnosis can usually be made with a thorough history and physical examination. Frequently, therapy can be initiated with no laboratory data.

Screening tests may include a nasal smear for eosinophils. A result of greater than 10% eosinophils is considered confirmatory data for allergic rhinitis. Although serum IgE levels are sometimes performed, they are not sensitive or specific and have limited value. A multiallergen screening test, which gives reliable results when checking for the presence of allergic disease, is currently available.

Skin testing for specific antigens should be performed if desensitization shots or environmental changes are being considered in the management plan. Skin tests are sensitive and accurate. Positive tests indicate the presence of an antigen-specific IgE. Prick tests are used initially. They may be followed by intradermal tests for allergens that are negative on prick testing. Although skin testing may be less reliable in infants because their skin is less reactive, the tests have been performed in children as young as 4 months of age.

Radioallergosorbent testing (RAST) of sera, which is also available for the laboratory assessment of allergies, provides a semiquantitative measure of the amount of IgE specific for individual allergens. RAST is much more expensive than skin testing and has no advantage unless skin testing cannot be performed.

Objective testing with skin tests by the prick method may be helpful in diagnosing food allergies. Negative tests are accurate for excluding food allergies, but positive tests may occur in patients without symptoms related to a particular food. Intradermal skin tests are not indicated. They do not give additional information, and they increase the risk of a serious reaction. RAST of sera may be used for specific foods.

MANAGEMENT

The first line of therapy for all allergic diseases is **avoidance of any precipitants.** For allergic rhinitis, this begins with environmental control, because the most frequent precipitants are inhalant allergens. Reducing exposure to the dust mite, a common allergen, can help control allergic rhinitis. Environmental humidity, which increases the dust mite population, should be decreased. Specifically, parents should be instructed to remove carpets, drapes, and upholstered furniture, which can harbor dust mites, from the house. They should cover mattresses with plastic covers and remove furry pets. Decreasing humidity also helps reduce mold counts, another important allergen, and air-conditioning units can lower pollen and mold counts. Nonspecific irritants such as smoke should be avoided because they can also precipitate any allergic symptom.

Anaphylaxis is considered a **medical emergency.** The first step in management is to establish an airway. Oxygen therapy should be instituted, and intravenous access established. Epinephrine is the drug of choice because of its potent vasoconstrictive and myocardial stimulating effects. The dose is 0.01 mL/kg of 1:1000 aqueous solution, up to 0.5 mL, given subcutaneously. If the blood pressure is decreased, epinephrine may be given intravenously, with normal saline fluid boluses to expand intravascular volume. Intravenous administration of an antihistamine, such as diphenhydramine, is used as well as a steroid, such as methylprednisolone, at 2 mg/kg.

The management of urticaria should begin with the **identification of the causal agent** and its elimination. Children who have experienced anaphylaxis should be instructed to avoid future exposure to the precipitating allergen. In addition, they should be instructed to wear a Medic Alert tag that notifies others of the potential for a severe allergic reaction and carry an epinephrine kit for immediate treatment.

A maintenance diet that does not contain the allergen is the basis for management of food allergies. It is essential that the prescribed diet be nutritionally sound. Families should be instructed by a nutritionist and taught to read food labels appropriately to avoid all exposure to the antigen. They should also be advised about what foods children can consume.

Medications should be used when additional management is indicated by persistent symptoms. H$_1$-receptor antagonists or **antihistamines** are frequently indicated in the treatment of allergic rhinitis. Diphenhydramine, chlorpheniramine, and brompheniramine have all been useful in relieving symptoms but may be very sedating. The newer antagonists, terfenadine, astemizole, and loratadine, do not readily cross the blood-brain barrier and are less sedating, but they are not yet approved for use in children under the age of 12 years. Oral decongestants have been effective in decreasing nasal congestion. Pseudoephedrine has been used in children. Topical nasal decongestants, which can cause dependence and rebound swelling, should not be used on a long-term basis.

Antihistamines are also used in the symptomatic treatment of urticaria and angioedema. These agents can relieve the rash as well as the itching of the rash. Diphenhydramine, 5–7 mg/kg/day in four doses, and hydroxyzine, 2–4 mg/kg/day in four doses, are both used. If the urticaria is extensive or severe, epinephrine or Sus-Phrine (epinephrine in oil) may be used subcutaneously. This often provides immediate relief of symptoms and is diagnostic as well as therapeutic.

Cromolyn sodium nasal spray is the next line of treatment for allergic rhinitis in children over the age of 6 years. A very effective mast cell stabilizer, it suppresses mediator release. Cromolyn spray should be used prophylactically on a regular basis two to six times per day, one spray per nostril, to prevent symptoms.

Steroids have an anti-inflammatory effect and work well topically for allergic rhinitis. Beclomethasone, triamcinolone, and flunisolide are available as nasal sprays. None of these agents is recommended in children under the age of 6 years, and all three agents may cause stinging and nasal irritation. Systemic steroids may also be utilized for treatment of urticaria, angioedema, and anaphylaxis.

Immunotherapy should be considered for children with allergic rhinitis or a history of anaphylaxis, depending on the allergen. This treatment has been effective in relieving symptoms due to dust mites, pollens, animal dander, molds, insect stings, and drug reactions. Immunotherapy involves a series of injections with extracts of allergens specific for individual patients, producing tolerance to particular antigens. The results of skin testing dictate which allergens to use. Initially, injections are given weekly. Then they are tapered and given on a maintenance schedule. Although immunotherapy can be performed at any age, the injections are painful and expensive. They necessitate frequent visits. Patients risk an allergic reaction with each injection.

PREVENTION

The cost of medical care, lost school and work days, disability from complications, and actual lives lost from allergic disease takes a great toll on the population. Many investigators have questioned whether the symptoms of allergies can be prevented.

No research indicates that maternal avoidance of allergens during pregnancy has any effect on subsequent development of allergies in children. Evidence currently suggests that sensitization to certain pollens and foods is more likely to occur in the first 6 to 12 months of life. Avoidance of these allergens at this age may decrease the subsequent development of allergic disease. For children at high risk for the development of allergic disease, which is usually determined by family history, the following steps are recommended:

- Keep the home free of dust.
- Keep pets out of the home.
- Keep humidity below 35% in the home.
- Prevent smoking in the environment.
- Limit infectious exposures.

To reduce the incidence of food allergies, it is recommended that mothers breast-feed infants exclusively for the first 6 months of life. When infants are 6 months old, foods can gradually be introduced. Cow's milk, wheat, corn, and citrus should be avoided until after the age of 1 year. Peanuts, eggs, fish, and shellfish should be delayed until 24 months. Postponing the introduction of food allergens may reduce the rate of sensitization in high-risk infants, but this is a controversial issue. Recent studies demonstrate that such postponement may only delay the sensitization.

PROGNOSIS

The prognosis for children with allergic disease is good when the diagnosis is made correctly. Allergic rhinitis, urticaria, and anaphylactic reactions tend to persist throughout life on exposure to antigens. However, with appropriate management with medication and avoidance of allergens, children with allergic disease can thrive and live a normal life without restrictions on activity. Immunotherapy can be effective in alleviating the allergic response to inhalants in allergic rhinitis and to bee venoms in anaphylaxis. The chance for resolution of food allergies is very good. Many foods that initially elicit an allergenic reaction can be tolerated

after the age of 3 to 4 years, presumably as a result of maturation of the GI mucosa.

Case Resolution

In the case presented at the beginning of the chapter, the girl's symptoms of rash, swelling, and wheezing after exposure to an antigen suggest a systemic allergic reaction of angioedema and asthma. Treatment with epinephrine and antihistamines is clearly indicated. Because of the presence of pulmonary symptoms, admission for observation is warranted. The child and family should be counseled to avoid peanut butter in the future.

Selected Readings

Burks, A. W., and H. Sampson. Food allergies in children. Curr. Probl. Pediatr. 23:230–252, 1993.

Ferguson, A. Definitions and diagnosis of food intolerance and food allergy: consensus and controversy. J. Pediatr. 121:S1–S11, 1992.

Rooklin, A. R., and S. M. Gaqchik. Allergic rhinitis—it's that time again. Contemp. Pediatr. 11:19–41, 1994.

Rosen, F. S. Urticaria, angioedema, and anaphylaxis. Pediatr. Rev. 13:387–390, 1992.

Simons, F. E. R. Allergic rhinitis: recent advances. Pediatr. Clin. North Am. 35:1053–1074, 1988.

Solomon, W. R. Prevention of allergic disorders. Pediatr. Rev. 15:301–309, 1994.

Virant, F. S. Allergic rhinitis. Pediatr. Rev. 13:323–333, 1992.

Wood, R. A. Diagnosing allergies: when to test, when to refer. Contemp. Pediatr. 11:13–28, 1994.

CHAPTER 55

WHEEZING AND ASTHMA

James S. Seidel, M.D., Ph.D.

H$_x$ ·A seven-year-old boy is referred to the office after being seen in the emergency department for wheezing. He has been treated in the emergency department for wheezing four times in the past month and was once hospitalized for three days. The boy's father and paternal grandmother both have asthma.

The child's physical examination is remarkable for end-expiratory wheezing on forced expiration.

Questions

1. What are the most common causes of wheezing in infants and children?

2. What are the causes of reversible bronchospasm?
3. What is the pathophysiology of reversible bronchospasm?
4. How should children with asthma be managed?

Recurrent wheezing is a frequent symptom of obstructive airway disease in children that may be caused by intrinsic or extrinsic compression of the airway, bronchospasm, inflammation, or defective clearance of secretions. Reactive airway disease (asthma) is the most common cause of wheezing in childhood. This is a chronic illness and requires longitudinal care by a pri-

TABLE 55–1. Causes of Wheezing

Infection

Bronchiolitis
Pneumonia
Toxocariasis
Ascariasis

Foreign Body
Reactive Airway Disease

Asthma
Exercise-induced asthma
Anaphylaxis
Nighttime cough, asthma
Toxic exposure (smoke, organophosphate poisoning)
Allergic aspergillosis

Congenital Structural Anomalies

Vascular rings
Bronchiectasis
Lung cysts
Laryngotracheoesophageal cleft
Tracheobronchomalacia

Cardiac Disease
Defective Secretion Clearance

Cystic fibrosis
Immotile cilia syndrome

Tumor

Mediastinal tumors (lymphoma, teratoma, neuroblastoma, thymoma)

Chronic Aspiration

Gastroesophageal reflux
Bulbar palsy
Tracheoesophageal fistula

Other Causes

Bronchopulmonary dysplasia
α_1-antitrypsin deficiency
Pulmonary hemosiderosis
Sarcoidosis

---

mary care provider to ensure optimum treatment and reduction in costly emergency department visits and hospital admissions.

The site of the airway obstruction may be in the large or small bronchioles, and the audible "musical or squeaking sounds" noted with obstruction are caused by the turbulence of the air as it is forced through a narrowed airway. Infants and young children are more prone to wheezing when they have airway obstruction because air forced through smaller airways is more turbulent than air forced through the larger airways of older children and adults. Wheezing in children under one year of age is most commonly due to bronchiolitis, an infectious disease caused by RSV; pneumonia; and asthma. Less common causes include congenital structural anomalies, gastroesophageal reflux and aspiration, cardiac failure, cystic fibrosis, and foreign bodies (Table 55–1).

Infants may present with apnea, inspiratory and expiratory wheezing, fever, and respiratory distress. Treatment is symptomatic, including hospitalization for apnea and severe respiratory distress. Infants with "recurrent bronchiolitis" may have reactive airway disease.

In older children, asthma is the most common cause of persistent or recurrent wheezing, although foreign body aspiration should also be considered in children who present with new onset wheezing. Asthma is a lung disease with the following characteristics: (1) increased airway responsiveness to a variety of stimuli, (2) reversible airway obstruction (reversibility may be incomplete in some children), and (3) inflammation of the airways. Less common causes of wheezing include α_1-antitrypsin deficiency, tumors, and pulmonary hemosiderosis. Most children with recurrent reversible bronchospasm have asthma.

EPIDEMIOLOGY

Asthma is the most common chronic childhood illness. The disease affects 5 to 15% of all children and has increased by 29% in recent years. One third of patients first experience symptoms in the first year of life, and 80% are diagnosed by the time they reach school age. One percent of all outpatient visits (6.5 million visits per year) are for asthma; the condition is the fourth most common reason for visits to emergency departments by children. In the United States, asthma is the most frequent admitting diagnosis to children's hospitals. Hospitalization for children under 15 years of age with asthma has increased by 10% in the last several years. In addition, asthma is a major cause of school absence; 23% of school days missed can be attributed to asthma.

In recent years more serious disease in younger children and adolescents has increased. Inner-city African Americans are most at risk. At present, about 4500 individuals die annually from asthma in the United States, which represents an increase of over 30% from a decade ago.

CLINICAL PRESENTATION

Children with asthma may present with acute symptoms of cough and shortness of breath. Wheezing may be audible and detected by the parent or not appreciated until the child is examined by a physician. There may be no wheezing in children with severe bronchoconstriction, because the flow of air is impeded. Some children have cough, which may be nocturnal or recurrent as a predominant symptom. Some pediatric patients have symptoms such as cough or wheezing that are precipitated or exacerbated by exercise (D_x Box).

PATHOPHYSIOLOGY

Asthma is characterized by exaggerated bronchoconstriction in response to a variety of physical, chemical,

---

D_x Asthma

- Recurrent wheezing
- Shortness of breath
- Exercise intolerance
- History of allergies
- History of atopic dermatitis
- Nasal polyps
- History of nighttime cough

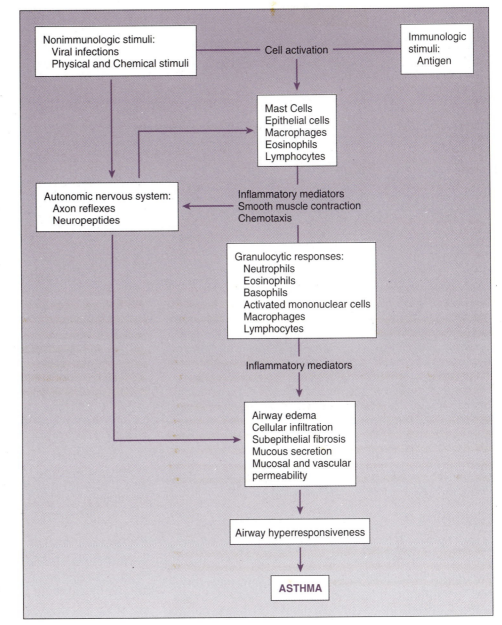

FIGURE 55–1. *Proposed pathways in the pathogenesis of bronchial inflammation and airway hyper-responsiveness.* (Reproduced from the National Asthma Education Program Expert Panel Report, Guidelines for Diagnosis and Management of Asthma, NIH Publication No. 91-3042, 1991.)

and pharmacologic agents. Environmental changes such as wind or temperature changes or increased exposure to air pollutants or allergens may precipitate clinical attacks. Emotional stress may also play a role in the exacerbation of asthma. The changes associated with airway obstruction are now thought to be due primarily to inflammatory changes in the airways. Bronchospasm is the result of complex interactions between inflammatory cells and mediators and the target cells of the airway. Damage to epithelial cells that varies from mild loss of cilia to total destruction of the lining of the bronchioles results.

The physiologic changes involved in asthma occur in two phases. An immediate response to the offending agent causes edema and bronchial smooth muscle constriction that lead to narrowing of the airway and plugging with secretions. Air is trapped behind the narrowed airways, resulting in altered gas exchange,

increased respiratory rate, decreased tidal volume, and increased work of breathing. The late response, which occurs four to eight hours after the initial symptoms, primarily involves infiltration of the airways with inflammatory cells. The end pathway in the disease process is obstruction to airflow. The pathophysiology of asthma is reviewed in Figure 55–1.

DIFFERENTIAL DIAGNOSIS

An extensive differential diagnosis is listed in Table 55–1. Most conditions are differentiated from asthma by the presence of associated symptoms or the child's response to bronchodilators.

Asthma may be classified as mild, moderate, or severe. **Mild asthma** is characterized by relatively few clinical attacks (no more than 1–2 per week) with no symptoms evident in between clinical attacks. Exercise

TABLE 55–2.   **Parameters Used to Estimate the Severity of Acute Asthma**

Sign/Symptom	Classification		
	Mild	*Moderate*	*Severe*
Respiratory rate	Normal	Increased	Increased > 2 S.D.
Breath sounds	Normal (some end-expiratory wheezes)	Wheezing in inspiration and expiration	Decreased ± wheezing
Shortness of breath	None (can speak in sentences)	Can speak in phrases	Speaks only single words
Skin color	Normal (pink)	Pale	Pale to cyanotic
Work of breathing	Normal	Moderate retractions; some use of accessory muscles	Severe retractions; nasal flaring; use of accessory muscles
Pulse	Normal	Normal or increased	Increased
Level of consciousness	Normal	Normal	Diminished; may be lethargic or combative
Pulsus paradoxus	< 10 mm Hg	10–20 mm Hg	20–40 mm Hg
Oxygen saturation	> 95%	90–95%	< 92%
Pulmonary function	80% of predicted	50–70% of predicted	< 50% of predicted

Abbreviations: S.D., standard deviation.

tolerance is good, and pulmonary function is only moderately affected (usually > 80% of predicted values). Individuals with **moderate asthma** have more frequent exacerbations and have cough or wheezing between acute exacerbations. Affected children usually require treatment at an urgent care facility or emergency department several times per year. Exercise tolerance is decreased, and school attendance is usually affected. Pulmonary function testing is usually below normal. **Severe asthma** is associated with daily wheezing and cough. Children with severe asthma make frequent visits to the emergency department and are hospitalized at least two times per year. Sleep interruption, poor exercise tolerance, and chronic school absence may occur. Pulmonary function is less than 60% of baseline and can vary markedly with acute attacks.

EVALUATION

An acute asthmatic attack is always considered a medical emergency because it has the potential to deteriorate into respiratory failure. Initially only a brief history should be obtained. If children have recurrent asthma, critical interventions should be begun during the evaluation. The initial assessment should include an estimation of the severity of the attack. This can be accomplished by a rapid assessment of the ventilation, oxygenation, and perfusion of the patient (Table 55–2). Signs of respiratory distress include rapid respiratory rate, decreased breath sounds, shortness of breath, use of accessory muscles of respiration, retractions (intercostal, sternal, and supraclavicular), nasal flaring, altered mental status, increased expiratory-inspiratory ratio, changes in skin color, and oxygen saturation. Pulsus paradoxus, the difference between systolic arterial blood pressure during inspiration and expiration, is normally less than 10 mm Hg. During an acute asthmatic attack this difference may be increased; however, this measurement may be difficult to obtain in young children. Children who are older than 6 years of age and are not in extreme respiratory distress should have their pulmonary function measured; this may include an estimation of peak expiratory flow rate or forced expiratory volume in one second (FEV_1).

If signs of a moderate or severe attack are present, children need to be monitored continuously. A severe attack may be heralded by the signs of respiratory distress listed above. In addition, patients may be unable to speak in sentences or have altered mental status. Therapy includes placing patients in a position of comfort and giving oxygen by mask, nasal prongs, or having oxygen blown in front of the face. Initiation of drug therapy may also be indicated.

History

If children are not in respiratory distress, a history should be taken (Questions Box). Practitioners should also find out how children and their families perceive the illness.

Physical Examination

Vital signs should be obtained and breath sounds, work of breathing, and the inspiratory-expiratory ratio should be carefully assessed. The nose and associated

---

Questions: Asthma

- What symptoms (e.g., wheezing, exercise intolerance) does the child experience?
- Does the child experience any nocturnal awakening or cough?
- What time of day and year do the symptoms occur?
- When did the symptoms begin? How old was the child?
- Are the symptoms associated with any particular activity? Does anything seem to trigger the symptoms?
- Are the child's activities limited in any way?
- How often do the asthma attacks occur?
- What is the child's living situation? Are there pets in the home?
- Do the asthma attacks cause the child to be absent from school?
- Does the child manage the condition at home with any particular treatments or medications?
- Has the child visited any urgent care and emergency departments for treatment for asthma or related episodes in the past? Has the child had any hospitalizations?
- Does the child have a history of allergies?

nasal passages should be examined for secretions, edema, pallor, and polyps. The skin should be assessed for eczema and other rashes. The chest should be carefully checked for increased anteroposterior diameter of the chest wall, use of accessory muscles, presence of retractions, decreased quality of breath sounds, and presence of prolonged expiration.

Laboratory Tests

The laboratory assessment of children with recurrent wheezing is still somewhat controversial. In older children air flow should be assessed by some objective measure such as peak expiratory flow or FEV_1. A CBC with a differential count may suggest infection or allergies. Nasal swabs for eosinophils and serum IgE antibodies may identify patients with asthma who may benefit from management of specific allergies. Pulse oximetry assesses the degree of oxygen saturation. Arterial blood gases are indicated for children with acute asthma attacks who are not improving with therapy or who may have possible respiratory failure. Extensive laboratory testing should be reserved for children with severe disease who may benefit from consultation with an allergy specialist.

Imaging Studies

Although some physicians recommend routine chest radiographs in children with asthma, such films are probably not indicated unless there is clinical evidence of infection or a foreign body or if another cause of wheezing is suspected. Sinus radiographs should be obtained in children with clinical evidence of acute sinusitis.

MANAGEMENT

Both immediate and long-term management of asthma are indicated.

Short-Term Management

Acute attacks can be managed in the office if the staff is prepared to deal with children in respiratory distress. Otherwise children can be referred to the emergency department. Equipment and supplies for resuscitation of infants and children must be available in offices that care for children with asthma.

The goal of therapy is to relieve airflow obstruction and prevent respiratory failure. All children with moderate or severe asthma should be placed in a **position of comfort** and given **oxygen** by nasal prongs or mask as tolerated. Assessment of work of breathing and the use of pulse oximetry help guide oxygen therapy. Nebulized β_2-agonists such as albuterol are used until symptoms subside. Children may require drug therapy every 20 to 30 minutes. β_2-agonists may also be given as a continuous nebulized treatment for severe acute attacks. Not only are nebulized beta-adrenergic agonists more effective than oral medications, they are associated with fewer side effects. Methylprednisolone, which helps reduce the inflammation associated with clinical attacks, is indicated in most moderate and severe cases. Response to therapy is determined by clinical assessment of work of breathing, respiratory rate, objective changes in pulmonary function, and pulse oximetry. Children with incomplete responses to initial therapy may require several hours of treatment or hospitalization.

Long-Term Management

Asthma is a chronic condition with a varying number of acute exacerbations. The goals of long-term management are shown in Table 55–3.

Continuous and longitudinal primary care of children with asthma can profoundly affect the course of their disease. Primary care practitioners, children, and their families must work together to achieve good control of symptoms. Prevention of exacerbations may be accomplished by **removal of offending allergens,** giving **appropriate medications,** and participation in **home pulmonary function testing.** Periodic assessment ensures appropriate therapy and compliance with treatment. Practitioners should make sure that families can afford the necessary medications. During routine visits, home monitoring and therapy as well as any diaries and records should be reviewed, children's and families' expectations about the course of the disease should be discussed, and all parties should be allowed to express their concerns regarding the development of a treatment plan.

Home therapy can be directed by assessment of pulmonary function and respiratory status. Family members and children should be instructed in the use of peak flow meters to indicate when medical treatment is necessary. Some meters have three color zones: a green zone, which indicates good air flow; a yellow zone, which signals the need for treatment; and a red zone, which suggests that a visit to the emergency department may be indicated.

The most effective form of drug therapy is nebulized beta-adrenergic drugs that can be delivered by a metered-dose inhaler (MDI) or by a nebulizer. The psychomotor skills required to use an MDI are complex, but this barrier may be overcome by the use of spacers that come with a mask or mouthpiece; even infants can be treated with spacers. Devices that deliver a dry powder of albuterol have recently become available and are preferred by some patients. Cromolyn sodium, which also may be given via an MDI, inhibits the release

---

TABLE 55–3. Therapeutic Goals for Children With Chronic Asthma

To maintain a normal, age-appropriate activity level
To maintain near-normal pulmonary function
To prevent symptoms such as exercise intolerance, chronic cough, and shortness of breath
To prevent acute exacerbations of the disease that require acute therapy
To minimize adverse effects of the drugs used to treat the disease
To promote self-esteem and a sense of well-being

of vasoactive triggers from mast cells and is used to prevent bronchospasm and inflammation. The use of xanthines such as theophylline has recently fallen out of favor. Theophylline is a bronchodilator but may not be as effective as nebulized drugs. Steroids, which are reserved for the most severe asthmatics, can be given systemically or via an MDI.

PROGNOSIS

Asthma can result in significant morbidity and mortality if children are not managed appropriately. Children without longitudinal primary care generally require expensive therapy in emergency departments or inpatient settings. A significant number of individuals with asthma have fatal outcomes because of lack of timely and appropriate care. Practically all of these deaths are preventable.

Case Resolution

The 7-year-old boy in the case history who visits the office for asthma requires not only medication but also education and longitudinal primary care. It is particularly important to assess possible environmental factors (e.g.,

pets) and poor compliance with previous recommendations, which have contributed to his recurrent symptoms.

Selected Readings

American Academy of Pediatrics, Provisional Committee on Quality Improvement. Practice parameters: the office management of acute asthma exacerbations in children. Pediatrics 93:119–127, 1994.

Buist, A. S., and W. M. Vollmer. Preventing deaths from asthma. N. Engl. J. Med. 331:1584–1585, 1994.

Hickey, R. W., et al. Albuterol delivered via a metered-dose inhaler with spacer for outpatient treatment of young children with wheezing. Arch. Pediatr. Adol. Med. 148:189–194, 1994.

Leturneau, M. A., S. Schuh, and M. Gausche. Respiratory disorders. *In* Barkin, R. (ed.). Pediatric Emergency Medicine. Concepts and Clinical Practice. St. Louis, Mosby-Year Book, 1992, pp. 969–1037.

National Asthma Education Program Expert Panel Report, Guidelines for the Diagnosis and Management of Asthma. U.S. Department of Health and Human Services, Publication No. 91-3042, 1991.

Rosenthal, B. W. Wheezing. *In* Fleisher, G. R., and S. Ludwig (eds.). Textbook of Pediatric Emergency Medicine, 3rd ed. Baltimore, Williams & Wilkins, 1993, pp. 518–525.

Schuh, S., et al. High- versus low-dose, frequently administered nebulized albuterol in children with severe asthma. Pediatrics 83:513–518, 1989.

Silverstein, M. D., et al. Long-term survival of community residents with asthma. N. Engl. J. Med. 331:1537–1541, 1994.

Stempel, D. A., and S. J. Szelfer (eds.). Asthma. Pediatr. Clin. North Am. 39, 1992.

CHAPTER 56

COUGH

Julie E. Noble, M.D.

H$_x$ A 3-year-old boy presents with a cough that he has had for four weeks. In the past he has had coughs with colds, but this cough is persistent and deeper in quality. The cough seemed to develop suddenly when he was playing at a friend's house. It occurs all day and disrupts his sleep at night. The boy has had no nasal congestion, fever, or sore throat. No one at home is coughing, and the boy has not traveled recently. Neither the boy nor his family have a history of allergies or asthma. Over-the-counter cough preparations have not helped relieve his symptoms.

On examination, growth parameters are normal. The child has a persistent cough with no respiratory distress. Chest examination reveals a normal respiratory rate, no retractions, no use of accessory muscles, but diffuse expiratory wheezing is noted in the right lower lobe. The remainder of the examination is normal.

Questions

1. What are common parental concerns regarding cough?
2. What diagnoses in children with persistent cough should be considered?
3. What historical factors and physical findings are important to determine the etiology of cough?
4. What diagnostic workup is appropriate?
5. How should children with chronic cough be managed?

Cough is an essential protective reflex to ensure airway patency. Its persistence can generate much parental anxiety because of concern about its etiology and frequently associated disruption of sleep patterns.

Cough is either acute or chronic. Acute cough, which may persist up to two weeks, is often associated with respiratory tract infections in children. It is important to remember that always chronic cough begins acutely. When the duration is prolonged, cough is considered chronic and etiologic possibilities are expanded. Chronic cough is defined as a cough lasting for more than two to four weeks. Parental sensitivity as well as accessibility to medical care influence when in the course of disease children present with this problem.

EPIDEMIOLOGY

Cough is a very common complaint initiating pediatric office visits. In the National Ambulatory Medical Care Survey, 6.7% of pediatric office visits involved children who presented with cough. Typically, preschool children have up to eight URIs with associated cough in a winter season. Many other diseases, including cystic fibrosis, congenital heart disease, asthma, and immunodeficiency disorders, may result in cough.

CLINICAL PRESENTATION

The presentation varies greatly depending on the etiology of the cough. Children may present in severe respiratory distress or have no evidence of respiratory compromise. They may have conditions such as FTT or appear totally healthy (D_x Box).

PATHOPHYSIOLOGY

Coughing is a complicated reflex process initiated through irritation of one of the multiple cough receptors. These receptors are located in the nose, paranasal sinuses, posterior pharynx, larynx, trachea, bronchi, and pleura. They can also be found outside of the respiratory tract in the ear canal, stomach, pericardium, and diaphragm. Stimulation of any of these receptors by an irritant, whether mechanical, chemical, thermal, or inflammatory, can initiate the cough reflex. The lung parenchymal tissue contains no cough receptors, so pneumonia may not produce a cough. The receptors send the cough message along the vagal and laryngeal nerves to the upper brain stem, where the cough center receives the message and coordinates the cough mechanism. The cough center can be voluntarily stimulated or suppressed.

TABLE 56–1. Causes of Cough

Congenital Anomalies
Tracheoesophageal fistula
Laryngeal cleft
Vocal cord paralysis
Mediastinal tumors
Pulmonary malformations
Tracheobronchomalacia
Congenital heart disease

Infections (e.g., upper respiratory infection, sinusitis, pneumonia)
Viral
 Adenovirus
 Influenza
 Parainfluenza
 Respiratory syncytial virus
 Rhinovirus
Bacterial
 Pertussis
 Pneumococcal
 Staphylococcal
 Tuberculosis
Fungal
 Coccidioidomycosis
Other
 Chlamydial
 Mycoplasmosis

Chronic Disease
Cystic fibrosis
Human immunodeficiency virus infection
Immunodeficiency syndrome
Dyskinetic cilia

Allergic Conditions
Allergic rhinitis
Asthma
Serous otitis media

Foreign Body Aspiration
Gastroesophageal Reflux
Environmental Irritants
Psychogenic Cough
Drug-Induced Conditions

The actual cough experienced by patients may be broken down into three phases. First, the glottis opens with an inspiratory gasp. Second, the glottis closes with forceful contraction of the chest wall, diaphragm, and abdominal muscles. Third, the glottis again opens with release of airway pressure in an expiratory phase. This process expels mucus or irritants from the airways, clearing the passages for normal air flow.

DIFFERENTIAL DIAGNOSIS

The list of differential diagnoses of cough is long (Table 56–1). Narrowing the list of causes can be accomplished by paying attention to several factors.

As with any pediatric symptom, the child's **age** influences the diagnostic possibilities and management of the cough. Congenital anomalies, which are most likely to present in the first few months of life, include tracheoesophageal fistula, laryngeal cleft, vocal cord paralysis, and tracheobronchomalacia. Congenital heart disease can produce a cough from heart failure and pulmonary edema. Congenital mediastinal tumors cause infants to cough if the tumor presses on the bronchial tree.

The **duration of the cough** also determines its possible cause. Most acute coughs are infectious in origin.

D_x Cough

- Dry, productive, brassy cough
  - Duration: acute, chronic, recurrent
  - Timing: during day, at night, on awakening, with exercise
- Fever or URI associated with infectious origin
- Allergic findings of rhinorrhea, sneezing, wheezing, atopic dermatitis associated with asthma or allergic rhinitis
- FTT (indicates chronic disease)

URIs can initiate an acute cough through stimulation of the cough receptors in the nose and posterior pharynx. If nasal congestion and cough persist, a diagnosis of allergic rhinitis or sinusitis should be considered. Serous otitis media can also cause a persistent cough and may occur in children with chronic congestion. Children with pneumonia may present with either acute or chronic cough.

The presence of a **nighttime cough** can be important. Pathologic coughs, including those caused by sinusitis with postnasal drip, gastroesophageal reflux, and asthma, are more likely to occur at night.

The **character of the cough** is a fourth factor to consider in the differential diagnosis. Some causes produce a very specific type of cough. A barking cough is consistent with laryngeal edema and croup, whereas an inspiratory whoop is characteristic of pertussis or parapertussis. The psychogenic cough is a strange, honking sound.

Pneumococcus is the most probable causal agent in acute cough with pneumonia, but when the cough becomes chronic, other infectious agents are more likely. Adenovirus and RSV, which occur more commonly in infants, and influenza and parainfluenza, which affect children of all ages, are common viral agents that produce chronic cough. *Bordetella pertussis*, mycoplasma, and chlamydia also cause chronic cough. Other infections such as tuberculosis and coccidioidomycosis should also be considered in endemic areas or high-risk populations. Chronic infectious coughs, such as those associated with influenza and pertussis, can last up to six months. Host factors that may predispose to chronic cough should also be investigated. Children with cystic fibrosis, BPD, HIV and other immunodeficiency syndromes, and congenital pulmonary malformations may present with chronic, recurrent cough.

The most common cause of chronic cough is reactive airway disease (asthma) (see Chapter 55, Wheezing and Asthma). In fact, cough with no notable wheezing may be the only manifestation of asthma. In infants or neurologically impaired children, chronic cough may indicate gastroesophageal reflux with recurrent aspiration. An unexplained persistent cough, primarily in toddlers, may be the result of foreign body aspiration if the initial aspiration was not observed. The foreign object acts as a chronic airway irritant that stimulates coughing, and it may be the cause of recurrent infections. Other irritants that initiate cough include dust, smoke, and chemicals. A psychogenic cough should also be considered, especially if the cough is absent at night. Such a cough may be a habit or an expression of anxiety. Drugs such as beta-adrenergic receptor antagonists and angiotensin-converting enzyme inhibitors can also induce a chronic cough, probably by increasing the sensitivity of the cough reflex.

EVALUATION

History

A complete history should be obtained when children present with cough (Questions Box). All symptoms should be noted. Vomiting with cough can indicate

---

Questions: Cough

- How old is the child?
- How long has the child had the cough?
- How frequent is the child's cough?
- Does the cough occur at night?
- Does exercise make the cough worse?
- Do any factors such as environmental irritants seem to precipitate the cough?
- Does the child have any related infectious symptoms, including fever and nasal congestion?
- Does the child have any other symptoms?
- Has the child had any previous episodes of coughing or associated symptoms?
- Has the child lost weight recently?
- What is the child's birth history?
- Has the child had any pulmonary injuries?
- What is the child's immunization status?
- Does the child have a history of recent travel?
- Has a family member had similar symptoms?
- Does the family have a history of pulmonary disease or allergies?
- Has the child been treated with any medications for the cough? Have they helped?
- Is the child taking any other medications?

---

phlegm production. In fact, some children present with a chief complaint of vomiting when it is actually the cough that precipitates the vomiting.

Physical Examination

A complete physical examination should be performed on all children who present with cough. Growth parameters and vital signs should be assessed. Skin should be examined for evidence of cyanosis or atopy. Facial petechiae or subconjunctival hemorrhage indicates particularly forceful coughing. Extremities should be evaluated for fingernail clubbing, which is a sign of chronic pulmonary disease. The nose should be assessed for evidence of congestion. Allergic disease produces pale, cyanotic mucosa, whereas infection results in more inflammatory mucosa. TMs should be examined and mobility tested.

The effort of respiration, including the use of accessory muscles, should also be noted. Careful attention should be paid to breath sounds; whether abnormal sounds are in the inspiratory or expiratory phase of respiration should be determined. Stridor is classically an inspiratory sound (see Chapter 37, Stridor and Croup), whereas wheezing is usually an expiratory sound. Prolongation of the expiratory phase also indicates wheezing. Abnormal breath sounds should be localized if possible. Because the character of the cough can establish the diagnosis, listening to the cough is probably the most important part of the physical examination. A parental description of the cough may be less diagnostic.

Laboratory Tests

After a thorough history and physical examination, laboratory data may not be necessary. Laboratory tests should be ordered when more information is needed to help make a reasonable diagnosis. The laboratory data should be directed at proving or disproving the most likely diagnosis in a specific patient.

If after the history, physical examination, and chest x-ray, an infectious etiology for cough is suspected, a CBC with differential and a PPD test should be ordered. Appropriate cultures should be obtained, if possible. Most children swallow their phlegm, so sputum cultures may be difficult to obtain. Gastric aspirates can sometimes yield a reasonable sputum specimen for culture. Nasopharyngeal cultures are useful for diagnosing pertussis and viral etiologies.

Imaging Studies

The chest x-ray (anteroposterior and lateral), the mainstay of the laboratory evaluation of cough, should be the first test ordered in the evaluation of a chronic cough or if definite findings are evident on physical examination. A lateral decubitus film can provide additional information about pleural fluid or air trapping. Inspiratory and expiratory films can be obtained if a foreign body is suspected. If a pulmonary lesion is found on x-ray, bronchoscopy may be the next step to further define the lesion. If sinusitis is suspected, x-rays of the sinuses can be performed. An upper GI series of x-rays which helps define gastroesophageal reflux is warranted if the cough occurs after recurrent episodes of vomiting or at night.

In children with asthma, the chest x-ray may be totally normal. Further laboratory testing with peak flow measurements in children over the age of 4 can be done to demonstrate restricted expiratory flow. The most helpful test to diagnose asthma may be a trial of a bronchodilator (see Chapter 55, Wheezing and Asthma).

MANAGEMENT

Cough should not be treated until the cause has been identified by a thorough consideration of the differential diagnoses. Therapy should then be directed toward treating that etiology. If the cough is secondary to a URI or allergic rhinitis, an **antihistamine/decongestant** combination may help decrease postnasal drip and relieve the cough. If the cough is keeping children awake at night, a **cough suppressant** may be indicated so that children and their families can rest. Cough syrups containing dextromethorphan are efficacious. Cough syrups with codeine can also be used. Such medications can be very helpful in interrupting the cough cycle generated by constant irritation of the cough receptors. Expectorants and mucolytic agents in cough syrups have little effect on relieving coughs.

PROGNOSIS

With thoughtful evaluation, it is usually possible to identify the causes of both acute and chronic cough. Most symptoms resolve with appropriate therapy. If the cough persists with treatment, then alternate diagnoses should be considered.

Case Resolution

In the case presented at the beginning of this chapter, the child's cough began acutely and developed into a chronic cough. The boy has no history of allergies or symptoms consistent with an infectious process. Physical examination reveals localized wheezing. A chest x-ray should be ordered to gain more information. His symptoms and presentation are most consistent with foreign body aspiration.

Selected Readings

Hatch, R. T., G. B. Carpenter, and L. J. Smith. Treatment options in the child with a chronic cough. Drugs 45:367–373, 1993.

Kamei, R. K. Chronic cough in children. Pediatr. Clin. North Am. 38:593–605, 1991.

Morgan, W. J., and L. M. Taussig. The child with persistent cough. Pediatr. Rev. 8:249–253, 1987.

Parks, D. P., et al. Chronic cough in childhood: approach to diagnosis and treatment. J. Pediatr. 115:856–862, 1989.

Richards, W. What's causing that child's chronic cough? Compr. Ther. 19:256–260, 1993.

Rojas, A. R., E. J. O'Connell, and M. I. Sachs. Chronic cough in children: what to do, and why. J. Respir. Dis. 12:891–903, 1991.

HEMATOLOGIC DISORDERS

C H A P T E R   5 7

ANEMIA

Pamela S. Cohen, M.D.

Hx   An 18-month-old girl is brought to the office with a 36-hour history of increasing scleral icterus and pallor, which are accompanied by symptoms of a viral upper respiratory tract infection (e.g., coughing, nasal discharge, low-grade fever). During her first week of life, the girl had hyperbilirubinemia of unknown etiology that required "bililights." Her family history is significant for mild anemia in her father; the cause of his condition is also unknown. A paternal aunt and grandfather had cholecystectomies while in their thirties.

On physical examination, the girl has tachycardia and mild tachypnea (no respiratory distress), in addition to the scleral icterus and pallor. Except for a spleen palpable 3 cm below the midcostal margin, the rest of the examination is normal.

Questions

1. What hemoglobin/hematocrit values are associated with anemia?
2. What is the appropriate initial evaluation of children with anemia?
3. When should children receive transfusions of red blood cells?
4. What emergency situations in children who present with anemia should be recognized by the primary pediatrician?

Anemia, a very common condition encountered by every pediatrician, is characterized by a hemoglobin or hematocrit value that is less than two standard deviations below the mean normal value for age. These values vary widely during the first year of life as newborn infants' hematopoiesis changes from fetal to adult-type (see Table 57–1 for normal age-related values). From the age of about 6 months through 8 years, a value of hemoglobin less than 11 g/dL or a hematocrit below 33% is considered consistent with the diagnosis of anemia. When evaluating children with suspected anemia, it is very important to ascertain whether only anemia is present or whether the WBC count or platelet count is also affected by the underlying disorder. This informa-

tion greatly helps determine the diagnosis and dictates the treatment plan.

EPIDEMIOLOGY

Iron deficiency anemia is the leading cause of anemia among infants and children in the United States. The overall incidence of anemia has decreased markedly in the past 15 years as a result of iron supplementation of infant formula and food products. The incidence of iron deficiency anemia in particular, and anemia in general, appears to depend on socioeconomic status, and is about 3% in children under 2 years of age seen in a suburban pediatric office, compared to about 8% among inner-city children not taking iron-fortified formula.

Other epidemiologic factors that contribute to anemia are presented in Table 57–2. Most of the nonimmune hemolytic anemias are inherited. Dietary factors, such as oxidants (e.g., fava beans), can trigger hemolysis in glucose-6-phosphate-dehydrogenase (G6PD) deficiency or can cause suppression of hematopoiesis as in iron, folate, or vitamin B_{12} deficiency. Ingestion of toxins such as lead can also result in impaired hematopoiesis.

CLINICAL PRESENTATION

Children who have anemia present with pallor, fatigue, and decreased exercise tolerance. Other signs and symptoms that suggest anemia or its underlying causes include scleral icterus, jaundice, hepatosplenomegaly, and in severe cases, shortness of breath due to congestive heart failure (CHF) (D_x Box).

PATHOPHYSIOLOGY

RBCs develop from pluripotent stem cells in the bone marrow that also give rise to myeloid cells and platelets. These stem cells ultimately differentiate into mature, enucleated RBCs through interaction with various hematopoietic growth factors, including erythropoietin (whose synthesis requires functioning kidneys), interleukin-3, and stem cell factor. RBCs, which are then extruded through the bone marrow into the

TABLE 57–1.   Age-Related Normal Values for Hemoglobin, Hematocrit, and Mean Corpuscular Volume

Age	Hemoglobin (g/dL)		Hematocrit (%)		MCV (fL)	
	Mean	*22 S.D.*	*Mean*	*22 S.D.*	*Mean*	*22 S.D.*
1 day	18.5	14.5	56	45	108	95
2 wk	16.5	12.5	51	39	105	86
1 mo	13.9	10.7	44	33	104	85
2 mo	11.2	9.4	35	28	96	77
6 mo–2 yr	12.5	11.0	37	33	77	70
2–4 yr	12.5	11.0	38	34	79	73
5–7 yr	13.0	11.5	39	35	81	75
8–11 yr	13.5	12.0	40	36	83	76
12–14 yr						
Female	13.5	12.0	41	36	85	78
Male	14.0	12.5	43	37	84	77
15–17 yr						
Female	14.0	12.0	41	36	87	79
Male	15.0	13.0	46	38	86	78
Adult						
Female	14.0	12.0	42	37	90	80
Male	16.0	14.0	47	40	90	80

Abbreviations: MCV, mean corpuscular volume; S.D., standard deviation.
Reproduced, with permission, from Green, M., and R.J. Haggerty (eds.). Ambulatory Pediatrics, 4th ed. Philadelphia, W.B. Saunders, 1990. p. 377.

peripheral circulation, normally have a life span of about 120 days. They become deformed with age and eventually are trapped in the spleen and destroyed. Iron from RBCs is then recycled via binding to transferrin and returned to the marrow for further use.

Anemia can occur as a consequence of perturbation of any of these steps. Pathophysiologically, it can result from conditions leading to **decreased production** or **increased destruction** (i.e., hemolysis) of RBCs or **increased blood loss.** Deficient production may be caused by either marrow infiltration (e.g., leukemia), bone marrow failure (Blackfan-Diamond syndrome), or dietary factors (iron deficiency anemia). Increased destruction of red cells (hemolysis) can be either intracorpuscular (RBC cytoskeleton defects, RBC enzyme deficiencies, or hemoglobinopathies) or extracorpuscular (immune or nonimmune etiologies). Anemia results when the rate of red cell loss exceeds the rate of red cell production.

DIFFERENTIAL DIAGNOSIS

The differential diagnosis of anemia can be assessed on either the basis of etiology or size of RBCs. The clinician can determine whether the anemia is associated with decreased or increased production of red cells or increased blood loss. A differential diagnosis of anemia based on this classification is shown in Table 57–3. A reduced reticulocyte count indicates decreased marrow production in children with suspected anemia. In general, an elevated indirect bilirubin along with a high reticulocyte count is highly suggestive of hemolysis. Various tests indicate increased destruction, depending on the extent and the chronicity of the hemolysis. Excessive blood loss can occur at any mucosal site. Blood may be lost into the stool or urine as well as through menorrhagia or nosebleeds.

RBC size, as assessed by mean corpuscular volume (MCV), is useful for determining the cause of anemia. Table 57–4 lists the acute anemias of childhood by cell

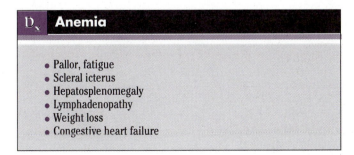

Dx **Anemia**

- Pallor, fatigue
- Scleral icterus
- Hepatosplenomegaly
- Lymphadenopathy
- Weight loss
- Congestive heart failure

TABLE 57–2.   Epidemiologic Factors Related to Anemia

Genetic
Autosomal dominant: hereditary spherocytosis
Autosomal recessive: most Embden-Meyerhof pathway enzyme deficiencies (e.g., pyruvate kinase deficiency), most hemoglobinopathies (e.g., sickle cell anemia, beta-thalassemia)
X-linked: glucose-6-phosphate dehydrogenase (G6PD) deficiency
Ethnicity
  Northern European Caucasian: hereditary spherocytosis, pyruvate kinase deficiency
  Mediterranean (Italian, Greek, North African): beta-thalassemia
  African: sickle cell anemia, malaria, hemoglobin C, D
  Asian: alpha-thalassemia, hemoglobin E
Dietary
Ingestion of oxidants (e.g., fava beans in G6PD deficiency)
Poor dietary intake (e.g., iron, folate, or vitamin B_{12} deficiency)
Poor gastrointestinal absorption (e.g., vitamin B_{12} deficiency)
Toxins (e.g., lead)
Socioeconomic
Living near highways: increased incidence of lead poisoning
Poverty: associated with pica and lead poisoning

TABLE 57–3. Differential Diagnosis of Anemia Based on Pathophysiology

Pathophysiologic Mechanism	General Diagnostic Features	Specific Diagnostic Features
Decreased Production of Red Blood Cells	Evidence of decreased production: ↓ reticulocytes	*Pancytopenia due to bone marrow infiltration with:*
Marrow infiltration		
Secondary to tumor infiltration		Leukemia, neuroblastoma, etc.
Secondary to infiltration with nonmalignant cells		
Lipidoses		Lipid-filled macrophages
X-linked lymphoproliferative disorder		Erythrophagocytosis
Decreased production of hematopoietic elements (bone marrow failure)		Hepatosplenomegaly
Decreased RBC production only		
Constitutional: Blackfan-Diamond Syndrome		Multiple physical deformities
Acquired		
Acquired pure red cell aplasia		Associated with thymoma
Transient erythrocytopenia of childhood		Associated with parvovirus infection
Decreased RBC and WBC production		
Constitutional		
Fanconi's anemia		Multiple physical deformities
Shwachman's syndrome		Pancreatic insufficiency
Decreased production of RBC, WBC, and platelets		
Constitutional		
Fanconi's anemia		Multiple physical deformities
Shwachman's syndrome		Pancreatic insufficiency
Acquired: aplastic anemia (idiopathic or secondary to toxins, drugs, or infection [e.g., hepatitis B]		History of hepatitis B, toxin exposure
Dietary deficiency		
Iron deficiency		↓ MCV, ↓ MCH, ↑ RDW, ↓ serum iron, ↓ serum ferritin, excessive milk intake
Folic acid deficiency		↑ MCV, ↑ RDW, megaloblastic marrow, low serum and RBC folate
Vitamin B_{12} deficiency		↑ MCV, ↑ RDW, megaloblastic marrow, low serum B_{12} levels, + Schilling test
Vitamin C deficiency		Clinical scurvy
Protein deficiency		Kwashiorkor
Hypothyroidism		Low T_4, elevated TSH
Increased Production (Hemolysis)	Evidence of hemolysis: ↑ Reticulocytes	
Intrinsic RBC defects		
RBC Membrane defects (spherocytosis, elliptocytosis)	Hyperbilirubinemia	+ Osmotic fragility, spectrin deficiency (HS)
RBC Enzyme defects (G6PD deficiency, pyruvate kinase)	↑ LDH (RBC)	+ enzyme assays
Hemoglobin defects	MCV may be ↑ if reticulocytes high	
1. Qualitative defects (sickle cell anemia, Hb C, Hb E)		Hb electrophoresis
2. Quantitative defects (thalassemia)		↑ Hb A2 (beta-thalassemia), targets cells, basophilic stippling
Extrinsic RBC disorders		
Immune		
Isoimmune hemolytic anemia (e.g., ABO, Rh incompatibility)		+ Coombs' test
Autoimmune hemolytic anemia		
Idiopathic		
Secondary: postviral, autoimmune disorders, Evan's syndrome		+ ANA
Nonimmune (e.g., DIC, HUS)		Concomitant renal disease (HUS)
Blood Loss	Reticulocytes normal (acute loss)	
Overt (e.g. splenic sequestration, gastrointestinal, or nasal bleeding)	↑ Reticulocytes (chronic loss, not iron deficient)	Sickle cell anemia (splenic sequestration)
Occult (e.g. bleeding Meckel's diverticulum, pulmonary hemosiderosis)	↓ Reticulocytes (chronic loss, iron deficient) May have rapidly falling hematocrit	Pulmonary infiltrates + iron deficiency (pulmonary hemosiderosis)

Abbreviations: RBC, red blood cell; WBC, white blood cell; MCV, mean corpuscular volume; MCH, mean corpuscular hemoglobin; RDW, red cell distribution width; TSH, thyroid-stimulating hormone; LDH, lactate dehydrogenase; HS, hereditary spherocytosis; G6PD, glucose-6-phosphate dehydrogenase; DIC, disseminated intravascular coagulation; HUS, hemolytic-uremic syndrome; ANA, antinuclear antibodies.

Adapted from Lanzkowsky, P. Manual of Pediatric Hematology-Oncology. New York, Churchill Livingstone, 1989, pp. 2–3.

size with pertinent clinical and laboratory features. Low MCV anemias usually result from iron deficiency or thalassemia trait. High MCV anemias are usually of nutritional origin (vitamin B_{12} or folate deficiency). The many other causes of anemia commonly fall into the normal MCV category.

Etiology and RBC size, the two systems for classification of anemia, are not mutually exclusive and are not

TABLE 57–4.   Differential Diagnosis of Childhood Anemias Based on Red Blood Cell (RBC) Size

Hypochromic, Microcytic Anemia (low MCV)
Iron deficiency anemia
Thalassemia trait (alpha-, beta-)
Lead poisoning
Anemia of chronic disease (juvenile rheumatoid arthritis)
Normochromic, Normocytic Anemia (normal MCV)
Caused by intrinsic RBC defects
  Hemoglobinopathies (e.g., SS)
  Enzymopathies (e.g., G6PD deficiency, PK deficiency)
  RBC membrane abnormalities
    Nonimmune (e.g., HS, HE [not readily apparent])
    Immune (e.g., autoimmune hemolytic anemia)
  Decreased RBC production (e.g., aplastic anemia)
Caused by extrinsic RBC defects
  Microangiopathic hemolytic anemia (e.g., hemolytic-uremic syndrome)
Hyperchromic, Macrocytic Anemia (increased MCV)
Folate deficiency
Vitamin B_{12} deficiency
Preleukemia

Abbreviations: MCV, mean corpuscular volume; G6PD, glucose-6-phosphate dehydrogenase; PK, pyruvate kinase; SS, sickle cell anemia; HS, hereditary spherocytosis; HE, hereditary elliptocytosis.

equally helpful in all situations. Simultaneous application of these two systems enables the physician to make a primary diagnosis of the anemia and determine its probable causes.

EVALUATION

History

It is important to take a good history from patients with anemia to obtain etiologic clues relating to their condition (Questions Box). Anemia based on marrow failure can be congenital or acquired. Historical clues consistent with all marrow failure syndromes include a prolonged (months) history of increased fatigue and pallor, with occasional history of previous transfusions of RBCs prior to diagnosis. In acquired marrow failure states such as aplastic anemia, the history is occasionally consistent with antecedent hepatitis, a viral syndrome, exposure to toxins such as benzene- and toluene-containing compounds, or oral chloramphenicol use (commonly available over-the-counter in Latin America).

A clinical history consistent with anemia secondary to hemolysis includes hyperbilirubinemia with scleral icterus in the newborn period. If hemolysis is acute, red urine due to hemoglobinuria is evident. If the cause is genetic, a positive family history for anemia as well as for cholecystectomy is often elicited.

Physical Examination

In addition to historical features, physical findings can often give the clinician strong clues concerning the pathophysiologic process that has caused the anemia. Severe anemia (hemoglobin < 3 g/dL) secondary to chronic causes and moderate anemia (hemoglobin of 3–7 g/dL) in more acute conditions (e.g., blood loss) can cause CHF regardless of etiology owing to insufficient oxygenation of the anemic blood. Aplastic anemia occurs with concomitant neutropenia and thrombocytopenia. Symptoms consistent with concomitant neutropenia (absolute neutrophil count < 1000 /mL), including fever or focal infection, especially pneumonia and perirectal abscesses, may be elicited. Symptoms associated with thrombocytopenia include bruises, petechiae, and mucosal bleeding from the mouth, nose, and GI tract. Absent or bifid thumbs are often indicators of both Fanconi's anemia and amegakaryocytic thrombocytopenia. Children with either Fanconi's anemia or Blackfan-Diamond syndrome may exhibit several other physical deformities, including short stature, cardiac anomalies, and mental retardation. Thinning hair that falls out and koilonychia (nail spooning) may result from chronic, severe iron deficiency.

Some physical findings are particular to individual diseases that lead to increased destruction of RBCs. In infants, sickle cell disease may present as hand-foot syndrome, a form of painful crisis that manifests as swelling of one to four digits associated with pain and sometimes fever. Splenomegaly, a feature of sickle cell anemia in younger children prior to autosplenectomy, thalassemia major, and thalassemia intermedia, is also characteristic of RBC membrane disorders, most commonly hereditary spherocytosis. In children with severe chronic hemolysis, regardless of etiology, classic facies (often called "thalassemia facies") can develop, with frontal bossing and flattened nasal bridge, because of the thinning of the facial bones as a result of brisk intramedullary hematopoiesis.

Laboratory Tests

Initial laboratory tests for patients with suspected anemia include hemoglobin, hematocrit, MCV, and blood smear examination. Screening laboratory findings consistent with hemolysis, regardless of etiology, include an elevated reticulocyte count (if secondary to chronic disease), and mildly to moderately elevated indirect and total bilirubin. If the anemia is secondary to immune causes, Coombs' test is positive. All children with anemia secondary to marrow failure have decreased reticulocyte counts in the peripheral blood. Further tests specific for individual hemolytic diseases or particular diseases secondary to marrow failure are summarized in Table 57–3.

Questions: Anemia

- Does the child eat meat?
- Does the child drink too much milk (> 32 oz/day)?
- Has the child lost a lot of blood recently?
- Have the child's eyes appeared "yellow"?
- Does the child have a family history of anemia, jaundice, or gallstones?
- Did the child need phototherapy at birth for hyperbilirubinemia?

Imaging Studies

Few children routinely require imaging studies to determine the cause of their anemia. Hemolysis is reflected on x-ray by the "hair-on-end" appearance of bones. Patients who have anemia associated with lead poisoning may have lead deposition in their long bones.

MANAGEMENT

Two anemia-related conditions constitute emergencies. Prompt recognition of these conditions is vital if proper treatment is to be initiated. **Splenic sequestration** occurs in patients, usually infants, with sickle cell anemia who sequester large volumes of sickling blood within the spleen over a period of hours. This results in rapidly dropping hemoglobin, clinically resembling anemia due to massive blood loss. The blood pooled in the spleen is not available to the circulation, and affected children are subject to fatal splenic rupture. The clinician should suspect this condition in young African-American or Hispanic infants with severe Coombs-negative anemia, rapidly dropping hemoglobin, tachypnea, tachycardia, and an enlarged spleen, even in the absence of a history of sickle cell anemia. Treatment involves transfusion or exchange transfusion.

Severe autoimmune hemolytic anemia is the second anemia-related emergency. Children with this disorder can occasionally present with severe Coombs-positive anemia and clinical evidence of rapid hemolysis; their hemoglobin may fall as much as 1 g/dL/hr. These patients generally require hospitalization, transfusion, and treatment with prednisone, 2 mg/kg/day.

The treatment of anemia varies depending on the etiology. In **iron deficiency anemia,** the single most common cause of anemia in children, administration of **supplemental iron** may be all that is necessary. In physically normal children with a history of poor iron intake, a therapeutic trial of iron, 6 mg/kg/day divided into two doses, is justified before proceeding with further laboratory tests. Normal-appearing children who drink excessive amounts of milk or eat no meat and have a CBC consistent with iron deficiency (i.e., microcytic anemia with a hemoglobin concentration less than the 10th percentile for age with absent reticulocytes) should be treated with iron supplementation. They should demonstrate a brisk reticulocytosis within seven days of starting iron. An increase of 1.0 g/dL or more in the hemoglobin concentration in one month is considered diagnostic of iron deficiency anemia; this justifies the continuation of therapy for an additional two to three months. The therapeutic trial should not be continued if the hemoglobin concentration does not increase. Other diagnoses, particularly those related to microcytic anemia, should be entertained and evaluated with appropriate laboratory tests at this point.

The use of **blood transfusions** in patients with anemia is a complex topic that ultimately should be decided after careful consideration by the physician responsible for the patient's care. Because of the risk of acquisition of blood-borne infection, including hepatitis, CMV, and HIV, blood transfusions should never be given to a patient unless it is deemed necessary. "Necessary" reasons for transfusion include (1) patients who are unable to make their own RBCs (e.g., patients with aplastic anemia) and (2) patients whose cardiovascular status is compromised because of the anemia (e.g., patients with orthostatic hypotension or poor tissue perfusion) or who suffer congestive heart failure.

Before children with acute anemia receive transfusions, the clinician must be sure that all blood tests necessary for making the diagnosis have been obtained. This is very important because in several conditions, such as sickle cell anemia, thalassemia, and RBC enzyme disorders such as G6PD and pyruvate kinase deficiency, transfusion obscures the diagnosis until transfused cells have diminished in number. Packed RBCs should be used slowly in conditions in which anemia has occurred slowly to avoid fluid overload. In children with hemoglobin over 7 g/dL, packed RBCs can be given at 10 mL/kg over three to four hours; in children with less than 7 g/dL of hemoglobin, 5 mL/kg of packed RBCs can be given over three to four hours and then repeated until the desired hemoglobin level is reached. Children with anemia secondary to acute rapid blood loss should receive whole blood to both expand the intravascular volume and treat the anemia.

PROGNOSIS

The prognosis depends on the underlying cause. Children with some conditions (e.g., thalassemia trait) require no treatment. Some children, such as those with thalassemia major, Blackfan-Diamond syndrome, and aplastic anemia, have a lifelong dependency on transfusions that may result in premature death at age 30 to 40 years from iron overload. Some conditions normalize after splenectomy (e.g., hereditary spherocytosis).

Case Resolution

The girl described in the case history at the beginning of the chapter has hereditary spherocytosis. Her history is highly suggestive of a hereditary hemolytic disorder, and the combination of spherocytes in the peripheral smear, a negative Coombs' test, and a positive, incubated, osmotic fragility test is diagnostic of the condition. At the age of 5 years, she undergoes a splenectomy and has no more hemolytic episodes that require transfusions.

Selected Readings

Charache, S., B. Lubin, and C. D. Reid (eds.). Management and Therapy of Sickle Cell Disease. NIH Publication No. 89-2117, 1989.

Gaston, M. H., et al. Prophylaxis with oral penicillin in children with sickle cell anemia. N. Engl. J. Med. 314:1593, 1986.

Giardina, P. J., and M. W. Hilgartner. Update on thalassemia. Pediatr. Rev. 13:55–62, 1992.

Oski, F. A. Iron deficiency in infancy and childhood. N. Engl. J. Med. 329:190–193, 1993.

BLEEDING DISORDERS

Pamela S. Cohen, M.D.

H$_x$ An 8-year-old girl who has been healthy is brought to the office with a two-week history of increased bruises and nosebleeds. On physical examination, hypertension, petechiae, and ecchymosis are evident, but no lymphadenopathy or hepatomegaly is seen. Dried blood is present around the nares. The initial laboratory evaluation includes a CBC, which is normal, except for a platelet count of 7000/mL. The ESR is 105 mm/hr, and a urinalysis is 2+ for protein.

Questions

1. What conditions should be considered when easy bruisability is the chief complaint?
2. What is the appropriate laboratory workup for children with clinical signs of bleeding disorders?
3. What management is appropriate for the most common pediatric bleeding disorders?

Bruises are a common finding in children and usually reflect their activity level. However, bruises as well as mucosal bleeding may be indicative of a clotting disorder. Such disorders most commonly involve disturbances in number or function of platelets or in one or more of the factors essential in the formation of normal clots.

EPIDEMIOLOGY

HEMOPHILIA A   HEMOPHILIA B

Classic hemophilia, a hereditary deficiency of factor VIII, is the most commonly diagnosed coagulation factor deficiency. Factor IX deficiency, or Christmas disease, another sex-linked disease, is second in terms of prevalence. Other factor deficiencies are quite rare.

Genetics control the occurrence of factor deficiencies. Infections, most often viral, can precede the development of acute ITP and aplastic anemia. Dietary deficiency of vitamin K, caused by intestinal disease or malabsorption, or failure to provide the breast-fed neonate with exogenous vitamin K, can give rise to a bleeding diathesis.

CLINICAL PRESENTATION

Bleeding disorders can manifest themselves in various ways, depending on etiology. Children with deficiencies of clotting factors that cause diseases such as hemophilia often present with ecchymosis (often multiple), bleeding from mucous membranes (e.g., nasal, oral, vaginal), and bleeding into large joints (e.g.,

elbows, knees, hips). CNS hemorrhage or retroperitoneal bleeding may also occur. Newborn males with hemophilia who undergo circumcision first come to medical attention because of unceasing bleeding after the procedure. Bleeding disorders involving platelet number or function are also characterized by mucous membrane bleeding but usually lead to petechiae rather than large ecchymoses (D$_x$ Box).

PATHOPHYSIOLOGY

Normally, hemostasis occurs following vascular injury. Platelets adhere via von Willebrand's factor to the exposed vascular endothelium and release thromboxane A$_2$, causing local vasoconstriction and further platelet aggregation. The activated platelets then release granules containing adhesive factors (factor V) and serve as a template for the coagulation factor cascade. This ultimately leads to the formation of thrombin and fibrin (Figs. 58–1 and 58–2). This platelet-fibrin collection, called the hemostatic plug, becomes a permanent barrier to further blood loss at the site of vessel injury.

Effective hemostasis depends on blood platelets, plasma proteins with coagulation factors, and components of the vessel wall. Changes in either the number or function of any of these elements can result in hemorrhaging.

DIFFERENTIAL DIAGNOSIS

Disorders involving coagulation factors can be either hereditary or acquired. **Hereditary deficiencies** include the various factor deficiencies such as factor VIII deficiency (hemophilia), factor IX deficiency (Christmas disease), and other rare factor deficiencies, such as defects or dysfunctional production of factors I (fibrinogen), II (prothrombin), V, VII, X, XI, XIII, α_2-antiplasmin, and α_1-antitrypsin.

Acquired deficiencies may result from vitamin K-dependent conditions, liver disease, blood transfusions, or the presence of certain factor inhibitors.

D$_x$ Bleeding Disorders

- Easy bruising with minimal or no trauma
- Ecchymosis, petechiae
- Mucosal bleeding (e.g., oral, nasal, vaginal, urinary)
- Anemia (if bleeding has been extensive or chronic)

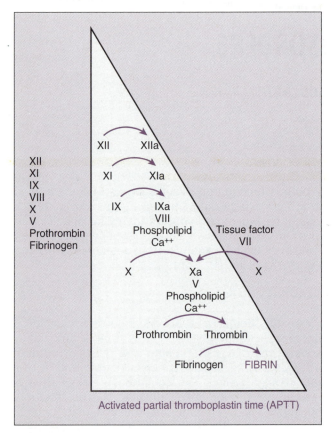

FIGURE 58-1. *Activated partial thromboplastin time (APTT).* The portion of the coagulation mechanism measured by the APTT is enclosed within the triangle, with the clotting factor to which the APTT is sensitive to the left. (Redrawn, with permission, from Nathan, D.G., and F.A. Oski [eds.]. Hematology of Infancy and Childhood, 4th ed. Philadelphia, W.B. Saunders, 1993, p. 1194.)

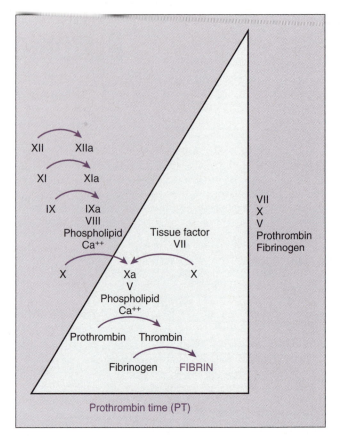

FIGURE 58-2. *Prothrombin time (PT).* The portion of the coagulation mechanism measured by the PT is enclosed within the triangle, with the clotting factors to which the PT is sensitive listed to the right. (Redrawn, with permission, from Nathan, D.G., and F.A. Oski [eds.]. Hematology of Infancy and Childhood, 4th ed. Philadelphia, W.B. Saunders, 1993, p. 1195.)

Factors II, VII, IX, and X depend on vitamin K for appropriate synthesis in the liver. Causes of the depletion of vitamin K–dependent factors include antibiotic use (especially for "bowel preps"), obstructive jaundice, malabsorptive states, parenchymal liver disease, and vitamin K deficiency in the newborn and exclusively breast-fed infant, especially if the mother is a lacto-ovo-vegetarian. The liver makes the vitamin K–dependent factors II, VII, IX, and X, as well as I and V. In addition, fibrin split products are normally cleared by the liver and therefore may be elevated in parenchymal liver disease, making the coagulation profile difficult to differentiate from DIC. It should be noted that because factor VIII is not made by the liver, normal factor VIII measurement is a way to distinguish liver disease from DIC, in which all factors are consumed.

Massive blood transfusions may also result in acquired factor deficiencies. Children who receive large volumes (35 mL/kg) of blood may have low levels of platelets and factors V and VIII.

Acquired factor inhibitors are usually only seen in children with hemophilia who receive regular transfusions with factor replacement and in children with autoimmune disorders. These inhibitors are rare in children with lymphoma.

Platelet disorders may be classified into two groups: disorders of platelet number (thrombocytopenia) (Table 58–1) and disorders of platelet function (thrombasthenia).

Thrombocytopenia is defined as a platelet count less than 150,000/mL. Spontaneous clinical bleeding does not usually occur until the platelet count is 20,000/mL or

---

**TABLE 58–1. Causes of Most Cases (95%)
of Thrombocytopenia in Children**

Destructive Thrombocytopenias
Primary platelet consumption syndromes (immunologic)
  Idiopathic thrombocytopenic purpura
  Infection-induced thrombocytopenia
  Autoimmune or lymphoproliferative disorders
  Allergy and anaphylaxis
            Impaired or Ineffective Production
Acquired disorders
  Aplastic anemia
  Marrow infiltrative processes
Sequestration
  Hypersplenism

Adapted, with permission, from Nathan, D.G., and F.A. Oski (eds.). Hematology of Infancy and Childhood, 4th ed. Philadelphia, W.B. Saunders, 1993.

less, in the absence of trauma. **Acute idiopathic thrombocytopenic purpura (ITP),** which occurs primarily in young children under 5 years of age, usually follows an intercurrent infection, often viral. Unless children bleed substantially, no abnormalities except thrombocytopenia should be evident on the CBC on initial evaluation. Except for petechiae and bruising, the physical examination should be normal. Enlargement of the liver, spleen, or lymph nodes should prompt a search for alternative etiologies (e.g., leukemia, HIV infection). **Chronic ITP** occurs in older, usually female children, and is not ordinarily preceded by a viral illness. Chronic ITP can be either preceded or followed by the development of SLE. By definition, the designation of chronic ITP is not made until patients have had thrombocytopenia for at least six months.

Hemolytic-uremic syndrome is associated with acute hemolytic anemia, thrombocytopenia, and renal failure in infants and young children. Despite the frequent occurrence of thrombocytopenia, bleeding is uncommon. HIV infection can often present as isolated thrombocytopenia in children. This occurs because of the production of antiplatelet antibodies and is often associated with concomitant autoimmune hemolytic anemia (Evans' syndrome).

Von Willebrand's disease (vWD), an autosomal-dominant disease, is a disorder of platelet function. Pathophysiologically, the plasma von Willebrand's factor (vWF), which is responsible for the adherence of platelets to damaged endothelium, is defective or deficient. In addition, vWF also serves as a carrier protein for factor VIII, so that vWD also results in an effective factor VIII deficiency. Thus in most forms of vWD, the PTT as well as the bleeding time is prolonged. As with factor VIII deficiency, the bleeding diathesis in vWD may be mild, moderate, or severe, depending on the genetic mutation and the extent of deficiency. A large majority of cases of vWD (70–80%) involve a quantitative genetic mutation resulting from a heterozygous deficiency of vWF, resulting in vWF levels between 20 and 40% of normal.

Three other disorders of platelet function are Glanzmann's thrombasthenia, Bernard-Soulier syndrome, and Wiskott-Aldrich syndrome. **Glanzmann's thrombasthenia** results from a defect in Gp IIb/IIIa, the fibrinogen receptor on the surface of platelets that is required for normal platelet aggregation. Patients with this rare disorder can be symptomatic at birth or experience life-threatening bleeding after minor injury. Platelet count is normal in affected individuals, and diagnosis is made by assessment of the platelet Gp IIb/IIIa protein levels.

Bernard-Soulier syndrome results from a defect in platelet glycoprotein Ib, the receptor for vWF, and, like vWD, manifests as a deficiency of platelet aggregation. Platelet counts are slightly lower, but platelet size is somewhat larger than normal.

Patients with **Wiskott-Aldrich syndrome,** which is sex-linked, have severe eczema, a predisposition to opportunistic and pyogenic infections, thrombocytopenia with small platelets, and severe bleeding. The gene affected in this disorder is unknown.

Questions: Bleeding Disorders

- Has the child ever had any episodes of abnormal bleeding? If so, what sites were involved?
- How long has the child experienced bleeding problems?
- Has the child experienced any recent trauma?
- Has the child had any recent infections?
- Do any other family members have bleeding problems?
- (If appropriate) Is menstrual flow heavy? Is it heavier than usual?
- Is the child taking any drugs that might cause bleeding problems?

Disorders of vascular endothelium, such as diseases of elastic tissue formation (e.g., Ehlers-Danlos syndrome, Marfan's syndrome, pseudoxanthoma elasticum), can also give rise to an increased bleeding diathesis because of disruption of the integrity of vascular endothelium.

Children who are victims of **child abuse** may present with ecchymoses suggestive of a coagulopathy. The laboratory assessment fails to reveal clotting deficits in these children (see Chapter 96, Physical Abuse).

EVALUATION

History

It is important to determine whether children have had abnormal bleeding in the past (Questions Box). A family history of easy bruisability suggests the presence of certain diseases (vWD, deficiencies of factor VIII or IX). In addition, physicians should find out if children are taking any medications that can cause platelet dysfunction, as measured by abnormal bleeding time. The list is extensive (Table 58–2); aspirin and other NSAIDs are notorious for this side effect.

Physical Examination

Children with bleeding disorders may have any of the following physical findings: petechiae, multiple ecchymosis, oral mucosal bleeding or oozing, nasal bleeding, vaginal bleeding, hematuria, swollen joints (hemorrhagic), or limitation of movement in the joints if the condition has been chronic.

Patients with findings related to other organ systems, such as organomegaly, may have a systemic disorder with an associated coagulopathy (e.g., lupus, lymphoma, leukemia). Children with chronic bleeding prior to coming to medical attention may have concomitant iron deficiency anemia from ongoing blood loss. Wiskott-Aldrich syndrome should be considered in male infants with severe eczema and thrombocytopenia. Children with abnormal or absent thumbs may have thrombocytopenia with absent radii (TAR) syndrome or other congenital thrombocytopenic syndromes (amegakaryocytopenic thrombocytopenia, Fanconi's anemia).

Laboratory Tests

Screening tests for children who present with a history of severe bleeding include PT, PTT, fibrinogen,

TABLE 58–2. Some Drugs That Inhibit Platelet Function*

Nonsteroidal Anti-inflammatory Drugs
Aspirin†
Beta-Lactam Antibiotics
Penicillins
  Ticarcillin (Ticar, Timentin)
Cephalosporins
  Cefotaxime (Claforan)
Other Drugs
Antibiotics
  Nitrofurantoin (Furadantin, Macrodantin)
Drugs that increase platelet cAMP concentration
  Prostacyclin
Anticoagulants
  Heparin
Cardiovascular drugs
  Propranolol (Inderal)
Psychotropic drugs
  Tricyclic antidepressants
    Imipramine (Tofranil)
  Phenothiazines
    Chlorpromazine (Thorazine)
Anesthetics
  Local
    Dibucaine (Lidocaine)
Narcotics
  Heroin
Oncologic drugs
  Mithramycin
Miscellaneous drugs
  Antihistamines
Foods and Food Additives
Chinese black tree fungus

*This list is by no means exhaustive. Only one drug has been given in each category.
†Used as a therapeutic antithrombotic agent.
Adapted, with permission, from Hoffman, R., et al. Hematology: Basic Principles and Practice. New York, Churchill Livingstone, 1991, p. 1530.

bleeding time, and CBC with platelet count (Tables 58–3 and 58–4). The bleeding time measures duration of bleeding in vivo and assesses platelet function, platelet number, and vascular endothelial integrity. A platelet number of less than 50,000/mL is abnormal. This may be the only abnormal screening result in children with vWD or bleeding due to uremia.

Mixing studies (i.e., mixing patient plasma 1:1 with normal plasma) are the next step if the PT or PTT is abnormal. If patients have a factor deficiency, the addition of 1:1 of normal plasma to patient plasma corrects a prolonged PT or PTT. If patients have a factor inhibitor, such an addition does not shorten the PT or PTT. Consultation with a pediatric hematologist and the hematology laboratory at this point is necessary to best determine what additional studies are necessary.

To avoid treating an unidentified leukemia, a bone marrow aspirate and biopsy is indicated in children with ITP if treatment with intravenous immune globulin (IVIG) has failed and prednisone is being considered. It is also useful in children in whom a marrow failure state (Fanconi's anemia, amegakaryocytic thrombocytopenia) is a possibility.

Imaging Studies

In general, imaging studies are not indicated. Bone films may be taken of the hands and feet in patients with thrombocytopenia to rule out Fanconi's anemia and TAR syndrome.

MANAGEMENT

Management of bleeding disorders in children depends on the diagnosis. In children with classic histories, physical findings, and laboratory features of acute ITP with platelet counts less than 20,000/mL, a trial of IVIG is warranted and is the treatment of choice where it is readily available and cost is not a concern. **Prednisone** is a good alternative but should be given only after leukemia is ruled out with bone marrow aspiration and biopsy. The use of **platelet transfusion** is not generally indicated in autoimmune thrombocytopenia (acute and chronic ITP), because the pathophysiology involves the generation of antibodies that recognize all platelets. In children with chronic ITP, **splenectomy** is indicated if severe thrombocytopenia persists, or treatment is prednisone-dependent. Other treatment modalities include **vinblastine.**

In newborn infants with alloimmune thrombocytopenia, washed irradiated maternal platelets can be transfused to correct bleeding.

HIV-associated thrombocytopenia is also immune-mediated and responds well to IVIG at ITP doses. Sometimes repeated, chronic IVIG is necessary to control the condition.

Nonimmune thrombocytopenia secondary to either decreased production (e.g., aplastic anemia) or increased destruction (DIC) can be treated with platelet transfusions.

For children with factor deficiencies, treatment requires **factor replacement.** Factor VIII replacement for children with hemophilia A can be in the form of cryoprecipitate (for young infants) or purified factor (recombinant or pooled-human). Factor IX replacement can only be in the form of concentrated factor IX (recombinant or pooled-human). HIV infection due to exposure to the blood of large numbers of donors has effectively been eliminated with new purification procedures. Recombinant factor replacement, the ideal choice, is still prohibitively expensive for use by all patients.

Correction of the coagulopathy of vWD depends on the type of vWD (Table 58–5).

In children in whom vitamin K deficiency is strongly suspected as the cause of bleeding, one dose of

TABLE 58–3. Major Screening Tests in Hemostasis

Test	Hemostatic Functions Measured
Prothrombin time	Extrinsic and common pathways of coagulation: factors I, II, V, VII, X
Partial thromboplastin time	Intrinsic and common pathways of coagulation: factors I, II, V, VIII, IX, XI, XII
Bleeding time	Platelet function and number; vascular endothelial integrity
Platelet count and examination of blood smear	Platelet number and morphology

Reproduced, with permission, from Miller, D.R., and R.L. Baehner. Blood Diseases of Infancy and Childhood, 6th ed. St. Louis, C.V. Mosby, 1990, p. 764.

TABLE 58–4. Screening Test Profiles and Diagnostic Procedures Used in Selected Disorders of Hemostasis

Disorder	Screening Test				Diagnostic Procedures
	PC	BT	PT	PTT	
Vascular Disorders					
Henoch-Schönlein purpura	N	N	N	N	Clinical diagnosis only
Ehlers-Danlos syndrome	N	N*	N	N	Clinical diagnosis only
Platelet Disorders					
Idiopathic thrombocytopenic purpura (ITP)	L	P	N	N	Clinical diagnosis supported by bone marrow examination and, if available, tests for platelet antibodies (positive)
Glanzmann's disease (thrombasthenia)	N	P	N	N	Clot retraction (abnormal) and platelet aggregation studies (defective first-phase aggregation)
Aspirin effect	N	P	N	N	Platelet aggregation studies (defective second-phase aggregation)
Coagulation Disorders					
Classic hemophilia	N	N	N	P	Factor VIII assay (deficient activity)
Christmas disease	N	N	N	P	Factor IX assay (deficient activity)
von Willebrand's disease	N	P	N	P	Assays of factor VIII activity, VIII antigen, and ristocetin cofactor activity (all low in typical cases)
Factor VII deficiency	N	N	P	P	Factor VII assay (deficient activity)
Factor X deficiency	N	N	P	P	Factor X assay (deficient assay)
Vitamin K deficiency	N	N*	P	P	Assay of factors II, VII, IX, X (specific deficiencies with other factors normal)
Disseminated intravascular coagulation	L	P	P	P	Assays of factors I, II, V, and VIII (deficient activities) and FDP titer (increased)

*Bleeding time may be prolonged.
Abbreviations: PC, platelet count; BT, standard bleeding time; PT, prothrombin time; PTT, partial thromboplastin time; N, normal result; L, low; P, prolonged.
Reproduced, with permission, from Miller, D.R., and R.L. Baehner. Blood Diseases of Infancy and Childhood, 6th ed. St. Louis, C.V. Mosby, 1990, p. 771.

vitamin K should correct the coagulopathy within 12 to 36 hours.

The coagulopathy of DIC involves both **platelets and coagulation factors** as well as factors regulating thrombosis such as **antithrombin II, protein C,** and **protein S.** Children with DIC should be given fresh-frozen plasma, cryoprecipitate (titrate the use of this to the fibrinogen level), and platelets as needed, while the underlying etiology of the DIC (e.g., infection, shock) is treated. In instances where thrombosis also occurs, continuous infusion of heparin may be indicated.

PROGNOSIS

The prognosis of bleeding disorders in children depends on the diagnosis. The most common cause of bleeding, acute ITP, is a time-limited condition that usually resolves uneventfully, although children with platelet counts under 10,000/mL are at risk of life-threatening CNS hemorrhage. Two thirds of patients with chronic ITP go into remission with splenectomy, but one third continue to be at high risk for severe bleeding.

In some cases, children with factor deficiencies now have access to recombinant factor replacement, which eradicates the problem of HIV and chronic hepatitis in this population, making their prognosis much better. Acquired factor inhibitors develop in patients who do not use recombinant factor replacement, making hemostasis difficult; chronic arthritis from repeated joint hemorrhage and hepatitis remain problems in this group.

TABLE 58–5. Therapeutic Alternatives in the Treatment of von Willebrand's Disease (vWD)

Type of vWD	DDAVP	vWF or FVIII Concentrate	Platelets
I	Preferred treatment if DDAVP proves effective in therapeutic trial	If DDAVP is not effective or if higher levels are required	Not indicated
IIA	Not usually effective; may cause improvement for 1 or 2 hr	Preferred treatment	Not indicated
IIB	May cause further decrease in platelet count	Preferred treatment	Not usually effective
III (platelet-type vWD)	May cause further decrease in platelet count	May cause further decrease in platelet count	Preferred treatment
Untyped vWD	Use with caution; follow platelet count and vWF levels	Preferred treatment in untyped patient with vWD	Not usually required unless patient has platelet-type vWD

Abbreviations: vWF, von Willebrand's factor; DDAVP, desmopressin.
Reproduced, with permission, from Nathan, D.G., and F.A. Oski (eds.). Hematology of Infancy and Childhood, 4th ed. Philadelphia, W.B. Saunders, 1993.

Selected Readings

Beardsley, D. B. Platelet abnormalities in infancy and childhood. *In* Nathan, D. G., and F. A. Oski (eds.). Hematology of Infancy and Childhood, 4th ed. Philadelphia, W.B. Saunders, 1993, pp. 1561–1604.

Blanchette, V. S., et al. A prospective, randomized trial of high-dose intravenous immune globulin G therapy, oral prednisone therapy and no therapy in childhood acute immune thrombocytopenic purpura. J. Pediatr. 123:989–995, 1993.

Hawiger, J., and R. I. Handin. Physiology of hemostasis: cellular aspects. *In* Nathan, D. G., and F. A. Oski (eds.). Hematology of Infancy and Childhood, 4th ed. Philadelphia, W.B. Saunders, 1993, pp. 1494–1533.

Jones, P. K., and O. D. Ratnoff. The changing prognosis of classic hemophilia (factor VIII "deficiency"). Ann. Intern. Med. 114:641–648, 1991.

Montgomery, R. R., and J. P. Scott. Hemostasis: diseases of the fluid phase. *In* Nathan, D. G., and F. A. Oski (eds.). Hematology of Infancy and Childhood, 4th ed. Philadelphia, W.B. Saunders, 1993, pp. 1561–1604.

Pramanik, A. K. Bleeding disorders in neonates. Pediatr. Rev. 13:163–173, 1992.

Soff, G. A., and Rosenberg, R. D. Physiology of hemostasis: the fluid phase. *In* Nathan, D. G., and F. A. Oski (eds.). Hematology of Infancy and Childhood, 4th ed. Philadelphia, W.B. Saunders, 1993, pp. 1534–1560.

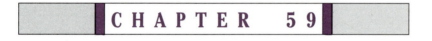

CHAPTER 59

LYMPHADENOPATHY

Pamela S. Cohen, M.D.

Hx An eight-year-old girl is brought to the office with swelling of the anterior cervical nodes, which she has had for four weeks. Intermittent fever with temperatures as high as 38.3° C (101° F) and decreased appetite have been associated with the condition. The girl appears pale. On examination, her temperature is 38.0° C (100.4° F), and her other vital signs are normal. Three to four nontender nodes 1–2 cm in diameter are present bilaterally. The remainder of the examination is normal.

Questions

1. When is lymphadenopathy of medical concern?
2. What are the clinical features of childhood diseases that present as cervical lymphadenopathy?
3. What are the diagnostic approaches to the evaluation of children with lymphadenopathy?
4. What is an appropriate therapeutic approach to cervical adenopathy in children?

Lymphadenopathy is a common physical finding in pediatric patients, because lymph node swelling frequently follows the many infections, most often viral, that affect children. Significant lymphadenopathy, which is indicative of a pathologic process requiring diagnosis and intervention, can be defined on the basis of the characteristics of the affected lymph nodes. The nodes must be: (1) greater than 1.0 cm in diameter in children younger than 12 years of age and greater than 0.5 cm in older children; (2) tender, warm, or erythematous; (3) hard, fixed, or matted; and/or (4) located in the supraclavicular area. Lymphadenopathy refers to enlargement of nodes, and adenitis to inflammation. Lymphadenitis is characterized by tenderness, warmth, and erythema.

EPIDEMIOLOGY

Physicians must be able to distinguish significant lymphadenopathy from benign conditions in order to detect underlying causes such as serious bacterial, viral, and protozoal infections; autoimmune disorders; and malignancy. Infections are the most likely cause of tender or unilateral adenopathy. Eighty percent of neck malignancies in children are the result of non-Hodgkin's lymphoma.

CLINICAL PRESENTATION

Cervical lymphadenopathy is the most common type of lymphadenopathy. Most frequently the cause is viral, and the lymphadenopathy is often **bilateral** in the cervical area, or it may be **generalized.** Cervical or generalized adenopathy may be associated with **hepatosplenomegaly** in children with CMV or EBV. Bacterial invasion of lymph nodes produces lymphadenitis, which is often **unilateral.** Bacterial lymphadenopathy may be accompanied by fever, respiratory symptoms, pharyngitis, and skin lesions. Other clues that may

---

Dx   Lymphadenopathy

- Enlarged lymph nodes
- Fever
- Tenderness or warmth over the lymph nodes (lymphadenitis)
- Pallor
- Weight loss
- Bone pain
- Antecedent infection (e.g., pharyngitis, URI, otitis media)

---

suggest bacterial infection include fluctuance, duration greater than seven days, and dental abnormalities. Lymphadenopathy related to malignancy is often nontender but accompanied by other signs and symptoms such as fever, pallor, and weight loss (Dx Box).

PATHOPHYSIOLOGY

Lymph nodes are the sites at which lymphocytes are exposed to antigens, such as pathogens (e.g., viruses,

bacteria, fungi, etc.), which may provoke a cellular or humorally mediated lymphocyte response. Normally, this response involves proliferation of lymphocytes within the nodes; this can result in clinical lymph node enlargement.

Occasionally, lymph nodes themselves become infected, as in tuberculosis (scrofula). Malignancy, most commonly lymphoma and leukemia, can also occur in or invade lymph nodes. This can cause lymph node enlargement and destruction of the normal lymph node architecture, which is a pathognomonic finding in malignant nodal invasion due to lymphoblasts.

DIFFERENTIAL DIAGNOSIS

Cervical lymphadenopathy may be either inflammatory or noninflammatory. Inflammatory lymphadenopathy, which can be infectious, is most commonly either viral or bacterial in etiology. Most cervical adenopathy is viral in etiology, in which case it is often bilateral, or generalized (Table 59–1).

Staphylococcus aureus is the causative agent in 30 to

TABLE 59–1. Differential Diagnosis of Lymphadenopathy

Diagnostic Category	Clinical Features	Epidemiologic Features	Laboratory Features
Neoplastic Conditions			
Hodgkin's lymphoma	Often associated with "B" symptoms (i.e. fever, weight loss, +/– splenomegaly)	Common among higher socioeconomic groups, only children	↑ ESR (can be >100), ↑ LDH, anergy
Non-Hodgkin's lymphoma	See Hodgkin's lymphoma		
Solid tumors (e.g., rhabdomyosarcoma, neuroblastoma)	Depends on underlying malignancy		
Langerhans cell histiocytosis	Eczema, failure to thrive, bony lesions, diabetes insipidus, proptosis, hepatosplenomegaly all possible		
Sinus histiocytosis with massive lymphadenopathy			
Autoimmune Disorders			
JRA	Generalized lymphadenopathy seen in systemic form (Still's) (i.e., fever, hepatosplenomegaly, evanescent rash, arthritis)	Equal incidence in males and females	↑ ESR, anemia, negative ANA and rheumatoid arthritis in Still's JRA
Lupus	Arthritis, butterfly facial rash, effusions (lung, joint, cardiac), CNS, nephrotic syndrome	Increased incidence in girls, Jewish heritage	↑ ESR, positive ANA, anti-ds DNA, ↓ C3, C4, or CH50, anemia, ↑ platelets, proteinuria
Autoimmune hemolytic anemia	Scleral icterus, splenomegaly +/– hepatomegaly, hemoglobinuria (dark red urine)		Positive Coombs' test, evidence of hemolysis (↑ bilirubin, reticulocytosis)
Infections			
Viral (EBV, CMV, rubella, HIV, cat-scratch disease)	Usually generalized, except for cat-scratch, not purulent or tender		
Mycobacterial (TB, atypical mycobacteria)	Usually localized; often tender, red, flocculent		
Bacterial (staphylococcal and streptococcal infections, tularemia, plague, diphtheria)	Usually localized; often tender, red, flocculent		
Protozoal (toxoplasmosis)	Generalized		
Spirochete (syphilis)			
Fungal (histoplasmosis, coccidioidomycosis)	May be generalized	Suspicion should be raised based on regional incidence	
Granulomatous Disease			
Sarcoidosis	Bilateral hilar lymphadenopathy, noncaseating granulomas (lung, liver)	↑ in those of black and Irish heritage	↑ serum angiotensin-1 converting enzyme (ACE), ↑ serum lysozyme
Chronic granulomatous disease		X-linked	Positive nitroblue tetrazolium test

Abbreviations: ANA, antinuclear antibody; CMV, cytomegalovirus; CNS, central nervous system; EBV, Epstein-Barr virus; ESR, erythrocyte sedimentation rate; JRA, juvenile rheumatoid arthritis; TB, tuberculosis; HIV, human immunodeficiency virus; LDH, lactate dehydrogenase.

40% of cases of bacterial adenitis, followed by group A *Streptococcus pyogenes,* anaerobes, and other species. When the condition appears subacute, cat-scratch disease, tuberculosis, atypical mycobacteria, toxoplasmosis, tularemia, and the more uncommon diseases such as histoplasmosis, brucellosis, and syphilis should be considered.

The cellulitis-adenitis syndrome seen in newborns is consistent with immunodeficiency, especially HIV. HIV, as well as EBV, CMV, and toxoplasmosis, may be associated with diffuse lymphadenopathy.

The noninfectious inflammatory causes of cervical lymphadenopathy include collagen-vascular diseases (e.g., juvenile rheumatoid arthritis, SLE) or other diseases such as chronic granulomatous disease and Kawasaki's disease. Noninflammatory causes of cervical lymphadenopathy include congenital causes (e.g., thyroglossal duct cyst, branchial cleft cyst, cystic hygroma) and neoplasms. Such neoplasms include Hodgkin's and non-Hodgkin's lymphoma; leukemia and other solid tumors that metastasize to the neck lymph nodes such as neuroblastoma, rhabdomyosarcoma, and fibrosarcoma; and thyroid carcinoma. In both types of lymphomas, nontender, rubbery nodes are usually characteristic. In Hodgkin's disease, the nodes enlarge sequentially, with involvement spreading from one chain to the next, rather than bilaterally. Nodes in Hodgkin's disease are often matted, whereas in non-Hodgkin's disease, the nodes may be large, but they are usually bilateral and not always matted.

EVALUATION

History

In patients with lymphadenopathy, physicians should always inquire about the duration of the lymphadenopathy, the rapidity of node enlargement, and the occurrence of associated fever and other constitutional symptoms such as weight loss, itching, or coughing. A history of distant travel; recent travel to areas with endemic histoplasmosis (southeastern United States) or coccidioidomycosis (San Joaquin Valley, CA); a detailed history of pet contact (cats, which transmit toxoplasmosis and cat-scratch disease); and exposure to ill contacts, particular individuals known to have tuberculosis, are also important (Questions Box).

Questions: Lymphadenopathy

- For how long have the nodes been enlarged?
- Was the child sick before the swelling began?
- Does the child have any symptoms now, such as fever, weight loss, pallor, or anorexia?
- Does the child come in contact with any animals, particularly cats?
- Has the child traveled anywhere?
- Is the child taking any medications?
- Has the child been in contact with anyone who is ill?

Physical Examination

The enlarged nodes should be measured and examined at their widest diameter and evaluated for evidence of redness, tenderness, and increased warmth, which are suggestive of infection. The extent of the lymphadenopathy should be assessed, as well as whether there is enlargement of the liver or spleen. Other physical findings depend on the underlying etiology (see Table 59–1).

Laboratory Tests

Laboratory tests used in the evaluation of lymphadenopathy depend on the location and distribution of the adenopathy (unilateral, bilateral, or diffuse). Needle aspirate for Gram's stain and culture is often helpful. CBC, ESR, liver function tests (elevated in EBV and CMV), a throat culture, and a PPD are appropriate screening studies. Viral studies (e.g., EBV, CMV, HIV) and skin tests for fungal disease may be indicated. In lupus and rheumatoid arthritis, antinuclear antibody (ANA) may be positive and complement levels may be reduced.

Lymph node biopsies are needed to diagnose lymphoma. Physicians should consult the pathologist about whether needle or excisional biopsy technique is preferred for two reasons: (1) in 13 to 35% of cases in which biopsy is performed, nodes are ultimately malignant; and (2) most pathologists insist on visualizing the entire lymph node to make the diagnosis of lymphoma. In patients with lymphoma, a bone marrow aspirate and biopsy may also be positive.

Imaging Studies

A chest x-ray should be performed in any child with suspected scrofula or malignancy. Other imaging studies are not routinely used, unless the diagnosis of malignant lymphoma is made. In these cases, CT scans of the neck, chest, abdomen, and pelvis, as well as gallium scan, are performed to stage the disease.

MANAGEMENT

Infection is the most common cause of cervical adenopathy. A trial of **antibiotics** with antistaphylococcal coverage is appropriate for tender, unilateral cervical node enlargement. **PPD testing** should also be carried out. If the adenopathy is unresponsive and the PPD is negative, a lymph node biopsy should be considered. Other indications for node biopsy include (1) supraclavicular adenopathy of unexplained etiology, (2) fixation of a node to overlying skin, (3) persistent adenopathy with nodes over 3 cm if cat-scratch disease is believed unlikely and cultures and PPD are negative.

Underlying fungal and mycobacterial diseases should be treated with appropriate **antifungal or antibacterial agents,** with the exception of cervical adenopathy due to atypical mycobacteria, which requires **surgical removal.** Malignant disorders such as lymphoma and leukemia require **multimodal therapy** with surgery, chemotherapy, or radiation, depending on the specific disorder and the extent of disease (see Chapter 105, Cancer in Children). Children with HIV are often managed by a multidisciplinary team, with primary care practitioners usually acting as key players in the day-to-day management of these children (see Chapter 106, Pediatric HIV Infection).

PROGNOSIS

The outcome of lymphadenopathy depends entirely on the underlying disorder (see Table 59–1). In the vast majority of cases, the cause is infectious, and the lymphadenopathy resolves completely with the use of appropriate antibiotics.

Case Resolution

In the case history, the bilateral nature of the swelling and the lack of tenderness of the nodes are very worrisome and suggest a noninfectious etiology. The girl had a throat culture, an intermediate PPD, and a chest x-ray, all of which were negative. A CBC reveals leukocytes with 28,000 WBCs/μL (60% lymphocytes), with a normal hemoglobin and platelet count. A heterophil test for infectious mononucleosis is positive. Bed rest is recommended, and the child makes a complete recovery in three weeks.

Selected Readings

Filston, H. C. Common lumps and bumps of the head and neck in infants and children. Pediatr. Ann. 18:180–186, 1989.

Gilchrist, G. S., and R. G. Evans. Contemporary issues in pediatric Hodgkin's disease. Pediatr. Clin. North Am. 32:721–734, 1985.

Hicks, R. B., and M. E. Melish. Kawasaki syndrome. Pediatr. Clin. North Am. 33:1151–1176, 1986.

Huebner, R. E., et al. Usefulness of skin testing with mycobacterial antigens in children with cervical lymphadenopathy. Pediatr. Infect. Dis. 1:450–456, 1992.

Knight, P. J., A. F. Mulne, and L. E. Vassy. When is lymph node biopsy indicated in children with enlarged peripheral nodes? Pediatrics 69:391–396, 1982.

Knight, P. J., and C. B. Reiner. Superficial lumps in children: what, when and why? Pediatrics 72:147–153, 1983.

Kurtzberg, J., and M. L. Graham. Non-Hodgkin's lymphoma: biologic classification and implications for therapy. Pediatr. Clin. North Am. 38:443–456, 1991.

Lake, A. M., and F. A. Oski. Peripheral lymphadenopathy in childhood. Am. J. Dis. Child. 132:357–359, 1978.

Leventhal, B. G., and G. J. Kato. Childhood Hodgkin and non-Hodgkin lymphomas. Pediatr. Rev. 12:171, 1990.

Marcy, S. M. Infections of lymph nodes of the head and neck. Pediatr. Infect. Dis. 2:397–405, 1983.

Pollock, B. H., J. P. Krischer, and T. J. Vietti. Interval between symptom onset and diagnosis of pediatric solid tumors. J. Pediatr. 119:725–732, 1991.

Zitelli, B. J. Evaluating the child with a neck mass. Contemp. Pediatr. 7:90–112, 1990.

CHAPTER 60

HEART MURMURS

Robin Winkler Doroshow, M.D.

H$_x$ A six-year-old girl is brought to the office for a physical examination for school. Her past medical history is unremarkable, and her growth and development have been normal. She is entirely asymptomatic. Her physical examination is normal except for a grade II/VI low-pitched vibratory systolic ejection murmur that is loudest at the left lower sternal border, with radiation to the apex and upper sternal border. The murmur increases to III/VI in the supine position.

Questions

1. What is the significance of a heart murmur in asymptomatic children? How reassuring are negative findings and history?
2. What workup should be done by primary care physicians?
3. What are the costs of excessive tests and unnecessary consultation? What are the costs of inadequate workup?
4. When should physicians refer children to specialists for consultation?

Asymptomatic children with heart murmurs are commonly encountered by physicians. Murmurs are a finding rather than a medical sign or symptom because they are detected incidentally at an examination conducted for another purpose.

Correct assessment of the significance of a heart murmur is important to ensure appropriate management of children with heart disease. Complications of undiagnosed cardiac disease in children include progressive hemodynamic impairment, endocarditis, and even sudden death.

The misinterpretation of an innocent murmur as organic in nature can also take its toll, primarily on parental anxiety. Unnecessary restriction of activities may result, which can have a negative impact on children's school life and social life as well as self-image. As adults these children may be denied health insurance, life insurance, and certain types of employment. In addition, misdiagnosis costs money and utilizes limited resources, with unnecessary tests and doctor visits, as this "non-disease" is evaluated and followed.

EPIDEMIOLOGY

An estimated 50% of healthy children have heart murmurs. The overall incidence of congenital heart disease (CHD), including symptomatic cases, is just under 1%, and some children with CHD have no murmur. Therefore, about 99 out of 100 murmurs are innocent.

CLINICAL PRESENTATION

Heart murmurs are usually detected on routine examination for well child care or on evaluation for an unrelated problem. Innocent murmurs are not associated with signs or symptoms because they are normal findings. The majority of the complaints sometimes associated with organic murmurs (i.e., murmurs of heart disease) are related to the presence of congestive heart failure (CHF) (see Chapter 62). Some children with murmurs come to medical attention with complaints of exercise intolerance or chest pain. It is necessary to determine whether these problems are actually referable to the heart.

PATHOPHYSIOLOGY

A murmur is a sustained sound that can be detected with a stethoscope placed on the chest. This sound is produced by turbulence of blood flow in the heart or great vessels. This turbulence may be due to structural abnormalities (e.g., aortic valve stenosis), benign or normal flow patterns (see below), or exaggeration of normal flow patterns (seen in high output states such as fever, exercise, or anemia, and sometimes termed "functional").

Not all significant heart disease in children is heralded by a murmur. Structural heart disease may be "silent" and be indicated by other findings. For example, transposition of the great arteries results in cyanosis, anomalous pulmonary venous return in CHF, hypoxia

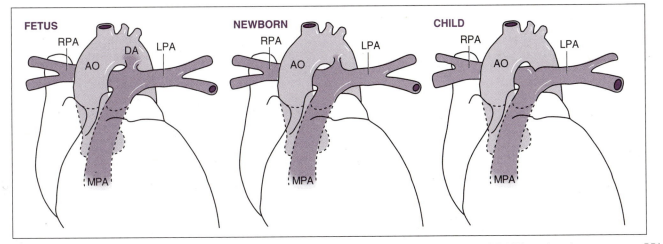

FIGURE 60–1. *Configuration of the central pulmonary arteries in the fetus, the newborn, and the child.* MPA, *main pulmonary artery;* RPA, *right pulmonary artery;* LPA, *left pulmonary artery;* DA, *ductus arteriosus;* AO, *aorta.*

and anomalous origin of the left coronary artery in CHF. Acquired heart disease such as Kawasaki's syndrome, myocarditis, or cardiomyopathy often produces no murmur.

The common innocent murmurs are better recognized than understood. Because they occur in normal, healthy individuals, there are few hemodynamic or anatomic data to correlate with the murmur, and pathophysiology is in some cases conjectural. **Still's murmur**, which was once thought to be due to easily appreciated aortic valve flow, is now believed to result from vibration of normal fibrous bands that cross the left ventricle. This murmur may also be heard in children who have undergone spontaneous closure of a membranous ventricular septal defect, with a small residual aneurysm in the septum. The **pulmonary flow murmur** appears to be caused by normal flow across the pulmonary valve, perhaps made more apparent because of high cardiac output, close proximity to the chest wall, and (in adolescent females) mild anemia. The **venous hum** is attributed to turbulence at the confluence of the innominate veins, which is exacerbated in the upright position by gravity.

The **physiologic peripheral pulmonic stenosis (PPPS) murmur** in newborns is produced by turbulence at the origins of the left and right pulmonary arteries. Because less than 10% of the combined ventricular output of the fetus goes to these branches, they are small and arise at a sharp angle from the main pulmonary artery. When postnatal circulation abruptly requires the entire cardiac output to enter these vessels, a relative stenosis is encountered (Fig. 60–1). This physiologic stenosis resolves gradually with remodeling of the pulmonary artery tree by two to three months of age.

DIFFERENTIAL DIAGNOSIS

In healthy children, the differential diagnosis of a heart murmur includes innocent murmurs and murmurs resulting from structural lesions (Table 60–1). The specific features of a particular murmur usually provide the clue to the diagnosis.

Some features may alert examiners to the organic nature of a murmur. Although very loud murmurs (grades IV–VI) are usually not innocent, some innocent murmurs may be as loud as grade III. Diastolic murmurs and continuous murmurs, other than the easily recognizable venous hum, are usually pathologic, as are high-pitched and harsh murmurs.

The common innocent murmurs of childhood are recognizable on auscultatory examination. **Still's murmur**, or the **innocent vibratory murmur**, is a low-pitched, vibratory, or musical murmur that sounds like a groan. Because of its low frequency, the murmur is better heard with the bell. It is loudest at the left lower sternal border but is often distributed widely over the precordium. This murmur is often quite loud and is extremely common in school-age children. The characteristics of the murmur are diagnostic, although the absence of other findings is supportive.

The **pulmonary flow murmur**, usually heard in older children, is a short, blowing systolic ejection (i.e., crescendo-decrescendo) murmur localized to the left upper sternal border. It may be louder in the supine position.

The **venous hum** is a soft continuous murmur, similar to the sound heard in a seashell. Because of its constancy, it is often overlooked. This murmur is very commonly heard in preschool and school-age children. Loudest in the right infraclavicular area, it may also be heard on the left. This murmur is highly variable with head and neck position and compression of the neck

TABLE 60–1.   Common Organic Murmurs in Asymptomatic Children

Lesion	Other Clues
Atrial septal defect	Fixed split S_2
Ventricular septal defect (small to moderate)	Loud heart sounds
Patent ductus arteriosus (small to moderate)	Full or bounding pulses
Pulmonic stenosis	Systolic ejection click (SEC)
Aortic stenosis	SEC; suprasternal thrill
Coarctation of the aorta	Weak or absent femoral pulses

veins, which may increase or diminish it. It usually disappears in the supine position.

The **PPPS** murmur is an innocent murmur found in newborns. Best heard at the upper sternal border, this blowing systolic ejection murmur radiates strikingly over the lung fields into the back and both axillae.

EVALUATION

History

The history may be helpful in assessment of children with a murmur. If a thorough history shows that children have no symptoms, this suggests the absence of severe heart disease and helps exclude many major or complex defects as well as CHF.

The most common symptom reported by children or parents is easy fatigability (Questions Box). This is difficult to quantitate. Determining exercise intolerance on the basis of history is very subjective; it may be due, of course, to noncardiac causes and may be unrelated to the murmur. Chest pain, a common symptom in adults with heart disease, is rarely cardiac in origin in children. A history of rapid breathing, excessive sweating, and other complaints referable to CHF suggests organic heart disease. Central cyanosis (i.e., involving the oral mucosa rather than the perioral area or the fingers) may be reported by parents of children with cyanotic CHD but is often not recognized.

Physical Examination

The physical examination often gives strong clues to the cardiac diagnosis beyond the murmur itself. Even in children with known CHD, the nonauscultatory portions of the examination are critical in assessing the cardiac status (i.e., how the patient is tolerating the defect).

Vital signs, preferably obtained with the child at rest or sleeping, yield more information regarding cardiac status than specific diagnosis. Tachypnea and tachycardia are present in CHF. A normal resting respiratory rate (i.e., < 60/minute in infants) argues strongly against CHF. Blood pressure is normal in most patients with CHD. It is necessary to measure blood pressure in the legs especially if coarctation of the aorta is suspected because of diminished pulses in the lower extremities.

The **growth pattern** may reflect the presence of any chronic illness, including hemodynamically significant congenital heart disease. Affected patients, particularly

infants and children with large left-to-right shunts (with or without CHF) gain weight poorly. Height and head circumference are usually normal, although in more severe or prolonged situations, height may also be affected.

A complete **cardiac examination** should be performed. Is the chest asymmetric, a sign of long-standing cardiomegaly? Is the precordial impulse hyperdynamic? Are extra sounds (e.g., clicks, rubs, gallops) heard? Is the second sound normal in intensity and in width and motion of splitting?

Additional pertinent findings include lethargy, dysmorphic features suggestive of a genetic syndrome, central cyanosis, and clubbing. Hepatomegaly is found in children with CHF. The peripheral pulses should be normal in volume, neither diminished (e.g., pedal pulses in coarctation) nor bounding (e.g., in patent ductus arteriosus), and equal in all extremities. The temperature and capillary refill of the extremities in children who are not overexposed reflect adequacy of the peripheral circulation.

Diagnostic Studies

Routine laboratory studies are not warranted in the evaluation of most murmurs. An **ECG** is indicated when heart disease is known or strongly suspected. In some cases, such as with echocardiography, the manner in which the examination is actually carried out may vary depending on the suspected diagnosis. Such tests are not suitable for screening purposes.

MANAGEMENT

If a heart murmur is suspected of being organic in origin because of its features or associated findings, referral to a pediatric cardiologist is indicated. In the case of asymptomatic children there is no urgency, but parental and physician anxiety can best be allayed by proceeding to consultation promptly (i.e., within weeks). In some cases, a repeat examination may be useful before deciding whether to consult a specialist, particularly if the murmur is initially heard under nonphysiologic conditions such as fever. Tests are usually best utilized if selected and ordered by specialists. Not all cardiologists perform all tests on all patients.

Management of organic heart disease in infants or children is also best handled by specialists. Treatment may include **medications, interventional catheterization,** or **cardiac surgery.** Communication with pediatricians, however, is essential to delivery of optimal patient care.

If the murmur is innocent, physicians must complete the following steps:

1. Children and their families must be informed about the presence of the murmur. Even if the murmur is benign, children have a right to know that it was heard. In addition, they are likely to be examined by other practitioners who will report it, which may lead to the suspicion of either a new murmur or negligence on the part of the first examiner.

Questions: Heart Murmurs

- Is the child easily tired?
  - Does the child keep up with others of his or her age?
  - If the child is having a good time—for example, at a park or a party—how is the child's endurance?
- Does the child have a family history of CHD?
- Was the child exposed antenatally to possible teratogens?
- Does the child ever complain of chest pain? At rest or with activity?
- Does the child ever appear blue?
- Does the child perspire excessively?

2. The diagnosis must be clearly explained to parents and children (depending on the age). It is essential that they understand that this is a normal finding rather than a minor abnormality. In some cases, notification of teachers or athletic coaches may be appropriate. Physicians must stress that no further evaluation is needed and no restrictions are indicated. Printed brochures that explain innocent murmurs are available from organizations such as the American Heart Association.

3. The description of the murmur and the diagnosis itself must be documented in the medical record. A murmur that is clearly and unequivocally innocent, with no evidence of heart disease, should not affect the child's access to insurance, participation in sports, etc. Medical documentation also helps protect patients from unnecessary reevaluations in the future.

4. Physicians should proceed no further. No laboratory studies or consultations need be performed. If the evaluation has been completed by a specialist because of suspicion of CHD by the referring physician, no follow-up with the specialist is indicated. Patients are referred back to their primary practitioners.

PROGNOSIS

The prognosis for children with heart murmurs depends on the cause of the murmur. Children with an innocent murmur, who by definition have normal hearts, have a normal prognosis—with one exception. If children or their parents mistakenly believe children to have heart disease, parents may treat the children inappropriately (e.g., unnecessary testing, restriction of activities). As a result, children may develop sedentary habits and inferior self-image.

With appropriate medical attention, the prognosis is normal or near-normal in the majority of cases of CHD. Children with minor defects not requiring intervention

(e.g., small ventricular septal defect, mild pulmonic stenosis) need only endocarditis prophylaxis (e.g., for dental procedures) and infrequent cardiology follow-up. With the development of refined cardiac surgery and interventional catheterization, even children with the most complex cardiac anomalies now have a good outlook with respect to both daily living and life expectancy.

Case Resolution

In the case presented, a healthy girl with no history of cardiovascular symptoms has a heart murmur and otherwise unremarkable physical examination. The murmur is a typical Still's (innocent vibratory) murmur, which is identifiable by its low-pitched, vibratory quality. No further evaluation is necessary. The diagnosis is explained, the girl and her parents are reassured, and the murmur and diagnosis are noted in the medical record.

Selected Readings

Bergman, A. B., and S. J. Stamm. The morbidity of cardiac nondisease in school children. N. Engl. J. Med. 276:1008–1013, 1967.
Danford, D. A., et al. Cost assessment of the evaluation of heart murmurs in children. Pediatrics 91:365–368, 1993.
Helfant, R. H., et al. Role of cardiac testing in an era of proliferating technology and cost containment. J. Am. Coll. Cardiol. 9:1194–1198, 1987.
Hohn, A. R. Congenital heart disease—the first test. West. J. Med. 156:435–436, 1992. (Editorial.)
Kimball, T. R., et al. Effect of digoxin on contractility and symptoms in infants with a large ventricular septal defect. Am. J. Cardiol. 68:1137–1382, 1991.
Liebman, J. Diagnosis and management of heart murmurs in children. Pediatr. Rev. 3:321–329, 1982.
Linde, L. M. Assessing chest pain in children and adolescents. Prim. Cardiol. 19:55–58, 1993.
Moss, A. J. Clues in diagnosing congenital heart disease. West. J. Med. 156:392–398, 1992.
Smythe, J. F., et al. Initial evaluation of heart murmurs: are laboratory tests necessary? Pediatrics 86:497–500, 1990.

CHAPTER 61

CYANOSIS IN THE NEWBORN

Robin Winkler Doroshow, M.D.

Hx A 3500-gram, term male infant born to a 29-year-old, gravida II para II, healthy mother by spontaneous vaginal delivery is well until 24 hours of age when a nurse notes that he is cyanotic. On examination, he appears blue but in no distress. The vital signs are temperature (axillary), 37° C (98.6° F); pulse, 130; respirations, 40; and blood pressure, 80/60 in the right arm. His general appearance is normal except for the cyanosis. His heart sounds are normal, and no murmur is heard. His liver is not palpable, and the peripheral pulses are normal and equal in all extremities. Capillary refill is normal. Oxygen saturation is 65% by pulse oximetry.

Questions

1. What are the causes of cyanosis in newborns?
2. What is the appropriate evaluation of cyanosis in newborns?
3. How urgent is the assessment? What are the risks and benefits of further evaluation?
4. Which aspects of management should be initiated by a primary physician at a community hospital?
5. Which types of treatment should be undertaken by the consulting pediatric cardiologist at the referral center?

Cyanosis is a bluish appearance of the skin due to the presence of reduced hemoglobin in the tissues. Central cyanosis, which is detected initially in the oral mucosa and nailbeds but is generalized when severe, indicates at least 4–5 grams of reduced hemoglobin per 100 mL blood. Hypoxemia is usually the cause. This condition is frequently present in neonates with pulmonary pathology but is also one of the most common presentations of severe congenital heart disease (CHD).

Because cyanotic CHD in newborns may be life-threatening, it must not go undiagnosed. Most diagnostic studies have minimal risk. Even the risk of cardiac catheterization in this setting is relatively low. Most of the lesions that cause cyanotic CHD can be palliated or corrected, and the prognosis is good.

EPIDEMIOLOGY

Cyanotic CHD occurs in about two to three of every 1000 live born infants. Approximately 80 to 90% of these cases, usually the most severe ones, are detected in the first 30 days of life. Infants with low pulmonary blood flow or lesions causing poor mixing present most often with obvious cyanosis, although initially they otherwise appear well and comfortable. Those with high pulmonary flow are less blue and often present first with congestive heart failure (CHF) or a murmur.

Most cyanotic CHD is not diagnosed before birth. The antenatal history, gestational age, birth weight, and delivery room examination are unremarkable. CHD is more likely in some situations that can be anticipated prenatally (Table 61–1). In these settings, increased suspicion may lead to antenatal detection using echocardiography.

TABLE 61–1. Settings With Increased Risk of Congenital Heart Disease

Genetic syndromes (e.g., trisomies, diGeorge's syndrome)
Certain extracardiac anomalies (e.g., omphalocele, forearm anomalies)
Maternal diabetes poorly controlled during first trimester
Exposure to cardiac teratogen (e.g., lithium, isotretinoin)
High incidence of congenital heart disease in family
Fetal or neonatal arrhythmia

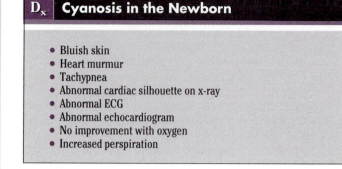

Dx Cyanosis in the Newborn

- Bluish skin
- Heart murmur
- Tachypnea
- Abnormal cardiac silhouette on x-ray
- Abnormal ECG
- Abnormal echocardiogram
- No improvement with oxygen
- Increased perspiration

CLINICAL PRESENTATION

Children with cyanotic CHD often present within the first week of life with blueness of the oral mucosa. In more severe cases, generalized blueness occurs. The abnormal color may be more apparent with effort (e.g., feeding, passing stool) or crying. Respiratory distress is a minor or absent finding in cyanotic CHD. The condition does not have a respiratory cause. In cases of severe hypoxia, metabolic acidosis leads to poor perfusion and compensatory tachypnea. Additional findings depend on the nature of the causal lesion (Dx Box).

PATHOPHYSIOLOGY

Cardiac cyanosis is due to **right-to-left shunting** so that systemic venous blood bypasses the pulmonary circulation and enters the systemic circulation. Two conditions are necessary to produce this type of shunting: communication, such as a septal defect, for the blood to shunt across; and some cause, such as pulmonic stenosis, for the blood to be shunted away from the lungs. Most cyanotic lesions are complex but they are usually named by the most prominent abnormality (e.g., tricuspid atresia). The most notable exception is simple transposition of the great arteries (TGA), where the fundamental connections are abnormal, and all venous blood is directed to the systemic circulation. Lesions associated with cyanosis may be divided into three groups.

1. The **low pulmonary blood flow (LPBF) group** consists of tetralogy of Fallot, pulmonary atresia with intact ventricular septum, and virtually any combination of defects that includes pulmonary atresia or severe stenosis. Pulmonary flow is diminished and may derive entirely from the ductus arteriosus while it remains patent. Aside from obvious cyanosis, infants often appear well.
2. The **high pulmonary blood flow (HPBF) group** includes truncus arteriosus, single ventricle, and combinations of defects that involve mixing of oxygenated and unoxygenated blood and little or no obstruction to pulmonary flow. Although a right-to-left shunt is present, the left-to-right shunt is even greater. Pulmonary venous return is therefore voluminous and contributes disproportionately to sys-

TABLE 61–2.   Noncardiac Causes of Neonatal Cyanosis

Pulmonary infection (e.g., group B streptococcal infection)
Aspiration (e.g., meconium aspiration syndrome, tracheoesophageal fistula)
Pulmonary hypoplasia (e.g., Potter's syndrome, diaphragmatic hernia)
Respiratory distress syndrome (e.g., in prematurity)
Thoracic hypoplasia (e.g., thanatophoric dwarfism)
Hypoventilation (e.g., neurologic depression)
Persistent fetal circulation

temic output. Cyanosis is less apparent. Pulmonary flow increases as the pulmonary vascular resistance falls and CHF develops, as in patients with isolated shunt lesions (e.g., ventricular septal defect). Some children with HPBF lesions also have obstruction to systemic blood flow (e.g., coarctation of the aorta, hypoplastic left heart syndrome) and may depend on the ductus arteriosus to carry some or all of this flow.

3. The **poor mixing group** is limited to TGA and its variants. The right and left circuits are in parallel rather than in series, and survival depends on interchange of oxygenated and unoxygenated blood between them. Most newborns with poor mixing present with marked cyanosis, like patients in the LPBF group.

Severe hypoxia ($pO_2 < 35$ mm Hg for the average newborn) is not compatible with prolonged survival. Death ensues in a matter of hours. Infants experience tissue hypoxia, anaerobic glycolysis, and metabolic acidosis. Respiratory compensation may occur at first. Even with a normal pH, however, the presence of metabolic acidosis indicates life-threatening hypoxia, necessitating immediate intervention.

DIFFERENTIAL DIAGNOSIS

The major causes of cyanosis are respiratory and cardiac (Table 61–2). Diagnoses in the former group include problems of the lung, chest, or airway, or of the respiratory drive.

The syndrome of **persistent fetal circulation** is perhaps most often confused with cyanotic CHD. In this syndrome the heart and great vessels are structurally normal, but high pulmonary resistance, which is often seen in postterm infants with perinatal distress or pulmonary disease, causes blood to shunt away from the lungs at the foramen ovale and ductus arteriosus. Profound cyanosis that is unresponsive to supplemental oxygen may be the only abnormal finding, and echocardiography is required to exclude CHD.

Pulmonary cyanosis may be due to **infection** (e.g., group B streptococcal pneumonia), **aspiration** (e.g., meconium, tracheoesophageal fistula), **pulmonary hypoplasia** (e.g., Potter's syndrome, diaphragmatic hernia), **respiratory distress syndrome** (e.g., prematurity), or a host of other problems of the lung, chest, or airway. Neurologic depression may produce hypoventilation with resultant hypoxia.

EVALUATION

Evaluation of cyanotic newborns must be expeditious so that management is not delayed. In some cases, therapy may be initiated before the evaluation is complete. All available information, the statistical likelihood of CHD, and the risk-benefit ratio of the treatment must be taken into account.

History

Review of the history may be helpful, particularly in certain situations, such as in children with pulmonary disease (Questions Box). It is important to note that a negative response to any or all of the questions does not make cyanotic CHD unlikely; in fact, negative responses are noted in most cases.

Physical Examination

Cyanosis may be the only abnormal physical finding in cardiac patients, but a careful, thorough examination often yields information about the underlying cardiac defect and the overall circulatory status.

External anomalies or abnormal phenotypic appearance may indicate a genetic disorder with associated cardiac anomalies. Dyspnea (grunting, nasal flaring, intercostal retractions) is more often seen with lung disease, but tachypnea (rapid respiration) is common with both severe heart disease and pulmonary problems. Tachypnea results either from CHF in HPBF lesions or from metabolic acidosis in severe hypoxia or impaired perfusion. Poor perfusion is also manifested by abnormal color (pallor or a gray or ashen appearance if combined with cyanosis), cool extremities, delayed capillary refill, and generally diminished pulses.

The peripheral pulses are palpated in all extremities. Abnormalities or discrepancies between extremities must be confirmed by measuring blood pressure. Weak pulses may be found in cardiogenic shock, and bounding pulses may be noted with diastolic runoff lesions such as patent ductus arteriosus or aortic insufficiency. Pulse quality and blood pressure may differ in different extremities if an aortic arch abnormality such as coarctation is present. The abdominal examination may reveal hepatomegaly (in CHF) or abnormal situs (as in

> **Questions: Cyanosis in the Newborn**
>
> - Has the infant been in any distress?
> - Has the infant had difficulty feeding?
> - Was the infant suspected of having a heart problem prior to birth (e.g., fetal arrhythmia, abnormal heart on ultrasound)?
> - Is the mother diabetic?
> - Did the mother take any drugs (prescribed or not) during the pregnancy?
> - Was the mother ill during the first trimester?
> - Is there a positive family history of CHD or other birth defects?
> - Did any perinatal problems (e.g., meconium staining) occur?

asplenia syndrome, usually associated with complex cyanotic CHD).

The cardiac examination may disclose a loud murmur if an obstruction such as pulmonary stenosis is present. The physician should note, however, that atresia, being a total obstruction, produces no murmur. Heart sounds may be loud and the precordium hyperdynamic, particularly in children with HPBF. Splitting of the second sound confirms that two patent semilunar valves are present, but this finding is often difficult to appreciate even in normal newborns.

Laboratory Tests

A number of laboratory studies are available (see Chapter 62, Congestive Heart Failure; Table 62–2). As in CHF, it is initially more important to determine whether patients have heart disease than to obtain a precise, complete diagnosis. In cyanotic CHD, sophisticated studies such as echocardiography and catheterization are usually needed to make a detailed diagnosis.

The suspicion of arterial hypoxia should be confirmed by **pulse oximetry,** an indirect measurement. It is readily available and noninvasive but has shortcomings. Perfusion must be adequate to obtain a reading. Accuracy is diminished at saturations below 75%, although the presence of profound hypoxia can still be confirmed. Cyanotic CHD cannot be ruled out by pulse oximetry, however, because readings of 100% saturation may reflect pO_2 values that range anywhere between 75 and 250 mm Hg (Fig. 61–1). **Arterial blood gases** are more accurate and give important additional information about ventilation and acid-base status. Arterialized capillary gases may suffice if perfusion is adequate.

Oxygenation of the extremities may differ in infants with certain lesions (e.g., coarctation). The site of sampling should be noted. If possible, the saturation should be measured both proximal and distal to the ductus arteriosus (i.e., from the right arm and either leg).

FIGURE 61–1. *Comparison between PO_2 by arterial blood gas measurement and oxygen saturation by pulse oximetry. (Reproduced, with permission, from Neihoff, J., et al. Efficacy of pulse oximetry and capnometry in postoperative ventilatory weaning. Crit. Care Med. 16:701, 1988.)*

FIGURE 61–2. *Oxyhemoglobin dissociation curve. Note that the position of the curve itself may vary with temperature, pH, pCO_2, and 2,3-diphosphoglycerate (2,3-DPG).*

A **shunt study,** also known as a hyperoxia challenge, should be performed to determine whether a right-to-left cardiac shunt is present. In patients with LPBF or TGA, increasing the inspired oxygen does not affect the oxygenation of the blood because it is unable to enter the lungs; this is a positive result. In patients with pulmonary disease or hypoventilation, oxygenation increases strikingly, often to a pO_2 exceeding 200 mm Hg; this negative result rules out cyanotic CHD.

A "blunted" shunt study, characterized by a rise in pO_2 but rarely to levels above 150 mm Hg, is seen in patients with severe pulmonary disease and in those with HPBF lesions. With such lesions the pulmonary venous blood is high in volume, and the rise in its saturation causes a definite rise in arterial oxygenation. This effect is exaggerated by the further increase in pulmonary flow due to the vasodilating effect of oxygen.

A positive shunt study may be identified with pulse oximetry. It is difficult or impossible, however, to distinguish between a blunted study and a negative one with this tool. The oxyhemoglobin dissociation curve is flattened at the upper end, and the saturation changes very little over a wide range of pO_2 (Fig. 61–2). Capillary gases may be equally inaccurate in this range, but directly measured arterial blood gases are highly reliable. In addition, they may reveal hypercapnia, with or without respiratory acidosis, suggesting a pulmonary cause for the hypoxia.

ECG, a fairly inexpensive test, is readily available and noninvasive. However, it does not often help distinguish cyanotic CHD from other causes of cyanosis, particularly for those practitioners who lack experience with neonatal ECGs. The normal range is large in neonates, with much overlap between normal and CHD. Care must also be taken in placing the leads correctly and minimizing artifacts.

Imaging Studies

The **chest x-ray,** a relatively inexpensive and readily available test, is often extremely helpful in differentiating between cardiac and noncardiac disease. Pulmonary disease is often readily apparent on chest x-ray.

The x-ray also helps define the cardiac diagnosis broadly but not precisely. Patients with LPBF lesions have small hearts and diminished pulmonary flow. In contrast, patients with HPBF lesions have large hearts and increased flow, such as is seen in infants with simple left-to-right shunts. With many cyanotic lesions, the cardiac silhouette is abnormal in configuration (e.g., boot-shaped heart in tetralogy of Fallot) or position (e.g., dextrocardia in patients with heterotaxia syndromes). TGA may be more misleading; pulmonary flow may be increased despite the severe cyanosis, and the heart size may be normal. An apparently normal x-ray does not exclude TGA.

Under optimal conditions, **echocardiography** enables the physician not only to recognize CHD but to identify details of anatomy and physiology. Conversely, a properly performed, complete, negative echocardiogram rules out CHD. The performance of a high-quality study requires the appropriate equipment (with high-resolution imaging), an experienced sonographer, and an experienced cardiologist for interpretation. In the absence of these elements, echocardiography may be used cautiously as a screening device as part of the initial assessment to confirm heart disease prior to referral to a specialist. However, referral should not be delayed until echocardiography can be performed.

MANAGEMENT

Initial management prior to cardiac consultation (often with transfer to another institution) includes surveillance, assistance, direct medical management, and supportive care.

Close **surveillance,** including transfer to the highest level of neonatal care available, use of a cardiopulmonary monitor and continuous pulse oximetry, frequent monitoring of vital signs, and repeat physical examinations, is begun as soon as cyanotic CHD is identified. Even if infants are feeding well, it is best to suspend feedings because of the likelihood of invasive procedures or spontaneous deterioration in the near future. A secure intravenous line should be placed for administration of fluids, glucose, and medications.

While undertaking these measures, the physician should make every effort to seek **assistance** from a pediatric cardiologist. A neonatologist may be consulted if a pediatric cardiologist is not immediately available. Much advice may be obtained over the telephone. In addition, plans for immediate consultation or transfer of patients may be discussed in this way.

The need for **supportive care** depends on the case. In the absence of metabolic acidosis or impaired perfusion, no special care is indicated. In some cases, intravenous fluid boluses, inotropic agents, and other treatments may be needed as part of the early management. Mechanical ventilation should be used in patients with metabolic acidosis, whether compensated or uncompensated, because of the increased oxygen requirement produced by hyperventilation and the tendency for tiring, leading to superimposed respiratory acidosis.

The temptation to give supplemental oxygen is great but must be resisted. Oxygen is rarely helpful and may be harmful. In infants with TGA or LPBF lesions, oxygenation is not affected. In infants with HPBF lesions, oxygenation is usually adequate in room air (saturation: > 80%), and an increase in F_{IO_2} may exacerbate the CHF. Oxygen may also constrict the ductus arteriosus on which the patient may depend.

The possibility of ductal dependency should prompt consideration of administering the ductus dilator, **prostaglandin E-1 (PGE-1).** The definitive diagnosis of cyanotic CHD need not be made prior to institution of this lifesaving treatment. In infants who remain adequately oxygenated (no acidosis) and perfused, the drug can be prepared but administration deferred pending consultation. The benefits of giving PGE-1 to severely hypoxic infants or infants with compromised perfusion far outweigh the risks, which include apnea and fever. A dramatic improvement is often seen within seconds to minutes, confirming the diagnosis of a ductal-dependent lesion, and enabling the physician to stabilize the patient until more definitive intervention can occur.

PROGNOSIS

If untreated, LPBF lesions and TGA are usually fatal during infancy, most often during the neonatal period, because of severe hypoxia. Untreated HPBF lesions may lead to death in infancy from either CHF or complications such as pneumonia. If the systemic blood flow is ductus-dependent (e.g., interruption of the aortic arch), death occurs shortly after ductal closure, usually during the first week of life.

With prompt recognition and intervention, however, the prognosis for infants with cyanotic CHD is surprisingly good in the absence of a genetic syndrome (e.g., trisomy 18) or a major complicating extracardiac malformation (e.g., neural tube defect). If diagnosed before the onset of severe circulatory compromise, infants can be stabilized and evaluated promptly, and palliative or corrective procedures can be performed. The large majority of such patients can survive for decades with fair-to-good quality of life. Infants with lesions with all four chambers adequate in size (e.g., tetralogy of Fallot) have a better lifetime prognosis than those with a hypoplastic chamber (e.g., tricuspid atresia). Even infants with anatomic abnormalities such as asplenia syndrome or hypoplastic left heart syndrome now have a reasonable outlook with complex reconstructive surgery or heart transplantation.

Case Resolution

In the case presented at the beginning of the chapter, marked hypoxia is present in the absence of other cardiac findings such as a heart murmur. The oxygen saturation does not rise after the infant breathes 100% oxygen for 10 minutes. The chest x-ray shows a small, boot-shaped heart and diminished pulmonary blood flow, and the ECG is normal. Transport is arranged. Because of the marked cyanosis, infusion of PGE-1 is begun, and saturation increases to 80%, with the pO_2 rising from 33 to 48 mm Hg. The infant is transferred to a tertiary care center, where consultation is obtained. An echocardiogram is also performed, which demonstrates tetralogy of Fallot with pulmonary atresia. A Blalock-Taussig shunt is placed in the newborn period, and complete repair using a pulmonary artery homograft is performed at 5 years of age.

Selected Readings

DiMaio, A. M., and J. Singh. The infant with cyanosis in the emergency department. Pediatr. Clin. North Am. 39:987–1006, 1992.

Driscoll, D. J. Evaluation of the cyanotic newborn. Pediatr. Clin. North Am. 37:1–23, 1990.

Freed, M. D., et al. Prostaglandin E-1 in infants with ductus arteriosus dependent congenital heart disease. Circulation 64:899–905, 1981.

Jones, R. W. A., et al. Arterial oxygen tension and response to oxygen breathing in differential diagnosis of congenital heart disease in infancy. Arch. Dis. Child. 51:667–673, 1976.

Lees, M. H., and D. H. King. Cyanosis in the newborn. Pediatr. Rev. 9:36–42, 1987.

Niehoff, J., et al. Efficacy of pulse oximetry and capnometry in postoperative ventilatory weaning. Crit. Care Med. 16:701–705, 1988.

Tateishi, K., and I. Yamanouchi. Noninvasive transcutaneous oxygen pressure diagnosis of reversed ductal shunts in cyanotic heart disease. Pediatrics 66:22–25, 1980.

Victorica, B. E. Cyanotic newborns. In Gessner, I. H., and B. E. Victorica. (eds.). Pediatric Cardiology: A Problem Oriented Approach. Philadelphia, W.B. Saunders, 1993.

CONGESTIVE HEART FAILURE

Robin Winkler Doroshow, M.D.

H$_x$ A 2-month-old infant is brought to the office by his mother, who complains that her son has been eating poorly and breathing oddly for the past few days. The perinatal history is unremarkable. A heart murmur was noted at the one-month checkup.

The infant is scrawny and irritable. Physical examination shows that the boy's weight, which was at the 50th percentile at birth, is now at the fifth percentile; his height, which was at the 50th percentile, is now at the 25th percentile. He is afebrile, and his heart rate is 165/min, with respirations 60/min and shallow but without respiratory distress. The skin is pale and diaphoretic, and the mucous membranes are pink. Examination of the head and neck is normal; likewise, no jugular distention is present. The lungs are clear. The precordium is hyperdynamic, and the heart sounds are loud; a prominent systolic murmur is audible at the left lower sternal border. The liver edge is palpable 4 cm below the right costal margin in the right midclavicular line, and the spleen is not palpable. The extremities are thin, with normal pulses and no edema. Capillary refill is slightly delayed.

Questions

1. What are acute and chronic signs of cardiac disease in children?
2. What are the signs of congestive heart failure (CHF) in children? How do signs in children differ from those in adults?
3. What underlying disorders can cause CHF in young infants?
4. What is the appropriate emergent management for infants with CHF? What are the risks of treatment if the diagnosis is incorrect?

Congestive heart failure (CHF) is the most common presentation of serious heart disease in infants. Although this condition also occurs in older children, an estimated 90% of cases of CHF in the pediatric population begin in the first year of life. In children CHF is most often caused by structural congenital heart disease. Compensatory mechanisms are fewer and less successful in small infants. Other causes of CHF are listed in Table 62–1.

EPIDEMIOLOGY

The precise incidence of CHF in children is unknown; it is approximately 0.1%. Most cases result from con-

---

TABLE 62–1. Causes of Congestive Heart Failure in Children

Volume Overload
Left-to-right shunts (e.g., ventricular septal defect)
Bidirectional shunts (e.g., truncus arteriosus)
Valvular insufficiency (e.g., mitral regurgitation)
Extracardiac conditions (e.g., anemia, arteriovenous malformation)

Pressure Overload
Outflow obstruction (e.g., coarctation of the aorta)
Inflow obstruction (e.g., obstructed anomalous pulmonary veins)
Vascular resistance (e.g., hypertension, chronic pulmonary disease)

Myocardial Dysfunction
Intrinsic conditions (e.g., cardiomyopathy, anthracycline toxicity)
Inflammatory conditions (e.g., viral myocarditis, rheumatic fever)
Coronary insufficiency (e.g., anomalous left coronary artery)

Arrhythmias
Tachyarrhythmia (e.g., paroxysmal supraventricular tachycardia)
Bradyarrhythmia (e.g., third-degree atrioventricular block)

genital heart disease (CHD), which occurs in 0.8% of live births. The incidence of CHD varies little with geography, ethnic group, or gender. It is far more common in children with recognizable genetic syndromes (e.g., trisomy 21 [Down's syndrome], Turner's syndrome).

CLINICAL PRESENTATION

Most commonly, complaints about CHF take the form of queries about an infant's feeding. Comments are often vague (e.g., "my baby is not a good eater") but may be more precise (e.g., "he is taking less formula with each feeding," "he is taking longer to nurse"). Parents may also describe rapid breathing, excessive sweating, or decreased activity, but usually only on specific questioning.

CHF is also often detected on examination for routine infant checkups or for unrelated complaints. Careful assessment of the physical findings, including vital signs, reveals **tachypnea, tachycardia,** and **hepatomegaly** and frequently signs of underlying structural heart defects, such as a murmur (D_x Box).

PATHOPHYSIOLOGY

High cardiac output may lead to CHF in infants with large left-to-right shunts. Myocardial contractility is relatively normal, and children remain on the "normal" line of the Frank-Starling curve (also called preload), which relates cardiac output to diastolic volume or pressure (Fig. 62-1). The shunt requires a very large volume of output, primarily to the pulmonary bed. Although the heart may be able to meet this demand, preload is high, leading to "congestive" signs and symptoms (e.g., tachypnea, hepatomegaly). In more severe cases, systemic output may be compromised, resulting in hypotension, renal failure, and metabolic acidosis.

Left-sided failure caused by elevated pulmonary venous pressure produces increased lung water. Initially, this fluid is interstitial, and it does not interfere with gas exchange but does trigger reflex tachypnea. Minute volume is kept normal by decreasing tidal (breath-to-breath) volume, leading to shallow as well as rapid breathing. Only when the ability of the pulmonary lymphatics to drain this fluid is overcome by large volume does fluid accumulate in the alveoli. Rales and respiratory distress, or dyspnea, result.

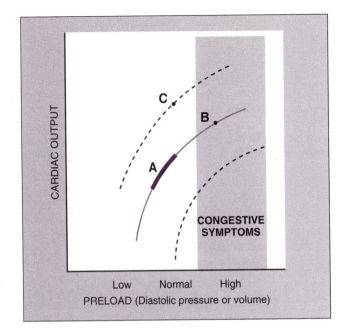

FIGURE 62-1. *Graph showing relationship of cardiac output to preload. The solid curve represents normal myocardial contractility, and the dotted curves represent impaired function (shifted downward) and the positive inotropic state (shifted upward). A: Normal range (no heart disease). B: Left-to-right shunt with congestive heart failure (CHF). Note that overall output is high but most of it is shunted. C: Same situation as B but after treatment for CHF. Cardiac output is the same or better, but preload is now out of the range that results in congestive symptoms.*

Right-sided failure caused by an elevated systemic venous load usually produces more volume than pressure load on this system, possibly as a result of the greater venous compliance in infants as compared with adults. The liver becomes very distended and is easily palpated. As long as the liver can absorb the increased venous volume, the portal pressure does not rise, and splenomegaly does not occur. Because the venous pressure rises very little, jugular distention, which is difficult to detect in young infants in any case, is rarely seen. Edema is also rare.

The left and right (systemic and pulmonary) circulations are more interdependent in infants and younger children than they are in older children or adults. As a result, **bilateral heart failure** is much more common than right-sided or left-sided failure alone. Although this means that recognition of bilateral heart failure may be easier, determination of the underlying condition may be more difficult because the clues are less specific. For example, in an adult with left-sided failure, the differential diagnosis includes mitral, but not tricuspid, valve disease.

DIFFERENTIAL DIAGNOSIS

When tachycardia, tachypnea without dyspnea, and hepatomegaly are present, the diagnosis of CHF is straightforward. CHF is most commonly confused with major respiratory infections such as bronchiolitis or pneumonia. Pulmonary infections are frequently associated with dyspnea as well as tachypnea, impaired

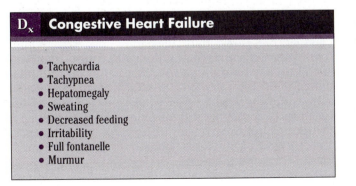

D_x Congestive Heart Failure

- Tachycardia
- Tachypnea
- Hepatomegaly
- Sweating
- Decreased feeding
- Irritability
- Full fontanelle
- Murmur

gas exchange, and other respiratory findings. Rhinorrhea, cough, fever, or wheezing may also be present. Rales may accompany pneumonia but are rare in CHF in infancy or early childhood. Hyperinflation due to lung disease may lead to a false impression of hepatomegaly. In some children, CHD, CHF, and respiratory infections coexist.

Clues to the presence of structural heart disease, such as a murmur or absent femoral pulses, may support the diagnosis of CHF. Severe CHF, with low cardiac output or even shock, has a broader differential diagnosis. In addition to cardiac causes, sepsis, hypovolemia, and disorders associated with inborn errors of metabolism should be considered.

EVALUATION

History

The history should include specific questions about feeding and growth (Questions Box). Poor feeding, often a nonspecific complaint in chronically or subacutely ill infants, results from tachypnea and fatigability in infants with heart disease. Growth failure may result from poor feeding and increased cardiopulmonary work. The physician should specifically query parents about possible excessive sweating or rapid breathing in infants, because parents may not volunteer this information.

Physical Examination

The diagnosis of CHF is primarily based on clinical findings, and physical examination is essential. The resting respiratory rate must be counted precisely, because infants in CHF most often have tachypnea without dyspnea. The liver edge is palpable more than 1 cm below the right costal margin in the midclavicular line, and the degree of enlargement mirrors the severity of the CHF.

Diagnostic Studies

Many laboratory tests can be performed to assess infants' hearts (Table 62–2), including ECG and echocardiogram. However, some procedures are very costly, and some are invasive and therefore carry risk. The value of most of these tests depends on the expertise of the individual who interprets them. It is important to remember that although test results and consultation with a pediatric cardiologist may be invaluable in the identification of the underlying lesion, *these procedures are not usually required in the diagnosis of CHF.*

Questions: Congestive Heart Failure

- How has the infant been feeding? Does he or she get out of breath or appear exhausted?
- Has the child's growth pattern changed recently?
- Does the child tire easily? With eating? With playing?
- Does the child perspire excessively, especially with efforts such as feeding?
- Does the infant breathe rapidly, even at rest?

TABLE 62–2. Laboratory Tests Used in the Evaluation of Heart Disease in Children

Test	Information
Chest x-ray	Presence and direction of shunt
	Hints concerning specific diagnosis (possible pulmonary disease ruled out)
Electrocardiogram (ECG)	Heart rhythm
	Chamber overload
	Coronary insufficiency
Ambulatory ECG (24-hour ECG)	Subacute rhythm assessment
	Correlation of symptoms with rhythm
Oximetry	Presence and degree of hypoxia
Arterial blood gases	Hypoxia
	Acid-base status
Hematocrit	Anemia
	Polycythemia
Exercise test	Quantitation of exercise tolerance
	Provocation of symptoms or arrhythmia
Echocardiogram	Specific structural diagnosis and hemodynamics
	Chamber enlargement and function
Cardiac catheterization	Specific structural diagnosis and hemodynamics

In children with severe CHF, further studies are indicated. **Arterial blood gases** show evidence of metabolic acidosis due to tissue anoxia, with respiratory compensation in early stages and superimposed respiratory acidosis in later stages. A **CBC** shows leukocytosis due to stress. It may not differentiate between heart disease and sepsis.

The most useful supportive study is a **chest x-ray**, preferably in anteroposterior and lateral projections. The x-ray shows cardiomegaly, due not to myocardial dysfunction, but to the volume overload from the shunt. In the absence of cardiac enlargement, the diagnosis of CHF must be seriously questioned. (However, CHF may occur in total anomalous pulmonary venous return with obstruction, which usually presents in the first week of life in association with hypoxia.) Pulmonary venous congestion occurs in left heart failure, but increased pulmonary arterial flow from a left-to-right shunt often obscures the congestion. Hyperinflation resulting from peribronchial edema is also a common finding.

MANAGEMENT

Inotropes and **diuretics** are used in the initial management of CHF in children. Inotropic support results in a shift to a higher Frank-Starling curve (see Fig. 62–1), which allows affected patients to maintain the high volume output necessitated by the underlying CHD at lower diastolic pressures, thus alleviating congestive symptoms. **Digoxin**, a form of digitalis, is the drug of choice in such cases, where cardiac output is not severely impaired. This agent is readily available, easily absorbed, safe in the therapeutic range, and easy to administer (elixir for oral administration). If digoxin is initially given at the maintenance dose (10 µg/kg/day), therapeutic levels are not attained for about a week; therefore loading is preferable (Table 62–3). Digoxin is well tolerated and rarely causes side effects. Because of the safety and reliability of absorption, blood levels need not be

TABLE 62–3. Digoxin: Total Oral
Loading Dose in Children*

Age	Dose (μg/kg)
Preterm newborns	20–30
Term newborns and infants	25–35
1–5 years	30–40
5–10 years†	20–30
10 years to adult†	10–15

*IV loading dose = 75–80% of PO dose. Usually given ½, followed 8 hours later by ¼, followed 8 hours later by ¼, followed 12 hours later by initiation of maintenance dose. Assumes normal renal function; dose must be adjusted downward for renal failure.

†In children over 5 years of age, loading dose can be calculated by surface area (0.5–1.0 μg/m²).

checked unless overdose is suspected (e.g., history of overadministration, toxic ingestion, unexplained vomiting, or second- or third-degree heart block).

The elevated diastolic preload of CHF is the result of renally mediated sodium and water retention. **Diuretics** reverse this phenomenon. **Furosemide**, a potent loop diuretic that is available in an oral suspension and is fairly well absorbed, is the most frequent drug of choice. The starting dose is 1 mg/kg once or twice daily. Initially, furosemide may be given intravenously or intramuscularly rather than orally, which reduces the time to onset of action, and is more effective. Such treatment also supports the patient while digoxin loading is in progress.

Fluid and sodium restriction, often used in adults with CHF, is difficult to achieve with infants because their diet is predominantly or exclusively liquid. High-calorie diets using concentrated formulas, complex carbohydrate additives, or medium-chain triglyceride oils may reduce the intake of free water and the effort of feeding without compromising caloric intake.

Breast milk and most proprietary formulas have a low sodium load. In older infants and children, salt intake is more easily modified and should be minimized.

Children with severe or refractory cases of CHF may require additional medications or interventions. These include **intravenous inotropes** (e.g., dopamine), **vasodilators** for afterload reduction (e.g., angiotensin-converting enzyme inhibitors), **correction of anemia** (e.g., transfusion), **treatment of fever** (e.g., antipyretics), and **reduction of metabolic demands** (e.g., ventilatory support, bed rest, sedation).

Ultimately, the best management for CHF is **treatment of the underlying disorder.** The degree of urgency depends on the nature of the disorder and the severity of the CHF. For example, in neonates with supraventricular tachycardia, conversion to normal sinus rhythm is often the only treatment necessary. CHF caused by severe anemia responds dramatically to correction of hemoglobin levels. When CHF is due to structural CHD (the most common situation), surgery to palliate the problem (e.g., pulmonary artery banding in left-to-right shunts) or correct the defect (e.g., repair of ventricular septal defect [VSD]) usually resolves the CHF. It is rarely necessary to "tolerate" prolonged, uncontrolled CHF in children or to treat the condition aggressively at the expense of a major change in life-style.

Family counseling, which should begin when CHF is identified, is essential. Several important points should be included, in addition to a general description of both the cardiac defect and CHF. The term "heart failure," which is commonly thought to refer to a sudden deterioration of heart function or even heart stoppage, must be clarified. It is also important to stress that affected infants should be treated as normally as possible, with the exception of administration of medicines and keeping medical appointments. Contrary to popular belief, infants with cardiac conditions are not fragile. Addressing parental concern, assuaging guilt, and normalizing existence are key quality-of-life issues.

PROGNOSIS

In the vast majority of young infants and children with CHF, the prognosis is excellent. CHF responds well to treatment, and the underlying defect can usually be corrected or at least palliated. Without cardiac surgery for CHD, CHF often remits spontaneously over months or years as a result of maturation of compensatory mechanisms, spontaneous improvement in the defect (e.g., decrease in the size of a VSD), or increase in pulmonary vascular resistance because of long-standing high pulmonary artery pressure and flow (Eisenmenger's syndrome). "Catch-up" growth occurs with remission of CHF, and children have the potential to reach their genetically determined height and weight.

Case Resolution

The case presented at the beginning of the chapter is typical of an otherwise normal infant with a large VSD who becomes symptomatic after the development of CHF. The boy's growth failure can be attributed to the chronicity of his illness.

The loud murmur and presentation in infancy strongly suggest the existence of underlying structural CHD as the cause of CHF. The time of onset of CHF also suggests a specific mechanism. When the onset is slightly delayed after birth, a lesion with changing postnatal hemodynamics, such as left-to-right shunt, which has increased as pulmonary resistance has fallen, is suggested. (Note that a ductus-dependent defect would have presented more acutely and severely in the first week of life.)

Selected Readings

Artman, M., and T. P. Graham. Congestive heart failure in infancy: recognition and management. Am Heart J. 103;1040–1055, 1982.

Friedman, W. F., and B. L. George. Medical progress–treatment of congestive heart failure by altering loading conditions of the heart. J. Pediatr. 106:697–706, 1985.

Kimball, T. R., et al. Effect of digoxin on contractility and symptoms in infants with a large ventricular septal defect. Am. J. Cardiol. 68:1377–1382, 1991.

Soyka, L. F. Pediatric clinical pharmacology of digoxin. Pediatr. Clin. North Am. 28:203–216, 1981.

Talner, N. S. Heart failure. In Emmanouilides, G. C., et al. (eds.). Moss and Adams' Heart Disease in Infants, Children, and Adolescents, 5th ed. Baltimore, Williams & Wilkins, 1995, pp. 890–911.

CHAPTER 63

HYPERTENSION

Sudhir K. Anand, M.D.

H$_x$ A 10-year-old girl is seen in the emergency department with a history of severe headache and generalized seizures lasting two minutes. Her past medical history is remarkable for a history of several episodes of unexplained fever as an infant and an episode of urinary tract infection at age 3 years; no radiologic studies were done. She also has a history of headaches for the past two years, which have been treated primarily with acetaminophen. There is no known history of drug ingestion or hypertension in the patient or family members.

The physical examination is remarkable for a pulse of 100 and a blood pressure of 210/130 mm Hg in the right arm in supine position. Equal pulses are palpable in all four extremities. Blood pressure is 216/134 mm Hg in the lower extremities. The funduscopic examination reveals evidence of petechial hemorrhages and mild papilledema. Chest examination finds normal breath sounds and an active precordium with the apical impulse shifted to the left; no murmurs are heard. The liver is palpable one centimeter below the right costal margin. The neurologic examination is remarkable for altered sensorium with lethargy; no focal neurologic deficit is present. A routine urinalysis shows 2+ protein and normal urinary sediment. The hemoglobin is 11.2g/dL and hematocrit is 33%. Sodium is 139 mEq/L, potassium 3.8 mEq/L, chloride 102 mEq/L, and bicarbonate 22 mEq/L. BUN is 35 mg/dL and serum creatinine is 1.8 mg/dL. An electrocardiogram shows left ventricular enlargement. CT scan of the head is normal.

Questions

1. What is the definition of hypertension in children?
2. What are the causes of hypertension in children?
3. What is the appropriate evaluation of hypertension in children?
4. What acute and long-term management is used in hypertensive children?
5. What is the appropriate emergency treatment of symptomatic hypertension?

Hypertension is a major public health problem in the adult population. Because of its effects on the heart, central nervous system, kidneys, and eyes, it is one of the leading causes of increased mortality and morbidity. Hypertension is frequently identified in children. As with adults, the etiology of elevated blood pressure in children may be idiopathic (i.e., essential hypertension); or, more often it may signify the presence of an underlying disorder, especially renal disease.

NORMAL BLOOD PRESSURE

Both systolic and diastolic blood pressures (BP) in children gradually increase, from the newborn period through adolescence; therefore, age-appropriate norms should be used to classify a given BP reading as normal or hypertensive. For example, a BP reading of 132/84 mm Hg would be regarded as normal for a 16-year-old adolescent, but it would signify severe hypertension in a 2-year-old child. BP measurements should be part of routine physical examinations in all children over 3 years of age and in all hospitalized children. Also, an appropriately sized blood-pressure cuff should be used; the cuff width should cover approximately 75% of the upper arm and nearly completely encircle the arm (D$_x$ Box).

EPIDEMIOLOGY: DEFINITION AND INCIDENCE OF HYPERTENSION

BP values in children are a continuum, with no clear dividing line between normal and high. Despite this limitation, the report of the second Task Force on Blood Pressure Control in Children recently defined hypertension to be an average systolic or diastolic BP equal to or greater than the 95th percentile for age and sex, with measurements obtained on at least three occasions (Table 63–1). Readings between the 90th and 95th percentile were regarded as high-normal, and it was suggested that such children should be monitored more closely for future development of hypertension. The Task Force further classified hypertension into two categories: (1) significant hypertension (BP persistently between the 95th and 99th percentiles for age and sex) and (2) severe hypertension (BP persistently at or above the 99th percentile for age and sex). BP values that qualify as significant or severe hypertension in newborn infants and children are described in Table 63–2. As would be obvious from the above definition of hypertension, 5% of all children (those with BP readings > 95th

---

D$_x$ **Hypertension**

- BP elevated > 95th percentile for age on at least 3 consecutive occasions with the child in a quiet, nonapprehensive state and with BP cuff of appropriate size
- BP check in both upper and at least one lower extremity
- Fundus examination: vascular changes, exudates, and papilledema
- Abnormal urinalysis

TABLE 63–1. Definitions of Hypertension

Term	Definition
Normal BP	Systolic and diastolic BPs < 90th percentile for age and sex
High-normal BP*	Average systolic and/or average diastolic BP between 90th and 95th percentiles for age and sex
High BP (hypertension)	Average systolic and/or average diastolic BPs ≥ 95th percentile for age and sex with measurements obtained on at least three occasions

*If the BP reading is high-normal for age, but can be accounted for by excess height for age or excess lean body mass for age, such children are considered to have normal BP.

Reproduced, with permission, from the Report of the Second Task Force on Blood Pressure Control in Children–1987. Pediatrics 79:1, 1987.

percentile) have hypertension, with 4% having significant hypertension and 1% having severe hypertension. However, most pediatricians and health care workers screening healthy children identify hypertension in only 1 to 2% (or less) of children and not the expected 5%.

CLINICAL PRESENTATION

Hypertension in most children with mildly elevated BP is usually asymptomatic; the symptoms of headache, dizziness, and nosebleeds occur probably no more frequently in children with hypertension than in those without it. However, when children with severe hypertension complain of headaches, dizziness, and nosebleeds, these symptoms may be superimposed upon symptoms of primary disorders that led to the hypertension. Children with severe hypertension, especially malignant hypertension, may have signs of heart failure (tachycardia, tachypnea, or enlarged liver), experience seizures, and infrequently suffer seventh nerve paralysis.

TABLE 63–2. Classification of Hypertension by Age Group

Age Group	Significant Hypertension (mm Hg)	Severe Hypertension (mm Hg)
Newborn		
1–7d	Systolic BP ≥ 96	Systolic BP ≥ 106
8–30d	Systolic BP ≥ 104	Systolic BP ≥ 110
Infant (<2 yr)	Systolic BP ≥ 112	Systolic BP ≥ 118
	Diastolic BP ≥ 74	Diastolic BP ≥ 82
Children (3–5 yr)	Systolic BP ≥ 116	Systolic BP ≥ 124
	Diastolic BP ≥ 76	Diastolic BP ≥ 84
Children (6–9 yr)	Systolic BP ≥ 122	Systolic BP ≥ 130
	Diastolic BP ≥ 78	Diastolic BP ≥ 86
Children (10–12 yr)	Systolic BP ≥ 126	Systolic BP ≥ 134
	Diastolic BP ≥ 82	Diastolic BP ≥ 90
Adolescents (13–15 yr)	Systolic BP ≥ 136	Systolic BP ≥ 144
	Diastolic BP ≥ 86	Diastolic BP ≥ 92
Adolescents (16–18 yr)	Systolic BP ≥ 142	Systolic BP ≥ 150
	Diastolic BP ≥ 92	Diastolic BP ≥ 98

Reproduced, with permission, from the Report of the Second Task Force on Blood Pressure Control in Children–1987. Pediatrics 79:1, 1987.

Also, a fundus examination may show vascular changes, exudates, and papilledema.

ETIOLOGY AND PATHOPHYSIOLOGY

An increase in BP results from an increase in peripheral resistance or cardiac output (usually caused by excess extracellular fluid volume) or a mixture of the two. The exact cause of hypertension in 90 to 95% of adults is still uncertain; hence, the name essential, primary, or idiopathic hypertension. In the past, it was often stated that in more than 80% of children hypertension was secondary to an underlying disorder and that fewer than 20% of cases were idiopathic; however, this is true only in children with severe hypertension. In the majority of children, especially in adolescents, with mild increases in blood pressure (i.e., slightly beyond the 95th percentile), no etiology of hypertension is found, and they are classified as having idiopathic or essential hypertension.

Many factors play a role in the development of essential hypertension; these include **heredity, stress response, salt sensitivity,** and **obesity**. In addition, during investigations of hypertension, alterations to a variable degree have been found in cardiac output, extracellular fluid volume, peripheral resistance, renin-angiotensin system, aldosterone, balance of sodium, potassium, calcium, and chloride ions, catecholamines, sympathetic nervous system, natriuretic hormones, prostaglandins, kinins, antidiuretic hormone, insulin response, endothelins, nitric oxide (endothelium-derived relaxation factors), and others. Whether these abnormalities are primary or secondary and what their exact role is in the pathogenesis of essential hypertension is still uncertain.

The etiology of secondary hypertension varies with the age of the patient and with the nature of the hypertension—i.e., whether the condition is acute or chronic (Tables 63–3 and 63–4). Renal abnormalities account for 70 to 80% of secondary hypertension in children, the pathogenesis of which may be related to either an increase in extracellular fluid volume (e.g., acute glomerulonephritis or chronic renal failure) or an increase in renin-angiotensin II activity (e.g., renal artery stenosis, renin-producing tumor, or reflux nephropathy) or a combination of both mechanisms (e.g., a patient with chronic renal failure caused by reflux nephropathy).

DIFFERENTIAL DIAGNOSIS

In any child in whom hypertension is confirmed, all reasonable effort should be made to identify the cause of hypertension (see Tables 63–3 and 63–4). Even though in children with mild increases in blood pressure, essential hypertension is common, essential hypertension must remain a diagnosis of exclusion. The cause of hypertension is often obvious from a detailed history, complete examination, and simple laboratory tests. However, extensive evaluation is sometimes necessary to determine the etiology of hypertension, especially in cases of renovascular hypertension.

TABLE 63–3. Causes of Acute or Intermittent Increases in Blood Pressure in Children

Renal Causes

Acute glomerulonephritis
Hemolytic-uremic syndrome
Henoch-Schönlein purpura nephritis
Renal trauma
Renal artery or vein thrombosis
After renal biopsy
Acute obstructive uropathy
Post genitourinary surgery
Blood transfusions in patients with renal failure
After kidney transplant or with transplant rejection

Drug-Induced Causes

Corticosteroids
Amphetamine overdose
Phencyclidine overdose
Cocaine overdose
Anabolic steroids
Oral contraceptives
Excessive erythropoietin use in patients with end-stage renal disease
Cyclosporine A and FK506

Central Nervous System Causes

Increased intracranial pressure (e.g., subdural hematoma, meningitis, tumors)
Encephalitis
Poliomyelitis
Guillain-Barré syndrome
Porphyria
Familial dysautonomia

Miscellaneous Causes

Wrong blood pressure cuff size
Anxiety, apprehension (white coat hypertension)
Pain
Fractures
Orthopedic procedures (especially leg lengthening)
Burns
Leukemia
Stevens-Johnson syndrome
Bacterial endocarditis
Hypernatremia
Hypercalcemia
Heavy metal poisoning

TABLE 63–4. Causes of Chronic Hypertension in Children

Renal

Scarred kidney: due to pyelonephritis and/or vesicoureteral reflux nephropathy
Chronic glomerulonephritis
Connective tissue disease: systemic lupus erythematosus, HS purpura
Hydronephrosis
Congenital dysplastic kidneys, multicystic kidney
Polycystic kidney disease
Solitary renal cyst
Tumors: Wilms', pericytoma (renin-producing tumor)

Renal Vascular Lesions

Renal artery stenosis (fibromuscular dysplasia)
Renal artery thrombosis (especially in the newborn following umbilical artery catheterization)
Renal vein thrombosis
Renal artery lesions with neurofibromatosis, tuberous sclerosis

Other Vascular Lesions

Coarctation of aorta: thoracic, abdominal
Polyarteritis nodosa and other vasculitides

Endocrine

Corticosteroid treatment
Neuroblastoma or other neural crest tumors
Pheochromocytoma
Congenital adrenal hyperplasia with 11β- or 17α-hydroxylase deficiency
Cortisol II-β hydroxysteroid dehydrogenase deficiency
Liddle's syndrome
Primary hyperaldosteronism
Dexamethasone—suppressible hyperaldosteronism
Hyperthyroidism
Hyperparathyroidism
Cushing's syndrome

Central Nervous System

Intracranial hemorrhage
Intracranial mass

Essential (Primary) Hypertension

EVALUATION

When a child is identified as having an elevated BP on any occasion, the finding should be verified with at least two additional measurements. The physician should also verify that an appropriately sized cuff is being used to take the measurements and that efforts have been made to put the child at ease. Many children develop mild increases of BP (which can extend into the hypertensive range) when they visit a doctor's office because of anxiety or apprehension ("white coat hypertension"). Sometimes 24-hour ambulatory BP readings are necessary to confirm whether hypertension is present or not. An isolated finding of a mild increase in BP with normal subsequent readings does not indicate hypertension. Once hypertension is confirmed, a detailed history, complete physical examination, and appropriate laboratory evaluation should be performed.

History

Information should be obtained about the child's symptoms associated with hypertension, such as head-

aches and visual difficulties (Questions Box). Inquiry should also be made about the child's history of renal disease, especially previous urinary tract infections, unexplained fevers during infancy and early childhood, edema, hematuria, enuresis, or nocturia, and the use of umbilical artery catheterization during the newborn period. Information regarding the child's physical growth, BP recordings during previous physical examinations, eating habits–especially salt intake, use of drugs–especially illicit drugs, and the family's history of hypertension and renal disease should be obtained.

Questions: Hypertension

- Does the child have any symptoms associated with hypertension, e.g., headache, dizziness, nosebleed, visual difficulty, or shortness of breath?
- Have BP readings been taken during previous routine physical examinations?
- Has the child had any hematuria, generalized swelling of the body (edema), enuresis (nocturia), burning urination, previous urinary tract infection, or other kidney problems?
- How much salt does the child take? Does he or she love to put extra salt on most foods and frequently like to eat salty foods?
- How has the child been growing?
- Is there a history of use of illicit drugs or contraceptives?
- Is there a family history of hypertension or renal disease?

Physical Examination

A thorough examination is essential for determining the etiology of hypertension and the extent of target organ damage caused by hypertension. Poor physical growth or short stature may indicate the presence of some disorder, such as Turner's syndrome or chronic renal disease with or without renal failure; it may also be the consequence of long-standing severe hypertension. Tachycardia may signify heart failure or thyrotoxicosis. The child's pulses should be felt in both the upper and lower extremities, and the BP should be measured in all four extremities to determine whether coarctation of the aorta or other vascular lesions exists. Fundus examination is essential to determine if hypertension has been severe and chronic leading to arterial changes, exudate, hemorrhages and/or papilledema. Presence of café-au-lait spots or depigmented spots on the skin may signify hypertension secondary to neurofibromatosis or tuberous sclerosis, respectively.

Heart murmur may be present in hypertension due to coarctation of aorta, and heart failure may be present in patients with severe hypertension or in patients with renal disease and fluid retention. The abdomen should be carefully examined for presence of renal or other masses caused by, for example, cystic kidneys, Wilms' tumor, or neuroblastoma, and for tenderness especially in the costovertebral angle (CVA). Bruits sometimes may be heard over the CVA in patients with renal artery stenosis.

Laboratory Evaluation

The extent of laboratory evaluation depends upon the clinical findings; the nature of the hypertension (e.g., mild or severe, acute or chronic); and whether an etiology is apparent or obscure. Table 63–5 outlines suggested laboratory workups for a patient with asymptomatic mild hypertension and for a patient with severe hypertension. Presence of hematuria, heavy proteinuria and leukocyturia, and/or elevated BUN or plasma creatinine would clearly signify a renal disorder as the cause of hypertension (unless it is superimposed upon some other disorder) and require appropriate renal evaluation, including renal Doppler ultrasonography, nuclear scans, or renal biopsy to identify scarred kidneys,

hydronephrosis, cystic kidneys, renal or other tumors, or glomerulonephritis. The presence of electrolyte abnormalities such as hypokalemia, hypochloremia, or metabolic alkalosis would indicate the presence of an increased mineralocorticoid hormone either on a primary basis (primary hyperaldosteronism, adrenogenital syndrome with 11β- or 17α-hydroxylase deficiency, Liddle's syndrome, cortisol 11β-hydroxysteroid deficiency, etc.) or secondary to increased renin activity in renovascular hypertension, renin-producing tumor, or reflux nephropathy; these values would also indicate a need to measure plasma renin activity and urinary or plasma aldosterone levels. Endocrine-based causes of hypertension in children are uncommon, and tests like plasma or urinary catecholamines, plasma cortisol, and T_3 are measured on an individual basis depending on the clinical evaluation of the patient.

Although ECGs and chest x-rays are often requested to evaluate the effects of hypertension on the heart, they reveal normal results until the patient enters the late stages of severe hypertension. Echocardiography showing cardiac hypertrophy is much more sensitive for detecting target organ damage caused by hypertension.

In any child with severe hypertension in whom no etiology is apparent based upon clinical evaluation and the above-mentioned tests, the physician must consider renovascular disease and the necessary tests for it: renal Doppler ultrasonography, captopril-enhanced ^{131}I-MAG-3 renal scan, renal vein renin measurements, and selective renal arteriography (sometimes MRI-angiography may be used as a substitute).

MANAGEMENT

In all children with hypertension, an effort should be made to identify a remediable cause, so that an appropriate medical or surgical treatment can be offered that allows the child to avoid a lifelong regimen of drug treatment.

Patients with mild hypertension should be initially managed with nonpharmacologic measures, including supportive care, reduction in sodium intake to about 80–100 mEq/d, and weight reduction if the child is obese. Some physicians find teaching relaxation and biofeedback techniques helpful in reducing BP. If after a 3–6 month observation period, BP remains persistently elevated or if target organ damage is present, drug treatment should be initiated and a decision should be made whether or not the child needs a more thorough laboratory evaluation. Drug therapy may begin with a beta blocker (e.g., atenolol), an ACE inhibitor (e.g., enalapril) or a diuretic (e.g., hydrochlorothiazide).

Patients with severe hypertension may require combination therapy of the above drugs or additional drugs, such as calcium channel blockers (e.g., nifedipine), alpha blockers (e.g., prazocin), combined alpha-beta blockers (e.g., labetalol), peripheral vasodilators (e.g., hydralazine, minoxidil), or centrally acting drugs (e.g., clonidine). The use of one or more of these drugs can control BP in most patients within a satisfactory range and has a limited number of side effects.

TABLE 63–5. Laboratory Evaluation of Hypertension

A. Mild hypertension
1. Urinalysis (urine culture if indicated)
2. CBC, serum electrolytes, BUN, and creatinine
3. Plasma renin activity along with 24-hour urinary sodium excretion may sometimes be indicated
4. Sometimes echocardiography, ECG, chest x-ray

B. Severe hypertension (in addition to tests for mild hypertension listed above)
1. Chem-20 panel
2. 24-hour urine for creatinine, catecholamines, and aldosterone
3. Renal Doppler ultrasonography
4. Captopril-enhanced ^{131}I-MAG-3 renal scan
5. Renal vein renins
6. Renal arteriography (selective if necessary)

Patients with renal artery stenosis can be successfully treated with balloon dilatation of the stenosis. If this procedure is unsuccessful or restenosis occurs, surgical correction of the stenosis is usually successful.

Depending upon their clinical condition, patients with malignant hypertension may be treated initially with oral (sublingual) nifedipine or labetalol. However, if the condition warrants, they may be started on intravenous labetalol, diazoxide, or sodium nitroprusside. The aim is not to lower BP urgently to a normal range, but to lower BP by about 20 to 25% of the presenting values. Over the following days to weeks, BP can gradually be controlled to come within normal values for age.

PROGNOSIS

The long-term outcome of hypertension in children depends upon the underlying etiology. In children with severe hypertension, BP control improves growth and overall well-being. The very long-term (30–50 years) prognosis of children with persistent, mild essential hypertension is largely unknown; however, one would anticipate that adequate BP control would prolong life and reduce cardiovascular, central nervous system, renal, and retinal morbidity.

Case Resolution

In the case presented above, the child clearly has signs of malignant hypertension. The history of previous urinary tract infection and the laboratory findings of proteinuria and elevated plasma creatinine suggest chronic pyelonephritis or reflux nephropathy with hypertension and chronic renal failure. The elevated creatinine also suggests that both kidneys are affected either by the primary process or as a consequence of severe hypertension. After controlling the initial severe increase in BP, a renal Doppler ultrasound is the appropriate test to determine the kidney size, the extent of kidney damage, and possibly the etiology.

Selected Readings

Adelman, R. D. The hypertensive neonate. Clin. Perinatol. 15:567–584, 1988.

Calhoun, D. A., and S. Oparil. Treatment of hypertensive crisis. N. Engl. J. Med. 323:1177–1183, l990.

Dillon, M. J., and J. R. Ingelfinger. Pharmacological treatment of hypertension. In Holliday, M. A., T. M. Barratt, and E. D. Avner (eds.). Pediatric Nephrology, 3rd ed. Baltimore, Williams and Wilkins Company, 1994, pp. 1165–1174.

Gruskin, A. B., S. Dabbagh, and L.E. Fleischmann. Mechanisms of hypertension in childhood diseases. In Holliday, M. A., T. M. Barratt, and E. D. Avner (eds.). Pediatric Nephrology, 3rd ed. Baltimore, Williams and Wilkins Company, 1994, pp. 1096–1115.

Ingelfinger, J. R., and M. J. Dillon. Evaluation of secondary hypertension. In Holliday, M. A., T. M. Barratt, and E. D. Avner (eds.). Pediatric Nephrology, 3rd ed. Baltimore, Williams and Wilkins Company, 1994, pp. 1146–1164.

Report of the Second Task Force on Blood Pressure Control in Children—1987. Pediatrics 79:1–25, l987.

Yetman, R. J., M. A. Bonilla-Felix, and R. J. Portman. Primary hypertension in children and adolescents. In Holliday, M. A., T. M. Barratt, and E. D. Avner (eds.). Pediatric Nephrology, 3rd ed. Baltimore, Williams and Wilkins Company, 1994, pp. 1117–1145.

GENITOURINARY DISORDERS

C H A P T E R   6 4

AMBIGUOUS GENITALIA

Monica Sifuentes, M.D.

Hx   A term infant is being evaluated in the newborn nursery. The mother received prenatal care from the eighth week of gestation, reportedly had no problems during the pregnancy, and took no medications except prenatal vitamins with iron. She specifically denies taking any progesterone-containing drugs. Her previous pregnancy was uneventful, and her three-year-old son is healthy.

On physical examination, the infant is active and alert, with normal vital signs. Aside from a minimum amount of breast tissue bilaterally, the physical examination is unremarkable, except for the genitalia. The labia are swollen bilaterally and slightly hyperpigmented with what appear to be rugae. No masses are palpable in the labioscrotal folds. The clitoris is 1 cm in length. The introitus is difficult to visualize, but a vaginal opening and urethra are apparent.

Questions

1. What conditions should be considered in newborns with ambiguous genitalia?
2. What should families of such infants be told regarding the gender of the newborns?
3. What key historical information should be obtained from families of such newborns?
4. What laboratory studies must be obtained to aid in the diagnosis?
5. What psychosocial issues should be addressed with families while infants are in the newborn nursery?

Ambiguous genitalia result from an intersex abnormality in newborns and are classified according to the gonads present. This classification includes: female and male pseudohermaphroditism, true hermaphroditism, and mixed gonadal dysgenesis. Individuals with pure gonadal dysgenesis, another intersex disorder, present during adolescence rather than in infancy and are not discussed in this chapter.

Several health care practitioners are often involved in the care of infants with ambiguous genitalia. In addition to the general pediatrician, nurses, social workers, neonatologists, pediatric endocrinologists, geneticists, and surgeons are all significant members of the health care team. The role of primary care physicians, however, cannot be underestimated since they are always involved in the initial evaluations of the newborns and often have already developed relationships with the families.

EPIDEMIOLOGY

The prevalence of ambiguous genitalia in newborns is approximately one in 3,000–4,000 live births. Female pseudohermaphroditism is characterized by female chromosomes (46,XX), normal ovaries and müllerian structures, and virilized external genitalia. The commonest intersex disorder, female pseudohermaphroditism is most often caused by congenital adrenal hyperplasia (CAH). Neonatal screening studies suggest that the incidence of CAH is 1 in 5000 to 1 in 15,000.

Male pseudohermaphroditism occurs in genetic males (46,XY) who have testes but abnormal masculinization of the external genitalia. This disorder most commonly results from androgen insensitivity.

True hermaphroditism is a rare condition in which both ovarian and testicular tissues are present. Seventy to 80% of affected individuals have the 46,XX karyotype, and the morphology of the external genitalia varies widely.

Mixed gonadal dysgenesis is characterized by one testis and an abnormal streak gonad. Reports indicate that this condition is the second most common form of ambiguous genitalia. Affected newborns often have chromosomal mosaicism (45,X/46,XY).

CLINICAL PRESENTATION

Variability in the phenotypic as well as clinical presentation of these disorders is considerable (D_x Box). The newborn with ambiguous genitalia may have an enlarged phallus and varying degrees of labioscrotal fusion. Signs of virilization in the female infant might include hyperpigmented labia and the presence of labial rugae. Other findings suggestive of an intersex disorder in a female are perineal hypospadias or an inguinal hernia. More dramatic presentations, such as severe

Dx Ambiguous Genitalia

- Indeterminate or ambiguous genitalia
- Enlarged phallus
- Hyperpigmented, rugated labia majora that may be fused
- Blind-ending or completely absent vaginal pouch
- Phenotypic male neonate with hypospadias and cryptorchidism
- Phenotypic female neonate with an inguinal hernia or mass

dehydration and shock in a neonate, are associated with CAH of the salt-losing form.

PATHOPHYSIOLOGY

In order to appropriately evaluate and interpret laboratory results of neonates with ambiguous genitalia, it is important to understand the physiology of sexual differentiation and how deviations from this process lead to intersex disorders.

Normal Sexual Differentiation

Normally, before embryos are six weeks old, undifferentiated bilateral gonads into which germ cells migrate from the yolk sac have developed. Both wolffian and müllerian duct systems are present at this time.

If a Y chromosome is present, a histocompatibility-Y (H-Y) antigen is produced, which blocks female development and induces differentiation of these gonads into testes. This process involves the formation of seminiferous tubules that surround the germ cells. Leydig cells begin to produce testosterone, which in turn acts on the wolffian duct to result in the male internal genitalia: vas deferens, epididymis, and seminal vesicles. Concurrently, regression of the müllerian ducts occurs. For normal male external genitalia to form, testosterone must be converted to dihydrotestosterone (DHT) via 5-alpha-reductase. DHT then combines with a specific androgen receptor, which allows formation of the phallus and scrotum from the previously undifferentiated external genitalia. The process primarily involves growth and fusion. Later in gestation, the testes migrate into the scrotum.

For the undifferentiated gonads to develop into female organs, the Y chromosome must be absent and two X chromosomes must be present. Because androgens are not produced, the wolffian duct degenerates, and the müllerian duct develops into these internal female structures: fallopian tubes, uterus, and upper vagina. Fusion of undifferentiated external genitalia does not occur, so folds and swellings become the labia, and the genital tubercle becomes the clitoris.

Development of Ambiguous Genitalia

The adrenogenital syndrome, or CAH, is the most common cause of female pseudohermaphroditism and is a recessively inherited defect. CAH is the result of an enzymatic deficiency in the synthesis of cortisol as well as aldosterone from cholesterol. The most common of these enzymatic defects is 21-hydroxylase deficiency. Prenatally, circulating levels of androgens are abnormally high from the overproduction of intermediate steroids. Hence, the external genitalia of the fetus, which are controlled by androgens, are virilized in the female. Internal female organs, however, are normal, because their development is not influenced by androgens.

The salt-wasting form of 21-hydroxylase deficiency is found in approximately two thirds of patients with classic CAH. As a result of low levels of aldosterone, sodium resorption in the renal tubules is reduced, leading to hyponatremia and hyperkalemia. If this salt-wasting condition goes undiagnosed and untreated, shock and death may result in the first few weeks of life.

Male pseudohermaphroditism is secondary to insufficient testosterone production or insensitivity at the cellular level.

Androgen insensitivity, the most common cause of this disorder, is the result of either an abnormality or a reduction in the number of androgen receptors. Not all affected individuals present with ambiguous genitalia at birth because the spectrum of sensitivity is broad. If the androgen receptor is completely nonfunctional or absent, the external genitalia are those of a normal female (complete testicular feminization). This is a recessive condition. In the incomplete forms, which are X-linked recessive, genital ambiguity does occur.

Other causes of male pseudohermaphroditism are (1) inadequate testosterone production secondary to low levels of fetal gonadotropins; (2) defects in testosterone synthesis from enzyme deficiencies; (3) failure to convert testosterone to DHT as a result of 5-alpha-reductase deficiency; (4) deficient müllerian-duct inhibiting substance, which can be autosomal recessive or X-linked recessive; and (5) intrauterine loss of both testes secondary to torsion or another prenatal event.

Although most causes of ambiguous genitalia are related to chromosomal abnormalities and inherited enzymatic defects, exogenous sources of hormones can affect the differentiation of sexual organs. In most cases, the effect is minimal, and no ambiguity develops. Masculinized female external genitalia can occur, however, depending on the timing and duration of prenatal exposure to androgens or other virilizing drugs. Currently, the most commonly used androgens are probably anabolic steroids. Birth control pills do not contain sufficient androgens to cause a problem.

DIFFERENTIAL DIAGNOSIS

The differential diagnosis of ambiguous genitalia depends on the classification of the intersex disorder (Table 64–1). Some causes of this condition can be life-threatening and therefore must be recognized immediately (e.g., salt-losing CAH).

EVALUATION

History

The general obstetric history should be reviewed, although it may not be helpful in all cases. Probably the

**TABLE 64–1.   Classification and Causes of
Ambiguous Genitalia in the Newborn**

Classification of Intersex Disorder	Causes
Female pseudohermaphroditism	Congenital adrenal hyperplasia
	Maternal androgen ingestion
	Maternal virilizing hormones
	Idiopathic, associated with dysmorphic syndromes
Male pseudohermaphroditism	Biochemical defects in testosterone biosynthesis (enzyme deficiencies)
	Androgen insensitivity (receptor defects)
	5α-reductase deficiency
	Persistent müllerian duct syndrome
	Gonadotropic failure
	Dysgenetic testes
	Bilateral vanishing testes syndrome
True hermaphroditism	Chimerism
Mixed gonadal dysgenesis	Chromosomal mosaicism

most important source of information on family history can be derived from family pedigrees (Questions Box). Undiagnosed chromosomal disorders, consanguinity, and recurrent medical conditions may be established or inferred from the family background.

Physical Examination

A complete physical examination of newborns must be performed in the nursery, in addition to a detailed assessment of the genitalia. In particular, the presence of dysmorphic features (e.g., microcephaly, low set ears, micrognathia), which suggests the presence of a chromosomal abnormality, should be appreciated. The areola should be examined for any evidence of hyperpigmentation, and the inguinal area should be palpated for any masses or hernias.

A thorough genital examination should then be performed. The appearance and size of the labioscrotal folds should be noted in terms of pigmentation, presence of rugae, and size. Physicians should keep in mind that normal female labia majora may not completely cover the labia minora. Practitioners should determine whether any masses are palpable in what appear to be the labia and whether the testes are palpable in what

---

Questions: Ambiguous Genitalia

- Did the mother take any medications containing estrogen, progestins, or androgens during the pregnancy? Did she use any other virilizing drugs, such as danazol, during pregnancy?
- What is the mother's prior obstetric history?
- Did she have any problems with any previous pregnancies?
- Is there a history of any unexplained neonatal deaths?
- Are her other children growing and developing normally?
- Is there a family history of ambiguous genitalia, including microphallus, hypospadias, and cryptorchidism?
- Is there a family history of sterility, female hirsutism, or amenorrhea?
- Are the parents or other family members consanguinous?

---

appears to be the scrotum. The size of the phallus/clitoris should be measured; a normal stretched phallus is at least 2.5 cm long, whereas a normal clitoris should not exceed 1 cm in term infants. The labioscrotal folds should then be spread apart to look for a vaginal introitus. The presence of inferior labioscrotal fusion, which may preclude this, confirms the suspicion of indeterminate genitalia. Finally, the location of a urethral meatus should be noted, because if hypospadias and cryptorchidism occur together, the chance of an intersex disorder is approximately 50%. A rectal examination may help detect the presence of a uterus or prostate but may be difficult.

Laboratory Tests

Certain biochemical studies such as a serum 17-hydroxyprogesterone and a measurement of 17-ketosteroids and pregnanetriol in the urine are mandatory in newborns with ambiguous genitalia. If these initial studies are normal, other intermediate metabolites, such as 11-deoxycortisol and dehydroepiandrosterone sulfate (DHEA-S), and sex steroids (e.g., testosterone and dihydrotestosterone) can also be measured at a later date. In addition, serum electrolytes and a karyotype should be ordered in the nursery. Electrolytes should continue to be monitored closely if CAH is suspected. Karyotypes can be performed in 24 hours by many laboratories. Examination of Barr bodies in a buccal smear is not recommended because this test is unreliable.

A human chorionic gonadotropin stimulation test may be performed when male pseudohermaphroditism is suspected.

Imaging Studies

Pelvic ultrasonography is effective in determining if müllerian structures are present, but this technique is not as useful for locating the gonads. If the gonads are not palpable, computed tomography or magnetic resonance imaging of the pelvis may be considered. Genitography can aid in visualizing the duct structures under fluoroscopy.

MANAGEMENT

An interdisciplinary team consisting of a pediatrician, endocrinologist, medical geneticist, urologist, and psychologist or psychiatrist should be involved in the care of infants with ambiguous genitalia. All aspects of treatment can then be addressed in an efficient and comprehensive manner.

Initial Phase: Delivery Room and Newborn Nursery

If the sex of newborns is uncertain, it should not be assigned in the delivery room. Parents and nursing staff should be notified immediately of the ambiguity, and a unisex name should be assigned such as "Baby Smith" instead of "Baby Boy Smith" or "Baby Girl Smith." Physicians should then reassure parents that they will soon discuss the issue with them and tell them that until confirmatory tests are done, it is best not to speculate on the sex of the infant.

During the initial hours after birth, parents may have difficulty comprehending the condition. An open line of communication must be maintained with the family, however. Parents should be assured that gender assignment will be made as soon as possible—definitely within three to five days. Gender can be assigned even earlier in some institutions because most preliminary laboratory results are reported in 24 to 48 hours. Necessary radiographic studies should be ordered as soon as possible.

Intermediate Phase: Psychological Issues

Several psychological issues should be addressed at the time of diagnosis. Alleviation of parental anxiety regarding the cause of the condition should be the priority; general questions can also be answered. For example, parents may be unclear about what to tell others about the sex of the infant and find this process very awkward. In addition, parents should be educated about the normal sexual differentiation. Pediatricians must emphasize that during the first six to eight weeks of gestation, sexual organs are undifferentiated. Ambiguous genitalia should be explained as overdevelopment or underdevelopment rather than as freaky or highly unusual.

Primary care physicians must also assess parents' level of sophistication and their beliefs about gender identity and sexuality. The gender preference for newborn infants should be addressed. Were the parents hoping for a boy or girl? Do they feel strongly about one gender? The medical team can also help families establish a plan for newborns regarding what they want to tell the extended family and in what detail they want to disclose the information. After the initial meeting and while awaiting laboratory data, other questions regarding sexual orientation, puberty, fertility, and self-esteem may arise.

Final Phase: Gender Assignment

After karyotypes have been confirmed and types of intersex disorder have been considered, team members should meet with families to discuss gender assignment before discharge from the hospital. Possible male sex assignment based on factors such as size of the phallus, presence of corporal tissue, and the response to androgen stimulation must be considered. Otherwise, female sex assignment should probably be made regardless of the cause of the intersex disorder. Parents must be involved in this decision and must agree with the final outcome.

Detailed information should be given once again regarding the origin of the condition. The timing and nature of any future hormonal treatment and surgical procedures should be addressed as well. Parents should be urged to move beyond the issue of ambiguous genitalia once a decision regarding gender has been made. They must then deal with activities such as birth announcements and inquiries regarding gender from extended family, siblings, and baby-sitters. The entire medical team should offer parents encouragement concerning their parenting ability.

TREATMENT

Hormonal supplementation is indicated for some newborns with ambiguous genitalia. Cortisol replacement is mandatory in infants with CAH at daily physiologic doses of 10–20 mg/m^2/day. In infants with salt-wasting or classic 21-hydroxylase deficiency, mineralocorticoid replacement is indicated. Oral fludrocortisone should be administered at doses that suppress plasma renin activity to normal levels without causing hypertension.

Testosterone or estrogen replacement is needed at puberty in certain intersex disorders. Injections of testosterone cypionate at regular intervals may be used in certain cases to increase the length and width of the phallus. Recombinant human growth hormone replacement may also be considered for short stature in mixed gonadal dysgenesis.

Surgical procedures may be necessary in some cases. Although laparoscopy or laparotomy may be indicated for a gonadal biopsy, this is generally not needed in the neonatal period for gender assignment. A gonadectomy is indicated prophylactically in all phenotypic females with all or part of a Y chromosome because of the potential for malignancy. Clitoral recession, vaginoplasty, and labioscrotal reduction are usually performed if infants are to be raised as females. For children to be raised as males, orchiopexy, hypospadias repair, and chordee release are often indicated, but these surgical procedures may be difficult. In some specific cases, however, surgical procedures should be delayed until response to medical treatment is evaluated. For example, in CAH, clitoral size may decrease with glucocorticoid replacement.

PROGNOSIS

The prognosis for most infants with ambiguous genitalia is excellent. Problems arise with undiagnosed CAH, which may lead to shock and death in the neonatal period if unrecognized and untreated. Otherwise, children should be able to live long healthy lives once their families have come to grips with the diagnosis. Amenorrhea and sterility will need to be addressed with phenotypic females during adolescence, at which time psychological services should be provided.

Case Resolution

In the case described at the beginning of the chapter, the infant has ambiguous genitalia. The parents should be informed immediately of this finding, and all references related to gender should be avoided. A karyotype, in addition to serum electrolyte and 17-OH progesterone analyses, should be performed immediately. The physician should then meet with the family to further discuss intersex disorders and explain the diagnostic workup. General psychological services should also be provided.

Selected Readings

Donahoe, P. K. The diagnosis and treatment of infants with intersex abnormalities. Pediatr. Clin. North Am. 34:1333–1348, 1987.

Hadjiathanasiou, C. G., et al. True hermaphroditism: genetic variants and clinical management. J. Pediatr. 125:738–744, 1994.

McCauley, E. Disorders of sexual differentiation and development. Pediatr. Clin. North Am. 37:1405–1420, 1990.

McGillivay, B. C. Genetic aspects of ambiguous genitalia. Pediatr. Clin. North Am. 39:307–317, 1992.

Pagon, R. A. Diagnostic approach to the newborn with ambiguous genitalia. Pediatr. Clin. North Am. 34:1019–1032, 1987.

Rubenstein, S. C., and J. Mandell. Ambiguous genitalia in newborns. Contemp. Pediatr. 10:83–94, 1993.

White, P. C., M. I. New, and B. Dupont. Congenital adrenal hyperplasia. N. Engl. J. Med. 316:1519–1524, 1987.

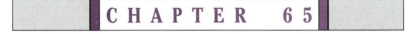

CHAPTER   65

HEMATURIA

Elaine Kamil, M.D.

H$_x$ A five-year-old boy is brought to the office for a school entry examination. He was the full-term product of an uncomplicated pregnancy, labor, and delivery. Although the boy has had four or five episodes of otitis media, he has generally been in good health. He has never been hospitalized or experienced any significant trauma. He has no known allergies, has been fully immunized, and is developmentally normal.

In addition, the physical examination is completely normal. The boy's height and weight are at the 75th percentile, and his blood pressure is 100/64. Screening tests for hearing and vision are completely normal. The boy's hematocrit is 42. His urinalysis comes back with a specific gravity of 1.025, pH 6, 2+ blood, and trace protein. Microscopic examination shows 18–20 RBCs per high-power field, 0–1 WBC per high-power field, and a rare, fine, granular cast.

Questions

1. What disease entities cause hematuria?
2. How should hematuria be evaluated?
3. How does the approach to hematuria differ in children who complain of "dark" or red urine?
4. What is the appropriate follow-up of children with asymptomatic microscopic hematuria?

Hematuria is a common problem in pediatrics, and primary care physicians should have a clear understanding of its pathophysiology, etiology, evaluation, and therapy. Hematuria can be caused by a serious medical problem, or it may only be an incidental finding with no potential for impairment of patients' health.

In general, hematuria is categorized as either gross or microscopic (microhematuria). The etiology and approach to hematuria vary with its severity. Gross hematuria is defined as red or brown urine caused by the presence of RBCs. Microhematuria is defined as three or more consecutive urine samples with a positive dipstick and six or more RBCs per high-power field in a fresh, spun urine sample.

EPIDEMIOLOGY

The incidence of **gross hematuria** is about 1.3 per 1000 patient visits (Table 65–1). In about half of these patients, the causes are readily apparent from the intake

TABLE 65–1.   Etiology of Gross Hematuria in an Unselected Pediatric Population

Causes	Percent (%) of Patients
Readily Apparent Causes	
Documented urinary tract infection (UTI)	26
Perineal irritation	11
Meatal stenosis with ulcer	7
Trauma	7
Coagulopathy	3
Stones	2
Total	56
Other Causes	
Suspected UTI	23
Recurrent gross hematuria	5
Acute nephritis	4
Ureteropelvic junction obstruction	1
Cystitis cystica	< 1
Epididymitis	< 1
Tumor	< 1
Unknown	9
Total	44

Modified, with permission, from Ingelfinger, J.R., et al. Frequency and etiology of gross hematuria in a general pediatric setting. Pediatrics 59:557–561, 1977.

history or physical examination. The incidence of this type of hematuria may increase in the community as a result of an epidemic of a disease, such as acute glomerulonephritis, that causes hematuria.

Microscopic hematuria is a more common pediatric problem. Prevalence rates for persistent, microscopic hematuria range from 0.5 to 2.0%, but 4 to 5% of school-age children have microhematuria on a single voided specimen. The incidence is artificially increased in late summer, because at that time children tend to visit pediatricians for school physicals that typically include a screening urinalysis.

CLINICAL PRESENTATION

Children with gross hematuria present with a sudden appearance of red or brown urine, which may be associated with flank or urethral pain or with a history of trauma.

Children with microscopic hematuria may have urinary complaints (e.g., dysuria). In children who appear well, microhematuria is usually detected on screening dipstick examination.

PATHOPHYSIOLOGY

Gross Hematuria

Gross hematuria occurs because of the presence of large numbers of RBCs in the urine. Blood may enter the urine because of rupture of blood vessels following trauma or inflammation in the glomeruli or interstitial regions of the kidney. It may also occur as a result of severe inflammation of the bladder wall.

Causes of gross hematuria are listed in Table 65–2. The presence of casts in the urine suggests the diagnosis of glomerulonephritis. The most common causes of glomerulonephritis in children include acute poststreptococcal glomerulonephritis, anaphylactoid purpura, IgA nephropathy, membranoproliferative glomerulonephritis (MPGN), and SLE.

Common causes of gross hematuria in the absence of RBC casts include **UTI, renal trauma, bleeding diathesis** (e.g., hemophilia or idiopathic thrombocytopenic purpura), **renal tumors, obstruction of the urinary tract, renal stones**, or perhaps **hemolytic-uremic syn-**

TABLE 65–2. Common Causes of Gross Hematuria in Pediatric Patients

Glomerulonephritis	*Structural Causes*
IgA nephropathy	Renal trauma
Acute poststreptococcal GN*	Tumor
Lupus nephritis	Obstruction
Membranoproliferative GN*	Renal stones
Anaphylactoid purpura GN*	Vascular abnormality
Hematologic Causes	*Infectious Causes*
Sickle cell disease	Bacterial urinary tract infection
Hemophilia	Viral cystitis
Thrombocytopenia	
Thrombosis (renal arterial or venous)	

*GN, glomerulonephritis.

drome (HUS). A hemangioma in the urinary tract is an extremely rare cause of gross hematuria.

Microhematuria

Microhematuria occurs when small numbers of RBCs enter the urine via tiny ruptures in the glomerular capillary walls or in the capillaries of the tubular or bladder lining. For purposes of discussion, the following causes of microscopic hematuria are considered: infectious, structural, traumatic, glomerular, and interstitial. Separate consideration of the causes of microscopic and gross hematuria is often helpful, although significant overlap exists.

UTI is one of the most common **infectious causes** of hematuria. Bacterial infections of the bladder or kidney occur much more frequently than viral cystitis. Adenovirus is the most common viral cause of hemorrhagic cystitis and is usually associated with dysuria. Vaginitis in girls and prostatitis in teenage boys may also result in hematuria.

Any type of congenital obstructive uropathy may lead to massive dilatation of the urinary tract, which makes the urinary tract more susceptible to bleeding, even with trivial trauma. **Chronic urinary tract obstruction** in children (e.g., posterior urethral valves or congenital ureteropelvic junction obstruction) is often asymptomatic. In the past these conditions were typically diagnosed when children presented with UTIs. Now they are commonly diagnosed after a prenatal ultrasound reveals hydronephrosis. Nevertheless, urinary tract obstruction may be detected during an evaluation for asymptomatic microhematuria.

Any **tumor** of the genitourinary tract may be associated with both gross and microscopic hematuria. Pelvic tumors rarely cause urinary obstruction in children, although such tumors frequently cause obstruction in adults. Children with Wilms' tumor, the most common childhood renal tumor, usually present with an abdominal mass, but it may cause hematuria.

Congenital renal malformations are quite common. Any of these may be associated with hematuria and include polycystic kidney disease, renal dysplasia, medullary sponge kidney, and simple cysts. Patients with polycystic kidney disease may even have severe, painful hematuria.

Vascular problems may also lead to hematuria. Hemangiomas of the kidney, bladder, or ureter are very rare. Arteriovenous malformations also occur infrequently. Hematuria may be a sign of a renal artery or vein thrombosis, particularly in sick neonates.

Young children are more susceptible to **renal injury,** which may result in hematuria, than older children or adults because their kidneys are relatively less protected by the rib cage. In addition, children may insert foreign objects into the urethra and bladder that cause pain and hematuria. Microhematuria has also been described after extremely vigorous exercise such as marathon running. Child abuse should be considered if any suspicions are raised on the basis of the history or physical examination.

TABLE 65–3. Normal Values for Urinary Calcium-Creatinine Ratios*

Age	Urine Calcium-Creatinine	24-Hour Urine Calcium
Preterm	≤ 0.82	≤8.9 mg/kg/day†
< 7 months	≤ 0.86	
7–18 months	≤ 0.60	
19 months–6 years	≤ 0.42	
6 years–adult	≤ 0.22	<4 mg/kg/day

*Samples for calcium-creatinine ratio should be obtained on a fasting, first voided morning specimen. The calcium and creatinine concentrations must be in the same units (e.g., mg/dL) before the ratio is calculated.

†For healthy preterm infants taking no medications. Calcium excretion varies with diet and phosphorus intake, and it is higher if patients are treated with furosemide, xanthines, or glucocorticoids.

TABLE 65–4. Distinguishing Hematuria From Pigmenturia*

Problem	Urine Color	Hemastix	Microscopic Appearance
Hematuria	Red, brown, or red-brown	Positive	Red blood cells
Hemoglobinuria	Red, brown, or red-brown	Positive	Negative
Myoglobinuria	Red, brown, or red-brown	Positive	Negative
Porphyrins	Red	Negative	Negative
Exogenous pigments	Red or orange	Negative	Negative

*Some common exogenous pigments include phenytoin, beets, rifampin, nitrofurantoin, sulfas, amitriptyline, methyldopa, phenothiazine, and chloroquine.

Hypercalciuria is another cause of microscopic hematuria. Children with hypercalciuria often have a family history of urinary calculi. Calcium oxalate crystals may be present on the microscopic examination of the urine. A urinary calcium-creatinine ratio is best obtained on a first morning, fasting urine sample. Calcium excretion varies with age. Normal values are listed in Table 65–3.

There are two types of hypercalciuria: absorptive and "renal leak." Children with absorptive hypercalciuria overabsorb calcium from the GI tract, probably because of an exquisite sensitivity to vitamin D, and can be treated with a reduced calcium diet. Children with renal leak hypercalciuria have an inherently higher rate of urinary calcium excretion and may require thiazide diuretics to reduce urinary calcium excretion.

Interstitial nephritis, usually from drug exposure, may also cause hematuria. Generally patients with interstitial nephritis may exhibit other signs of tubular disease such as glucosuria or proteinuria.

DIFFERENTIAL DIAGNOSIS

When children complain of gross hematuria or "red" urine, practitioners must first determine if they have hematuria or pigmenturia by using a urine dipstick. If the dipstick is negative for blood, then the dark urine is due to dyes, drugs, or pigments (Table 65–4). If the dipstick is positive for blood, the red color is caused by intact RBCs, hemolyzed RBCs, or myoglobin; the clarification is based on microscopic examination of a fresh, spun urine.

Children whose dipsticks are positive for blood but show no RBCs may have hemoglobinuria or myoglobinuria. Hemoglobinuria may be seen with acute autoimmune hemolytic anemia, drug-induced hemolysis, paroxysmal nocturnal hemoglobinuria, a mismatched blood transfusion, cardiopulmonary bypass, freshwater drowning, and in some cases, HUS. Myoglobinuria is seen in individuals with rhabdomyolysis. Acute rhabdomyolysis can occur after a crush injury or a very prolonged seizure and in certain susceptible individuals with an inborn error of muscle metabolism. Both free hemoglobin and myoglobin are toxic to the renal epithelial cells, mandating a generous fluid intake and close monitoring.

EVALUATION

Gross Hematuria

History

The history is crucial to an accurate, efficient, and cost-effective evaluation of patients with hematuria (Questions Box). The family should be questioned carefully about trauma (to trunk or perineum), recent skin infection or pharyngitis, dysuria, and abdominal or flank pain. Parents should be asked whether their children appear "puffy." A family history of kidney disease, bleeding diathesis, hemolytic anemia, or inborn error of muscle metabolism may be important.

Physical Examination

A complete physical examination is also essential. Blood pressure should be measured accurately. The skin should be examined thoroughly for rashes or petechiae; the abdomen should be checked carefully for renal masses or tenderness; the genitalia should be examined thoroughly for signs of trauma, masses, or rashes (see Chapter 97, Child Sexual Abuse); and the joints should be checked carefully for signs of arthritis. Fundi should be examined for any hypertensive

---

Questions: Hematuria

- Has the child suffered any recent trauma?
- Has the child had fever or dysuria?
- Does the child have any flank or abdominal pain?
- Does the child have any rashes, joint pains, or edema?
- Does the child have a family history of hematuria, kidney disease, kidney stones, or gross hematuria?
- Is there a family history of bleeding disorders or inborn errors of muscle metabolism?

changes. Children should be assessed for the presence of edema.

A careful cardiac and chest examination is necessary to detect signs of congestive heart failure, a finding seen in acute glomerulonephritis.

Laboratory Tests

Recent studies have shown that careful microscopic examination of a urine sample can help determine whether bleeding originates from the upper urinary tract or the lower urinary tract. The first morning urine sample is the most reliable but is not appropriate in some settings, such as after an automobile accident. Sometimes the gross hematuria is so substantial that spinning the urine results in a large pellet of debris that is difficult to examine. In such instances, it is prudent to examine an unspun sample. The presence of RBC casts indicates glomerulonephritis, but the absence of such casts does not rule out this condition.

If the urine shows RBC casts, then the evaluation should include an antistreptolysin-O (ASO) titer, antinuclear antibody (ANA), C3, CBC and differential with platelet count, BUN and creatinine, serum albumin, and a random urine for a urinary total protein-creatinine ratio.

If the urine shows only large numbers of RBCs, no RBC casts, and no bacteriuria, a CBC with differential and platelet count, a urine culture, and a PT and PTT should be obtained. A sickle cell test should be considered as well.

Imaging Studies

If the urine has large numbers of RBCs and no bacteriuria, a renal ultrasound should be obtained. With gross hematuria and a history of serious trauma, an abdominal CT scan should be performed. Children with RBC casts should also have a chest x-ray to evaluate for signs of congestive heart failure.

Microhematuria

The evaluation of microscopic hematuria is similar to that of gross hematuria. Figure 65–1 outlines an approach to the evaluation of microscopic hematuria.

History and Physical Examination

Because many conditions may cause either gross or microscopic hematuria, the same historical questions apply to both conditions, and the same careful physical examination is indicated.

Laboratory Tests

Generally, the initial evaluation includes a urine culture and a careful microscopic examination of the urine. If the culture is negative, the hematuria is minimal, and children are otherwise healthy, the urinalysis should be repeated once or twice over the following two weeks.

RBC casts always signify a glomerular origin. Casts are best preserved in acidic, concentrated urine. Thus, the first morning urine is the best sample to examine for casts. RBC morphology should be assessed. RBCs originating in the glomerulus are **dysmorphic** and of smaller caliber, whereas those that come from lower downstream appear like normal **biconcave** disks. Although RBC morphology is best appreciated with the use of a polarizing microscope, with experience, dys-

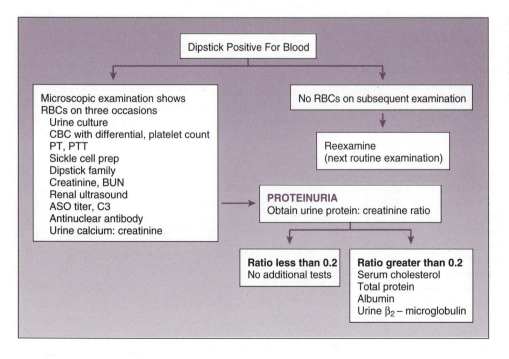

FIGURE 65–1. Evaluation of asymptomatic, microscopic hematuria. ASO, antistreptolysin-O; BUN, blood urea nitrogen; CBC, complete blood count; PT, prothrombin time; PTT, partial thromboplastin time; RBCs, red blood cells.

morphic RBCs can be recognized using an ordinary microscope. RBCs of glomerular origin have a mean cell volume of 50 μL or less. In contrast, RBCs of nonglomerular origin have a mean cell volume of 80 to 90 μL.

Clotting ability should be determined with a platelet count, PT, and PTT. A sickle cell test should be performed. Renal function should be screened with a BUN and creatinine, and a urine calcium-creatinine ratio should be determined. A C3, ANA, and ASO titer should also be checked. If a urine dipstick shows more than a trace of protein, a urinary protein:creatinine ratio should also be determined. If there is a family history of renal disease, a hearing screen should be ordered. All immediate family members should have their urine checked for blood.

If a bloody urine sample is analyzed with a Coulter counter, characteristic distribution curves are seen for glomerular and nonglomerular hematuria. This test is not readily available, however.

Imaging Studies

A renal ultrasound should be performed to rule out structural abnormalities and tumors. Chest x-rays should be obtained if acute glomerulonephritis is suspected.

GLOMERULAR DISEASES ASSOCIATED WITH HEMATURIA

Glomerulonephritis

Both acute and chronic glomerulonephritis are associated with hematuria. The diagnosis of acute poststreptococcal glomerulonephritis requires a "nephritic" urine sediment (RBCs, RBC casts), a low serum complement, and an elevated streptococcal titer (ASO titer, anti-DNAase B, or positive streptozyme). It is important to document that the serum complement returns to normal, because MPGN may present in a similar way. The serum complement is chronically depressed in MPGN.

The most common form of glomerulonephritis in children is **acute poststreptococcal glomerulonephritis**. Many cases are asymptomatic, however, and do not come to the attention of physicians. The resulting hematuria, which may be gross or microscopic, is rarely seen before the age of two years. The condition is most commonly diagnosed in preschool-age children, who typically present with gross hematuria, often with some edema and hypertension. The hypertension may be severe, and occasionally children even have hypertensive seizures. The edema results from transient, acute renal failure with salt and fluid retention.

The majority of children with acute poststreptococcal glomerulonephritis recover completely and have an excellent long-term prognosis. Proteinuria is rarely severe enough to cause nephrotic syndrome, and renal failure is rarely serious enough to require dialysis. If hypertension occurs, the chest x-ray often shows some degree of pulmonary edema, even in the absence of overt signs of congestive heart failure. Any hypertension requires treatment.

Other infections cause postinfectious glomerulonephritis, but they are less common and less well characterized. The most common form of chronic glomerulonephritis that affects children is **IgA nephropathy**. On kidney biopsy, patients have mesangial proliferation with mesangial deposits of IgA as the dominant immunoglobulin. In the later stages, glomerulosclerosis and interstitial fibrosis are apparent. More than one-third of adults with IgA nephropathy develop end-stage renal disease; the percent of children who progress to this point is less well known. Gross hematuria in IgA nephropathy is occasionally so severe that patients may pass clots and have flank pain. The presence of persistent proteinuria is considered a poor prognostic sign.

Other forms of primary chronic glomerulonephritis include **MPGN, mesangial proliferative glomerulonephritis,** and **membranous nephropathy**, which is technically not a form of glomerulonephritis because it usually lacks a significant proliferative component. Children with these diseases present with hematuria, almost always associated with heavy proteinuria.

Secondary forms of glomerulonephritis include the nephritis of SLE, anaphylactoid purpura, and the nephritis associated with various vasculitides such as Wegener's granulomatosis and pauci-immune crescentic glomerulonephritis. Children with lupus tend to present with multisystem disorders but may have only renal manifestations of the disease. ANA is a good screening test for lupus. If ANA is positive, C3, C4, antidouble-stranded DNA, and a Coombs test should be checked.

Anaphylactoid Purpura

This disease is almost always accompanied by the classical cutaneous vasculitis rash, which is prominent over the lower arms and lower extremities. Abdominal pain may be severe, and affected patients are at risk for the development of intussusception. Children with anaphylactoid purpura have microscopic hematuria, which usually clears, but is occasionally associated with heavy proteinuria and nephrotic syndrome. These children are at risk for developing progressive renal disease. All children with anaphylactoid purpura should have their urine monitored for cessation of hematuria or development of proteinuria. Children with heavy proteinuria and suspected anaphylactoid purpura should have a diagnostic renal biopsy.

Hemolytic-Uremic Syndrome

HUS is a disease characterized by microangiopathic hemolytic anemia, thrombocytopenia, and acute renal failure. It typically follows a prodrome of bloody diarrhea from acute colitis caused by a verotoxin-producing strain of *Escherichia coli* (O157/H7). The verotoxin is believed to be toxic to human endothelial cells. The damaged endothelial cells incite the deposition of fibrin within the glomerular capillaries. These fibrin thrombi lead to the shearing of RBCs and consumption of platelets. Several other organisms, such as pneumococcus and *Shigella*, may precipitate HUS. In atypical cases of HUS, the precipitating event may be a URI. Some cases are familial. Children present with pallor and severe abdominal pain. Urine output may be diminished as a result of renal failure, and in many cases dialysis is required. Hypertension may be severe.

Other Glomerular Diseases

Alport's syndrome, thin basement membrane disease (benign familial hematuria), focal segmental glomerulosclerosis (FSGS), minimal change disease (MCD), and nephrosclerosis are also associated with hematuria. **Alport's syndrome** is a disease of the glomerular basement membrane, where thinning and duplication of the basement membrane occur. The renal involvement eventually leads to end-stage renal disease. Patients or their family members often have nerve deafness or keratoconus. The inheritance of Alport's syndrome varies by kindred; it may be either autosomal dominant or sex-linked. Thin basement membrane disease also is characterized by thinning of the glomerular basement membrane, but the glomeruli are otherwise normal, and the clinical course is benign. Patients with MCD and FSGS present with nephrotic syndrome but may also have microscopic hematuria.

MANAGEMENT

Gross Hematuria

The management of gross hematuria depends on the underlying cause. Children with a history of trauma should be placed on bed rest pending surgical consultation (see Chapter 40, Abdominal Trauma). If the evaluation indicates acute glomerulonephritis and if children are not hypertensive, they can be followed carefully as outpatients with monitoring of blood pressure and renal function with consultation with a pediatric nephrologist. Children with coagulopathies require specific treatment of their bleeding disorders (e.g., intravenous gamma globulin for idiopathic thrombocytopenic purpura).

If some degree of renal insufficiency is present, then children should be referred to a pediatric nephrologist to rule out more unusual causes of glomerulonephritis, for consideration of renal biopsy, and for treatment.

Microhematuria

Laboratory tests other than urinalysis may be negative in otherwise healthy children with microscopic hematuria. Some of these children may be recovering from subclinical cases of poststreptococcal glomerulonephritis, which can cause microscopic hematuria for up to one year. Others may have early IgA nephropathy and not yet have significant proteinuria, and some may have thin basement membrane disease. As long as children have normal renal function, normal blood pressure, and no significant proteinuria, and all other tests are normal, it is safe to monitor them every three to six months until the problem resolves. Healthy children with an otherwise negative workup who show no change in their clinical state for a period of one year may subsequently be monitored annually. If hypercalciuria is detected, a low-calcium diet or treatment with thiazide diuretics may be tried.

PROGNOSIS

The prognosis for children with hematuria depends on the underlying cause. Gross hematuria is more often associated with serious renal disease such as acute glomerulonephritis, HUS, or renal trauma. Even so, most children with gross hematuria have a good prognosis, provided the diagnosis is rapidly discovered and appropriate specific therapy is given. Children with persistent microscopic hematuria who have no family history of the condition, have a negative evaluation, and do not develop hypertension or proteinuria have an excellent long-term prognosis.

> ### Case Resolution
>
> The boy in the opening scenario shows no worrisome clinical signs such as hypertension or significant proteinuria. His urine should be rechecked twice more, and if the hematuria persists, his evaluation should follow the algorithm in Figure 65–1.

Selected Readings

Adams, N . D., and J. C. Rowe. Nephrocalcinosis. *In* Bailie, M. D. (ed.). Clinics in Perinatology. Philadelphia, W. B. Saunders, 1992, pp. 179–195.

Boineau, F. G., and J. E. Lewy. Evaluation of hematuria in children and adolescents. Pediatr. Rev. 11:101, 1989.

Ingelfinger, J. R., A. E. Davis, and W. E. Grupe. Frequency and etiology of gross hematuria in a general pediatric setting. Pediatrics 59:557–561, 1977.

Kitagawa, T. Lessons learned from the Japanese nephritis screening study. Pediatr. Nephrol. 2:256–263, 1988.

Lieu, T. A., and H. M. Grasmeder, III. An approach to the evaluation and treatment of microscopic hematuria. Pediatr. Clin. North Am. 38:579–592, 1991.

Sargent, J. D., et al. Normal values for random urinary calcium to creatinine ratios in infancy. J. Pediatr. 123:393–397, 1993.

Tsukahara, H., et al. Urinary erythrocyte volume analysis: a simple method for localizing the site of hematuria in pediatric patients. J. Pediatr. 115:433–436, 1989.

CHAPTER 66

PROTEINURIA

Elaine Kamil, M.D.

Hx A 14-year-old boy is brought to the office for a preparticipation sports physical examination. He has been previously healthy but had one hospital admission at the age of two years for treatment of a fractured humerus. He has no acute complaints. The family history is positive for diabetes mellitus in the paternal grandfather and lung cancer in the maternal grandfather. It is negative for renal disease or hypertension. The boy's height and weight are at the 75th percentile for age, and his blood pressure is 110/70.

On physical examination he is a well-developed, well-nourished, athletic teenager. No abnormal findings are present. The CBC reveals a hemoglobin of 14.8 g/dL, a hematocrit of 48.3%, and a WBC of 8400/mm^3 with a normal differential. The urine has a pH of 5, a specific gravity of 1.025, and a 3+ protein on dipstick. The rest of the dipstick is negative. Microscopic examination shows 0–1 WBC per high-power field and 0–2 hyaline casts per low-power field.

Questions

1. What conditions cause proteinuria?
2. When should children with proteinuria undergo further evaluation?
3. What type of evaluation should be carried out to assess proteinuria?
4. When should children with proteinuria be referred to a pediatric nephrologist?

A small amount of protein is normally present in the urine. Protein levels increase somewhat in certain conditions such as vigorous exercise, febrile illnesses, accidental trauma, and congestive heart failure. Most of the protein in the glomerular filtrate is reabsorbed by the tubular cells. Pathologic amounts of protein are present in the urine when the glomerular leak of protein is increased, when the tubules fail to reabsorb the protein filtered by the glomerulus, or if inflammation in the renal interstitium leads to the addition of globulins to the urine.

Urinary protein is initially detected by urine dipstick, but this method is unreliable in alkaline urine. Dipstick protein is also affected by urine concentration. A dipstick for protein of 1+ in a concentrated urine may not correlate with an abnormal 24-hour urinary protein excretion, whereas a dipstick of 1+ in a very dilute urine may be associated with an abnormal 24-hour urinary protein excretion. Proteinuria may be more accurately determined by performing a timed urine collection or a random sample for chemical determination of the total protein concentration.

EPIDEMIOLOGY

The prevalence of proteinuria depends on how the condition is defined. In a Texas study, 10 mg/dL of proteinuria was found consistently in the urine of 2 to 3% of children in three consecutive urine samples. When 50 mg/dL was used as the cutoff for proteinuria, however, only 0.4 to 0.7% of boys and 0.4 to 2.5% of girls had proteinuria in two of three consecutive samples. The prevalence of proteinuria increased with age. In Finland, about 11% of school-age children had at least one episode of proteinuria of 25 mg/dL by dipstick when the urine was tested four times. Approximately 2.5% of the children had proteinuria on two of four occasions.

CLINICAL PRESENTATION

Proteinuria is a laboratory finding that may present incidentally on a screening urinalysis or be detected during the evaluation of a complaint, such as edema, that may be caused by renal disease. When proteinuria is detected as an incidental finding in otherwise normal children, the laboratory evaluation of the proteinuria should be delayed until its persistence is confirmed on repeat dipstick (D_x Box). Edematous children with proteinuria certainly have renal lesions. Additional findings on examination could include the presence of hypertension, ascites, pleural effusions, or the rash of SLE or anaphylactoid purpura.

PATHOPHYSIOLOGY

The glomerular capillaries are adapted to permit the filtration of minimal amounts of plasma proteins, particularly those with a small molecular radius. Approximately 320 mg of albumin and 360 mg of lower molecular weight proteins are filtered by the glomerular capillaries each day. Ninety-five percent of this is reabsorbed by the proximal tubular cells. Normally, children may

---

D_x Proteinuria

- Presence of dipstick proteinuria (> 1+ confirmed on three occasions)
- Random urine total protein-creatinine ratio greater than 0.25 *or* 24-hour urine protein greater than 4 mg/m^2/hr
- Orthostatic proteinuria (assessed through separate measurement of afternoon and first-morning urines for total protein-creatinine ratios)

excrete up to 100 mg/m^2 of protein per day. Urinary protein excretion is increased in newborns to about 240 mg/m^2/day and in adolescents to about 300 mg/day. Adults may normally excrete up to 150 mg of protein per day. Only 10 to 15% of this is albumin; the rest of the proteins are other plasma proteins and urinary glycoproteins.

When increased proteinuria results from glomerular disease, higher levels of urinary proteins are primarily due to the enhanced filtration of albumin. Protein excretion may be increased transiently by any condition that raises intraglomerular capillary pressure such as congestive heart failure, strenuous exercise, epinephrine use, fever, or surgery.

Orthostatic proteinuria, which affects some children, is a poorly understood, benign condition. Individuals excrete pathologic amounts of protein in their urine while they are upright, but their urinary protein excretion returns to normal when they are recumbent. This condition seems to be more common in athletic individuals. Some investigators believe that orthostatic proteinuria is due to increased pressure in the renal vasculature while patients are upright.

DIFFERENTIAL DIAGNOSIS

The proteinuria may be physiologic (secondary to fever, congestive heart failure), orthostatic, tubular (as seen in allergic interstitial nephritis), or glomerular. Aminoaciduria may occur, as is seen in certain inborn errors of metabolism.

EVALUATION

History

It is important to elicit a complete history (Questions Box) in children with proteinuria. When asking about a history of swelling, the practitioner should note that subtle periorbital edema may be present only in the early morning hours. If the proteinuria is detected at a routine screening examination, the conditions under which the urine was obtained should be

---

Questions: Proteinuria

- Was the mother's pregnancy remarkable in any way? What was the child's birth like?
- Did the child have any neonatal problems that may indicate possible renal damage?
- Is any swelling apparent in areas such as the ankles, the abdomen, or the periorbital region?
- Has the child had any recent illnesses, particularly pharyngitis or impetigo?
- Does the child have a history of joint pains and skin rashes, especially the adolescent patient who may be at greater risk of having a collagen-vascular disease?
- Has the child had any previous UTIs, urinary abnormalities, or dark urine?
- Does the child have a history of hypertension or weight loss or gain?
- Is there a family history of renal disease?
- Does the child have diabetes mellitus?

---

determined. Children may have been sick with a high fever or have just participated in an athletic event such as a track meet.

Physical Examination

The physical examination should include a determination of blood pressure and measurement of height and weight. A careful assessment for edema should be made. The skin should be examined for signs of rashes such as Henoch-Schönlein purpura or healing impetigo. The joints should be inspected for any signs of swelling or joint inflammation. The abdominal examination should include a careful search for ascites or organomegaly.

Laboratory Tests

The extent of the laboratory evaluation depends on the child's general health (e.g., is the child ill with another problem?), the amount of proteinuria on dipstick, and whether the child has edema. The suggested evaluation is outlined in Figure 66–1. In nonedematous, otherwise healthy children, it is prudent to examine the urine sediment, and if negative, recheck the dipstick in a few days. If proteinuria of 1+ is consistently present and no hematuria is evident, a first-stage evaluation is indicated. If children are ill with a fever or are hospitalized with a serious illness, it is often appropriate to delay the evaluation of the proteinuria until the acute illness is under control, providing no associated hematuria or azotemia is present.

In healthy ambulatory patients with persistent, isolated, dipstick proteinuria on three occasions, it is important to quantitate the proteinuria (Box 66–1). This may be done simply by ordering a urinary protein-creatinine ratio. If the ratio is abnormal (> 0.25), children need to be evaluated first for orthostatic proteinuria.

Orthostatic proteinuria can be ruled out in several ways. The simplest evaluation involves checking a urine dipstick on a first voided morning sample and again on an afternoon specimen. This procedure should be repeated on two different days. It is critical to be sure that children empty their bladders before going to bed, because urine produced when they are nonrecumbent may contain protein and give an inaccurate result. If the dipstick from the morning urine is negative on a concentrated, acid urine, and if the afternoon sample is positive on a concentrated, acid urine, children most likely have orthostatic proteinuria.

A more accurate way of checking for orthostatic proteinuria involves the determination of urine protein: creatinine ratios on the first-morning and afternoon urine samples. A diagnosis of orthostatic proteinuria can be made if the ratio is normal on the "recumbent" sample and elevated on the daytime sample. The most accurate way of diagnosing orthostatic proteinuria entails collecting two timed urine samples, one during the hours that children are up during the day and the other while they are in bed at night. In most instances of orthostatic proteinuria in children, the total urinary protein excretion is less than one gram. The urine collected

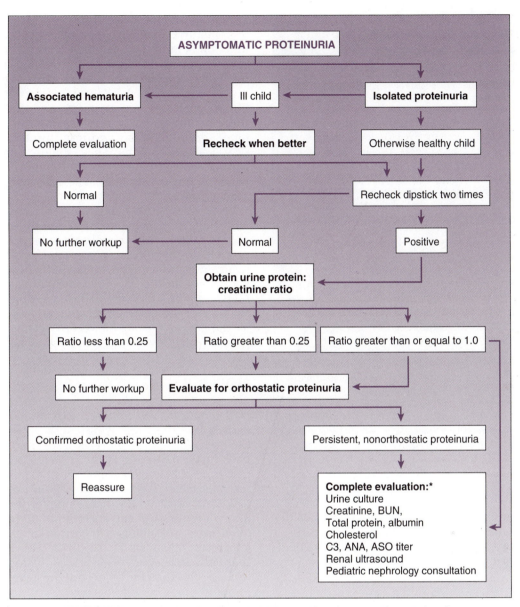

FIGURE 66–1. *Suggested evaluation of children with asymptomatic proteinuria.*

in the recumbent period should contain less than 50 mg/m^2 of protein. If these two timed samples meet the criteria for orthostatic proteinuria, they do not need to be repeated. It is important to remember that even in renal disease, proteinuria improves somewhat when patients are recumbent.

If children do not have orthostatic proteinuria, a 24-hour urine protein excretion should be determined. If the collection of a 24-hour urine sample is impractical, the urine protein:creatinine ratio is a reliable alternative. Blood chemistries (e.g., BUN, creatinine) should be obtained to determine renal function. Electrolyte status should be assessed with total carbon dioxide, total protein, albumin, and cholesterol. Serologies should be obtained for antinuclear antibodies, C3, antistreptolysin-O titer, and hepatitis B surface antigen if children come from a population at risk for hepatitis B.

Twenty-four-hour urine protein excretion should be less than 4 mg/m^2/hr. Neonates may excrete as much as 150 mg/m^2/12 hr, however. Table 66–1 gives a summary of normal urinary protein excretion. If children have nephrotic range proteinuria or nephrotic syndrome (heavy proteinuria accompanied by hypoalbuminemia and hypercholesterolemia), they require further evaluation for nephrotic syndrome (see Chapter 112, Nephrotic Syndrome). If they do not have nephrotic range proteinuria, abnormal tubular proteinuria should be ruled out. A normal urinary β_2-microglobulin rules out tubular proteinuria.

In general, consultation with a pediatric nephrologist is recommended if children have an abnormal 24-hour urinary protein excretion (see Table 66–1). If the proteinuria exceeds one gram per day or if any other minor signs of renal dysfunction or hematuria are

BOX 66–1 Methods for Assessment of Urinary Protein

Detection of proteinuria by dipstick is only semiquantitative. This examination is affected by urinary pH and concentration, and therefore more definitive tests are warranted if a patient's urine consistently shows dipstick proteinuria. The sulfasalicylic acid (SSA) turbidity test is also semiquantitative. When SSA is added to an aliquot of urine, it precipitates urinary proteins. The amount of turbidity is graded on a scale of 0 to 4+.

Urinary protein is most accurately quantitated by a chemical determination on a timed urine collection (usually 24 hours). The concentration (measured in mg/dL) is multiplied by the total urine volume to determine the milligrams of protein excreted in 24 hours. Twenty-four-hour urine samples are difficult to collect in young children. However, several studies have shown that a random urine sample for a protein:creatinine ratio correlates well with the 24-hour urinary protein excretion. The ratio is determined by dividing the urine protein concentration (mg/dL) by the urine creatinine concentration (mg/dL). The units must be the same for each component. The urinary protein:creatinine ratio is normally less than 0.25. A ratio of 3.5 or greater in an adult or greater than 1.0 in children indicates nephrotic-range proteinuria.

Occasionally it is important to determine whether proteinuria has a tubular or glomerular basis. In these instances, a urinary β_2-microglobulin is helpful. β_2-microglobulin, a very small protein that is freely filtered at the glomerular level, is nearly completely reabsorbed by the proximal tubules. In instances of tubular injury such as interstitial nephritis, acute tubular necrosis, or nephrotoxic renal injury, urinary β_2-microglobulin is increased. With glomerular proteinuria, urine protein electrophoresis shows a heavy preponderance of albumin.

present, a biopsy is warranted. Often, otherwise healthy children with small amounts of isolated proteinuria of less than 750 to 1000 mg/day are followed by the pediatric nephrologist without a kidney biopsy.

Imaging Studies

A renal ultrasound should be obtained to rule out any structural abnormalities.

MANAGEMENT

Most children with normal renal function and normal blood pressure whose evaluation reveals physiologic or orthostatic proteinuria should have repeat urinalysis on an annual basis. If the proteinuria worsens or if hematuria develops, a repeat evaluation of renal function is indicated. Children whose initial evaluation reveals persistent, significant proteinuria require careful follow-up to detect and monitor signs of serious renal disease. This follow-up should include repeat blood pressure measurement and urinalysis every three months and repeat chemistries (BUN, creatinine, serum albumin) and urine protein:creatinine ratios every six months. These children should be managed in consultation with the pediatric nephrologist, whose experience is helpful in reassessing the need for kidney biopsy.

Children with physiologic or orthostatic proteinuria who have minimal, persistent proteinuria should be able to follow a full school schedule and be allowed to participate in sports, provided there are no other contraindications. The usual immunization schedule should not be interrupted, and children should follow a regular diet. No increase in dietary protein is necessary to compensate for the minimal amounts of protein lost in the urine. Results of recent studies in nephrotic patients have even suggested that a high-protein diet may increase urinary protein losses.

PROGNOSIS

The outlook for children with proteinuria depends entirely on the underlying cause of the proteinuria. Children whose proteinuria is associated with edema or hematuria are more likely to have significant renal disease, such as glomerulonephritis, however, and the prognosis may be less favorable. If the proteinuria is due to a form of chronic glomerulonephritis, children may ultimately develop end-stage renal disease. If the proteinuria is physiologic or orthostatic, however, the long-term prognosis is excellent. The likelihood that these children will develop renal functional impairment is no greater than for the rest of the general population.

Case Resolution

In the case presented at the beginning of the chapter, odds are that the evaluation of the healthy teenage boy with isolated proteinuria will reveal that he has orthostatic proteinuria, and his long-term prognosis is good.

TABLE 66–1. Urinary Protein Excretion by Age

Age	24-hour Urine Protein (mg)	Urine Protein:Creatinine
Premature infant	14–60	—
Full-term infant	15–68	—
2–12 months	17–85	≤0.50
2–4 years	20–121	≤0.25
4–10 years	26–194	≤0.25
10–16 years	29–238	≤0.25

Selected Readings

Albitol, C., et al. Quantitation of proteinuria with urinary protein/creatinine ratios and random testing with dipsticks in nephrotic children. J. Pediatr. 116:243–247, 1990.

Dodge, W. F., et al. Proteinuria and hematuria in schoolchildren: epidemiology and early natural history. J. Pediatr. 88:327–347, 1976.

Ginsberg, J. M., et al. Use of single voided urine samples to estimate quantitative proteinuria. N. Engl. J. Med. 309:1543–1546, 1983.

Houser, M. T., M. F. Jahn, and A. Kobayashi. Assessment of urinary protein excretion in the adolescent: effect of body position and exercise. J. Pediatr. 109:556–561, 1986.

Kurtin, P. S. Hematuria and proteinuria. Acute and chronic medical disorders. Adolesc. Med. State Art Rev. 2:649, 1991.

Miltenyi, M. Urinary protein excretion in healthy children. Clin. Nephrol. 12:216–221, 1979.

Reuben, D. B., et al. Transient proteinuria in emergency medical admissions. N. Engl. J. Med. 306:1031–1033, 1982.

Vehaskari, V. M., and J. Rapola. Isolated proteinuria: analysis of a school-age population. J. Pediatr. 101:661–668, 1982.

Vehaskari, V. M., and A. Robson. Proteinuria. In Edelmann, C. M., et al. (eds.). Pediatric Kidney Disease. Boston, Little, Brown, 1992, pp. 531–551.

Yoshikawa, N., et al. Asymptomatic constant isolated proteinuria in children. J. Pediatr. 119:375–379, 1991.

CHAPTER 67

URINARY TRACT INFECTIONS

Sudhir K. Anand, M.D.

H$_x$ A seven-month-old girl is brought to the office with a one-day history of fever (temperature: 103° F [39.4° C]), vomiting, and questionable abdominal pain. The mother has not noticed any change in urination pattern or any unusual urine odor. The child has been somewhat irritable but fully alert.

Physical examination reveals an active infant. The temperature is 39.2° C (102.6° F), the heart rate is 122 beats/min, the respiratory rate is 30 breaths/min, and the blood pressure is 90/60. The neck is supple. The head, eye, ear, nose, throat, chest, heart, abdominal, and genital examination is normal. Urinalysis shows specific gravity 1.025, pH 6.0, leukocyte esterase and nitrite both strongly positive, protein trace, and blood trace; the sediment is 15–20 WBCs per high-power field and 2–4 RBCs per high-power field. Urine is sent for culture.

Questions

1. What are the possible diagnoses of children with positive leukocyte esterase or nitrite on urinalysis?
2. What are the indications for hospital admission of children with UTIs?
3. What antibiotics are used in the treatment of UTIs?
4. What is the appropriate diagnostic workup for children with suspected UTIs? When are renal ultrasound, IVP, 99m-Tc-DMSA renal scan, and voiding cystourethrogram included in the evaluation?
5. If workup reveals vesiculoureteral reflux, how should children be managed over the long term?

Urinary tract infection (UTI) is one of the most common infections that affect infants and children. The disorder may be asymptomatic, associated with urinary symptoms, or occasionally accompanied by sepsis. In most children UTIs resolve completely. In some young children, especially those with vesicoureteral reflux (VUR), obstructive uropathy, or delayed or inadequate antibiotic treatment, however, UTIs may lead to renal scarring and eventual hypertension or end-stage renal failure in later childhood.

UTI is a nonspecific, generic term implying significant bacteriuria, irrespective of the site of bacterial growth in the urinary tract, and includes the heterogeneous group of conditions listed below. In many young children with bacteriuria, clinical findings overlap and precise classification cannot be easily made.

Asymptomatic, covert, and **screening bacteriuria** are synonymous terms usually used when bacteriuria is detected during surveys of healthy children. The term "screening bacteriuria" is preferable because some affected children may have low-grade symptoms on close questioning.

Acute pyelonephritis is a symptomatic infection of renal parenchyma characterized by systemic symptoms (e.g., high fever, chills, flank pain, vomiting, and dysuria [burning urination]).

Chronic pyelonephritis is a term that has been used in various ways. Ideally, it should be used in renal biopsy specimens in conjunction with histologic lesions of renal scarring due to infection. Practically, the term often refers to scarred kidneys as demonstrated by radiologic techniques (IVP or nuclear scan) or kidneys with reduced function due to such scarring.

Cystitis implies infection of the bladder. Its major features are voiding symptoms (e.g., dysuria, frequency, urgency, enuresis, and foul-smelling urine). Fever, if present, is usually low-grade.

Recurrent UTI generally refers to reinfection with a new organism (often same species but different strain). This condition is a common problem, especially in the first year after initial infection. Reinfection with the same organism is infrequent and may indicate underlying structural problems of the urinary tract or the presence of stones.

Urethritis implies infection of the urethra, primarily, and is usually seen in adolescent children in the context of a venereal infection. The usual symptoms are burning urination and urethral discharge.

EPIDEMIOLOGY

Bacteriuria is detected in approximately 1% of girls and 2% of boys during screening of healthy newborns and young infants. Approximately 1% of girls continue to have screening bacteriuria throughout childhood. In boys over one year of age, however, bacteriuria is uncommon. In most affected infants and children, bacteriuria resolves spontaneously with time, and it does not lead to increased risk of renal damage.

Symptomatic UTI occurs in approximately 0.2% of newborns and young infants. In early infancy, UTI is about twice as common in boys than in girls and about 10 times more common in uncircumcised boys than circumcised boys. After the first six months of life, the incidence and prevalence of symptomatic UTI continue to be considerably higher in males than females; the difference between circumcised and uncircumcised males disappears. Among febrile infants, UTI is the source of fever in approximately 4 to 8% of patients, especially in those who do not have an apparent source of infection on physical examination.

CLINICAL PRESENTATION

Symptoms and signs of UTI in newborns and young infants are usually nonspecific and include fever, irritability, poor weight gain (or weight loss), diarrhea, vomiting, and jaundice. Occasionally, severe sepsis with temperature instability, cyanosis, and DIC may occur. Bacteremia may be present in neonates with UTI. In older children, symptoms include fever, abdominal or flank pain, vomiting, dysuria, frequency and urgency of urination, enuresis, foul-smelling or cloudy urine, and occasionally gross hematuria (D_x Box).

PATHOPHYSIOLOGY

The pathogenesis of UTI involves interaction between various bacterial factors and protective host factors.

Bacterial Factors

Escherichia coli accounts for 80 to 90% of first infections. The remainder are caused by other gram-negative enteric bacilli (*Proteus, Klebsiella, Enterobacter*) and gram-positive cocci (enterococci, *Staphylococcus epidermidis*). Most organisms that cause UTI originate from the fecal flora. *S. epidermidis* infections are primarily seen in adolescents with UTI.

D_x **Urinary Tract Infection**

- Abdominal pain
- Burning urination
- Fever
- Leukocyturia
- Positive urine culture

Microorganisms that cause UTI usually enter the urinary tract by an ascending route. To initiate colonization and induce UTI, these organisms must first adhere to uroepithelium; otherwise they will be swept away during voiding. Bacterial adhesion in *E. coli* is mediated by fimbriae, which are fine, hairlike proteins emanating from the bacterial cell wall. One important type of fimbriae, called P-fimbriae, adheres to receptors (Gal-Gal) on uroepithelium. In most young children, acute pyelonephritis is caused by *E. coli* with P-fimbriae. In the majority of patients with VUR and scarred kidneys, however, the *E. coli* do not have P-fimbriae. Other bacterial virulence factors include K and H antigens, colicin, and hemolysin, but their role in the pathogenesis of UTI is not clearly defined.

Host Factors

Host factors that contribute to the pathogenesis of UTI include age, sex, genetic makeup, VUR, abnormal voiding urodynamics leading to incomplete bladder emptying and residual urine, severe constipation, and immune response to infection. The uroepithelium of older girls and adult women who develop recurrent UTI binds *E. coli* more avidly than uroepithelium from nonsusceptible patients, perhaps because of higher density of receptors. In addition, individuals with certain P and Lewis blood groups develop more UTIs than others. Urinary obstruction or other anomalies may contribute to the development of UTIs in about 2% of girls and 10% of boys, especially infants.

VUR signifies retrograde passage of urine from the bladder to the ureter. After passage through the bladder wall, the normal ureter tunnels under the bladder mucosa before it opens into the bladder lumen. Under normal circumstances, when the bladder is filled and during voiding, the submucosal segment is compressed, preventing reflux of urine into the ureter.

Most VURs are primary and caused by a congenital abnormality of the ureterovesical junction, with the ureter having a short submucosal segment and more laterally placed openings. Transient VUR is sometimes believed to follow a UTI, but this finding has not been well substantiated. Reflux may also occur in the presence of normal ureteral anatomy when bladder pressures exceed 40 cm of water, as seen in patients with posterior urethral valves or neurogenic bladders. VUR is graded on a scale of I to V, with stage V being the most severe (Fig. 67–1).

The incidence of VUR in normal infants is less than 2%. In infants with UTI, the incidence of VUR is about 40 to 50%; in school-age children, about 25%; and in adolescents, about 10 to 15%. These figures suggest that with increasing age and maturation of the bladder wall, VUR spontaneously resolves in the majority of patients. VUR may also be a familial disorder and has been reported in 10 to 30% of siblings of index cases.

In the presence of VUR, the incidence of UTI is increased, probably because of incomplete emptying of the bladder; the refluxed urine (from the ureters) returns to the bladder at the end of voiding. Further-

FIGURE 67–1. *Grading of vesicoureteral reflux by vesicoureterogram based on international classification. I, ureter only; II, ureter, pelvis, and calyces, but without dilatation; III, mild or moderate dilatation of ureter and mild or moderate dilatation of renal pelvis, but no or slight blunting of fornices; IV, moderate dilatation or tortuosity of the ureter with moderate dilatation of renal pelvis and calyces and complete obliteration of the sharp angles of fornices, but maintenance of papillary impressions in the majority of calyces; V, gross dilatation and tortuosity of ureters, renal pelvis, and calyces; papillary impressions are no longer visible in the majority of calyces.*

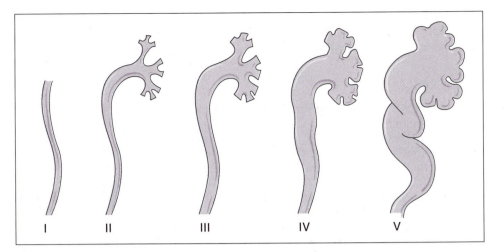

I   II   III   IV   V

more, VUR provides infected urine from the bladder direct access to the ureters and kidneys, leading to pyelonephritis and renal scarring, especially in infants and young children.

DIFFERENTIAL DIAGNOSIS

In infants and young children, findings of UTI are often nonspecific. Thus a high degree of suspicion for UTI must be maintained. Acute abdomen (e.g., appendicitis, glomerulonephritis, renal stones) may occasionally be confused with UTI. Some children with dysuria may have chemical irritation from exposure to materials such as bubble baths. In these cases, urine culture findings usually help differentiate the disorder.

EVALUATION

In all infants and young children with fever without an apparent source, urinalysis and urine culture must be obtained to verify the presence or absence of UTI.

History

In older children, a history of fever, dysuria, frequency, abdominal pain, and nausea and vomiting is suggestive of UTI (Questions Box). History of previous UTIs and abnormal urination should also be sought.

Physical Examination

The abdomen should be examined for masses and tenderness, the genitalia for local lesions, and the lumbosacral area for anomalies such as sinus tracts. Blood pressure should be measured to document the presence of hypertension.

Laboratory Tests

The diagnosis of UTI is established by documenting significant bacteria in a urine specimen sent for culture. In young infants the specimen should always be obtained by bladder puncture or catheterization. Because of the risk of contamination, a "bag urine" sample is

reliable only if the urine is sterile because of the risk of contamination. In older children with bladder control, a midstream urine collection is satisfactory. The diagnosis of UTI should never be based on the presence or absence of leukocyturia alone. Although most older children with symptomatic UTI have leukocyturia, many neonates and young infants with UTI (25–50%) may not manifest this finding. Furthermore, leukocyturia may occur in other renal disorders in the absence of UTI.

Most patients with UTI (> 85%) have urine bacterial counts greater than 100,000/mL on a voided specimen (i.e., significant bacteriuria). Some adult women and teenage girls with symptomatic recurrent UTI have catheterized or "clean catch" urine colony counts less than 1000/mL. In general, this has not been observed in young children. Colony counts between 10,000 and 100,000/mL are generally considered suspect (unlikely to be significant) in clean voided specimens unless children have symptoms of UTI, associated leukocyturia, and cultures that are pure growths of a single organism. Specimens are also considered significant if any growth of organisms is evident in urine samples obtained by suprapubic puncture or if there are more than 10,000 organisms/mL in samples obtained by catheterization.

Several laboratory studies, including ESR, C-reactive protein, urinary lactic acid dehydrogenase isoenzymes, urinary concentrating ability, and antibody-coated bacteria, have been used with varying success to differentiate upper (renal) from lower (bladder) UTI in older children and adults. Overall, the reliability of these studies in pediatric patients, especially infants and young children, is not adequate to recommend their routine use. Furthermore, in young children, both upper

---

Questions: Urinary Tract Infection

- Does it hurt when the child urinates? Does the child scream when urinating?
- Does the child void more frequently?
- Does the urine have an unusual odor?
- Has the child had previous urinary infections?
- Does the child have a good urinary stream? Or does the child dribble?

and lower tract infections mandate complete evaluation for urinary anomalies and VUR followed by the institution of adequate treatment.

Imaging Studies

All girls younger than five years of age and all boys (irrespective of age) should have renal ultrasonography and voiding cystoureterogram (VCUG) performed following detection of the first UTI. These two studies detect structural renal anomalies and VUR in most patients. In girls, nuclear VCUG instead of contrast VCUG is an acceptable alternative. Renal ultrasound can be performed as soon as feasible after diagnosis. VCUG is generally delayed four to six weeks to exclude the possibility of reflux secondary to UTI. This delay, however, entails antibiotic prophylaxis until completion of the study. An excretory urogram (IVP) is usually not indicated unless a ureteral duplication, a ureterocele, or some other anomaly is suspected.

In recent years, some authorities have recommended a routine 99m-Tc-DMSA renal scan to differentiate upper from lower tract infection. At present, the usefulness of this study has not been established during acute infection. It is helpful when used in follow-up to detect development of renal scars, especially in patients with VUR, however.

MANAGEMENT

All infants younger than two months of age with UTIs should be treated with parenteral **antibiotics,** starting with ampicillin and gentamicin (or cefotaxime), pending results of sensitivity studies. Children over two months of age who are not vomiting and who appear stable and nontoxic may receive oral antibiotics. Most physicians recommend trimethoprim-sulfamethoxazole for the first infection until the results of bacterial sensitivity tests are available. Treatment is continued for 10 days. Children over two months of age who have persistent vomiting and appear toxic should be admitted to the hospital and started on parenteral antibiotics until they show clinical improvement. They then can be switched to oral therapy.

In children with VUR, low-dose antibiotics (trimethoprim-sulfamethoxazole) are continued for one year following treatment for an acute infection. At the end of this period, a radionuclide VCUG is repeated to determine the disappearance of reflux. Development of new renal scars can be best detected by DMSA scanning.

Surgery is not necessary in most infants with VUR, including many with severe disease (grades IV and V), because most grade I to III and some grade IV to V reflux in infants disappears with increasing age. In older children (> 5 years of age) with grade IV or V reflux, the rate of disappearance with medical treatment is much lower (about 20–25%). The results of the International Vesicoureteral Reflux Study Group show no difference in the rate of renal scarring between prophylactic medical treatment and surgery. Surgical reimplantation of the ureter is usually recommended only for those patients

who have poor compliance or breakthrough infections, especially if the upper tract is involved. This latter group seems to have benefited the most from surgery. In Europe, endoscopic injection with Teflon has been used with equally good short-term results; the long-term safety of Teflon has not been established, however.

PROGNOSIS

In most children, UTI is a nuisance illness with no long-term or serious consequences. However, in 25 to 50% of children, a repeat UTI may occur, especially during the first year following the initial UTI. Repeat urine cultures should be made during follow-up assessments in all children, especially those with VUR, first at 1–2-month intervals and later at 3–4-month intervals for at least one year or until disappearance of reflux.

Newborn and young infants with UTIs, especially those with high-grade VUR, may potentially experience renal scarring, eventual hypertension, and renal failure. If repeat infection is prevented in these children, however, development of fresh scars is uncommon, and renal function and growth remain normal. The more episodes of acute pyelonephritis children have, the greater the likelihood of renal scarring. As a group, infants and children younger than three years of age with UTI and high-grade VUR are more likely to develop calyceal clubbing and renal scarring, whereas progressive renal scarring as a result of UTI or reflux after age five years is uncommon.

Case Resolution

In the case history, the young girl is hospitalized because of the vomiting. She is started on intravenous trimethoprim-sulfamethoxazole, and she improves in 48 hours. Renal ultrasound is normal. She is discharged and continued on oral antibiotics, and a radionuclide VCUG is planned in four weeks.

Selected Readings

Crain, E. F., and J. C. Gershal. Urinary tract infections in febrile infants younger than 8 weeks age. Pediatrics 86:363–367, 1990.

Hellerstein, S. Evolving concepts in the evaluation of the child with a UTI. J. Pediatr. 24:589–592, 1994.

Jodal, U., and S. Hansson. Urinary tract infection: clinical. *In* Holliday, M. A., T. M. Barratt, and E. D. Avner (eds.). Pediatric Nephrology, 3rd ed. Baltimore, Williams & Wilkins, 1994, pp. 950–962.

Rushton, H. G., and A. B. Belman. Vesicoureteral reflux and renal scarring. *In* Holliday, M. A., T. M. Barratt, and E. D. Avner (eds.). Pediatric Nephrology, 3rd ed. Baltimore, Williams & Wilkins, 1994, pp. 963–986.

Steele, B., and J. DeMaria. A new perspective on the natural history of vesicoureteral reflux. Pediatrics 90:30–32, 1992.

Uehling, D. T. Susceptibility factors in ascending urinary tract infection. *In* Holliday, M. A., T. M. Barratt, and E. D. Avner (eds.). Pediatric Nephrology, 3rd ed. Baltimore, Williams & Wilkins, 1994, pp. 986–993.

Weiss, R. A. Vesicoureteral reflux (VUR) in children. Kidney 25:1–6, 1993.

CHAPTER 68

VAGINITIS

Monica Sifuentes, M.D.

H_x An 11-year-old girl is brought to your office with vaginal itching that has lasted for one week. Her mother has noted a yellow discharge on her panties for the past four days. The girl reports no associated abdominal pain, vomiting, or diarrhea. She has no urinary problems and also denies any history of sexual abuse. Although she occasionally bathes with bubble bath, she usually takes showers. Except for the vaginal complaint, she is healthy, and she takes no medications.

The physical examination is remarkable for a soft, non-tender abdomen with no organomegaly. Bowel sounds are audible in all quadrants. The girl is at Tanner stage II. The labia majora and minora and the clitoris all appear normal, and the hymen is annular in shape with a smooth rim. A scant amount of yellow discharge, along with minimal perihymenal injection, is noted at the introitus. The anal examination is normal, with an intact anal wink.

Questions

1. What are the most common causes for vaginal discharge in prepubescent and adolescent females? How do they differ?
2. What basic historical information must be obtained from all females whose chief complaint is vaginal discharge?
3. What specific methods are used to perform a gynecologic examination in prepubescent and adolescent females?
4. What is the appropriate laboratory evaluation for prepubescent and adolescent females who complain of vaginal discharge? How does this evaluation differ in adolescent females who are sexually active?
5. What are the various treatment options for females with vaginitis?

Vulvovaginitis, which is often used interchangeably with vaginitis or vulvitis, signifies inflammation of the perineal area often accompanied by a vaginal discharge. The discharge may be bloody, malodorous, or purulent, depending on the etiology (Table 68–1).

EPIDEMIOLOGY

Vulvovaginitis is the most common gynecologic complaint in prepubescent girls. Most cases of vulvovaginitis in these girls result from **nonspecific inflammation;** vaginal cultures show normal flora in 33 to 85% of such cases. The incidence of more specific **bacterial causes,** such as group A beta-hemolytic streptococcus, has been reported in approximately 14% of patients. However, its occurrence appears to be seasonal and diagnosis depends on the use of proper culturing techniques and appropriate media. Other bacterial causes include respiratory pathogens such as *Haemophilus influenzae, Neisseria meningitidis, Streptococcus pneumoniae,* and enteric organisms such as *Shigella.* A positive culture for *Chlamydia trachomatis* or *N. gonorrhoeae* can be found in approximately 10 to 15% of children who are evaluated for sexual abuse. These organisms are not considered part of the normal flora in prepubescent girls. Vaginal and rectal infections with *C. trachomatis* can be acquired perinatally, however.

Parasitic infections may also lead to vaginal symptoms. Twenty percent of females with a rectal infestation of *Enterobius vermicularis,* the organism known as pinworm, have vulvovaginitis. Affected patients often complain of pruritus in addition to the vaginal discharge. **Mycotic infections** with organisms such as *Candida* may also cause symptoms in prepubescent

A vaginal discharge is not an uncommon occurrence in prepubescent and adolescent females. Practitioners are largely responsible for differentiating between a physiologic discharge, or leukorrhea, and a pathologic discharge, which occurs, for example, with a bacterial or yeast infection. In cases of an abnormal discharge, the possibility of abuse needs to be considered and investigated appropriately (see Chapter 97, Child Sexual Abuse). Therefore, primary care physicians should be familiar with the various causes of vaginal discharge in both prepubescent and adolescent females. In addition, they should be comfortable performing gynecologic examinations in these children. Appropriate treatment can then be initiated.

TABLE 68–1. Characteristics and Specific Causes of Vaginal Discharge

Color	Consistency	Amount	Cause
Clear/white	Thin	Variable	Physiologic
White	Cottage cheeselike	Moderate	*Candida*
White/yellow	Variable	Variable	Chemical irritation, *Chlamydia*
Yellow/green	Thick	Moderate-profuse	*Neisseria gonorrhoeae,* foreign body, *Trichomonas*
Bloody	Variable	Variable	*Shigella,* group A streptococcus, foreign body

---

Dx Vaginitis

- Nonphysiologic vaginal discharge
- Perineal erythema
- Pruritus
- Dysuria
- Malodorous vaginal discharge

---

girls, although many of these girls have a previous history of oral antibiotic use.

CLINICAL PRESENTATION

Prepubescent and adolescent females with vulvovaginitis most commonly present with a vaginal discharge, which may be white, purulent (i.e., yellow or green), or serosanguinous. Its consistency can range from smooth and thin to thick and cottage cheese-like. The discharge may also be malodorous. In addition, females may complain of associated pruritus, erythema, urinary problems such as dysuria and increased frequency, and abdominal pain (Dx Box). Sexually active adolescent females with vaginitis from an STD (e.g., gonorrhea) may have a more profuse, purulent discharge.

PATHOPHYSIOLOGY

Prepubescent girls are at risk for developing vulvovaginitis for both anatomic and physiologic reasons. Unlike pubertal adolescents and young women, young girls have no labial fat pad or pubic hair to protect the introitus. The labia minora are small and tend to open when girls are in a squatting position, thereby exposing the vaginal introitus. The relative proximity of the anus to the vagina in young girls also contributes to vaginal contamination with enteric organisms. More importantly, poor hygienic practices (i.e., wiping back to front after urination or defecation) can further compound the problem.

In addition, the normal physiology of the vaginal epithelium in prepubescent girls predisposes to vaginitis. The unestrogenized vaginal epithelium is relatively thin, immature, and easily traumatized. In addition, the pH of the vagina is neutral to alkaline, as compared to the acidic environment of the vagina in adults. Local antibody production is also believed to be lacking in the vagina of prepubescent girls.

DIFFERENTIAL DIAGNOSIS

A vaginal discharge is normal at two distinct times in prepubescent girls: shortly after birth, secondary to the effects of maternal estrogen, and approximately six months to one year before the onset of menarche, which occurs after Tanner stage III. The causes of other vaginal discharges in prepubescent and pubescent females are presented in Table 68–2.

TABLE 68–2. Causes of Vaginal Discharge in Prepubescent and Pubescent Females

Prepubescent Females

Estrogen withdrawal (neonates)
Chemical irritation secondary to soaps and detergents
Mechanical irritation from nylon panties or tight-fitting clothes
Foreign body in vagina
Poor hygiene
Pinworms
Yeast infection
Bacterial infection (e.g., group A streptococcus, *Shigella*)
Sexually transmitted disease (e.g., gonococcal infection, chlamydial infection, trichomoniasis)
Congenital abnormality (e.g., ectopic ureter [local inflammation])
Acquired abnormality (e.g., labial fusion [pooling of urine in vagina])
Urethral prolapse
Systemic illness (e.g., scarlet fever, Crohn's disease)

Pubescent Females

Physiologic leukorrhea
Foreign body in vagina (e.g., retained tampon)
Yeast infection
Bacterial infection (e.g., group A streptococcus, *Staphylococcus aureus*)
Sexually transmitted disease (e.g., gonococcal infection, chlamydial infection, trichomoniasis)
Chemical irritation (e.g., douches, spermicides)

EVALUATION

Prepubescent Females

History

A complete history should be obtained in all females with a vaginal discharge (Questions Box). Practitioners should learn about the appearance of the discharge, its

---

Questions: Vaginitis

Prepubescent Females

- What is the color of the discharge?
- What is the consistency of the discharge?
- How profuse is the discharge?
- How long has the discharge been apparent?
- How often does the discharge occur (i.e., is it found on the panties daily)?
- Are there any associated problems (e.g., abdominal pain)?
- What types of laundry soaps or detergents are used?
- Does the child take bubble baths?
- Has the child had any recent illnesses?
- Does the child clean herself after using the toilet, or does she require help?
- In what direction does she tend to wipe after a bowel movement?

Adolescent Females (all of the above questions plus the following):

- What is the reproductive history (menstrual and sexual)?
- If appropriate, is the adolescent using any form of contraception? When was the last episode of unprotected intercourse?
- If appropriate, how many sexual partners has the patient had?
- Does the patient or partner have any history of a previous STD, including hepatitis B?

duration, and the relative amount. A profuse discharge is probably more consistent with one specific etiology (e.g., *N. gonorrhoeae*). The existence of urinary problems should be determined. Pooling of urine in the vagina secondary to labial fusion can lead to vulvovaginitis in addition to a UTI. Changes in bowel or bladder habits and sudden changes in behavior such as nightmares or inappropriate stranger anxiety may also be noted. Such changes in behavior warrant a further inquiry into the possibility of sexual abuse, regardless of the practitioner's index of suspicion. Depending on the information disclosed, both children and parents should be interviewed independently.

Other points to discuss include the type of detergents or soaps used for laundry as well as for bathing, because these may be irritating. Any recent illnesses should also be documented as a possible source of autoinoculation or, if oral antibiotics were required, as a reason for the alteration of the normal vaginal flora. In addition, patients' hygienic practices should be reviewed.

Adolescent patients should always be interviewed alone (see Chapter 4, Talking to Adolescents). In particular, a reproductive history must be obtained, keeping in mind that puberty and sexual activity both alter vaginal flora.

Physical Examination

Although a genital examination is a priority, a complete physical examination should be performed. This not only allows clinicians to identify other abnormal physical findings, but it also alleviates some of the anxiety often associated with a genital examination. Because most vaginal discharges in prepubescent girls result from nonspecific vulvovaginitis, visualization of the cervix with a speculum is not indicated.

The overall demeanor of young girls at the onset of the genital examination should be noted. Overly cooperative, apathetic behavior in children may be a cause for concern regarding abuse, especially in the context of a chronic purulent discharge.

On physical examination, children's Tanner stage or sexual maturity rating must be noted and recorded. In addition, the external genitalia should be examined closely for the presence of any lesions or any evidence of erythema. Chronic changes in labial skin, such as those associated with constant scratching, should also be noted.

Girls should be placed in the modified lithotomy or "frog leg" position, and the labia majora should be gently spread apart to visualize the hymen. The knee-chest position can also be used, depending on the comfort of the practitioner as well as the patient. If the labia cannot be spread apart, the girl may have labial fusion. Perihymenal and periurethral erythema and injection should also be assessed, in addition to any evidence of edema, trauma, or abnormal masses such as urethral prolapse. Hymenal size and appearance should be carefully evaluated for any evidence of abuse (see Chapter 97, Child Sexual Abuse). The appearance, consistency, and amount of the vaginal discharge, including the presence or absence of an odor, should also be noted. These findings may vary depending on the characteristics and cause of the discharge. Finally, the anus should be inspected for tone and any evidence of trauma or abnormal lesions such as venereal warts. An anal wink may normally be elicited.

Laboratory Tests

Laboratory studies are often unnecessary in prepubescent girls with a nonspecific, nonbloody vaginal discharge, diffuse vulvar erythema, and no suspicion or history of sexual abuse. A vaginal culture for isolation of group A beta-hemolytic streptococcus is indicated in girls with an abrupt onset of a serosanguinous discharge and a history of a systemic illness. The cellophane tape test may be helpful in diagnosing a pinworm infection in girls with associated anal pruritus. A KOH wet mount reveals hyphae if a monilial infection is present.

If the discharge is purulent or malodorous or if abuse is suspected, vaginal cultures should be obtained for gonococcus and chlamydia. A chlamydia culture is preferred because of the risk of a false-positive result with the rapid assay. In certain cases, a normal saline wet mount to check for mobile trichomonads may be indicated.

Pubescent Females

History

In adolescent or pubescent females with vaginal discharge, physicians should inquire about a history of sexual activity or assault in addition to other information that relates to their condition (Questions Box). Questions concerning the possible acquisition of an STD must also be asked.

Physical Examination

In addition to an overall physical examination, a complete genital examination using a speculum is indicated. The purpose of the speculum examination is to visualize the cervix, properly obtain cervical specimens, and examine the vagina for lesions (i.e., condylomata acuminata). A bimanual examination must also be performed to check for cervical motion tenderness, which may be associated with pelvic inflammatory disease (PID).

Laboratory Tests

Adolescent females who are not sexually active should have a laboratory evaluation similar to that described for prepubescent girls. The approach to sexually active adolescents, however, warrants modification. A cervical culture for gonorrhea should be obtained in all sexually active adolescents with a vaginal discharge. In addition, a rapid assay for chlamydia should be performed. A Pap smear should also be done at this time, not only to screen for cervical dysplasia, but also to detect cellular changes consistent with HPV or trichomoniasis. A culture for herpes simplex is indicated only if the history of exposure is positive or ulcerative, or vesicular lesions are present.

A normal saline wet mount should be made, especially if a nonspecific discharge or bacterial vaginosis is a concern. A 10% KOH mount is appropriate in cases of suspected candidiasis. Mixing 10% KOH with the discharge may also produce a "fishy" odor (positive "whiff test"), which is consistent with bacterial vaginosis or trichomoniasis. A Gram's stain of any purulent material may lead to an early diagnosis of gonorrhea. Serologies for syphilis should also be obtained in adolescents with suspected or proven STDs. In addition, patients should be offered testing for HIV, with appropriate pretest and posttest counseling.

MANAGEMENT

Management of a **nonspecific vaginal discharge** is aimed at relieving the uncomfortable symptoms associated with this type of inflammation. Prepubescent females should be instructed to **discontinue use of all chemical irritants**, including bubble baths, in the genital area. Warm water **sitz baths** are also recommended twice daily for approximately one week or until patients feel better. In addition, females should be instructed in **proper hygiene** (e.g., wiping front to back after a bowel movement). The use of cotton or cotton-crotch panties should be recommended.

Antifungal medications such as **clotrimazole** (Lotrimin) or **miconazole** (Monistat) cream may be prescribed if a monilial infection is present. Empiric treatment may be warranted in children or adolescents with a previous history of oral antibiotic usage, diabetes mellitus, or other chronic conditions that may alter the normal vaginal flora.

Pinworms are treated with a single oral dose of **mebendazole** (Vermox), 100 mg, or **pyrantel pamoate** (Antiminth), 11 mg/kg/dose (to a maximum of 1 gram). Most authorities recommend repeat treatment after two weeks.

If a retained foreign body is suspected in prepubescent girls, then examination under general anesthesia may be necessary. Alternatively, practitioners can attempt vaginal irrigation in cooperative children by placing a small feeding tube at the hymenal opening and injecting warm saline. Toilet paper is the most commonly retrieved material in prepubescent girls.

Adolescent females who are not sexually active should be treated as outlined above. If the discharge is believed to be physiologic leukorrhea, practitioners should reassure patients and educate them about other issues related to puberty (e.g., menarche, body odor). Sexually active adolescents with positive vaginal cultures or highly suspicious vaginal discharges should receive treatment depending on the causal organism (see Chapter 69, Sexually Transmitted Diseases, for details concerning treatment). Table 68–3 briefly outlines current recommendations.

TABLE 68–3. Treatment Recommendations for Adolescents With Infectious Vaginitis

Organism	Treatment*
Neisseria gonorrhoeae	Ceftriaxone, 125 mg IM, once
Chlamydia trachomatis	Doxycycline, 100 mg PO, bid for 7 days
Trichomonas	Metronidazole, 2 g PO, once
Bacterial vaginosis	Metronidazole, 500 mg, bid for 7 days
Candida albicans	1% clotrimazole, cream, one applicatorful vaginally qhs for 7 days; 2% miconazole cream, 1 applicatorful vaginally qhs for 7 days; 0.8% terconazole cream, 1 applicatorful vaginally qhs for 3 days; fluconazole, 150 mg PO once

*For treatment options, refer to Centers for Disease Control and Prevention. 1993 Sexually Transmitted Disease Treatment Guidelines. M.M.W.R. 42:RR–14, 1–102, 1993.

Any disclosure of molestation by prepubescent or adolescent females must be reported to the appropriate authorities. In addition, abnormal physical findings and positive cultures of STDs in prepubescent females and adolescent females who have never been sexually active must be reported and investigated.

PROGNOSIS

In the majority of prepubescent females, vaginitis resolves spontaneously or after appropriate treatment with no permanent sequelae. In contrast, adolescent females treated for vulvovaginitis or uncomplicated cervicitis from an STD are at some risk for the development of PID, HIV, and pregnancy given their high-risk behavior.

Case Resolution

In the case presented at the beginning of the chapter, the girl and her parents should be assured that the discharge is consistent with a nonspecific process. She should be instructed to take sitz baths for one week, discontinue bubble baths and the use of soap in the genital area, and wear loose-fitting clothes with cotton underwear. The girl should be reexamined in one to two weeks.

Selected Readings

Blake, J. Gynecologic examination of the teenager and young child. Obstet. Gynecol. Clin. North Am. 19:27–38, 1992.

Elvik, S. L. Vaginal discharge in the prepubertal girl. J. Pediatr. Health Care 4:181–185, 1990.

Pierce, A. M., and C. A. Hart. Vulvovaginitis: causes and management. Arch. Dis. Child 67:509–512, 1992.

Porkorny, S. F. Prepubertal vulvovaginopathies. Obstet. Gynecol. Clin. North Am. 19:39–58, 1992.

Shafer, M. A., R. L. Sweet, and M. J. Ohm-Smith. Microbiology of the lower genital tract in postmenarchal adolescent girl: difference by sexual activity, contraception, and presence of nonspecific vaginitis. J. Pediatr. 107:974–981, 1985.

Straumanis, J. P., and J. A. Bocchini. Group A beta-hemolytic streptococcal vulvovaginitis in prepubertal girls: a case report and review of the past twenty years. Pediatr. Infect. Dis. J. 9:845–848, 1990.

Vandeven, A. M., and S. J. Emans. Vulvovaginitis in the child and adolescent. Pediatr. Rev. 14:141–147, 1993.

CHAPTER 69

SEXUALLY TRANSMITTED DISEASES

Monica Sifuentes, M.D.

Hₓ   A 17-year-old male presents with a small red lesion on the tip of his penis. He noticed an area of erythema a few weeks before, but it resolved spontaneously. He reports no fever, myalgias, headache, dysuria, or urethral discharge. He is sexually active and occasionally uses condoms. He did not use a condom during his last sexual encounter two weeks ago, however, because his partner uses oral contraception. The adolescent has never been treated for any sexually transmitted diseases (STDs) and is otherwise healthy.

On examination, he is a Tanner IV circumcised male with a 2–3-mm vesicle on the glans penis. Minimal erythema is present at the base of the lesion, and there is no urethral discharge. The testicles are descended bilaterally, and no masses are palpable. Shotty, nontender, inguinal adenopathy is evident.

Questions

1. What conditions are associated with vesicles in the genital area?
2. What screening tests should be performed in patients with suspected STDs?
3. What recommendations regarding partners of patients with STDs should be given?
4. What issues of confidentiality are important to address with adolescents who desire treatment for STDs?

A majority of teenagers in the United States have their first sexual experience before they graduate from high school. In a recent survey conducted by the Centers for Disease Control and Prevention (CDC), two-thirds of boys and approximately one-half of girls in high school reported having intercourse. More importantly, 27% of boys and 12% of girls in grades 9 to 12 reported having had four or more sexual partners.

The consequences of such sexual activity in adolescents include increased rates of bacterial and viral STDs, unintended pregnancy, and the emergence of acquired immunodeficiency syndrome (AIDS) as the sixth leading cause of death in the 15–24-year age group. Given the dramatic nature of these consequences, the physician must be skilled in obtaining a sexual history in teenage patients and in diagnosing and treating STDs.

Increasing levels of sexual activity affect STD trends in adolescents. Other influential factors include inconsistent use of condoms and other barrier methods; experimentation with drugs, including alcohol, which results in poor judgment concerning sexual activity; poor compliance with antibiotic regimens; and biologic factors, such as an earlier age of menarche and the presence of cervical ectopy in adolescent females. The feeling of invulnerability and the associated risk-taking behavior that occurs during adolescence make sexual activity "spontaneous" rather than premeditated. As a result, preventive measures are hindered, ignored, or simply unheard of, and adolescents deny the consequences of their actions. Other factors influencing STD trends are related to societal norms. Traditionally, educational materials and STD services have not been available to adolescents. In addition, the depiction of casual sexual relationships on television sitcoms, music videos, and motion pictures may play a major role in glamorizing sex.

EPIDEMIOLOGY

The overall prevalence of STDs in adolescents is difficult to estimate, because not all STDs are reportable, and collected data are often influenced by the particular population studied. It has been estimated, however, that approximately 4% of high school students have had at least one STD. **Chlamydia** remains the most common cause of cervicitis and urethritis in adolescents, with a prevalence rate of 5 to 40% in females and 8 to 35% in males. Complications of chlamydial cervicitis occur in 10 to 30% of cases. Epididymitis, a result of urethral infection, occurs in 1 to 3% of infected males.

Teenagers have the highest incidence of **gonorrhea** of any other population group, although this incidence is decreasing. The highest rates of gonorrhea reportedly occur in adolescent females, young men in their 20s, young adult inner-city minorities, homosexual men, and prostitutes. A large number of sexual partners, intravenous drug use, exposure to prostitutes, and casual sexual contacts also contribute to the risk of infection. In 1992, the CDC reported that the incidence of gonorrhea in the 15–19-year age group was 837 in 100,000.

CDC data also show that **syphilis** rates have been declining in recent years, a change in direction from the previous ten years. During 1992, the incidence of syphilis in the 15–19-year age group was 21 in 100,000. Studies have shown, however, that people with syphilis, as well as other STD-causing genital ulcers, are at increased risk for HIV acquisition.

Human papillomavirus (HPV) may infect 38 to 46% of adolescent females. The prevalence of HPV in adolescents varies widely for two reasons: (1) infection with HPV is often latent, and (2) HPV is not a reportable condition. Risk factors for HPV infections are similar to those for other STDs: multiple sexual partners, age greater than 25 years, lack of condom use, previous STD infection, pregnancy, sex with an infected partner, and altered immune response.

Infection with **herpes simplex virus type 2 (HSV-2)** is also underestimated. Reportedly, HSV-2 occurs in approximately 4% of whites and 17% of African Americans by the end of their teenage years.

As of June 1994, the number of **AIDS** cases reported in the United States in adolescents aged 13–19 years was 1,768; the number of cases in young adults between 20 and 24 years of age was 15,204. Because the incubation period for AIDS is believed to be from 8 to 10 years for adolescents, estimates of asymptomatic or early HIV infection are often based on reported cases of AIDS in young adults in their 20s. AIDS cases in adolescents occur primarily in males and minorities. Most of these individuals are infected through sexual contact or intravenous drug use.

CLINICAL PRESENTATION

Adolescents with a sexually transmitted disease may go to their physicians with specific complaints related to the genitourinary system, such as painful urination or vaginal discharge. They may also report more generalized complaints, like fever and malaise, especially in cases of primary HSV (Dx Box: STDs). In addition, some teenagers will use a vague complaint to see their primary care practitioner with the hope that the physician asks about sexual activity. It is only then that they will disclose their real concern.

PATHOPHYSIOLOGY

A number of biologic factors contribute to the increased prevalence rates of STDs in adolescents, particularly in females. At the onset of puberty, the columnar epithelial cells in the vagina transform to squamous

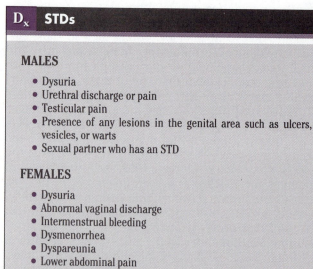

Dx STDs

MALES

- Dysuria
- Urethral discharge or pain
- Testicular pain
- Presence of any lesions in the genital area such as ulcers, vesicles, or warts
- Sexual partner who has an STD

FEMALES

- Dysuria
- Abnormal vaginal discharge
- Intermenstrual bleeding
- Dysmenorrhea
- Dyspareunia
- Lower abdominal pain
- Systemic symptoms such as fever, nausea, vomiting, malaise
- Presence of any lesions in the genital area such as ulcers, vesicles, or warts
- Sexual partner who has an STD

epithelium while columnar cells at the cervix persist (Fig. 69–1). With increasing age, the squamocolumnar junction recedes into the endocervix. In adolescent females, however, this junction is often located at the ectocervix and is relatively exposed, which places these females at particular risk for gonococcal and chlamydial infections. The infectious organisms preferentially attach to cervical columnar cells and infect them. Of note is that the use of oral contraceptives also prolongs this immature histologic state.

The cytologic changes seen in cervical cells of adolescents with HPV infection are also believed to be age-related. The immature cervical metaplastic or columnar cells appear to be more highly vulnerable to infection and neoplastic changes. In addition, exposure to other cofactors (e.g., tobacco use, multiple episodes of new HPV infections) is likely to promote the development of squamous intraepithelial neoplasia (SIN) and cervical carcinoma. Not all young women exposed to HPV develop lesions or progress to SIN, and most will not remain positive for HPV throughout their lifetime.

The presence of genital ulcers has been shown to facilitate both the transmission and the acquisition of HIV. Such ulcers provide a point of entry past denuded epithelium. In addition, it is hypothesized that many activated lymphocytes and macrophages are located at the base of the ulcer and are therefore "ripe" for infection by HIV.

Pelvic inflammatory disease (PID) usually develops from an ascending infection, often an untreated STD of the cervix and vagina, which spreads contiguously upward to the upper genital tract. Inflammation, scarring, and crypt formation in the fallopian tubes result. The most common causal organisms, which account for more than half of the cases of PID in most studies, are *Chlamydia trachomatis* and *Neisseria gonorrhoeae*. Other agents include *Escherichia coli;* other enteric flora; and microbes implicated in bacterial vaginosis, such as *Mycoplasma hominis, Ureaplasma urealyticum, Bacteroides* spp., and anaerobic cocci.

DIFFERENTIAL DIAGNOSIS

Most patients with STDs present with one of five clinical syndromes—urethritis/cervicitis, epididymitis, pelvic inflammatory disease, genital ulcer disease, or genital warts, all of which can be easily diagnosed (Table 69–1). Other conditions that mimic STDs, however, must be considered in certain cases where the adolescent denies sexual activity or where the disorder does not respond to routine treatment. These disorders include **mucocutaneous ulcers** associated with lupus erythematosus and Behçet's disease. Often, systemic disorders such as these can be ruled out historically. **Benign oral lesions** such as aphthous ulcers can also be confused with herpes ulcers. When evaluating an adolescent female with acute lower abdominal pain, surgical conditions such as **appendicitis** and **ovarian torsion** must be ruled out. In the sexually active male with testicular pain, **testicular torsion** must be considered before a diagnosis of epididymitis is made.

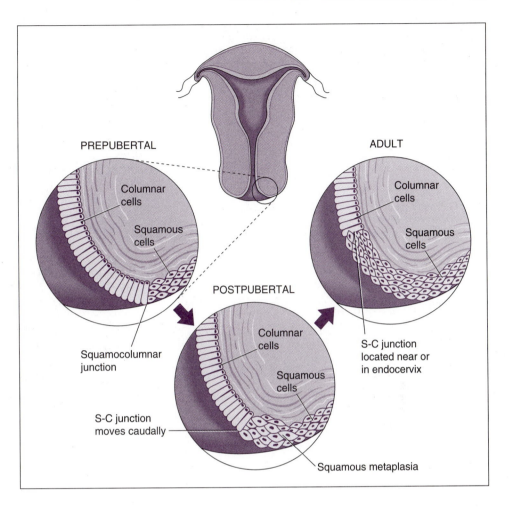

PREPUBERTAL

ADULT

POSTPUBERTAL

Columnar cells

Squamous cells

Squamocolumnar junction

Columnar cells

Squamous cells

S-C junction moves caudally

Squamous metaplasia

Columnar cells

Squamous cells

S-C junction located near or in endocervix

FIGURE 69–1. *Development of the cervical squamocolumnar junction, from puberty to adulthood.*

EVALUATION

In all sexually active adolescents, a complete history, including a sexual history, should be obtained (Questions Box). A detailed gynecologic history should also be taken in females. The rest of the history should then focus on the particular complaint and any associated symptoms. Sexually active female adolescents should have a complete speculum examination, whereas males should have a thorough genital examination. Diagnostic tests should be determined by the historical and physical findings.

URETHRITIS

History

Because urethritis is more common in young men, all sexually active adolescent males should be asked about the presence of dysuria, urethral discharge, and urethral pruritus. In females, symptoms such as dysuria may appear more gradually. Other symptoms like meatal edema or erythema should also be noted. General urinary symptoms such as acute urinary frequency or urgency are uncommon, especially in males, but all patients should be asked about such symptoms. More often, urethritis is asymptomatic, and the diagnosis is made by routine screening in sexually active adolescents or through known contact with a partner with an STD (e.g., *C. trachomatis*).

Physical Examination

In males, the urethra should be the focus of the genital examination. The presence of a urethral discharge and its consistency (i.e., mucoid or purulent) should be noted. Any other urethral or genital lesions should also be assessed.

In females, a full pelvic examination should be performed after careful examination of the external genitalia for any ulcerative or wartlike lesions. Urethritis is most often caused by *C. trachomatis,* but HSV can be another cause. The urethra should also be inspected for edema, erythema, or any evidence of a discharge. During the speculum examination, the presence or absence of a vaginal or cervical discharge should also be noted.

Laboratory Tests

A Gram's stain of the urethral discharge may confirm the diagnosis of urethritis in both males and females. The specimen should be obtained using a Dacron or

---

TABLE 69–1.   Differential Diagnosis of Sexually Transmitted Disease by Clinical Syndrome

---

Urethritis
  Neisseria gonorrhoeae
  Nongonococcal disease
    Chlamydia trachomatis
    Ureaplasma urealyticum
    Trichomonas vaginalis
    Herpes simplex virus
    Yeasts
Cervicitis
  C. trachomatis
  N. gonorrhoeae
  Herpes simplex virus
Pelvic Inflammatory Disease
  N. gonorrhoeae
  C. trachomatis
  Anaerobes
  Gram-negative rods
  Streptococci
  Mycoplasma hominis
  U. urealyticum
Vaginitis
  T. vaginalis
  Candida albicans and other fungi
  Gardnerella vaginalis
Genital Ulcers
  Treponema pallidum (syphilis)
  Herpes simplex virus, types 1 and 2
  Haemophilus ducreyi (chancroid)
  C. trachomatis (lymphogranuloma venereum)
Genital Warts
  T. pallidum (condyloma latum)
  Human papillomavirus (condyloma acuminatum)
Proctitis
  N. gonorrhoeae
  C. trachomatis
  T. pallidum
  Herpes simplex virus
  Particular to homosexual youth (in addition to the above)
    Hepatitis A and B virus
    Shigella spp.
    Campylobacter spp.
    Giardia lamblia
    Entamoeba histolytica
Pharyngitis
  N. gonorrhoeae
  C. trachomatis
  Herpes simplex virus, types 1 and 2

---

cotton swab because calcium alginate inhibits the growth of *Chlamydia*. The presence of gram-negative, intracellular diplococci with the typical "kidney-bean" morphology is indicative of an infection with *N. gonorrhoeae*. Five or more polymorphonuclear (PMN) leukocytes per high-power field but no organisms indicates the more common type of infection, nongonococcal urethritis, usually found in males. A culture for gonococcus (GC) and *Chlamydia* should still be obtained.

If no PMN leukocytes are seen on Gram's stain, assessment for leukocyte esterase with a urine dipstick should be made using the first 10–15 mL of a voided urine specimen. This specimen should also be examined under the microscope. A routine urine culture is generally not recommended in males and may be of little help in females.

CERVICITIS

History

Cervicitis in females is parallel to urethritis in males. Because cervicitis is a local infection, systemic symptoms may not occur. However, a variety of important historical points and associated complaints should be addressed. Is a vaginal discharge present? If so, does it have an odor? Is the patient experiencing any urinary frequency, urgency, or dysuria? Has she had any nonmenstrual vaginal bleeding? A known exposure to an STD must also be ascertained. Is the partner symptomatic or currently receiving treatment? Does the patient or her partner have a past history of an STD?

More generalized symptoms such as moderate lower abdominal pain (either acute or chronic) and fever may indicate a complication of untreated cervicitis such as PID.

Physical Examination

After completing the full physical examination, the physician should focus on the genitourinary examination. The Tanner stage should first be noted, then the presence of any lesions on the external genitalia or inflammation of the perineum. Any urethral erythema or discharge should also be noted. A vaginal discharge can be assessed more completely when performing the speculum examination, which should be performed in all sexually active adolescent females with vaginal or lower urinary tract complaints.

During the speculum examination, the vaginal mucosa should be inspected and the appearance of the cervical os should be noted. The physician should determine whether a purulent discharge is coming from the os and look for any evidence of cervical friability as opposed to normal adolescent ectopy. Mucopurulent cervicitis is diagnosed when there is a discharge from the cervical os, erosion, friability, and Gram's stain with more than 10 PMN leukocytes per high-power field. A bimanual examination must also be performed to check for

---

Questions: STDs

Questions to Ask the Patient

- Are you sexually active?
- How many partners have you had? When was your last contact?
- Do you or your partner(s) use contraception? What type?
- Have any of your sexual contacts ever been diagnosed with an STD?
- Do you have abdominal pain, dysuria, increased urinary frequency, or hesitancy?
- Have you noticed any ulcers, blisters, warts, or other bumps in the genital area?
- For females: Do you have a vaginal discharge or itching? Is sex uncomfortable or painful?
- For males: Do you have a discharge from your penis? Any testicular pain? Any associated burning or itching?

cervical motion tenderness (CMT) and adnexal masses or fullness.

Laboratory Tests

Cultures for GC and *Chlamydia* must be obtained in all sexually active females who, on speculum examination, show symptoms of vaginal discharge or evidence of cervicitis. In addition, a Gram's stain of the discharge should be performed to detect the presence of gram-negative diplococci or PMN leukocytes. The culture for gonococcus should be obtained before other cultures because the organisms can be found in the purulent discharge itself. After the cervix is cleaned, the specimen for the chlamydial enzyme immunoassay can be collected. Because *C. trachomatis* is an intracellular organism, the cytobrush should be used to rub the surface of the cervix, thus enhancing the recovery of organisms. A wet mount to diagnose associated STDs such as trichomoniasis may also be performed, especially if the discharge is foul-smelling or frothy.

PELVIC INFLAMMATORY DISEASE

History

When considering PID, the history should include a discussion of known risk factors such as sexual activity, including the number of sexual partners, especially new partners in the previous two months; a previous STD or recent episode of an STD; the type and consistency of contraceptive use; and the timing of the last menstrual cycle. The physician should also ask patients about the presence of symptoms associated with PID: the onset, duration, quality, and location of abdominal pain; urinary symptoms that may indicate concomitant urethritis; intermenstrual bleeding; dysmenorrhea or dyspareunia; abnormal vaginal discharge; and systemic symptoms such as nausea, vomiting, fever, and malaise. The classic symptoms of PID, which include lower abdominal pain, vaginal discharge, fever, and irregular vaginal bleeding, may not be present. More often symptoms are nonspecific, and the practitioner must maintain a high index of suspicion in any sexually active female with abdominal pain.

Physical Examination

Classic signs of acute PID include fever with tenderness of the lower abdomen, cervix, and adnexa. A thorough physical examination should be completed before performing the pelvic examination. Vital signs should be obtained, looking for fever or tachycardia. Blood pressure should also be taken, because hypotension can be seen with a ruptured ectopic pregnancy, which may present with abdominal pain and vaginal bleeding. The abdomen should be assessed for tenderness and guarding. The location of the pain is particularly important, because acute surgical conditions such as appendicitis or ovarian torsion are included in the differential diagnosis of PID.

The speculum examination should then be performed, looking for a purulent discharge or any evidence of cervicitis (cervical friability or erosion). The bimanual examination is the most important part of the physical examination. The cervix should be carefully palpated for any evidence of CMT and the adnexa for tenderness or masses.

Laboratory Tests

A cervical culture for *N. gonorrhoeae*, a cervical specimen for a chlamydial enzyme immunoassay, and Gram's stain of any cervical discharge should be performed. The specimen should be examined microscopically for PMN leukocytes as well as gram-negative, intracellular diplococci. The presence of five or more PMNs per oil immersion field is one of the clinical criteria for making a diagnosis of PID. (See D_x Box: Pelvic Inflammatory Disease for additional criteria.)

Other laboratory studies to be obtained include a complete blood count with differential and a sedimentation rate. A urine pregnancy test should also be completed.

Laparoscopy should be performed to make a definitive diagnosis or to obtain diagnostic cultures in cases where the diagnosis is questionable or patients are not responding to standard therapy.

Imaging Studies

A pelvic ultrasound may help exclude diagnoses such as ectopic pregnancy or ovarian torsion and can also aid in the detection of associated complications of PID such as tubo-ovarian abscess. Fluid in the cul-de-sac may also be seen on ultrasound.

GENITAL ULCERS

History

Probably the most important information to learn about genital ulcers is whether they are painful. A painless chancre on the penis, around the mouth, in the oropharynx, or on the external genitalia in females is

---

D_x **Pelvic Inflammatory Disease**

- Lower abdominal pain
- Adnexal tenderness
- Cervical motion tenderness

ADDITIONAL FINDINGS
- Fever > 38.3° C (101° F)
- Abnormal vaginal discharge
- Elevated erythrocyte sedimentation rate, C-reactive protein, or white blood cell count (> 10,500/mm^3)
- Culture proven infection with *N. gonorrhoeae* or *C. trachomatis*
- Inflammatory mass on palpation, ultrasound, or laparoscopy
- Endometritis on biopsy

consistent with syphilis. If the lesions are painful or are associated with a grouped vesicular eruption, HSV is the likely cause. The presence of systemic symptoms such as fever, chills, headache, or malaise is also important to determine because these symptoms are seen with a primary infection with either organism. Generalized complaints, however, are associated with secondary syphilis only 50% of the time. A history of adenopathy, either localized or generalized, must also be noted, and dysuria may be present in females with HSV. In addition, a history of a virus-like illness accompanied by a rash should be explored. A diffuse maculopapular rash, especially on the palms and soles, is a classic sign of secondary syphilis. Known exposure to STDs should be ascertained.

Physical Examination

All adolescents who present with chancres, or ulcers, should receive a complete physical examination. The skin, including the palms and soles, should be examined closely for any dull red to reddish-brown macular or papular lesions. The orophayrnx should be carefully checked for chancres or blisters. All lymph nodes should be palpated for pain, enlargement, or induration. Suppurative or fluctuant nodes are often associated with chancroid caused by *Haemophilus ducreyi*.

The genital examination should then focus on the appearance of the lesions. The following questions should be asked of the patient: Are the lesions ulcerative, clustered, and painful? (HSV or chancroid.) Are they associated with grouped vesicles on an erythematous base? (HSV.) Is tender inguinal adenopathy present? (HSV or chancroid.) Or is there a single, painless chancre with a clean base and a sharply defined, slightly elevated border? (Syphilis.) The lymph nodes associated with this syphilitic type chancre are often nontender, but enlarged. Other less common STDs produce venereal ulcers that are often painful, deep, and that may be accompanied by some purulence. Adenopathy is also quite impressive with chancroid and lymphogranuloma venereum (*C. trachomatis*).

Laboratory Tests

The necessary diagnostic tests depend on the patient's clinical picture. However, all adolescents who present with an ulcerative lesion should have darkfield microscopy performed for syphilis. Direct fluorescent antibody testing of the lesions is also available and is very specific. Nontreponemal serologic tests for syphilis, such as the Venereal Disease Research Laboratory (VDRL) or rapid plasma reagin (RPR) tests, should be done if direct examination is not available or the clinical appearance of the ulcer is nonspecific. In cases of early primary syphilis where the VDRL or RPR may not be reactive initially, the test should be repeated in one week. Treponemal tests, such as the fluorescent treponemal antibody absorption test (FTA-ABS), should be used only as confirmatory tests and not for screening purposes.

A viral culture for HSV should also be performed from the base of an unroofed vesicle. HSV monoclonal antibody can be performed in older lesions that may be culture-negative and can differentiate between types 1 and 2. HSV serology is generally not helpful.

Given the well-described correlation between genital ulcers and HIV, it is recommended that all patients with a diagnosis of syphilis be tested for HIV as well.

GENITAL WARTS

History

Risk factors for HPV infection should be assessed. These include a history of multiple sexual partners; age younger than 25 years; a previous history of an STD; lack of condom use; pregnancy; altered immune response; and tobacco use. Symptoms may include pruritus, pain, or dyspareunia, but often the condition is asymptomatic. Adolescents may inadvertently palpate a papule on the external genitalia and be concerned.

Physical Examination

A complete pelvic examination should be performed on all sexually active female adolescents. Before the speculum is inserted, the external genitalia should be carefully inspected for lesions. Genital warts, or condyloma acuminatum, most commonly appear on squamous epithelium as irregular polypoid masses that may coalesce into larger ones. They are usually located at the posterior introitus, labia minora, and in the vestibule in females, and they may be found on the cervix and vagina as well. In males, warts can be seen more commonly on the penile shaft, glans, or corona. They may also appear as flat, flesh-colored papules on the scrotum and anus. Because this is a common location for lesions, the anus should be inspected carefully in both males and females.

Condylomata planum are subclinical lesions that are not grossly visible but are apparent on colposcopy and histology. Condylomata lata are flat, flesh-colored warts associated with secondary syphilis.

Laboratory Tests

A Pap smear should be performed on all females with any evidence of condyloma acuminatum. Cytologic findings associated with HPV include atypia, koilocytosis, and dysplasia. When considering referral to a gynecologist, the grade of the lesion should be reviewed. Classification of HPV is often left to the discretion of the specialist, however.

Subclinical HPV infection can be detected using acetic acid, Schiller's iodine, and colposcopy. Suspicious areas of white epithelium or a specific vascular pattern consistent with HPV infection should be biopsied. Females may be referred to a gynecologist for this procedure. Subclinical lesions in males should also be evaluated using 3% acetic acid. Biopsy may be difficult to perform but is indicated if any findings are positive.

A culture for gonorrhea and an enzyme immunoassay for chlamydia should be obtained. A nontreponemal antibody test for syphilis (RPR or VDRL) should also be performed. An HIV antibody test should be offered to all adolescents who are deemed appropriately "at risk" after receiving pretest counseling.

A urinalysis for asymptomatic hematuria is indicated in males with visible condyloma. Its presence would indicate a urethral lesion.

MANAGEMENT

Although many states differ with regard to the details of health care delivery for adolescents, a universal policy allows health care providers to evaluate and treat adolescents for an STD without parental consent. Notification of partners is usually anonymous and carried out by local public health officials. Contacts are informed that a partner has been diagnosed with an STD and are instructed to be evaluated for treatment. For details regarding specific conditions and therapies, the reader may consult the selected readings at the end of the chapter.

In addition to antimicrobial therapy, management of an STD should include preventive services. Adolescents with a first-time STD as well as those with recurrent STDs should be educated about disease transmission, consequences of delayed treatment, and methods for prevention. Other associated STDs, such as HIV, should also be addressed. The physician should spend time with adolescents with recurrent STDs and explore the reasons why preventive methods have failed. Several factors are extremely important to consider, including an untreated partner, poor sexual judgment secondary to substance use or abuse, and noncompliance with the treatment regimen, because they are certain to influence current treatment.

PROGNOSIS

If diagnosed and treated in a timely manner, the prognosis for most STDs is good. Sequelae of PID, however, regardless of treatment, include tubo-ovarian abscess and Fitz-Hugh-Curtis syndrome (perihepatitis). Long-term consequences of PID are chronic abdominal pain, ectopic pregnancy, and infertility. Currently, there is no pharmacologic agent to eradicate HSV or HIV. Although acyclovir is useful in treating the signs of primary herpes and reducing the incidence of recurrences, long-term safety of using acyclovir is unknown. The prognosis for HIV is variable, depending on the individual's progression at the time of diagnosis.

Case Resolution

In the case presented at the beginning of the chapter, a diagnosis of HSV can be made clinically. The adolescent should be counseled with regard to the mode of transmission, the natural history of primary versus recurrent infection, and the role of antiviral agents. An RPR or VDRL test should be performed as well as a thorough assessment for HIV risk. HIV testing should be offered after appropriate pretest counseling has been performed.

Selected Readings

Anderson, M. M., and R. E. Morris. HIV and adolescents. Pediatr. Ann. 22:436–446, 1993.

Centers for Disease Control and Prevention. 1993 Sexually transmitted diseases treatment guidelines. M.M.W.R. 42:RR–14, 1–102, 1993.

Drugs for sexually transmitted diseases. Med. Lett. 36:1–6, 1994.

Ellen, J. M., A. B. Moscicki, and M. B. Shafer. Genital herpes simplex virus and human papillomavirus infection. Adv. Ped. Infect. Dis. 9:97–124, 1994.

Gittes, E. B., and C. E. Irwin. Sexually transmitted diseases in adolescents. Pediatr. Rev. 14:180–189, 1993.

McCabe, E., L. R. Jaffe, and A. Diaz. Human immunodeficiency virus seropositivity in adolescents with syphilis. Pediatrics 92:695–698, 1993.

McCormack, W. M. Pelvic inflammatory disease. N. Engl. J. Med. 330:115–119, 1994.

Rosenfeld, W. D. Sexually transmitted diseases in adolescents: update 1991. Pediatr. Ann. 20:303–312, 1991.

Schydlower, M., and Shafer, M. (eds.). AIDS and other sexually transmitted diseases. Adolesc. Med. State Art Rev. 1:409–642, 1990.

Shafer, M. B. Sexually transmitted diseases in adolescents: prevention, diagnosis, and treatment in pediatric practice. Adolesc. Health Update 6:1–7. 1994.

CHAPTER 70

MENSTRUAL DISORDERS

Monica Sifuentes, M.D.

Hx A 16-year-old female presents with a nine-day history of vaginal bleeding. She has no history of abdominal pain, nausea, vomiting, fever, dysuria, or anorexia, and she reports no dizziness or syncope. Her menses usually last six to eight days and occur every 21 to 25 days. Her last menstrual period was three weeks ago and was normal in duration and flow. Menarche occurred at 15 years of age. She is sexually active, has had two partners, and reportedly uses condoms. Neither she nor her current partner has ever been diagnosed with or treated for an STD. She has no family history of blood dyscrasias or cancer.

On physical examination, she is an obese adolescent female in no acute distress. Her temperature is 98.4° F (36.9 °C). Her heart rate is 100 beats/minute, and her blood pressure is 110/60. The physical examination, including a pelvic examination, is unremarkable except for minimal blood noted at the vaginal introitus.

Questions

1. What menstrual disorders commonly affect adolescent females?
2. What factors contribute to the development of menstrual disorders, particularly during adolescence?
3. What relevant history should be obtained in adolescents with menstrual or pelvic disorders?
4. What treatment options are currently available for primary dysmenorrhea?
5. What conditions must be considered in adolescents with abnormal uterine bleeding?
6. How is dysfunctional uterine bleeding managed in adolescent patients?

Gynecologic concerns and complaints are common reasons for visits by adolescent females to their primary care physicians. The challenge for practitioners is to differentiate between an organic etiology, functional condition, and psychogenic complaints. When this cannot be readily determined or if the physical examination is equivocal, multiple diagnostic procedures are performed, often with disappointing results. In addition, many pediatricians are uncomfortable dealing with adolescents and performing pelvic examinations, which contributes to this diagnostic problem. The purpose of this chapter is to review some of the more common gynecologic conditions affecting the adolescent female and to highlight the significant historical and physical findings associated with each problem. For a discussion of the infectious conditions that cause pelvic pain, the reader is referred to Chapter 69, Sexually Transmitted Diseases.

EPIDEMIOLOGY

The overall prevalence of menstrual disorders during adolescence is estimated to be 50%. The most common gynecologic complaint is dysmenorrhea, or painful menstruation. Dysmenorrhea has been found to be responsible for significantly limiting activity in 10 to 15% of females. At least 75% of women reportedly have some pain associated with menses regardless of the degree of discomfort. Prevalence estimates regarding premenstrual syndrome (PMS) are difficult to assess because most studies are retrospective and complaints can be exaggerated. Between 31 and 73% of older adolescents reportedly have significant PMS-type complaints. An estimated 20 to 40% of adult women experience PMS, and 5 to 10% have debilitating symptoms. Other problems include abnormal uterine bleeding, vaginal discharge, and amenorrhea.

Several factors contribute to the occurrence of gynecologic problems during adolescence. The average age of menarche in the United States is 12.5 years (range: 9–16 years). Bleeding may be irregular or prolonged initially because most early menstrual cycles are anovulatory. Once ovulatory cycles are established, bleeding problems may resolve, but menstrual symptoms such as pain may predominate. Early sexual activity among adolescents and associated STDs may also contribute to the presence of certain gynecologic conditions in this age group, particularly vaginitis and abnormal uterine bleeding.

CLINICAL PRESENTATION

Adolescents with menstrual disorders may present in a variety of ways. They may have specific symptoms, such as heavy bleeding, irregular periods, or painful menses, or more general complaints, such as fatigue, dizziness, and syncope (D_x Box). Adolescents or their parents may have questions or concerns about delayed pubertal development and amenorrhea.

D_x Menstrual Disorders

PRIMARY DYSMENORRHEA
- Painful menstruation
- Lower abdominal pain associated with menstruation, usually worse on the first few days of bleeding
- Associated back pain
- Pain sometimes accompanied by nausea, vomiting, fatigue, headache, and diarrhea
- Symptoms began six to twelve months after menarche

DYSFUNCTIONAL UTERINE BLEEDING
- Prolonged bleeding (> 8 days) *or*
- Excessive bleeding (> 6 tampons/pads per day) *or*
- Frequent uterine bleeding (≤ 21 days)
- No demonstrable organic etiology
- Normal laboratory studies, except for anemia

PRIMARY AMENORRHEA
- No spontaneous menstruation in a female of reproductive age
- Absence of menarche by age 16 to 18 in a female with normal pubertal development *or*
- Absence of menarche by age 14 to 16 in a female with no secondary sexual development *or*
- Absence of menarche within one to two years of reaching full sexual maturation (Tanner stage V)

PATHOPHYSIOLOGY

Puberty and the Normal Menstrual Cycle

Figure 70–1 depicts the menstrual cycle, which normally lasts for 21 to 45 days, with a mean length of approximately 28 days. Normal duration of menses is four days (± 2–3). Blood loss is usually 30 to 40 mL per cycle, and most women do not lose more than 60 mL per cycle. Regular ovulatory cycles usually do not occur until one to two years after menarche.

One-quarter of females begin menstruating when they reach Tanner stage III of sexual maturation, but approximately two-thirds do not menstruate until they reach Tanner stage IV. It is important to note that several other processes occur before the onset of menstruation. Thelarche, or the beginning of breast development, takes place approximately 2 to 2½ years before menarche, and growth acceleration usually begins about one year before thelarche.

Dysmenorrhea

This condition is often accompanied by other symptoms such as nausea, vomiting, diarrhea, and headaches. It can be classified as either primary or secondary. **Primary dysmenorrhea** occurs in the absence of any pelvic pathology and is most commonly seen in adolescents. **Secondary dysmenorrhea** refers to painful menses associated with some underlying pelvic pathology, such as PID, endometriosis, ovarian cysts or tumors, or cervical stenosis. A complete list of causes of secondary amenorrhea can be found in Table

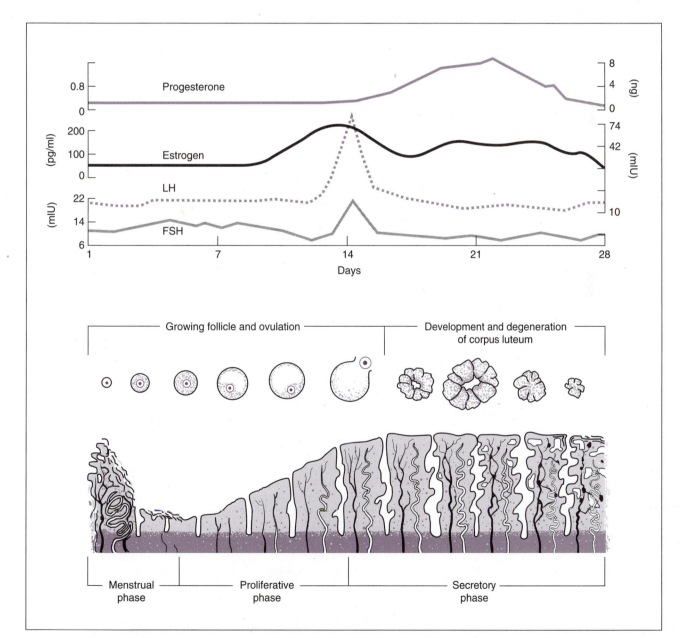

FIGURE 70–1. *The normal ovulatory menstrual cycle. FSH, follicle-stimulating hormone; LH, luteinizing hormone.*

TABLE 70–1. Differential Diagnosis of Common Menstrual Disorders

Dysmenorrhea

Primary
Secondary
Pelvic inflammatory disease
Endometriosis
Uterine myomas, polyps, or adhesions
Adenomyosis
Ovarian cysts or tumors
Presence of an intrauterine device
Cervical stenosis or strictures
Congenital malformations (i.e., septate uterus)

Abnormal Uterine Bleeding

Dysfunctional uterine bleeding: anovulation
Complications of pregnancy: threatened/spontaneous abortion, ectopic pregnancy, hydatidiform mole
Infections of the lower and upper genital tract: PID, cervicitis/vaginitis
Blood dyscrasias: vWD, ITP, leukemia, platelet defects
Endocrine disorders: hypothyroidism, hyperprolactinemia, late-onset 21-hydroxylase deficiency
Vaginal anomalies: adenosis (DES exposure), carcinoma
Cervical/uterine abnormalities: endometriosis, polyps
Ovarian abnormalities: polycystic ovary syndrome, tumors, cysts
Systemic illness: inflammatory bowel disease, malignancy
Foreign body: condoms, tampons, IUDs
Medications: aspirin, anticoagulants, oral contraceptives
Trauma or sexual assault

Abbreviations: DES, diethylstilbestrol; IUD, intrauterine device; ITP, idiopathic thrombocytopenic purpura; PID, pelvic inflammatory disease; vWD, von Willebrand's disease.

70–1. In adolescents, endometriosis is the most common cause of secondary dysmenorrhea.

Numerous studies have shown that endometrial prostaglandins play a role in the pathogenesis of primary dysmenorrhea. During menses, prostaglandin $F_{2\alpha}$ ($PGF_{2\alpha}$) is produced locally by the endometrium from arachidonic acid. $PGF_{2\alpha}$ is a potent vasoconstrictor and myometrial stimulant that causes uterine contractions and tissue ischemia. Another prostaglandin, $E_{2\alpha}$, causes hypersensitivity of the pain nerve terminals in the uterine myometrium. The cumulative effect of these prostaglandins may cause the pain of primary dysmenorrhea. Hormonal and endocrine factors may also play a role in the etiology of primary dysmenorrhea, because ovulatory cycles with estrogen and progesterone are necessary for development of the condition.

Most cases of primary dysmenorrhea begin 6 to 12 months after menarche, and symptoms gradually increase until patients reach their mid-20s. Parity and advancing age are associated with a decrease in symptomatology.

Dysfunctional Uterine Bleeding

Dysfunctional uterine bleeding (DUB) is defined as abnormal or excessive endometrial bleeding in the absence of any pelvic pathology. Menstruation is considered excessive if the cycles are short (< 21 days) and the bleeding is prolonged (8 days or more). Although DUB is relatively common in adolescents, it should be considered a diagnosis of exclusion. Other causes of abnormal bleeding should first be investigated by obtaining a thorough history and then excluded by performing a complete physical examination.

DUB is usually the result of anovulatory, immature menstrual cycles. In adolescents, 50% of menstrual cycles are anovulatory within the first two years of menarche. If menarche occurs later in adolescence (i.e., at Tanner stage V), this period of anovulation reportedly lasts even longer. The majority of cases of DUB in adolescence are thought to result from the delayed maturation of the hypothalamic-pituitary-ovarian axis. Normally, a positive feedback mechanism develops with rising estrogen levels, resulting in a surge in luteinizing hormone (LH) and follicle-stimulating hormone (FSH), which triggers ovulation. The progesterone-producing corpus luteum then stimulates development of the secretory endometrium, with subsequent shedding after approximately 14 days (menses). With anovulation, there is no progesterone-producing corpus luteum and therefore no development of a secretory endometrium. Thus, estrogen remains unopposed, and proliferative endometrium continues to accumulate. Finally, when the tissue can no longer maintain its integrity, it sloughs. In addition, without progesterone, the normal vasospasm that helps limit endometrial bleeding does not occur. Hence, bleeding is prolonged, frequent, and heavy.

Premenstrual Syndrome

PMS refers to a group of both physical and emotional symptoms that occur prior to menses and resolve following menstruation. A variety of mechanisms have been proposed, including fluctuations in steroid hormones and releasing factors, a deficiency of vitamin B_6, changes in salt and water balance, prostaglandin synthesis, and a release of endorphins and other neurotransmitters. Allergies to environmental agents and foods have also been implicated.

Amenorrhea

Amenorrhea is defined as the lack of spontaneous menstruation in women of reproductive age. Like dysmenorrhea, it can be considered primary or secondary. **Primary amenorrhea** can be further defined by the following criteria: (1) an absence of menarche by the age 16 to 18 years in females with otherwise normal pubertal development, (2) an absence of menarche by the age of 14 to 16 years in females with no secondary sexual development, and (3) an absence of menarche within 1 to 2 years of reaching Tanner stage V pubic hair. Causes of primary amenorrhea range from congenital anatomic anomalies to genetic and endocrine conditions. A detailed discussion of each of these etiologies is beyond the scope of this chapter (see the references listed at the end of this chapter for more information).

Secondary amenorrhea occurs in females who have already established menstruation but have had no periods for six months or the equivalent of three cycles. The most common cause of secondary amenorrhea is pregnancy, which must be ruled out in all adolescents presenting with this complaint, regardless of their acknowledgement of sexual activity. Other causes include infections, systemic illnesses, significant weight loss, stress, exercise, eating disorders (e.g., anorexia nervosa, bulimia nervosa), and certain medications.

Vaginal Discharge

Vaginal discharge can be normal. A thin, white discharge, known as leukorrhea, occurs approximately one year prior to the onset of menarche. A purulent, malodorous, or bloody discharge is considered abnormal, however. Etiologies are varied and may be infectious, inflammatory, or traumatic (see Chapter 69, Sexually Transmitted Diseases).

DIFFERENTIAL DIAGNOSIS

The differential diagnosis of the disorders described above can be found in Table 70–1. Other etiologies of pelvic pain include midcycle menstrual disorders (e.g., mittelschmerz), UTIs, abdominal conditions such as appendicitis, inflammatory bowel disease, and irritable bowel syndrome. Psychogenic pain should also be considered as a cause of recurrent pelvic pain and may be secondary to depression, anxiety, previous sexual abuse, or another psychological condition.

EVALUATION

History

A thorough history should be obtained in adolescent females with suspected menstrual disorders because many nongynecologic conditions can affect menses. A complete psychosocial assessment should also be performed. The acronym **HEADSSS** (**h**ome environment, **e**mployment and education, **a**ctivities, **d**rugs, **s**exuality/sexual activity, **s**uicide/depression, **s**afety) serves as a useful tool (see Chapter 4, Talking to Adolescents).

The majority of the interview should then focus on the gynecologic history (Table 70–2) and any specific problems (Questions Box). With primary dysmenorrhea, pain that radiates to the anterior thighs or the

---

Questions: Menstrual Disorders

Dysmenorrhea
- What is the pain like?
- When did the pain first begin?
- How frequently does the pain occur?
- How long does the pain last?
- Are any symptoms associated with the pain (e.g., nausea, vomiting, diarrhea, headache)?
- Does the adolescent miss a lot of school as a result of painful menses?
- Do the painful menses interfere with other activities?
- What does the adolescent do for the pain? Has she tried any medications or home remedies?
- Is there a maternal or sibling history of painful menses?

Abnormal Uterine Bleeding
- Does the adolescent have any symptoms of anemia?
  - Is she fatigued, easily tired, dizzy, or short of breath?
  - Has she experienced any syncopal episodes?
- Does the adolescent have any history of blood loss in the urine or stool?
- Is there any evidence of a bleeding disorder (e.g., easy bruisability, bleeding from the gums or nares)?
- Does the adolescent have any symptoms of pregnancy (e.g., breast tenderness, nausea, fatigue)?
- Is there any known exposure to STDs?
- Is there a marked change in the adolescent's weight? Has the adolescent been on any diets recently?
- Is the adolescent using any medications such as aspirin, oral contraceptives, or anticoagulants?
- Does the adolescent have a history of trauma?
- Is the bleeding cyclic in nature?
- Is there breakthrough bleeding throughout the cycle?
- Does the adolescent have a family history of bleeding disorders, thyroid disease, or exposure to DES?

---

lower back is not uncommon. The color of the blood may be helpful when assessing abnormal uterine bleeding. Brown or dark blood may be associated with a cervical obstruction or endometriosis, whereas red or pink blood is found with most other conditions. More importantly, the timing of the bleeding is extremely significant. Cyclical bleeding is more consistent with a blood dyscrasia. In contrast, breakthrough bleeding throughout the cycle may indicate an infection, endometriosis, or perhaps a polyp.

Physical Examination

A complete physical examination, including an evaluation for stigmata of a systemic illness, must be performed in adolescent females with suspected menstrual disorders. Patients' height and weight should be plotted on the growth chart and compared to previous measurements. Depending on the Tanner stage, physicians can then determine if they have experienced their expected growth spurt. Vital signs, including orthostatic measurements, are a screen for significant blood loss and are especially important in patients with abnormal uterine bleeding. The skin should be inspected for any evidence of androgen excess (e.g.,

---

TABLE 70–2.   Gynecologic History

Age at menarche
Last menstrual period
Regularity of menses
Duration of bleeding
Amount of flow (number of pads/tampons used per day and amount of saturation)
Associated symptoms such as bloating, headache, lower abdominal pain and cramping
Sexual activity
    Age at debut
    Number of partners and ages
    Consensual vs. nonconsensual sex
    Date of last encounter
    Protected vs. unprotected sex
    Current method of contraception
Maternal and sibling gynecologic history
    Ages at menarche
    Symptoms with menses
    Treatment of symptoms

hirsutism, acne), bruising, or petechiae. The thyroid gland should be palpated for masses or any evidence of hypertrophy, and the abdomen and suprapubic area should also be palpated for masses.

In addition, the Tanner stage of the breasts should be noted and compared to the pubic hair development, particularly in adolescents with primary amenorrhea. The external genitalia should then be carefully inspected for clitoral size and patency of the hymen. A bimanual or rectoabdominal examination should be performed in adolescents who are not sexually active. Depending on the findings, a speculum examination is often not necessary. In adolescents who are sexually active or desire contraception, however, a complete pelvic and bimanual examination are indicated.

Laboratory Tests

The performance of laboratory studies depends on the particular menstrual complaint. No laboratory studies are necessary for primary dysmenorrhea because the diagnosis is usually based on history and physical examination. The same is true for PMS. For a discussion of the diagnostic evaluation of amenorrhea, the reader is referred to the article by Neinstein listed in Selected Readings.

In the case of abnormal uterine bleeding, baseline studies mandate a hemoglobin or hematocrit. Initial laboratory studies should also include a CBC to evaluate the red cell indices and platelets, a reticulocyte count, and a pregnancy test. Further studies depend on the severity of the anemia and findings on history and physical examination. These may include coagulation studies (bleeding time, PT/PTT), liver function tests, ESR, and thyroid function tests. If the patient is sexually active, endocervical cultures for *Chlamydia trachomatis* and *Neisseria gonorrhoeae* should also be obtained. FSH, LH, prolactin, testosterone, and DHEA-S (dehydroepiandrosterone-sulfate) studies should be performed in patients with a history of chronic anovulation or in whom androgen excess is suspected.

Imaging Studies

A pelvic ultrasound or CT scan can be helpful in patients with abnormal uterine bleeding if a mass is suspected or palpated on physical examination.

MANAGEMENT

With each of these adolescent gynecologic conditions, effective treatment is multifaceted and includes patient and parent education, reassurance regarding the ease with which the condition can be treated, and medications. In general, a menstrual calendar or diary can be helpful to gain a more objective idea of the problem.

Dysmenorrhea

General measures in the treatment of dysmenorrhea include education about menstruation, proper diet,

TABLE 70–3. Nonsteroidal Antiinflammatory Drugs in the Treatment of Primary Dysmenorrhea

Generic Name	Trade Names	Dosage
Ibuprofen	Motrin, Advil	400 mg q4–6h for 24–72 h
Naproxen	Aleve, Naprosyn	500 mg at onset, then 250 mg q4–6h
Naproxen sodium	Anaprox	500 mg at onset, then 275 mg q6–8h
Mefenamic acid	Ponstel	500 mg at onset, then 250 mg q6–8h

application of heat, simple exercise, and psychological support.

For mild symptoms of dysmenorrhea, over-the-counter analgesics, such as ibuprofen, aspirin, or acetaminophen, are appropriate. Physicians most often suggest that patients use ibuprofen because it is probably the most efficacious. The dose is 400 mg every four to six hours. Ibuprofen should be taken at the onset of the menstrual cycle and continued for 24 to 72 hours.

For moderate to severe dysmenorrhea in patients who are not sexually active and do not desire birth control, a stronger **NSAID** is the treatment of choice (Table 70–3). The major mechanism of action of NSAIDs is the inhibition of prostaglandin synthesis. Side effects of these drugs, which most commonly relate to the GI tract, are nausea, vomiting, and dyspepsia. These reactions can be minimized by taking the medication with food or an antacid. Other adverse reactions include renal effects; skin reactions, such as erythema multiforme and urticaria; and CNS effects, including headache and dizziness. Contraindications to NSAID use include peptic ulcer disease, clotting disorders, and renal disease. All NSAIDs should be tried for three to four cycles before their efficacy is judged.

Low-dose combination oral contraceptives are indicated in adolescents with severe dysmenorrhea who are sexually active or in patients whose symptoms are not relieved by NSAIDs alone. Oral contraceptives decrease the production of prostaglandins by inhibiting ovulation as well as endometrial growth. Because the symptoms of dysmenorrhea are prevented only after several cycles, patients should be told not to expect complete resolution of symptoms during the first month of treatment.

Oral contraceptives should be used for a minimum of three to four months. If symptoms do not improve, then an NSAID can be added to the treatment regimen. Oral contraceptives are more than 90% effective in cases of severe dysmenorrhea, and physicians should emphasize this benefit to both patients and their parents.

Dysfunctional Uterine Bleeding (Table 70–4)

The management of DUB depends on the severity of the bleeding. The goal of treatment is threefold: (1) to control the bleeding, (2) to correct the anemia, and (3) to replenish iron stores. Patients with mild or moderate DUB can be treated as outpatients with weekly to monthly follow-up depending on how quickly the bleeding stops. Although **oral contraceptives** are

TABLE 70–4.   General Guidelines for the Management of Dysfunctional Uterine Bleeding (DUB) in Adolescents

	Mild DUB	Moderate DUB	Severe DUB
Hemoglobin (g/dL)	> 11	9–11	< 9
Management	Menstrual calendar, oral iron, OBCP (if sexually active)	OBCP (1/35) for minimum of 3 mo	OBCP (1/35) for 6–12 mo
Follow-up	2–3 mo	2–3 wk, then every 2–3 mo	1–2 wk, then every mo

Abbreviations: OBCP, oral birth control pill.

appropriate in the treatment of DUB if the condition is moderate or if birth control is desired, **other hormone regimens** such as estrogen (alone) or synthetic progestin (alone) can also be used.

Most adolescent females with severe bleeding require a more extensive evaluation, and such patients must be hospitalized for appropriate parenteral therapy. A high-dose combination estrogen and synthetic progestin pill (Enovid) is given simultaneously, and an antiemetic is often required during the first few days of therapy. Once bleeding has stopped, adolescents can continue Enovid for a total of 21 days and then switch to a low-dose combination oral contraceptive for at least three cycles. Studies have shown that 20 to 25% of adolescents who require hospitalization for severe anemia within the first year following menarche have an underlying coagulopathy. In cases of DUB where oral contraceptives are used but patients do not desire birth control, oral contraceptives should not be stopped until at least three months after the anemia has resolved to ensure restoration of iron stores.

Premenstrual Syndrome

Although various sources have advocated many different treatment regimens for the management of PMS, no single effective treatment has been found. Therapies include diet modification for patients who complain predominantly of bloating, regular exercise, vitamin supplementation with pyridoxine (B_6), and evening primrose oil. Other medications have been used, including the antihypertensive drug clonidine, alprazolam, diuretics such as spironolactone, danazol, and mefenamic acid (Ponstel).

Vaginitis

See Chapter 68, Vaginitis, and Chapter 69, Sexually Transmitted Diseases, for a discussion of the management of vaginal discharge in adolescents.

PROGNOSIS

Most adolescents with common menstrual complaints who receive aggressive, appropriate care are symptom-free after three to four months of continuous therapy. Complications associated with oral contraceptive use and NSAIDs are rare in this otherwise healthy population. Symptoms associated with immaturity, such as anovulatory bleeding and DUB, often resolve spontaneously. The prognosis for adolescents with amenorrhea depends in part on the underlying etiology.

Case Resolution

In the case presented at the beginning of the chapter, more information should be obtained to exclude the numerous other causes of abnormal uterine bleeding in the adolescent before a diagnosis of DUB can be made. Questions about breast tenderness, galactorrhea, weight loss, fatigue, and visual changes can be particularly important. If the adolescent has no other complaints, a hemoglobin or hematocrit as well as a CBC and a pregnancy test should be performed. Cervical cultures should also be taken to rule out infection. Depending on the degree of anemia and the desire for contraception, the adolescent should then be placed on iron supplementation and hormonal therapy if the bleeding is significant.

Selected Readings

Anderson, M. M., C. E. Irwin, and D.L. Snyder. Abnormal vaginal bleeding in adolescents. Pediatr. Ann. 15:697–707, 1986.

Bayer, S. R., and A. H. DeCherney. Clinical manifestations and treatment of dysfunctional uterine bleeding. J.A.M.A. 269:1823–1828, 1993.

Blythe, M. Common menstrual problems. Part 3, abnormal uterine bleeding. Adolesc. Health Update 4:1–5, 1992.

Cholst, I. N., and A. T. Carlon. Oral contraceptives and dysmenorrhea. J. Adolesc. Health Care 8:121–128, 1987.

Coupey, S. M., and P. Ahlstrom. Common menstrual disorders. Pediatr. Clin. North Am. 36:551–571, 1989.

Cowan, B., and J. Morrison. Management of abnormal genital bleeding in girls and women. N. Engl. J. Med. 324:1710–1715, 1991.

Hertweck, S. P. Dysfunctional uterine bleeding. Obstet. Gynecol. Clin. North Am. 19:129–149, 1992.

Neinstein, L. S. Menstrual problems in adolescents. Med. Clin. North Am. 74:1181–1203, 1990.

Polaneczky, M. M., and G. B. Slap. Dysmenorrhea and dysfunctional uterine bleeding. Pediatr. Rev. 13:83–87, 1992.

Polaneczky, M. M., and G. B. Slap. Menstrual disorders in the adolescent: amenorrhea. Pediatr. Rev. 13:43–48, 1992.

ORTHOPEDIC DISORDERS

C H A P T E R   7 1

DEVELOPMENTAL HIP DYSPLASIA

Geeta Grover, M.D.

H$_x$ A four-month-old girl is seen for her routine health maintenance visit. She is doing well and has no complaints. The results of the entire examination are within normal limits except for limited abduction of the left hip, which is approximately 45 degrees, in comparison to that of the right hip, which is almost 90 degrees.

Questions

1. What specific physical maneuvers help in the evaluation of infants with decreased range of motion of the hip?
2. What are the clinical findings of hip dislocation during and after the neonatal period?
3. What are some of the conditions often seen in conjunction with hip dysplasia that may be noted on physical examination?
4. What is the appropriate diagnostic workup of infants with suspected hip dysplasia?

Developmental hip dysplasia (developmental dysplasia of the hip, DDH) defines a range of hip pathology, from frank dislocation to instability. DDH may either exist at birth or develop during infancy. The term DDH has replaced the term congenital hip dysplasia (CHD), because hip dysplasia may not always be apparent or present during the newborn period. DDH is a common pediatric orthopedic concern. When DDH is recognized and treated appropriately, children potentially develop completely normally. If the diagnosis is missed or delayed, however, children may suffer significant morbidity, including severe degenerative hip disease.

EPIDEMIOLOGY

The incidence of neonatal hip instability is estimated to range from 11.5 to 17 per 1000 live births. Approximately 50% of these cases resolve by one week of age, and 90% resolve by two months of age, which gives a true incidence of hip dislocation of 1 to 1.5 per 1000 live births. Approximately 60% of affected infants are first born. Girls are affected six to eight times more fre-

quently than boys. Incidence is increased among Caucasians (compared to African Americans), with breech presentation (approximately 20% of all dislocations occur in infants born in the breech position), and with a positive family history. The left hip is involved in 60% of children with DDH and the right hip in 20% of cases, and 20% of the time DDH is bilateral. DDH has an increased association with lesions believed to be secondary to mechanical molding such as congenital torticollis (approximately 20% of affected children may have DDH) and metatarsus adductus (approximately 2–10% of these children may have DDH).

CLINICAL PRESENTATION

The clinical presentation and signs of DDH in children vary with age. Diagnosis is made primarily by physical examination (i.e., Ortolani and Barlow maneuvers) during the neonatal period. Asymmetric skin folds, limitation of hip abduction, and a positive Galeazzi's sign are the classic signs of DDH in older infants. Physical signs, which become more obvious once children are walking, include limping and toe-walking (D$_x$ Box).

PATHOPHYSIOLOGY

DDH encompasses a wide variety of conditions ranging from hip instability to dislocation. A dislocated hip is one in which there is complete loss of contact between the femoral head and the acetabulum. The

---

D$_x$ **Developmental Hip Dysplasia**

- Breech presentation
- Female sex
- Asymmetric skin folds
- Limitation of hip reduction
- Positive Galeazzi's sign
- Limp
- Toe-walking

dislocation may be reducible using the Ortolani test (see below) or nonreducible. Nonreducible dislocations are usually teratologic and associated with other serious malformations such as arthrogryposis or spina bifida. An unstable hip is one in which the femoral head is within the acetabulum but may be dislocated using the Barlow test (see below).

Dysplasia of the acetabulum is also associated with hip instability. The dysplastic acetabular cavity is shallower with a more vertical inclination than normal. An understanding of the pathophysiology that relates primarily to ligamentous laxity and bony abnormalities of the acetabular cavity enables one to see that although most dislocations occur at or near the time of delivery, they can occur later in infancy as well. Late hip dislocations are reported in 3 to 8% of affected infants.

The etiology of DDH involves mechanical, physiologic, and environmental factors. The primary **mechanical factors** are tight maternal abdominal and uterine musculature, breech presentation (especially frank breech presentation with the knees in extension), and positioning of the fetal hip against the mother's sacrum. In utero mechanical factors relate to molding and restriction of fetal movement. It is believed that the tight, unstretched maternal abdomen and uterine musculature of primigravidas may prevent fetal movement, thus predisposing first-born infants to DDH. The increased occurrence of other conditions thought to be secondary to molding (e.g., congenital muscular torticollis) with DDH supports this theory of space restriction. **Physiologic factors** relate to ligamentous laxity. Female infants may be more sensitive to maternal hormones such as estrogen and relaxin, which are present around the time of delivery, resulting in generalized ligamentous laxity, including laxity of the hip capsule. **Environmental factors** that may predispose infants to DDH include swaddling with the legs in extension and adduction, which is still practiced in some societies (e.g., those who use cradleboards, such as Navajos in North America), and muscle contractures secondary to neuromuscular disease such as cerebral palsy.

DIFFERENTIAL DIAGNOSIS

The differential diagnosis of hip dysplasia depends on the age of the child and the presenting complaint. Infants may have a "click" on abduction of the hip that represents the snapping of a ligament rather than the reduction of the dislocated hip into the joint. Infants who have limited abduction may have a neuromuscular disorder such as spastic diplegia. Older children who present with gait disturbances such as limp, waddling gait, or toe-walking may have neuromuscular conditions, fractures, or infection (e.g., osteomyelitis, septic arthritis).

EVALUATION

History

Family history of DDH should be reviewed. A careful neonatal history detailing the type of presentation (e.g.,

---

Questions: Developmental Hip Dysplasia

- Was the infant a breech presentation?
- Does the child have any muscular problems, such as torticollis?
- When did the gait disturbance begin?
- Does anything make the child's gait better or worse?
- Is the child in any pain?
- Did any member of the family have hip dysplasia?

---

breech versus vertex), type of delivery, history of prenatal problems such as oligohydramnios, and presence of congenital torticollis or metatarsus adductus should also be taken (Questions Box).

Physical Examination

It is important to evaluate the hip joint for instability or dislocation throughout the first year of life or until the child begins to walk. The **Ortolani and Barlow maneuvers** may be used in the neonatal period to evaluate for DDH (Fig. 71–1). Both tests are performed with infants in a supine position and the hips and knees flexed to 90 degrees. Infants should be quiet and relaxed. Adequate results are difficult to obtain with crying or fussy infants.

In the Ortolani maneuver, a palpable "thunk" or "clunk" as the examiner relocates a dislocated hip by gentle abduction and lifting of the femoral head anteriorly is a positive result. This "clunk" differs from the audible hip click, which is secondary to nonpathologic processes such as ligamentous snapping. Each leg should be examined separately, not simultaneously. The Barlow maneuver attempts to dislocate the hip by adduction and posterior axial pressure on the thigh. These tests are not useful after approximately six to eight weeks of age, because the surrounding soft tissues and muscles adapt to the dislocated hip, which makes it more difficult to reduce.

After the neonatal period, several tests can be used to assess hip stability (Fig. 71–2). Asymmetry of hip abduction is secondary to adductor muscle shortening and contracture on the affected side. This asymmetry is one of the simplest ways to evaluate for hip dislocation after the first several weeks of life. Children under the age of eight weeks should achieve full abduction (90 degrees) with both knees touching the examination table, often even in the presence of hip dysplasia. After this age, with children supine, hips and knees flexed, and both legs abducted simultaneously, abduction limited to less than 60 degrees or asymmetry between the two sides may indicate dislocation. This test, however, is difficult to interpret with bilateral dislocation because no side is "normal."

As the femoral head dislocates posteriorly, the thigh is shortened on the affected side, producing an asymmetry of skin folds or a discrepancy in knee heights. Asymmetric gluteal folds result from bunching of skin and subcutaneous tissue on the affected side, thus producing extra skin folds. Galeazzi's sign refers to the discrepancy in knee heights noted when infants are

FIGURE 71–1. *Ortolani and Barlow tests.* A. Ortolani (reduction) test. B. Barlow (dislocation) test.

supine with the sacrum flat on the examination table and hips and knees bent.

In children of walking age, the physician may notice a limp secondary to shortening of the leg on the affected side, leading to a leg length discrepancy. (Children may try to disguise the limp by toe-walking.) A Trendelenburg test may be positive. Normally, when a child stands on one leg, the hip abductors straighten the pelvis and keep the center of gravity over the femoral head. If the abductors are weak, the weight shifts to the opposite side, causing it to droop. Children with bilateral dislo-

cations display hyperlordosis of the lumbar spine with a waddling type of gait.

Imaging Studies

Radiologic and ultrasound evaluations may aid in the diagnosis. Ultrasonography in trained hands can be quite useful in the diagnosis of DDH, especially in the neonatal period when x-ray changes may not be evident because the femoral head is not calcified. Reliable x-ray

FIGURE 71–2. *Late signs in the diagnosis of developmental dysplasia of the hip.* A. Asymmetry of thigh folds. B. Asymmetry of hip abduction. C. Discrepancy of knee heights.

FIGURE 71–3. *Radiographic findings associated with developmental dysplasia of the hip.* The left hip is dislocated. The femur is lateral and proximal, and the acetabulum is shallow and flat.

changes begin to become evident at about six weeks of age (Fig. 71–3). A flat, shallow acetabulum and delayed ossification of the femoral head are the simplest, most easily recognized findings.

MANAGEMENT

The need for repeat examinations of the hips during the first year of life cannot be overemphasized. Children suspected of any hip instability or any children with less than 60 degrees of hip abduction should be evaluated with appropriate imaging studies and referred to an orthopedic surgeon for further evaluation and management. An orthopedic surgeon can aid the primary care physician in the management of DDH.

The goal of treatment is to return the femoral head to its normal position within the acetabulum and restore normal hip functioning. The common practice of triple diapering should be discouraged because it is unreliable and often delays definitive therapy. The **Pavlik harness** is the primary method of treating DDH during infancy. When properly used, the harness returns the hip to its normal position, and it allows infants to move their legs within safe limits of abduction and adduction until stability is achieved. The harness should be applied and monitored by an orthopedic surgeon, because inappropriate application may produce adverse outcomes (e.g., avascular necrosis of the femoral head). Treatment should be continued for about four weeks in newborns

and for a period equal to approximately one to two times the child's age at the time treatment is started in other children.

If this treatment method is ineffective or the diagnosis is not made until after six months of age, **traction** followed by either open or closed **reduction and spica cast immobilization** may be used. Good results are more difficult to obtain with increasing age, especially after children are walking. Operative treatment (e.g., open reduction) is usually required in children over the age of 18 months. Additional procedures may be required in older children, especially those over the age of 36 months, including (1) **femoral osteotomy** either to shorten the femur or to correct femoral antetorsion and (2) **pelvic osteotomy** to correct acetabular dysplasia.

PROGNOSIS

The prognosis of DDH depends on age at the time of diagnosis and severity of the deformity. The long-term prognosis for satisfactory hip function is good for children when DDH is recognized early and treated appropriately. Generally, children with DDH that is diagnosed after the first year of life have a poorer prognosis for satisfactory hip function than those with DDH that is diagnosed during infancy. Left untreated, DDH may result in significant disability, ranging from limp to pain and stiffness in the hip.

Case Resolution

The infant presented in the case history has less than 60 degrees of abduction of the left hip, a sign of DDH. An anteroposterior view of the pelvis may be ordered to confirm the diagnosis. Regardless of the radiographic findings, the infant should be referred to an orthopedic surgeon for further evaluation and management. If hip dislocation is confirmed, the initial treatment will probably involve bracing with the Pavlik harness.

Selected Readings

Aronsson, D. D., et al. Developmental dysplasia of the hip. Pediatrics 94:201–208, 1994.

Hensinger, R. N. Congenital dislocation of the hip: treatment in infancy to walking age. Ortho. Clin. North Am. 18:597–615, 1987.

Herring, J. A. Congenital dislocation of the hip. *In* Morrissy, R. T. (ed.). Lovell and Winter's Pediatric Orthopedics, 3rd ed. Philadelphia, J. B. Lippincott, 1990.

MacEwen, G. D., and C. Millet. Congenital dislocation of the hip. Pediatr. Rev. 11:249–252, 1990.

Staheli, L. T. Fundamentals of Pediatric Orthopedics. New York, Raven Press, 1992. pp. 7.7–7.13.

Westin, G. W., et al. Developmental hip dislocation. Contemp. Ortho. 16:17–24, 1988.

CHAPTER 72

ROTATIONAL PROBLEMS OF THE LOWER EXTREMITY: IN-TOEING AND OUT-TOEING

Geeta Grover, M.D.

H$_x$ A 3-year-old girl is brought to the office. Her mother is concerned because beginning a few months ago her daughter's feet appeared to "turn in" when she walked. The girl has never walked like this before, and she has no history of trauma, fever, pain, or swelling in the joints. The physical examination is within normal limits except for the in-toeing gait.

Questions

1. How can observation of children's gaits help determine the etiology of their in-toeing and out-toeing (rotational problems)?
2. What are the common causes of in-toeing and out-toeing?
3. Does evaluation of in-toeing and out-toeing require any laboratory or radiologic studies?
4. What is the natural history of most rotational problems?

Rotational problems of the lower extremities, especially in-toeing, frequently occur during the first several years of life. Although rotational problems that produce in-toeing and out-toeing rarely lead to physical limitations in children, they are a common cause of parental concern during infancy and childhood. The large majority of these problems can be managed adequately by primary care physicians and do not necessitate orthopedic referral. Clubfoot, which is not a rotational deformity but a pathologic one, is included in this discussion because it is often confused with conditions of the feet that produce in-toeing.

EPIDEMIOLOGY

In neonates or young infants, in-toeing is most likely the result of clubfoot (talipes equinovarus), isolated metatarsus adductus, or metatarsus varus. The incidence of clubfoot is 1 in every 1000 live births, with a male-to-female ratio of 2 to 1. The condition is bilateral in approximately 50% of cases. The incidence of metatarsus adductus, a much more common problem, is about 2 in every 1000 live births. It is often bilateral. Medial tibial torsion is the primary cause of in-toeing in the second year of life, and medial femoral torsion accounts for most cases of this condition during early childhood.

Physiologic out-toeing is classically evident in infants who have not yet begun to walk. This condition, which

is believed to be secondary to an external rotatory contracture about the hip due to intrauterine positioning, is the most common cause of out-turning in both feet. Lateral tibial torsion may result in out-toeing in older infants and children.

CLINICAL PRESENTATION

Children with congenital clubfoot, metatarsus adductus, and metatarsus varus present with in-toeing during infancy. Congenital clubfoot is usually readily evident at birth. A severe medial, midline, plantar crease is present, and the foot appears C-shaped, with both the heel and forefront turned inward. The affected foot is small, wide, and stiff, and the lower leg appears small due to hypoplasia of the calf muscles. In contrast to clubfoot, only the forefoot turns inward in metatarsus adductus and varus.

Medial tibial torsion is apparent during the second year of life. Children's feet turn inward as they walk, but their knees point straight. Medial femoral torsion is evident at 3 to 4 years of age. Affected children are usually girls; they can sit in the "W" position with both legs behind them. As children walk, both the knees and the feet appear to turn inward.

Physiologic out-toeing is seen in infancy. Classically, parents note that when they hold their children in a standing position, both feet turn outward. Approximately five degrees of out-toeing is normal after age 3. Further degrees of out-toeing may be due to lateral tibial torsion.

PATHOPHYSIOLOGY

Several factors are involved in the etiology of rotational conditions. The majority of these problems are deformities secondary to intrauterine positioning. Metatarsus adductus and medial tibial torsion result from intrauterine positioning, and certain sleeping and sitting positions may perpetuate these problems in infants and children. For example, sleeping in the prone position with the legs internally rotated may lead to continued internal tibial torsion or metatarsus adductus. Heredity is also believed to play a role in the development of rotational problems. Sometimes parents have the same rotational deformity as their children. In addition, **bony and neuromuscular abnormalities** are part of the etiology of clubfoot.

Specific terminology is used to describe the position

of the limb. **Version** is normal variation in limb rotation, whereas **torsion** refers to abnormal conditions (i.e., > 2 standard deviations above or below the mean). **Adduction** is movement toward the midline, in contrast to **abduction,** which is movement away from the midline. **Varus angulation** is deviation toward the midline, whereas **valgus angulation** is deviation away from the midline. An **inverted** foot is one turned toward the midline on its long axis. An **everted** foot is one turned away from the midline on its long axis.

Medial rotation of the lower extremity (internal) brings the big toe to the midline during the early intrauterine period, whereas lateral (external) rotation occurs during the later intrauterine period, infancy, and childhood. Alterations in this normal lateral process caused by either genetic or environmental factors (e.g., intrauterine molding, sleep positions) may lead to rotational problems. Conditions influenced by intrauterine position, such as metatarsus adductus and developmental hip dysplasia, are sometimes found in the same children.

The primary pathology of congenital clubfoot is related to deformity and hypoplasia of the bones of the foot, especially the talus and tarsal bones, and environmental factors such as intrauterine position and molding. In addition, hypoplasia of the calf muscles and thickening of the ligaments contribute to the deformity.

DIFFERENTIAL DIAGNOSIS

In-toeing and out-toeing may be classified according to anatomic level and usual age at presentation (Table 72–1). These conditions may be localized to one of four areas: toe, foot, tibia, and femur. If in-toeing problems are placed in chronological order by age of presentation, the affected area follows a toe-to-femur sequence (see Table 72–1).

IN-TOEING

Searching Toe

Children with a so-called searching toe have a big toe that points medially when they walk. Unlike the other causes of in-toeing, which are structural and present at rest, this condition is a dynamic deformity. Searching

FIGURE 72–1. *Congenital clubfoot.*

toe results from the contraction of the abductors of the big toe during the stance phase of gait, which pulls the toe toward the midline.

Clubfoot

Congenital **clubfoot,** a pathologic deformity of the foot, may be identified at birth (Fig. 72–1). Clubfoot may be either an isolated deformity or seen in association with other neuromuscular anomalies such as arthrogryposis, myelomeningocele, amniotic band syndrome, cerebral palsy, or poliomyelitis.

The diagnosis of congenital clubfoot is made at birth on the basis of three conditions: forefoot varus, heel varus, and ankle equinus. Clubfoot can range in severity from a rigid deformity, in which the forefoot cannot be brought into a neutral position by passive abduction, to nonrigid deformities, in which the forefoot can be gently brought toward the midline.

Metatarsus Adductus and Metatarsus Varus

These terms, which are often used synonymously to describe an incurving foot, are actually two distinct conditions. **Metatarsus adductus** is a functional deformity in which the forefoot is adducted with respect to the hindfoot. The forefoot can be brought into the neutral position either by stroking the lateral border of the foot or by gently straightening it.

Congenital **metatarsus varus** is a bony abnormality characterized by subluxation of the tarsometatarsal joint with adduction of the metatarsals. The forefoot is inverted and adducted with respect to the hindfoot. Metatarsus varus is a fixed deformity, unlike metatarsus adductus. The foot cannot be bought into the neutral position. The prominence of the base of the fifth metatarsal, the convexity of the lateral border of the foot, and a deep crease along the plantar surface of the tarsometatarsal joints are evident on examination. Normal dorsiflexion of the ankle helps distinguish severe forms of metatarsus varus from clubfoot.

TABLE 72–1.   Site and Age of Onset of Rotational Problems of the Lower Extremity in Children

Problem	Site of Problem	Age of Onset
In-toeing		
Searching toe	Toe	Infancy
Clubfoot	Foot	Birth
Metatarsus adductus/varus	Foot	Birth/infancy
Medial tibial torsion	Tibia	Toddler stage (12–24 months)
Medial femoral torsion	Femur	Early childhood (3–5 years)
Out-toeing		
Physiologic out-toeing	Hips	Infancy
Lateral tibial torsion	Tibia	Childhood

Medial Tibial Torsion

This condition is usually first noticed by parents when children begin to walk. Medial tibial torsion is often bilateral:when it is unilateral, it more commonly affects the left leg. Observation of children's gaits reveals that the knees point forward but the feet turn inward. Because the knees are straight, the site of the rotational deformity is below this joint. If the feet are normal and no metatarsus adductus or varus is present, the rotational deformity can be isolated to the lower leg.

Medial Femoral Torsion

This condition can be conceptualized in the following way: When children lie on their backs, the torsion causes the femoral head to protrude instead of lie flat within the acetabulum. The presence of medial femoral torsion causes the entire distal limb to turn inward when the femoral head articulates normally with the acetabulum. The condition is usually bilateral.

Children who are 3 to 4 years of age present with this classic story: Their parents report that children, who showed no previous in-toeing, have a problem that is becoming severe. Excessive medial femoral torsion, which may have been present at birth, has been masked by the external rotatory forces present during infancy. Thus, the condition is clinically appreciated only as these forces resolve.

OUT-TOEING

Physiologic Out-toeing

Out-toeing of infancy, which is most commonly seen in children who are just learning to walk, is caused by an external rotatory contracture of the soft tissues

FIGURE 72–2. *Physiologic out-toeing of infancy.* *(Reproduced, with permission, from Staheli, L.T. Torsional deformity. Pediatr. Clin. North Am. 24:799–811, 1977.)*

Questions: In-toeing and Out-toeing

- Is there any family history of in-toeing or out-toeing?
- What is the birth history? Was the child a breech presentation?
- At what age did the child begin walking?
- When did the rotational deformity appear? Is it getting better or worse?
- Does the rotational problem produce any disability (e.g., tripping or falling a great deal when walking or running)?
- Has any previous treatment been tried?
- In what position does the child sleep? In what position does the child sit?

surrounding the hip seconday to intrauterine position. This condition may be perpetuated in children who sleep in the prone, frog-leg position, which does not allow for stretching of the external rotators of the hips. Although both feet turn outward when infants stand, the lateral rotation of both hips is normal on examination (Fig. 72–2).

Lateral Tibial Torsion

This condition may be suspected in children who are 3 to 5 years of age and present with out-toeing that worsens with time. Because the tibia normally rotates laterally with development, the condition may become more severe with age. Malalignment between the knee and the direction of gait may produce knee pain.

EVALUATION

History

A family history of any rotational problems should be noted. The age at onset and severity of symptoms in the patient should also be obtained. A thorough developmental history is important, because developmental delays may be a sign of underlying neuromuscular or neurologic disorders (Questions Box).

Physical Examination

A careful, detailed physical examination, including assessment of gait and neurologic and musculoskeletal function, is essential for making the correct diagnosis. This evaluation should include examination of the hips for signs of hip dysplasia, which may be associated with metatarsus adductus (see Chapter 71, Developmental Hip Dysplasia). A rotational profile consisting of four components should be assessed (Fig. 72–3). A negative value indicates in-toeing in these measurements.

The foot progression angle is estimated by watching a child walk (Fig. 72–4). The normal range of the foot progression angle may vary, but more than five degrees of in-toeing at any age is considered abnormal. Normal adults walk with their feet externally rotated slightly (approximately 5 degrees). The tibia rotates laterally with growth. In infancy, it is internally rotated and becomes externally rotated at about age 3 to 5 years. The thigh-foot angle can range between −30 to 30 degrees during infancy and 0 to 30 degrees (average is 10 degrees) during most of childhood. Internal

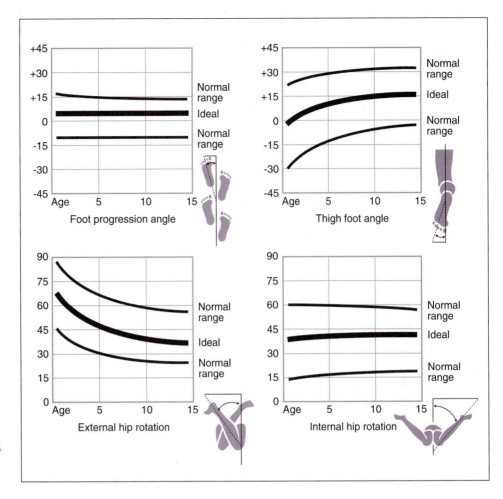

FIGURE 72–3. Rotational profile. *(Reproduced, with permission, from Wenger, D.R., and M. Rang. The Art and Practice of Children's Orthopedics. New York, Raven Press, 1993.)*

rotation of the hip is normally less than 60 to 70 degrees. It is greatest during early childhood and gradually declines after this time.

The examination of infants with clubfoot should include a careful examination of the back for signs of possible spinal dysraphism (e.g., skin dimples and hairy patches) and a thorough neurologic examination.

Medial tibial torsion may be diagnosed by having children sit at the end of the examination table with both knees flexed to 90 degrees and palpating the medial and

FIGURE 72–4. Evaluation of foot progression angle. *(Reproduced, with permission, from Staheli, L.T. Fundamentals of Pediatric Orthopedics. New York, Raven Press, 1992. pp. 4.6–4.7.)*

FIGURE 72–5. *Evaluation of the thigh-foot axis.* A. Observation with the child in the prone position is best. B. Determination of the thigh foot axis. C. Assessment of the shape of the foot. (Reproduced, with permission, from Staheli, L.T. Fundamentals of Pediatric Orthopedics. New York, Raven Press, 1992. pp. 4.6–4.7)

lateral malleoli with the thumb and index finger. Normally, the medial malleolus lies anterior to the lateral malleolus (approximately one fingerbreadth). If the lateral malleolus is on the same plane or anterior to the medial malleolus, internal tibial torsion is indicated.

The diagnosis of tibial torsion can also be made by measuring the thigh-foot angle (Fig. 72–5). Measurement of the thigh-foot angle involves having children lie prone on the examination table and observing the relationship of the long axis of the foot compared to the axis of the thigh as viewed from above. The shape of the foot itself can also be assessed with children

in this position. Slight internal rotation is normal as children first learn to walk.

Diagnosis of medial femoral torsion can be made by observing children's gaits and measuring hip rotation. The knees and the feet appear to turn inward when children with medial femoral torsion walk. Internal and external hip rotation are evaluated with the children in a prone position, the pelvis flat, and the knees flexed 90 degrees (Fig. 72–6). The degrees of normal rotation vary with age (see Fig. 72–3). During childhood, internal hip rotation greater than 70 degrees implies medial femoral torsion.

FIGURE 72–6. *Evaluation of hip rotation.* A. The child is prone and knees are flexed to 90°. B. Medial rotation is measured. C. Lateral rotation is measured. (Reproduced, with permission, from Staheli, L.T. Fundamentals of Pediatric Orthopedics. New York, Raven Press, 1992. pp. 4.6–4.7.)

Laboratory Tests

Such tests are generally not required in the assessment of rotational problems.

Imaging Studies

Routine imaging studies are not necessary for rotational deformities. Imaging studies may be considered by the orthopedic surgeon in severe deformities if operative correction is being considered. X-rays are used in clubfoot to assess the relationship and development of the bones of the foot and for monitoring cast correction.

MANAGEMENT

IN-TOEING

Metatarsus adductus generally resolves spontaneously, but stretching exercises for the foot can be ordered, particularly if parents are anxious to "do something." Parents are advised to manipulate the foot with each diaper change. Referral to an orthopedic surgeon for evaluation should be made if the deformity is still present at 3 to 4 months of age (the majority of cases resolve within the first 3 months of life). Cast correction may be required for rigid deformities or those that persist beyond 3 to 4 months. Shoe modifications (e.g., putting shoes on the wrong foot) should be avoided because they have not been shown to have any long-term benefits.

Because metatarsus varus may progress when children begin walking, referral to an orthopedic surgeon should be made as soon as the condition is detected. Serial casting followed by corrective shoes or inserts is the first line of treatment. Surgery is only rarely required.

Treatment for medial tibial torsion is rarely required, because this problem generally corrects with time when children learn to walk. If the deformity is severe or persists without improvement beyond the age of 18 months or after children have been walking for one year, referral to an orthopedic surgeon for evaluation should be made. Surgical correction (e.g., tibial rotational osteotomy) may be required if the deformity is severe or persists beyond 8 to 10 years of age.

Like the other conditions that produce in-toeing, medial femoral torsion generally does not require treatment. Even if it persists into adulthood, it usually produces no disability nor does it increase the risk for degenerative arthritis in the involved joint. Nonoperative treatment is ineffective. Surgical correction may be required if there is a history of repeated falls or severe gait problems. A derotational femoral osteotomy is the only effective method of treatment. It should not be performed until children are at least 8 to 10 years of age.

Clubfoot, unlike other problems, is a pathologic lesion that requires treatment. Treatment, which should begin during the first week of life, consists of serial manipulations of the foot and casting. Several months of casting

may be required to attain full correction. Surgery is often required for resistant or recurrent cases. As many as 50 to 75% of patients with clubfoot may eventually require surgery. Surgery is usually delayed until infants are 6 to 12 months of age.

OUT-TOEING

Physiologic out-toeing of infancy is a rotational problem that spontaneously resolves when children learn to walk. Most cases resolve by about 18 months of age. Severe lateral tibial torsion may require surgical correction with a tibial rotational osteotomy.

PROGNOSIS

Because the lower extremity rotates laterally with growth, the natural history of internal rotational problems, such as internal tibial torsion and medial femoral torsion, is resolution over time. In contrast, lateral tibial torsion may become worse with time.

The prognosis for the vast majority of rotational problems is excellent. Parental reassurance and education regarding the natural history of these deformities may decrease anxiety and prevent needless visits to specialists in search of treatments that may not be necessary. Functional disability or degenerative arthritis is not associated with these conditions.

Left untreated, clubfoot often leads to considerable pain and disability. The affected foot can be difficult to fit with shoes. And finally, clubfoot can be unsightly and cause children significant emotional distress.

Case Resolution

The girl described in the case history appears to have medial femoral torsion, because she has no history of rotational problems. Her entire leg turns in when she walks. Internal hip rotation greater than 70 degrees confirms the diagnosis. The mother can be reassured that this is a normal, age-related phenomenon that will most likely resolve over time. The child can be reevaluated in four to six months. Orthopedic referral is not required at this time.

Selected Readings

Craig, C. L., and M. J. Goldberg. Foot and leg problems. Pediatr. Rev. 14:395–400, 1993.

Scoles, P. V. Lower extremity development. *In* Pediatric Orthopedics in Clinical Practice, 2nd ed. Chicago, Year Book Medical Publishers, 1988.

Staheli, L. T. Fundamentals of Pediatric Orthopedics. New York, Raven Press, 1992, pp. 4.1–4.24.

Staheli, L. T. The lower limb. *In* Morrissy, R. T. (ed.). Lovell and Winter's Pediatric Orthopedics, 3rd ed. Philadelphia, J. B. Lippincott, 1990, pp. 741–766.

Staheli, L. T. Lower positional deformity in infants and children: a review. J Pediatr. Orthop. 10:559–563, 1990

Wenger, D. R., and M. Rang. The Art and Practice of Children's Orthopedics. New York, Raven Press, 1993.

CHAPTER 73

ANGULAR DEFORMITIES OF THE LOWER EXTREMITY: BOW LEGS AND KNOCK KNEES

Geeta Grover, M.D.

H$_x$ During the routine health maintenance examination of a 2-year-old child, you observe moderate to severe bilateral bowing of both legs. The child's mother reports that her son began walking at ten months. She has noticed no problems with his gait and says he does not trip or fall excessively. On examination, the boy's weight is greater than the 95th percentile for age, but otherwise he appears to be a healthy African-American child.

Questions

1. What types of angular deformities affect children's lower extremities?
2. How does children's age help determine whether they have physiologic or pathologic angular deformities?
3. What clinical measurements can help distinguish physiologic from pathologic angular deformities?
4. To what extent are x-rays used in the routine assessment of angular deformities?

With normal growth and development, the angular alignment of children's legs progresses through a series of developmental stages—from relative bow legs to knock knees and eventually straight legs. Rotational problems such as in-toeing and out-toeing are deformities in the transverse plane that occur when a bone rotates either internally or externally along its long axis (Fig. 73–1). Angular deformities such as bow legs and knock knees are deformities in the frontal plane. The legs distal to the knees are angled or tilted toward the midline in bow-leg deformity, whereas they are tilted away from the midline of the body in knock-knee deformity (Fig. 73–2). Variations in the knee angle that fall outside the normal range (e.g., more than plus-or-minus two standard deviations of the mean) are referred to as genu varum for bow legs and genu valgum for knock knees (D$_x$ Box). Appreciation of the normal developmental sequence in conjunction with a careful history and physical examination can help pediatricians identify pathologic cases of bow legs and knock knees and initiate prompt treatment.

EPIDEMIOLOGY

Bow legs and knock knees are common in infants and children. Knock knees occur less frequently than bow legs. Knock knees are seen more often in females and are commonly associated with generalized ligamentous laxity. Pathologic cases of bow legs and knock knees are uncommon.

CLINICAL PRESENTATION

Children with **bow legs** have a characteristic wide-based stance with increased distance between the knees. They may walk with a waddling gait. In-toeing may be noted as a result of associated internal tibial torsion. When the distance between the knees (intercondylar distance) is more than 10 cm when children are laying supine with their hips and knees in extension and their medial malleoli just touching, they require evaluation for pathologic bow legs.

Severe **knock knees** may produce an awkward gait with the knees rubbing. Children may walk with both feet apart in an effort to avoid knee-to-knee contact. They may need to place one knee behind the other to stand with both feet together. When the distance between the ankles (intermalleolar distance) is more than 10 cm when children are laying supine with their hips and knees in extension and their knees just touching, they warrant evaluation for pathologic knock knees.

PATHOPHYSIOLOGY

The normal variation in the angular alignment of the lower extremities changes with age. During the first two years of life, relative bowing of the legs is common. Although physiologic bowing of the lower leg may be appreciated at birth, it is most prominent during the second year of life when it most commonly involves both the tibia and the femur. When associated with internal tibial torsion, the deformity may appear more striking. Physiologic knock knees develop between three and four years of age. The knock-knee stage resolves somewhere between 5 and 7 years of age, when normal adult alignment develops. A slight knock-knee appearance remains in normal adults. Bow legs or knock knees that develop ouside of this sequence require further evaluation for pathologic causes.

The **tibiofemoral angle,** the angle between the long axis of the femur and the long axis of the tibia, is used to assess the angular alignment of the leg. At birth the tibiofemoral angle is approximately 15 degrees varus, and it decreases to 0 between the ages of 18 and 24 months. By 3 to 4 years, the angle peaks at about 10 degrees of valgus angulation. Then between 5 and 7

FIGURE 73–1. *Select body reference and rotational planes.* Rotational problems are deformities in the transverse plane. Angular deformities are in the frontal plane.

FIGURE 73–2. *Varus and valgus deformities of the lower extremities.*
A. *Bow-leg deformity.*
B. *Knock-knee deformity.*

years it decreases to the normal range of about seven to nine degrees in girls and four to six degrees in boys (Fig. 73–3).

DIFFERENTIAL DIAGNOSIS

The most common causes of genu varum and genu valgum are presented in Table 73–1. Physiologic bow legs and knock knees are usually bilateral, and they occur in a sequence that follows the normal developmental pattern. Lateral bowing of the tibia is commonly noted during the first year of life. Bow legs (involving both the femur and the tibia) are pronounced during the second year, and knock knees become prominent

Dx	**Pathologic Bow Legs and Knock Knees**

- Asymmetric deformity
- Inconsistency with the normal sequence of angular development
- Stature less than the fifth percentile for age
- Severe deformity (> 10 cm intermalleolar or intercondylar distance)
- History of rapid progression
- Presence of other musculoskeletal abnormalities

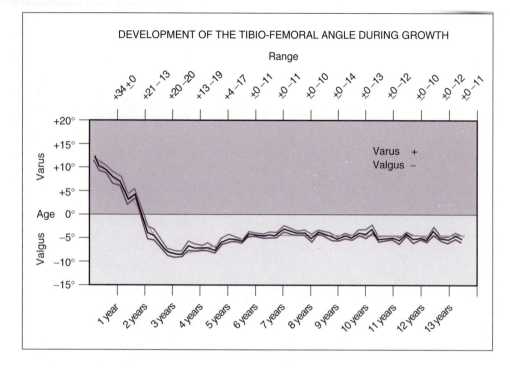

DEVELOPMENT OF THE TIBIO-FEMORAL ANGLE DURING GROWTH

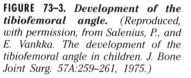

FIGURE 73–3. *Development of the tibiofemoral angle.* (Reproduced, with permission, from Salenius, P., and E. Vankka. The development of the tibiofemoral angle in children. J. Bone Joint Surg. 57A:259–261, 1975.)

between 3 and 4 years of age. This is the normal sequence of angular development. Most cases of bow legs are the result of normal physiologic processes, Blount's disease (tibia vara), and rickets. Common causes of pathologic knock knees are severe renal rickets and "old" fractures of the proximal tibia.

Blount's disease, a growth disturbance involving the posterior-medial aspect of the proximal tibia (physis, epiphysis, and metaphysis), is the most frequent cause of pathologic bow legs. Both infantile and juvenile forms of the disease are more common in African Americans. The infantile form affects children 1 to 3 years of age. Usually bilateral, it is associated with internal tibial torsion. The etiology is believed to involve mechanical stress on the growth plate, thus converting physiologic bow legs to pathologic varus. Affected children are often

obese and early walkers, which puts early stress on the growth plate. Blount's disease produces a sharp angulation at the proximal tibia, whereas physiologic bow legs lead to a gradual curvature of the legs involving both the femur and the tibia. Six stages of x-ray progression based on the degree of epiphyseal depression and metaphyseal fragmentation at the proximal tibia have been identified (Langenskiöld staging). It may be difficult to distinguish between early stages of Blount's disease and physiologic bow legs.

The less common, juvenile form of Blount's disease occurs in older children and adolescents. Knee pain, rather than deformity, is the most common presenting sign. Usually unilateral, it is more common in males than females. Affected children are generally obese and have a normal height. Although the etiology is unclear, it is believed that in predisposed obese adolescents, the decreased growth of the medial tibial physis is due to the repetitive trauma of excessive weight bearing.

Rickets, a disease of the growing skeleton, produces inadequate mineralization of the bone. The disorder is due to a disturbance in calcium and phosphorus metabolism. Rickets takes several forms, including vitamin D-deficient, or nutritional, rickets; vitamin D-resistant, or hereditary, rickets (the most common form); and severe renal osteodystrophy. Signs of rickets include short stature, poor muscle tone, joint pain, and angular deformities of the lower extremities. The alignment at the time of onset of disease determines the direction of angulation. For example, vitamin D-deficient or vitamin D-resistant rickets generally has an early onset and is more often associated with bow legs. Renal osteodystrophy, which usually has a later onset, results in a valgus deformity.

Pathologic processes, including trauma (fractures), infections, and tumors, involving the proximal tibia are additional potential causes of both bow legs and knock

---

TABLE 73–1. Common Causes of Genu Varum and Genu Valgum

Genu Varum

Physiologic bow legs
Rickets (vitamin D deficiency [nutritional] or vitamin D resistance [hereditary])
Blount's disease (tibia vara)
Achondroplasia
Metaphyseal dysplasia
Trauma, infection, or tumor of the proximal tibia (resulting in malunion or partial physeal arrest)
Excessive prenatal fluoride ingestion

Genu Valgum

Physiologic knock knees
Rickets (renal osteodystrophy)
Trauma, infection, or tumor of the distal femur or proximal tibia (resulting in malunion or partial physeal arrest)
Paralytic conditions (e.g., myelodysplasia, polio, cerebral palsy) leading to contracture of the iliotibial band
Osteogenesis imperfecta
Rheumatoid arthritis of the knee

knees. Overgrowth or malunion following fractures of the proximal tibial metaphysis most commonly results in genu valgum rather than genu varum.

EVALUATION

History

A family history, a description of the deformity and its progression, and an assessment of the child's growth and nutritional history (Questions Box) should be obtained from the parents or caregivers.

Physical Examination

Physical examination begins with a general screening of children's nutritional growth and developmental status. Children's growth parameters (height, weight, head circumference) should be measured and plotted on standard growth curves. The rotational status of the lower limb should be assessed, because internal tibial torsion is often associated with bow leg deformity (see Chapter 72, Rotational Problems of the Lower Extremity). Children should be observed both standing and ambulating to determine the alignment of the legs. The intercondylar and intermalleolar distances can be measured with the child supine to determine the presence of excessive bow legs or knock knees (see Clinical Presentation).

Laboratory Tests

Most children with physiologic angulation do not require any laboratory studies. A general metabolic screening, including hemoglobin, calcium, phosphorus, creatinine, and alkaline phosphatase, may be ordered if a systemic or metabolic abnormality is suspected.

Imaging Studies

X-rays are usually performed in the evaluation of bow legs or knock knees if pathology is suspected. If obtained, x-rays should include the entire leg so that the alignment of the femur and tibia may be assessed. Children should be standing, and a single radiograph of both legs should be taken, if possible. Pathologic

conditions such as rickets (osteoporosis, metaphyseal fraying, cortical thinning, widening of the growth plates), Blount's disease (beaking of the medial metaphysis of the femur and tibia), various bone dysplasias, and forms of dwarfism can usually be ruled out by x-rays. An increased uptake of the proximal medial aspect of the tibia on bone scan may help differentiate early infantile Blount's disease from extreme physiologic bow legs.

MANAGEMENT

Angular deformities within normal developmental limits should be managed with continual observation and reassessment. The severity of the deformity should be documented, and children should be followed at three- to six-month intervals until the condition resolves. Physicians should **reassure parents** that bow legs and knock knees are normal developmental variations that will correct spontaneously with time. Special diets, braces or shoe wedges, arch supports, and bars are generally best avoided; they have not been shown to affect the normal developmental sequence.

Children with physiologic varus may be followed clinically until 18 months to 2 years of age. Pathology should be suspected if correction has not begun by this time or if the lesion is progressive. Children with more than 10 degrees of valgus (or an intermalleolar distance > 10 cm) after eight to nine years of age may require further evaluation. Children with suspected cases of pathologic bow legs and knock knees require **referral to an orthopedist** for evaluation.

Treatment for children with Blount's disease may consist of **bracing** if the deformity is mild and identified early. **Surgery** may be necessary if the deformity is severe. Medical management, such as administration of vitamin D for nutritional rickets, is of primary importance in the treatment of the various forms of rickets. Surgical correction, such as osteotomies to correct varus or valgus deformities, should be reserved until medical management has been maximized, because even severe deformities may resolve with conservative management.

PROGNOSIS

Physiologic bow legs and knock knees spontaneously resolve without further sequelae. Although knock knees are primarily a cosmetic problem, degenerative arthritis may rarely be a late complication. Surgical correction may be required for adolescents with severe deformity to prevent such late complications.

Questions: Pathologic Bow Legs and Knock Knees

- When was the deformity first noticed?
- Has it changed? If so, how fast?
- Has the problem been treated in any way?
- Has the child had any recent illness or trauma in the affected leg?
- Does anyone else in the family have a similar problem?
- Aside from this condition, is the child growing and developing normally?
- Does the child eat a well-balanced diet?
- Does the child have any chronic medical problems such as kidney disease?

Case Resolution

The boy described in the case history should be evaluated for pathologic causes of genu varum, especially Blount's disease, for the following reasons: (1) his age is at the upper limit of normal for bow legs and his deformity is severe, (2) he is African American, (3) he has a history of early walking, and (4) he is obese. A standing x-ray of the lower extremities should be obtained, and the boy should be referred to an orthopedist for further evaluation and management.

Selected Readings

Henderson, R. C. Tibia vara: a complication of adolescent obesity. J. Pediatr. 121:482–486, 1992.

Kling, T. F. Angular deformities of the lower limbs in children. Orthop. Clin. North Am. 18:513–527, 1987.

McDade, W. Bow legs and knock knees. Pediatr. Clin. North Am. 24: 825–839, 1977.

Scoles, P. V. Lower extremity development. *In* Pediatric Orthopedics in Clinical Practice, 2nd ed. Chicago, Year Book Medical Publishers, 1988, pp. 82–121.

Staheli, L. T. Fundamentals of Pediatric Orthopedics. New York, Raven Press, 1992, pp. 4.19–4.24.

Wilkins, K. E. Bowlegs. Pediatr. Clin. North Am. 33:1429–1438, 1986.

CHAPTER 74

ORTHOPEDIC INJURIES AND GROWING PAINS

Geeta Grover, M.D.

H$_x$ A six-year-old boy has a one-week history of leg pains. He wakes up at night and cries because his legs hurt, yet during the day he is fine, with no pain or movement limitations. He has no history of trauma, fever, or joint swelling. The family history is negative for rheumatic or collagen-vascular disease. The boy's height and weight are at the 50th percentile for age, he is afebrile, and the physical examination is unremarkable.

Questions

1. What is the differential diagnosis of leg pains in school-age children?
2. What laboratory or radiographic studies are appropriate for children with leg pains?
3. How do musculoskeletal injuries in children differ from those in adults (e.g., the type of injury sustained, the location of the injury, the effect of age on injury, etc.)?

Children by nature are active and explorative. They experience cuts, scrapes, minor injuries, and pain routinely. Because primary care physicians are often the first to examine children with injuries, they play an important role in making the preliminary diagnosis and assessment regarding the need for further evaluation and treatment. The more common complaints and injuries seen in the pediatrician's office are discussed in this chapter: growing pains; nursemaid's elbow; and fractures, including growth plate injuries. The evaluation of children with limp is discussed in Chapter 76.

EPIDEMIOLOGY

The term **"growing pains"** is somewhat misleading, because there is no evidence that these pains are associated with growth. The period of middle childhood, when growing pains are diagnosed, is not the period of most rapid growth in the child. "Leg aches" or "idiopathic leg pain" may be better terms.

Growing pains occur in 15 to 30% of all children. They are seen most commonly in children between the ages of 3 and 12 years; the reported age range is infancy to 19 years. Girls are affected more frequently than boys.

Nursemaid's elbow or pulled elbow (subluxation of the radial head) is one of the most common ligamentous injuries seen in children. This condition occurs most often in children one to four years of age, with a peak incidence between the ages of two and three years.

Other ligament and tendon injuries are relatively uncommon in children due to the relative strength of these structures as compared to the growth plate of the developing bone. Type I fractures of the growth plate (discussed below) occur before ligamentous injury. When joint dislocations and ligamentous injury occur in children, they are usually secondary to significant trauma.

Trauma and injury, including child abuse or inflicted injury, are significant causes of morbidity and mortality in children. Injuries account for approximately 10 to 15% of all hospitalizations in children between 1 and 14 years of age and are the leading cause of death in children and adolescents beyond the first year of life. **Fractures,** which account for about 15% of all pediatric injuries, are perhaps the most common significant form of muscu-

Orthopedic Injuries and Growing Pains

GROWING PAINS
- Age between 3 and 12 years
- Normal growth and development
- Intermittent pain or aches in the legs
- Occurrence of symptoms at night
- Pain poorly localized to the anterior thighs, calves, and behind the knees; absence of joint involvement
- Absence of limp, disability, or inflammation
- Response to supportive measures such as heat and massage

NURSEMAID'S ELBOW
- Age between 1 and 4 years
- Elbow pain of acute onset
- History of sudden longitudinal traction on an extended and pronated arm
- Forearm held in a position of flexion and pronation
- Lack of spontaneous movement of the elbow

FRACTURES
- Obvious deformity
- Swelling or tenderness over the fracture site
- Limited range of movement or absence of movement of the affected extremity

loskeletal injury in children who present to physicians for evaluation and treatment.

CLINICAL PRESENTATION (D_x BOX)

Children with **growing pains** present with a history of intermittent night pain in the legs that awakens them from sleep. A feeling of restlessness is sometimes associated with the pain, which most commonly involves the front of the thighs, the calves, and the area behind the knees—never the joints. The pain is usually of short duration and typically bilateral, and it usually resolves after several minutes, with children going back to sleep. Pain may often occur at other sites, such as the abdomen and head. Pain is gone by morning, and children have normal activity during the day.

Nursemaid's elbow is characterized by a sudden onset of elbow pain and a reluctance to use the arm. Children usually cry briefly initially and then are fine except for inability to use the affected arm. Typically, children hold the injured arm close to the body in a position of flexion and pronation.

An underlying **fracture** is strongly indicated by obvious deformity or lack of spontaneous movement in the extremity in question. Localized swelling, tenderness, and limited range of movement may all be signs of a fracture.

PATHOPHYSIOLOGY

Growing pains are recurrent aches or pains localized to the muscles of the legs. The pain is located deep within the extremity and not in the joints. The etiology is unclear. Rapid growth, emotional and psychological stress, and myalgias secondary to excessive exercise have been implicated.

Nursemaid's elbow is a subluxation of the radial head caused by rapid extension and pronation of the arm. Typically, the injury occurs when parents suddenly pull children toward themselves, and children resist and want to go in the other direction (Fig. 74–1).

Because of anatomic and physiologic differences (e.g., presence of cartilaginous growth plate as well as thicker periosteum and greater plasticity of the skeleton), **fracture** patterns seen in children often differ from those in adults. Fractures may be more difficult to detect in children and may influence long-term growth and development of affected limbs.

Fractures are classified based on anatomic location, type of fracture, and degree of angulation or displacement. Fracture location may be described as diaphyseal,

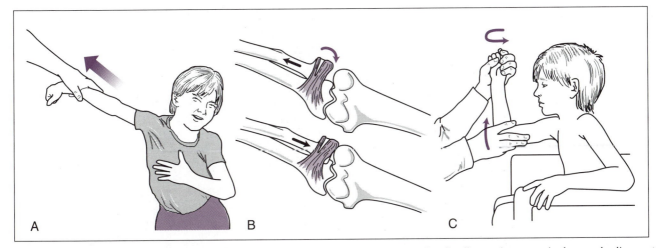

FIGURE 74–1. *Nursemaid's elbow.* The sudden traction on the outstretched arm pulls the radius distally, causing a tear in the annular ligament at its attachment to the radius. A portion of the ligament becomes trapped within the joint as the traction is released and the arm recoils. A. Mechanism of injury. B. Pathology. C. Method of reduction.

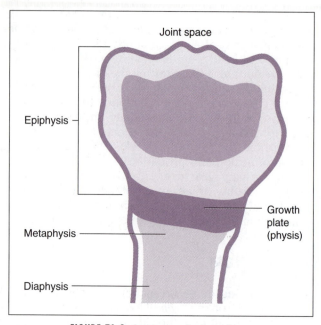

FIGURE 74–2. *Anatomy of a long bone.*

metaphyseal, or epiphyseal/growth plate depending on the portion of the bone involved (Figs. 74–2 and 74–3). Fractures may be either open or closed. In closed fractures, the skin over the fracture site is intact, whereas in open fractures, the skin is broken. Fractures in which the two bone fragments are displaced relative to each other are described as angulated or displaced; the direction and degree of displacement are based on the distal fragment.

The Salter-Harris classification is used most commonly to classify growth plate injury (Table 74–1, Fig. 74–4). Approximately 15% of all fractures in children involve the growth plate. Type I and type II are the most common fractures involving the growth plate. Type III

and IV fractures are intra-articular. Type V fractures are uncommon and are due to a crush injury to the growth plate. Initial x-rays in type I and type V fractures may appear normal, because bone fragments are not displaced. The likelihood of growth arrest associated with this type of injury is high.

DIFFERENTIAL DIAGNOSIS

The diagnosis of **growing pains** is one of exclusion. Leg pain in children has many causes (Table 74–2). If they are limited to vague pains in the legs at night with no associated limp or signs of inflammation, the differential diagnosis may be limited to growing pains, general systemic diseases such as leukemia, benign bone tumors such as osteoid osteoma, and perhaps fibromyalgia. Leukemic infiltration of the bones may cause leg pain before systemic signs such as fever, weight loss, and adenopathy are present. Osteoid osteoma, a benign bone tumor that most commonly occurs in adolescent boys, characteristically causes pain that is worse at night and is usually relieved by anti-inflammatory medications. The pain may be localized in one place, however, unlike with growing pains. Fibromyalgia, which is probably underdiagnosed in the pediatric population, is a well-recognized cause of chronic, generalized limb pain in adults without a clear, organic source. It is seen more commonly in adolescents than younger children. This benign, intermittent musculoskeletal pain syndrome is associated with multiple tender "trigger points," stiffness, fatigue, and a nonrestorative sleep pattern.

When evaluating for **nursemaid's elbow,** an elbow fracture should be ruled out.

Certain **fractures** and specific features of fractures deserve mention (see Fig. 74–3). Fractures that often occur during childhood include clavicular fractures and oblique fractures of the distal tibia, or the toddler's

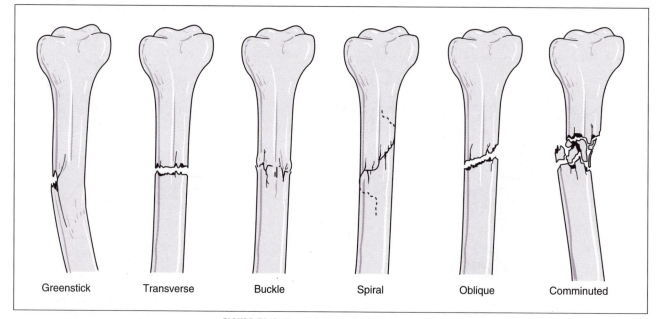

| Greenstick | Transverse | Buckle | Spiral | Oblique | Comminuted |

FIGURE 74–3. *Nonepiphyseal plate fractures.*

TABLE 74–1. Fracture Patterns Seen in Children

Nonepiphyseal Plate Fractures

Type	Description
Complete	Both sides of the bone fractured; type depends on direction of fracture line
Transverse	Perpendicular to long axis of the bone
Oblique	At an angle to long axis of the bone
Spiral	Zig-zag course around the bone
Comminuted	Fractures with three or more fragments (rare in children)
Buckle or torus	Bone compression causes it to bend or buckle rather than breaking
Greenstick	Cortex broken on tension side but intact on compression side
Bowing	Deformation of bone due to bending without fracturing

Epiphyseal Plate Fractures (Salter-Harris Classification)

Type	Description
Type I	Horizontal fracture through the physis
Type II	Fracture through the physis, extending into the metaphysis
Type III	Fracture through the epiphysis, extending into the physis
Type IV	Fracture through the epiphysis, physis, and metaphysis
Type V	Crush injury of the physis

fracture. This is seen most commonly in early walking children with unsteady gaits. Elbow fractures require careful attention to neurovascular status because of the risk of associated brachial artery injury, leading to Volkmann's ischemic contracture. A Monteggia fracture is a dislocation of the radial head in association with an ulnar shaft fracture. Spiral fractures of long bones, especially the femur, multiple rib fractures, and multiple fractures in various stages of healing are highly suggestive of child abuse (see Chapter 96, Physical Abuse).

Because of the relative weakness of the physis compared to the surrounding ligaments, trauma sus-

tained near joints may be more likely to cause a type I Salter-Harris growth plate fracture rather than ligamentous injury (e.g., sprain or strain). Therefore, it is important to include this type of fracture in the differential diagnosis of children with point tenderness near the end of a long bone, because this injury does require cast immobilization.

EVALUATION

Accurate diagnosis of pediatric orthopedic injuries is often challenging, because children may be not only poor "historians" but also uncooperative with examinations, especially in acute or emergency situations.

History

A thorough history is essential for the accurate diagnosis of growing pains and orthopedic injuries (Questions: Growing Pains; and Questions: Orthopedic Injuries). A complete history of the events related to the injury, including what happened after the injury was sustained, should be obtained.

Physical Examination

The physical examination of children with suspected **growing pains** should include evaluation for signs of systemic disease such as fever, abnormal growth, and generalized weakness or fatigue. Leg length and circumference should be measured. The legs should be palpated and joint range of motion assessed.

Children with suspected **nursemaid's elbow** should be observed for how they hold the affected arm compared to the unaffected arm. They should be evaluated for limited active motion at the elbow and resistance to attempts at passive movement, especially

FIGURE 74–4. *Salter-Harris classification of epiphyseal plate fractures.*

TABLE 74–2. Common Causes of Leg Pain in Children

Growing Pains
Trauma
Fracture
Compartment syndromes
Soft tissue injury
Muscle strain/sprain
Infection
Cellulitis
Soft tissue abscess
Myositis
Osteomyelitis
Septic arthritis
Neoplasia
Malignant bone tumors (e.g., osteogenic sarcoma, Ewing's sarcoma)
Leukemia
Metastatic disease (e.g., lymphoma, neuroblastoma)
Benign Bone Tumors
Osteoid osteoma
Bone cysts
Histiocytosis X
Collagen-Vascular Disease
Juvenile rheumatoid arthritis
Dermatomyositis
Fibromyalgia
Rheumatic fever
Other Musculoskeletal Causes
Legg-Calvé-Perthes disease
Slipped capital femoral epiphysis
Osgood-Schlatter disease
Transient synovitis of the hip
Osteochondritis dissecans
Patellofemoral stress/chondromalacia patellae
Generalized ligamentous laxity and joint hypermobility
Miscellaneous Causes
Sickle-cell disease pain crisis
Psychosomatic conditions

Questions: Orthopedic Injuries

- What led to the injury?
- How long ago was the injury sustained? When did the symptoms begin?
- Was the incident witnessed by an adult?
- How strong was the injuring force? What direction did it come from?
- What was the position of the affected extremity at the time of the injury?
- Did the child experience any loss of consciousness?
- What, if any, first aid was administered at the scene?
- Has the child been able to move the affected extremity since the injury occurred?

---

jury includes evaluation of capillary refill, peripheral pulses, and motor and sensory function.

Laboratory Tests

A CBC and ESR may be considered for children with growing pains that do not resolve. Rheumatologic screening tests can be ordered based on abnormalities in these tests (e.g., elevated ESR or WBC count). Routine laboratory studies are not necessary in the evaluation of nursemaid's elbow or fractures. However, because fractures of the femur are often associated with significant blood loss, it is important to monitor the hematocrit in these patients.

Imaging Studies

If growing pains persist and interfere with routine activity, x-rays or bone scans of the legs may be considered. Radiographic evaluation is not required for children with nursemaid's elbow if presentation is typical and reduction is successful. X-rays, if taken in such children, are usually completely negative because the dislocation is often corrected during positioning for x-rays. However, x-rays should be obtained in children with suspected fractures. Fractures involving the growth plate, especially type I and V Salter-Harris fractures, may be particularly difficult to diagnose radiographically because the growth plate is primarily cartilaginous and hence radiolucent. A bone scan may be used to diagnose suspected fractures when x-rays are negative.

MANAGEMENT

Parental education and reassurance regarding the benign nature of **growing pains** are important. The pains themselves usually respond to **supportive measures** such as heat, massage, and analgesia. Stretching exercises for the legs have also been recommended. Referral to an orthopedist should be considered if the pain is severe and persistent and physical examination and laboratory workup fail to reveal a specific diagnosis.

Nursemaid's elbow is one of the few medical conditions that has a dramatic, immediate cure. Rapid, firm **supination and flexion** of the arm with application of pressure over the radial head usually releases the

supination. No swelling or tenderness to palpation should be present.

It is important to undress children with suspected **fractures** and perform a complete physical examination. Simply examining the involved extremity is insufficient. The presence of a deformity, point tenderness, or limitation of motion supports the diagnosis of a fracture. All long bones should be palpated, and the presence of bruises and scars should be noted, because these may indicate child abuse. The examination of the involved extremity includes inspection of the overlying skin for swelling, lacerations, or punctures. The degree of active and passive motion and strength compared to the uninvolved side should be noted. In cases of suspected leg injuries, the child's gait should be observed, if possible. Assessment of neurovascular function distal to the in-

---

Questions: Growing Pains

- When (i.e., what time of day?) does the pain typically occur?
- Does the pain resolve and then recur in any predictable manner?
- Where is the pain? Does it change location?
- Does anything make the pain better or worse?
- Is the child sick in any other way?
- Does the pain interfere with the child's activities?

trapped tissues from the joint and allows for **reduction** of the radial head. A click may be heard or felt as the radial head is reduced. Relief of pain is usually immediate for children treated shortly after injury; return of function may require 15 to 30 minutes, however. If treatment is delayed, such rapid relief of pain and return of mobility may not be seen.

Following reduction, **immobilization of the arm** in a sling or splint permits healing of the soft tissues.

Most **fractures** should be referred to an orthopedic surgeon for evaluation and treatment unless the primary care physician is experienced in reducing and casting fractures. Several techniques are used in fracture management. **Closed reduction** is the nonoperative reduction or realignment of fracture fragments. Surgical reduction involves **open reduction** and **internal fixation** with pins to maintain reduction and provide stability. Indications for open reduction include failure of closed reduction; requirement for precise anatomic reduction; intra-articular fractures; Salter-Harris Type III or IV growth plate fractures; and complex, multisystem trauma or multiple fractures.

Certain fractures are common in pediatrics. Most clavicular fractures do not require reduction and can be treated with immobilization in a sling for four to eight weeks. Elbow fractures (e.g., lateral condyle and supracondylar humeral fractures) are serious and often necessitate open reduction to achieve anatomic reduction. Distal forearm fractures are usually managed with closed reduction and casting. Midforearm fractures may require open reduction, especially in adolescents. Stable metacarpal and phalangeal fractures can be either splinted in an aluminum splint or be taped to an adjacent finger ("buddy taping"). The metacarpophalangeal joints should be maintained in 50 to 90 degrees of flexion, and the interphalangeal joints should be in about 20 degrees of flexion to minimize stiffness. Unstable finger fractures may require open reduction and pin fixation.

Femoral shaft fractures in infants and children can be managed with either traction and spica cast immobilization or cast immobilization alone. Open reduction and intramedullary rod fixation can be used in adolescents. Closed reduction and cast immobilization are usually used in the management of tibial shaft fractures. Short-cast immobilization may be required for metatarsal fractures, and "buddy taping" is used for stable toe fractures.

Because of the potential for infection, open fractures are orthopedic emergencies that require immediate attention. Careful debridement of the wound is required. External pin fixation may be used to stabilize the fracture because the wound is usually left open. Antibiotics should be administered, and tetanus immunization may be given based on a review of the immunization history.

PROGNOSIS

Growing pains resolve over time without sequelae. Recurrence of nursemaid's elbow is common. Therefore, parents should be cautioned regarding pulling children's arms or lifting them by one hand.

Fractures in children generally heal and remodel (the spontaneous correction of deformity) better and faster than equivalent fractures in adults. Vascular and nerve injuries and growth disturbances are potential complications of fractures and their management. Growth plate injuries require special attention because of the potential for growth abnormalities. Compartment syndrome, a potentially serious vascular injury, may develop.

Prognosis of growth plate fractures depends on the type of injury sustained. Salter-Harris type I and II fractures generally have a good prognosis for long-term healing and growth. The severity of the injury and the accuracy of reduction determine the prognosis of type III and IV fractures; there is also a risk of future degenerative arthritis or growth disturbance. Growth arrest is common following type V fractures because the physis itself is injured.

Case Resolution

The child presented in the opening scenario has the benign condition commonly referred to as growing pains. Management involves parental education and reassurance.

Selected Readings

Conrad, E. U., and M. C. Rang. Fractures and sprains. Pediatr. Clin. North Am. 33: 1523–1539, 1986.

Grogan, D. P., and J. A. Ogden. Knee and ankle injuries in children. Pediatr. Rev. 13:429–434, 1992.

Jackman, K. V. Acute pediatric orthopedic conditions. Pediatr. Ann. 23:240–249, 1994.

Peterson, H. Growing pains. Pediatr. Clin. North Am. 33:1365–1371, 1986.

Rang, M. Other feet. In Wenger, D. R., and M. Rang. The Art and Practice of Children's Orthopedics. Raven Press, New York, 1993.

Scoles, P. V. Musculoskeletal trauma. In Pediatric Orthopedics in Clinical Practice, 2nd ed. Chicago, Year Book Medical Publishers, 1988, pp. 23–81.

Staheli, L. T. Fundamentals of Pediatric Orthopedics. New York, Raven Press, 1992, pp. 11.1–11.20.

Ward, W. T., H. W. Davis, and E. N. Hanley. Orthopedics: subluxation of the radial head. In Zitelli, B. J., and H. W. Davis. Atlas of Pediatric Physical Diagnosis, 2nd ed. Philadelphia, J. B. Lippincott, 1992.

CHAPTER 75

SPORTS-RELATED INJURIES

Monica Sifuentes, M.D.

Hx A 15-year-old male basketball player complains of six months of intermittent pain in his left knee. Occasionally the knee gives out while he is playing ball. The boy denies any associated swelling or erythema over the joint. He is able to walk with no problem and reports no history of direct trauma to the area. He is otherwise healthy.

Upon physical examination, he is a well-developed, well-nourished teenage male in no acute distress. The examination is normal except for mild pain to direct palpation of the left patella. No swelling or erythema of the joint is evident, and the left hip, knee, and ankle have full range of motion. The back is straight.

Questions

1. What is the purpose of the preparticipation sports physical examination?
2. What conditions disqualify adolescents from participation in competitive sports?
3. What are some of the most common orthopedic complaints in adolescent patients, and why do they occur in adolescents?
4. What is the pathophysiology of overuse syndromes?
5. What are the current recommendations for the treatment and rehabilitation of acute soft tissue injuries?

Many adolescents with varying degrees of athletic ability participate in sports during their junior high and high school years. Some choose to continue this participation on the college level. Regardless of the ultimate goal, team sports are an important means by which children and adolescents can experience both winning and losing. Individuals learn the importance of group participation and develop interactive skills with other team members. They are exposed to the concept of physical fitness, which can improve body image as well as self-esteem.

Participation in athletics carries significant risks, however. Accidental injuries, inappropriate coaching, and aggressive training sessions are not uncommon occurrences that have long-term sequelae for young athletes. Primary care practitioners are responsible not only for the evaluation of children prior to their participation in sports but also for diagnosis, treatment, and prevention of injuries if they occur.

EPIDEMIOLOGY

Estimates indicate that as many as seven million adolescents per year participate in organized sports activities in the United States. Several studies have attempted to quantify the overall injury rate associated with athletic participation. In general, the rate of injury for 13–19-year-olds is 7 to 11%. Approximately 20% of those injured sustain a significant injury. The sport with the highest injury rate in all age groups for boys is football, followed by basketball and soccer. Gymnastics leads to the most injuries in girls. Gender differences between boys and girls have been found in some studies depending on the sport. Overall, boys tend to have more shoulder-related injuries, whereas girls tend to have more knee and ankle injuries and more problems with overuse syndromes. Reports also indicate that girls tend to have more injuries requiring surgical correction.

PREPARTICIPATION SPORTS PHYSICAL EXAMINATION

The goal of the preparticipation physical examination (PPE) is the identification of any physical conditions or abnormalities that may predispose young athletes to injury. Examples include a history of syncope with exercise or an incompletely healed sprain.

The PPE consists of two parts: (1) a review of the patient's current health, past medical history, including sports injuries, and pertinent family history pertaining to participation in strenuous activities; and (2) a complete physical examination with a focus on the musculoskeletal system. Known as a "two-minute orthopedic examination," the musculoskeletal examination is a detailed assessment of all muscle groups, assessing their strength, tone, and function. Congenital or acquired deformities are also noted. The AAP has developed a form specifically for the PPE visit (see Chapter 7, Screening in Adolescents).

Disqualification from participation in specific sports is appropriate in certain situations. Competitive sports are classified according to their degree of contact or impact and how strenuous they are. Recommendations differ depending on the adolescent's medical condition and the type of sport the athlete desires to play. For details of these recommendations, the reader is referred to the AAP manual *Sports Medicine: Health Care for Young Athletes*. Fortunately, many young athletes are healthy and rarely need to be restricted from participation.

CLINICAL PRESENTATION

Older children and adolescents with sports-related injuries usually present to the practitioner with specific complaints of pain or swelling in a particular joint (Dx Box). In addition, they may complain of nonspecific musculoskeletal pain occurring in certain areas such as the lower back or shoulder. Other complaints may include a limp, decreased range of motion of an extremity, or an inability to participate in a desired activity.

PATHOPHYSIOLOGY

Adolescents, unlike adults, are particularly susceptible to injury because their bones and joints are developing. Most injuries during adolescence involve the epiphysis, which is the weakest point of the musculoskeletal system. In addition, the presence of congenital anomalies puts the young athlete at risk for injury.

Most orthopedic injuries are the result of either macrotrauma or microtrauma. Sprains are an example of macrotrauma, whereas overuse syndromes can be considered microtrauma. **Macrotrauma** occurs from complete or partial tearing of muscle, ligaments, or tendons, and is often associated with acute injuries. In contrast, **microtrauma** is usually produced by chronic repetitive trauma to a particular area, leading to inflammation and ultimately to pain. This most commonly occurs in soft tissues such as the muscle and tendon but can occur in the bone as well.

Definitions

A **sprain** is a stretching injury of a ligament or the connective tissue that attaches bone to bone. A **strain** is a stretching injury of a muscle or its tendon, which is the connective tissue that attaches muscle to bone. **Tendinitis** is an inflammation of the tendon. **Apophysitis** is an inflammation of the apophysis, which is the site of ligament or tendon attachment to growth cartilage (e.g., Osgood-Schlatter disease [apophysitis of the tibial tubercle], Sever's disease [calcaneal apophysitis]). A **stress fracture** is an incomplete fracture often occurring in the bones of the legs and feet from repetitive trauma to the area. It is believed that the pain associated with shin splints may be due in part to atypical stress fractures of the distal tibia.

Overuse syndromes occur from repetitive microtrauma to the musculoskeletal system secondary to excessive or biomechanically incorrect activity. They are usually the result of training errors in which athletes are "trying to do too much too fast." Common syndromes in adolescents include Osgood-Schlatter disease, shin splints, and patellofemoral syndrome (chondromalacia patellae).

Grading of Sports Injuries

Sprains can be classified according to the degree of injury and most commonly occur in the knee or ankle. Assigning a grade that describes the injury is useful when considering the prognosis of a particular injury. Consultants also find these grades helpful. Grade I through III is the usual classification used for sprains. Stability of the joint, range of motion, and degree of pain and swelling determine the grade of the sprain. The grading system for strains, on the other hand, is based on an assessment of strength. Because strains do not usually cause joint instability, criteria for grading strains are different than for sprains and may be more subjective. A general description of these two grading systems appears in Table 75–1.

DIFFERENTIAL DIAGNOSIS

The differential diagnosis of orthopedic conditions depends on the anatomic site of the injury or complaint and the mechanism of injury. Table 75–2 lists some of the more common orthopedic conditions by location. Anomalies of skeletal development such as congenital angular deformities of long bones and soft tissue abnormalities like Ehlers-Danlos syndrome should also be considered as possible etiologies for overuse syndromes. Other nonorthopedic conditions such as collagen-vascular diseases and infections may also present with joint or bone symptomatology.

TABLE 75–1.   General Classification of Sprains and Strains

	Joint	Range of Motion	Weight Bearing	Pain	Swelling
Sprains					
Grade I	stable	normal	normal	+	+
Grade II	± stable	↓	↓	++	++
Grade III	unstable	↓↓	↓↓	+++	+++

	Strength	Palpable Defect	Pain
Strains			
Grade I	$> \frac{4}{5}$	−	+
Grade II	$3\text{-}\frac{4}{5}$	+/−	++
Grade III	$< \frac{3}{5}$	+/−	+++

TABLE 75–2.   Differential Diagnosis Based on the Site of Injury

Back Injuries
Muscle strain
Spondylolysis
Epiphyseal injury
Herniated disks

Injuries to the Upper Extremity
Acromioclavicular sprains
Sternoclavicular sprains
Glenohumeral dislocation
Glenohumeral subluxation
Impingement syndrome
Acute elbow injuries
    Olecranon bursitis
    Lateral epicondylitis
    Flexor-pronator tendinitis
Wrist sprains
Navicular fractures
Hamate fractures
Finger injuries

Injuries to the Lower Extremity
Iliac crest contusion
Iliac apophysitis
Quadriceps contusion
Femoral stress fracture
Medial lateral ligament sprains
Anterior cruciate ligament sprain
Posterior cruciate ligament sprain
Patellar dislocation/subluxation
Prepatellar bursitis
Patellofemoral stress syndrome
Patellar tendinitis
Osgood-Schlatter disease
Shin splint syndrome
Ankle sprains
Achilles tendinitis
Calcaneal apophysitis
Plantar fasciitis

EVALUATION

History

The history should focus on the musculoskeletal system and how the injury occurred (Questions Box).

Questions: Sports-Related Injuries

- What activity or sport was the patient engaged in at the time of the injury?
- How often has the patient engaged in this sport or particular activity in the past?
- Were there any new additions to the routine this time?
- Did the pain begin after a single injury or after repetitive activity?
    - If the injury is related to a repetitive activity, does the pain occur at a specific time during this activity?
    - Is the pain incapacitating?
    - Has a similar injury ever occurred in the past?
    - How was the injury treated?
        - Was there any pain following the previous injury?
        - Does the patient feel as if he or she has completely recovered?
    - How was this current injury managed acutely?
    - Has the patient altered daily activity in any way to compensate for this problem?

Physical Examination

The physical examination should focus on the musculoskeletal system. If, however, teenagers have not had a physical examination within the past year, a complete physical examination should first be performed to exclude any systemic condition that might manifest itself initially as bone or joint pain. This is especially important in adolescents with chronic complaints.

In general, any pain or swelling of the affected joint or muscle should be noted. If adolescents have a history of acute trauma, an area of ecchymosis may be seen. The affected joint should be tested for range of motion and joint laxity that would differentiate a grade I from a grade II or III sprain. Various maneuvers for testing ligamentous laxity at each joint can be used (Figure 75–1).

FIGURE 75–1. *Maneuvers used to determine stability of the knee joint. **A.** Anterior drawer test: Anterior force is applied. **B.** Posterior drawer test: Posterior force is applied. **C.** Medical ligament stability: Lateral force is applied.*

The most common method is the "drawer test" for anterior and posterior movement of the knee joint. Muscle spasms and diminished range of motion in an adjacent joint should also be noted, because this may indicate a strain injury. Strength of the "strained" muscle(s) and any pain on palpation or contraction of the muscle(s) should be assessed. A palpable defect of the muscle suggests complete rupture of the muscle, whereas muscular contusions are associated with localized pain or hematoma. Pinpoint tenderness over a particular bone may indicate a fracture or, if at the site of a tendon insertion, inflammation. Reviewing the mechanism of injury is often helpful in differentiating between a fracture and tendinitis.

Laboratory Tests

A CBC and ESR may be helpful in adolescents with a history of chronic joint pain or swelling. If the results are abnormal, they suggest a collagen-vascular disease such as lupus or an infection such as osteomyelitis.

Imaging Studies

A radiograph of the involved joint or bone is often the only necessary diagnostic procedure. Other radiographs of joints above and below the symptomatic area are sometimes useful. See Chapter 76, Evaluation of Limp, for a discussion on of slipped capital femoral epiphysis and imaging studies.

MANAGEMENT

With acute soft tissue injuries, the aim of management is to limit the extent of bleeding and inflammation that occur in the first 48 to 72 hours following the injury. The mnemonic **RICE** (**r**est, **i**ce, **c**ompression, **e**levation) is helpful. The use of this plan for soft tissue injuries facilitates early healing and allows rehabilitation to proceed quickly.

Anti-inflammatory or analgesic medications such as ibuprofen, aspirin, and naproxen are useful in controlling the symptoms of pain and swelling. For adolescent patients, dosages are similar to those used in adults: aspirin, 650–1000 mg every six hours; ibuprofen, 400–800 mg every six to eight hours; naproxen, 500 mg twice daily. To minimize GI side effects, the medication should be administered with a snack or milk. Ideally, these drugs should be used on an as-needed basis, but occasionally chronic therapy is indicated.

After this acute phase, therapy is aimed at resolution of any edema and hematoma and at rehabilitation (Table 75–3). Athletes should slowly begin range-of-motion exercises as tolerated. Full tissue healing may take six to eight weeks, but most young athletes do not have to wait that long to return to athletic activity.

Complete rest or modified activity, depending on the degree of tissue damage, should initially be recommended in athletes who have suffered from overuse

TABLE 75–3.   Principles of Rehabilitation

Resolution of hematoma
Resolution of edema
Regain full range of motion or flexibility
Regain full muscle strength and endurance
Regain agility and coordination
Regain cardiovascular endurance

syndromes. Participation in another sport such as swimming is often preferable to complete immobilization. In addition to the use of anti-inflammatory agents, physical therapy is another important therapeutic modality. Cryotherapy, whirlpool, or alternate heat and ice treatments can be helpful. Reconditioning should be attempted after 3 to 12 weeks of modified activity, depending on the degree of recovery. This entails gradual strengthening and flexibility training as well as a reevaluation of previous modes of training to minimize the risk of reinjury (see Table 75–3).

PROGNOSIS

Orthopedic injuries in young athletes and active adolescents have a great capacity for healing if given the opportunity. Early medical intervention to prevent irreversible tissue damage assures complete recovery in most cases. Long-term sequelae are associated with repeated trauma, incompletely treated cases, and chronic inflammatory changes. Some conditions, however, such as Osgood-Schlatter disease, will resolve even without treatment and do not lead to any permanent damage to the joint.

Case Resolution

In the case presented at the beginning of the chapter, the teenager has symptoms and physical findings consistent with patellofemoral pain syndrome (traditionally referred to as chondromalacia of the patella). Since radiographs are usually not helpful in confirming the diagnosis, none are necessary at this time. Management should include strength training for the quadriceps muscles, activity modification, nonsteroidal anti-inflammatory medication, and ice compresses after activity. Orthotics such as an elastic cartilage brace may also be considered.

Selected Readings

American Academy of Pediatrics. Sports Medicine: Health Care for Young Athletes, 2nd ed. Elk Grove Village, IL, American Academy of Pediatrics, 1991.

Dyment, P. G., (ed.). Sports and the adolescent. Adol. Med. State of the Art Rev. 2:1–250, 1991.

Group on Science and Technology, American Medical Association. Athletic preparticipation examination for adolescents: Report of the Board of Trustees. Arch. Pediatr. Adolesc. Med. 148:93–98, 1994.

Risser, W. L. Sports medicine. Pediatr. Rev. 14:424–431, 1993.

CHAPTER 76

EVALUATION OF LIMP

Geeta Grover, M.D.

Hₓ A 6-year-old boy who has a two-day history of right knee pain and limp is brought to the office. No history of knee trauma, swelling, redness, or associated fever is present. The past medical history is unremarkable. The boy is afebrile, and his height and weight are at the 10th percentile for age. Examination of the right leg reveals decreased abduction and internal rotation of the hip; the knee is normal. The boy limps when he walks and favors his right leg.

Questions

1. What is the differential diagnosis of painful and painless limps in children?
2. What is the differential diagnosis of knee pain in children?
3. What laboratory and radiographic tests are indicated in the evaluation of children with limp?
4. What is the appropriate management of children with suspected infectious causes of limp?

A limp is an abnormal gait that minimizes weight bearing on the affected leg to reduce pain and instability. Limp may be secondary to muscle weakness, deformity, or pain. Because limp can be a sign of significant underlying disease, accurate diagnosis and appropriate management are essential to prevent potentially serious morbidity, including long-term disability.

EPIDEMIOLOGY

Limp, which is not uncommonly seen in children, may be due to pain originating in the leg or referred pain from the abdomen or spine. Age influences the number of diagnostic possibilities, because certain disorders are seen more frequently in one age group than another. Although septic arthritis occurs in children of all ages, it is seen most often in children under three years of age and in sexually active adolescents. Transient synovitis, the most common cause of hip pain in young children, is seen mostly in children 3 to 6 years of age.

Noninfectious causes of limp are more common in school-age children and adolescents than in younger children. Legg-Calvé-Perthes disease (LCPD) is seen primarily in children four to eight years of age with a male-to-female ratio of 4–5:1. LCPD has been associated with a history of low birth weight, delayed bone age, and short stature. Bilateral involvement is seen in about 10% of cases. Slipped capital femoral epiphysis (SCFE), the most common hip disorder in adolescents, is seen most often in the 11–15-year age group, with a male-to-female

ratio of about 2:1. It is bilateral about 20 to 25% of the time and has been associated with obesity. Osgood-Schlatter disease is seen most commonly in physically active males between the ages of 10 and 15 years.

CLINICAL PRESENTATION (Dₓ BOX)

Painful limp usually has an acute onset. It may be associated with systemic signs such as fever or irritability, especially when the etiology is infectious. Toddlers may simply refuse to walk or walk with a slow cautious gait (e.g., characteristic of diskitis) when they are in pain rather than limp. Nonpainful limp often has an insidious onset and is commonly due to weakness (e.g., muscular dystrophy) or deformity (e.g., leg length discrepancy).

PATHOPHYSIOLOGY

An understanding of normal gait and its development is essential to the evaluation of limp. Normal gait has two phases: stance and swing. During the stance phase, either one or both feet are on the ground, whereas during the swing phase, one foot is not touching the ground as the limb is moved forward. Stance phase is shortened in limp to decrease the amount of time spent in weight bearing on the affected side or to minimize instability.

Normal adult gait is smooth and efficient, requiring the coordinated actions of the muscles of the legs and pelvis. Normal gait in children varies according to age and developmental maturity. Toddlers typically walk with a broad-based, tiptoe, "bouncing" gait with arms abducted for balance; they may initiate the stance phase with either toe or heel strike. By 2 years of age, children should initiate the stance phase consistently with heel strike. Children who are three to four years of age should exhibit normal adult gait with reciprocating arm swing the majority of the time (Fig. 76–1).

Several types of abnormal gaits are recognized. A shortened stance phase due to pain is characteristic of

---

Dₓ **Evaluation of Limp**

- Decreased range of motion of involved extremity
- Knee pain or hip pain
- Abnormal gait (e.g., antalgic, Trendelenburg, toe-to-heel)
- Systemic signs (e.g., fever, irritability)
- Abnormal laboratory results (e.g., leukocytosis, elevated ESR)

FIGURE 76–1. *Phases of gait in a 4-year-old child.*

an **antalgic gait.** Weakness of the hip abductors (gluteus medius) leads to a **Trendelenburg gait,** where the pelvis dips down during stance phase, producing a swaying type of gait. A tiptoe or **toe-to-heel gait** is normal in children for several months after they learn to walk. Persistence of such a gait beyond 2 years of age is abnormal and may result from either idiopathic heelcord contracture or contracture secondary to cerebral palsy.

DIFFERENTIAL DIAGNOSIS

The differential diagnosis of limp may be classified by age group and the presence of associated pain (Table 76–1).

Children Aged One to Three Years

Infection is the most common cause of painful limp in toddlers. **Septic arthritis** is a significant cause. *Staphylococcus aureus* is the most common etiologic organism in septic arthritis. Before the use of *Haemophilus influenzae* type b (Hib) vaccine became widespread, Hib was the most frequently occurring pathogen in children younger than 2 years of age. *Neisseria gonorrhoeae* is a common pathogen in sexually active adolescents. The hip is involved, most commonly, followed by the knee. Acute onset of pain in the involved joint, fever, limited range of motion of the joint, and an antalgic gait or posturing are common. Often, children appear fine as long as the affected joint is not moved or touched. Children may lie perfectly still in an effort to minimize the characteristically exquisite pain associated with joint motion. In addition, the infected hip is usually kept in a position of flexion, abduction, and external rotation in an effort to lessen intraarticular pressure and pain.

Septic arthritis must be differentiated from **osteomyelitis** (see Chapter 110, Osteomyelitis) and **transient**

TABLE 76–1.   Differential Diagnosis of Limp in Children

Children Ages 1–3 Years
Painful Limp

Septic arthritis/osteomyelitis
Transient synovitis
Intervertebral diskitis
Juvenile rheumatoid arthritis (JRA)
Neoplasia (leukemia, metastatic disease)
Trauma (toddler's fractures)
Child abuse

Painless Limp

Developmental hip dysplasia
Neuromuscular disease (cerebral palsy)
Leg length discrepancy

Children Ages 4–10 Years
Painful Limp

Septic arthritis/osteomyelitis
Transient synovitis
Trauma
Legg-Calvé-Perthes disease (LCPD) (acute phase)
Intervertebral diskitis
JRA
Sickle cell pain crisis
Neoplasia (leukemia, primary bone tumor, metastatic disease)

Painless Limp

LCPD (chronic phase)
Developmental hip dysplasia
Neuromuscular disease (cerebral palsy, muscular dystrophy)
Leg length discrepancy

Children and Adolescents Ages 11 Years and Older
Painful Limp

Trauma
Septic arthritis/osteomyelitis
Slipped capital femoral epiphysis (SCFE)
Osgood-Schlatter disease
JRA
Sickle cell pain crisis
Neoplasia (leukemia, primary bone tumor, metastatic disease)

Painless Limp

SCFE
Leg length discrepancy
Neuromuscular disease (cerebral palsy, muscular dystrophy)
Scoliosis

synovitis. In theory, the absence of joint-specific symptoms (e.g., joint swelling, tenderness, limited range of motion) and the presence of swelling and tenderness localized to the metaphysis of the involved bone distinguish septic arthritis from osteomyelitis. In practice, this differentiation is often difficult. The clinician must maintain a high index of suspicion of simultaneous occurrence of both conditions, especially in joints such as the hip, ankle, shoulder, and elbow, where the metaphysis is intra-articular.

Transient synovitis is a self-limited, unilateral inflammation of the hip joint. Unlike septic arthritis and osteomyelitis, which are both characterized by the acute onset of severe pain, high fever, and systemic signs, transient synovitis is usually associated with a history of low-grade fever, insidious onset of pain, and antalgic limp or refusal to walk. As in septic arthritis, the hip is maintained in a position of flexion, abduction, and external rotation to minimize pain.

Other significant causes of limp in young children are **intervertebral diskitis, juvenile rheumatoid arthritis (JRA)** (see Chapter 111), and **toddler's fracture.** Diskitis is a benign, self-limited inflammation of the disk, often resulting from infection with *S. aureus.* Low-grade fever, back pain, irritability, and refusal to sit, stand, or walk are often present, depending on age. Although JRA may affect any synovial joint, it commonly begins in the large joints, especially the knee. The occurrence of morning stiffness that gradually resolves as the day progresses, which is characteristic of JRA, may help differentiate it from the other causes of antalgic limp. Occult fractures, especially the toddler's fracture or fracture secondary to child abuse (see Chapter 96), should also be entertained in the differential diagnosis. Toddler's fracture is a fracture of the mid or distal tibia, which usually develops after a fall or jump with a twist. Toddlers are prone to such injuries because of their unsteady gait.

Painless limp in toddlers may be due to **developmental hip dysplasia** (see Chapter 71), **cerebral palsy** (see Chapter 20, Needs of Children With Physical and Sensory Handicaps), or **leg length discrepancy** (anisomelia). As a result of developmental hip dysplasia, children may have a Trendelenburg gait secondary to leg length discrepancy or to weakness of the hip abductors. Children with spastic cerebral palsy often walk on their toes because of increased tone or heelcord contractures. Functional or apparent leg length discrepancies may result from pelvic obliquity or spinal deformity. Children with true leg length inequality compensate by either walking on tiptoe on the shorter side or bending the knee on the longer side; in either case, their gait is abnormal.

Children Aged Four to Ten Years

The differential diagnosis of painful limp in children in this age group includes **septic arthritis, osteomyelitis, transient synovitis, intervertebral diskitis, JRA, trauma, sickle cell disease pain crisis** (see Chapter 57, Anemia), and **neoplastic diseases** (see Chapter 105, Cancer in Children).

In addition, **LCPD** (idiopathic juvenile avascular necrosis of the femoral head) is an important cause of limp (both painful and painless). The etiology of LCPD is unclear, but it may result from disruption in blood supply to the femoral head, leading to avascular necrosis. Pain localized to the hip, inner thigh, or knee is usually insidious. The pain is aggravated by movement (i.e., especially internal rotation and abduction) and relieved by rest. Not uncommonly, LCPD is present for months before the diagnosis is made. Pain is especially prominent during the first stage because of synovitis. Later in the disease, painless limp may be more common. In LCPD the hip is kept in a position of flexion and slight external rotation.

Children and Adolescents Aged 11 Years and Older

The differential diagnosis of painful limp in older children and adolescents includes **trauma, septic arthritis, osteomyelitis, JRA, sickle cell disease pain crisis,** and **neoplastic disease.** Transient synovitis may develop a few weeks after rubella vaccination, especially in adolescent females. The small joints of the hands are involved more often than larger joints such as the ankles and knees. Other significant causes of painful limp in children aged 11 years and older are **SCFE** and **Osgood-Schlatter disease.**

SCFE is a displacement or slipping of the femoral head from the neck of the femur through the open growth plate. Affected children usually present with a history of dull, aching pain in the hip or knee that increases with activity. The onset of pain is insidious more often than it is acute. Children with SCFE walk with a Trendelenburg gait. The hip is held in extension and external rotation, and internal rotation is decreased.

Osgood-Schlatter disease, or traction apophysitis of the tibial tubercle, is an overuse syndrome in which repetitive microtrauma causes partial avulsion of the patellar tendon at its insertion on the tibia. Children with this condition present with localized prominence, swelling, and tenderness over the tibial tubercle at the insertion of the patellar tendon.

EVALUATION

History

The history should focus on the time of onset of the limp, its chronicity, and the degree of disability it produces (Questions Box). Delayed motor development

---

Questions: Evaluation of Limp

- How old was the child when the limp developed?
- Was the onset acute or chronic?
- Is the limp constant or intermittent (i.e., is it worse in the morning or at the end of the day)?
- Does the limp affect the child's regular activities in any way? How?
- Is the limp painful? Where does it hurt? Is the pain in one place?
- Does the child exhibit any other symptoms associated with the limp?
- Has the child lost any developmental milestones?
- Is there any history of trauma?

may be a sign of neuromuscular disease such as cerebral palsy, whereas a history of loss of motor milestones may indicate muscular dystrophy or spinal cord tumor. It is important to remember that pelvic pain may be referred to the hip, and hip pain is often referred to the knee.

Physical Examination

Physical examination begins with observation for any overt deformities (e.g., leg length discrepancy, fracture, joint swelling). All joints should be palpated, and the presence of swelling, tenderness, erythema, or warmth should be noted. A thorough evaluation of the hips is essential in children with knee pain. The type of gait (e.g., antalgic, Trendelenburg) may be determined by observing children walk or run (if possible) up and down corridors.

Children should also be examined both standing and supine, if possible. Standing children can be assessed for pelvic obliquity and spinal deformities. Range of motion of the hips, knees, ankles, and feet can be checked in supine children; one side can be compared to the other. Deep tendon reflexes and muscle strength should be assessed, and leg length measurements should also be made (Fig. 76–2). Children should be supine for a true measurement of leg length from the anterosuperior iliac spine to the medial malleolus. A discrepancy of more than 2 cm is considered significant in adults. The significance of discrepancies can be confirmed by imaging studies.

Laboratory Tests

Laboratory procedures are usually necessary in children with acute onset of limp and may be helpful. CBC and ESR are useful markers of systemic disease or significant inflammation. A normal CBC and ESR may help distinguish transient synovitis from septic arthri-

Imaging Studies

X-rays are the most commonly required imaging study. If LCPD or SCFE is suspected, x-rays of the hips should include both anteroposterior and frog-leg views. Early in the course of LCPD, x-rays may either be negative, or show widening of the joint space. In later stages, radiographic findings include an increased density and decreased size of the femoral head (necrosis), patchy areas of radiolucency near the epiphysis (fragmentation), and flattening of the femoral head (reconstitution). In SCFE, x-rays show the epiphysis slipping posteriorly and inferiorly with respect to the neck of the femur (e.g., like ice cream falling off a cone). In Osgood-Schlatter disease, knee x-rays may show soft tissue swelling over the tibial tubercle and a thickening of the patellar tendon. In children with knee pain, hip x-rays should be taken in addition to knee x-rays. X-rays are usually normal in transient synovitis.

In addition, bone scans may be useful in the early stages of certain diseases (e.g., osteomyelitis or toddler's fracture), when x-rays are typically normal.

MANAGEMENT

Management depends on the specific clinical diagnosis. **Immobilization** and **supportive care** are the backbone of treatment in transient synovitis, diskitis, LCPD, and Osgood-Schlatter disease. Symptoms of transient synovitis usually resolve within 7 to 10 days with no further intervention. Diskitis is generally a self-limited disease. Symptoms usually resolve within four to six weeks with immobilization and supportive care. Antistaphylococcal **antibiotics** may be used if *S. aureus* is suspected. The goals of treatment in LCPD are to maintain full joint mobility and prevent deformity of the femoral head. Bed rest and immobilization decrease the pain associated with synovitis and help restore range of motion. **Traction** and **abduction casts** are used to contain the femoral head within the acetabulum in an effort to maintain its spherical shape. Osgood-Schlatter disease, a self-limited condition, usually resolves when the proximal tibial epiphysis fuses. Symptoms generally resolve over a period of months. Supportive treatment consists of restriction of activity, use of analgesia, and stretching of the quadriceps and hamstring muscles. A knee immobilizer splint may be used.

Surgical treatment is required for SCFE and may be necessary in the management of septic arthritis and osteomyelitis. SCFE requires immediate operative fixation to prevent further slipping of the epiphysis. In septic arthritis, incision and drainage of the affected joint relieve the intraarticular pressure. A culture of the aspirate may allow identification of the organism. Empiric treatment with an antistaphylococcal penicillin (e.g., oxacillin, nafcillin) should be initiated until Gram's stain or culture results are available. Typically, 14 to 21 days of antibiotic treatment is required. Like septic

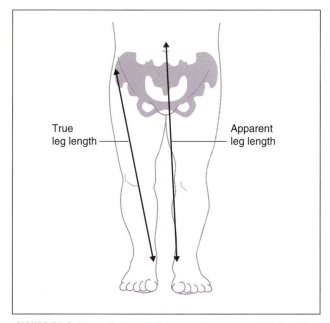

FIGURE 76–2. *Measurement of true and apparent leg lengths.*

True leg length

Apparent leg length

arthritis, osteomyelitis may also necessitate surgical decompression, followed by appropriate intravenous antibiotics (see Chapter 110, Osteomyelitis). Four to six weeks of treatment is usually required.

Management of leg length discrepancy depends on the predicted discrepancy at final adult height. Predicted differences less than 2 cm do not require treatment. Larger discrepancies may be managed either nonsurgically (e.g., heel lifts), especially when the predicted difference is less than 5 cm, or surgically. Surgical treatment may include leg lengthening procedures (e.g., Ilizarov method) of the shorter leg or shortening procedures (e.g., epiphysiodesis to produce growth arrest or osteotomy) of the longer leg.

If history, physical examination, laboratory tests, and imaging studies fail to reveal an abnormality, children should be reassessed weekly until a diagnosis is made or the limp resolves. If any uncertainty remains, **orthopedic consultation** should be promptly obtained, because missed or delayed diagnoses may result in long-term disability.

PROGNOSIS

Prognosis of LCPD is related to the degree of femoral head involvement and age at onset of the disease. Children less than 6 years of age have the best prognosis. The risk of development of degenerative arthritis in adulthood increases in children whose disease is more extensive and whose condition is diagnosed later (e.g., after 8 years of age).

If patients with SCFE are untreated, the potential for further slipping of the femoral head remains until the growth plate closes. Potential treatment-related complications of SCFE include chondrolysis of the femoral head and acetabulum, avascular necrosis, and fracture at the site of pin placement.

In about 5 to 10% of cases, Osgood-Schlatter disease may become chronic, with persistent swelling and tenderness. In such cases an x-ray may show the formation of an ossicle over the tibial tubercle; this ossicle may require surgical resection.

The prognosis is good in the majority of cases of septic arthritis and osteomyelitis if the infection is diagnosed early and treated appropriately.

Case Resolution

In the case described at the beginning of the chapter, the child's history and physical examination appear to be consistent with LCPD. The child's knee pain is actually secondary to hip pathology. The diagnosis may have been missed if the physician had not examined the hips and noted the abnormality in range of motion. Both anteroposterior and frog-leg x-rays of the hips were taken, which showed widening of the joint space. Orthopedic consultation was obtained, and hospitalization for bed rest and ensured immobilization was recommended.

Selected Readings

Henrickson, M., and M. H. Passo. Recognizing patterns in chronic limb pain. Contemp. Pediatr. 11:33–62, 1994.

Joffe, A. Limp. *In* R. A. Hoekelman, (ed.) Primary Pediatric Care, 2nd ed. St. Louis, Mosby-Year Book, 1992.

MacEwen, G. D., and R. Dehne. The limping child. Pediatr. Rev. 12:268–274, 1991.

Phillips, W. A. The child with a limp. Orthop. Clin. North Am. 18:489–501, 1987.

Sherry, D. D. Limb pain in childhood. Pediatr. Rev. 12:39–46, 1990.

Tunnessen, W. W. Limp. *In* Signs and Symptoms in Pediatrics, 2nd ed. Philadelphia, J. B. Lippincott, 1988.

C H A P T E R 7 7

DISORDERS OF THE SPINE

Geeta Grover, M. D.

Hₓ A 4-week-old male infant is brought to the office by his mother, who complains that her son always holds his head tilted to the right. She reports that he has held it in this position for about one week and prefers to look mainly to the left. The infant is the 8 lb, 8 oz product of a term gestation born via forceps extraction, and he had no complications in the neonatal period. He is feeding well on breast milk and has no history of fever, upper respiratory symptoms, or vomiting and diarrhea.

On examination, the head is tilted toward the right side with limited lateral rotation to the right and decreased lateral side bending to the left. Except for the presence of a small mass palpable on the right side of the neck, the examination is within normal limits.

Children with disorders of the spine can present with deformity, back pain, or occasionally both. Nontraumatic congenital and developmental deformities of the spine are frequently encountered in pediatric practice. Torticollis and scoliosis are two of the most common disorders in children that present as spinal deformity. **Torticollis,** or "wry neck," is a positional abnormality of the neck resulting in abnormal tilting and rotation of the head. **Scoliosis** refers to any lateral curvature of the spine. **Back pain** is a far less common complaint in children than in adults. When such pain occurs in children, it usually signals the presence of organic disease.

EPIDEMIOLOGY

Some degree of spinal asymmetry is seen in about 2 to 5% of the population.

The most common type of **torticollis** seen in children is congenital muscular torticollis. The incidence of this common neonatal orthopedic complaint is increased in breech presentations and difficult deliveries. It is associated with developmental dysplasia of the hip (DDH) in as many as 20% of affected infants. Family history may be positive in up to 10% of cases.

Acquired torticollis, usually secondary to infectious or traumatic causes, is much more common in older children. Episodes of benign paroxysmal torticollis, which often begin in the first year of life and generally resolve by five years of age, may have a familial basis. An association with benign paroxysmal vertigo and migraines has been noted.

The prevalence of **scoliosis** among school-age children is 3 to 5%. A right thoracic single curve is the most common curve seen by physicians. Seventy-five to 80% of cases of structural scoliosis are idiopathic, 10% are due to neuromuscular causes, 5% are congenital, and the remaining 5 to 10% are due to trauma or miscellaneous causes. Scoliosis that begins in childhood affects boys and girls equally, and affected boys actually outnumber girls during the first three years of life. Idiopathic scoliosis that develops after the age of 10 years is seen more frequently in girls than in boys, however. The ratio is approximately 5–7:1. In children with cerebral palsy, the incidence of scoliosis is increased and it is found in about 20% of all cases.

Back pain is quite uncommon in preadolescent children. In the majority of cases of back pain in children, it is possible to determine the etiology, unlike in adults, where it is often difficult to identify the cause.

FIGURE 77–1. *Torticollis.* *Infant with congenital muscular torticollis showing head tilt.*

CLINICAL PRESENTATION

Although **torticollis** may be noted at birth, it usually manifests at two to four weeks of age. Infants with congenital muscular torticollis present with a characteristic head tilt toward the affected side and the chin pointing toward the opposite side secondary to unilateral fibrosis and contracture of the sternocleidomastoid muscle (Fig. 77–1). Unrecognized or untreated cases of torticollis may present as plagiocephaly or facial asymmetry during infancy. Benign paroxysmal torticollis of infancy may present as recurrent episodes of head tilt that may be associated with vomiting, ataxia, agitation, or malaise (D_x Box).

No obvious deformity may be noted in mild **scoliosis.** Asymmetry of shoulder heights, scapular prominence or position, and waistline or pelvic levelness may all be

---

D_x Torticollis and Scoliosis

TORTICOLLIS
- Head tilt
- Limited range of motion of the neck
- Contracture of the sternocleidomastoid muscle
- Plagiocephaly (congenital torticollis)
- Firm, nontender, mobile mass within the body of the sternocleidomastoid muscle (congenital torticollis)

SCOLIOSIS
- Lateral curvature of the spine
- No pain
- Back or truncal asymmetry

signs of scoliosis (see D_x Box) (Fig 77–2A). Back pain is uncommon in adolescents with idiopathic scoliosis. When pain is present, further examination is warranted for some other cause (e.g., bone tumors, spondylolysis, spondylolisthesis).

Preverbal children with **back pain** may present with limp or refusal to bear weight or walk.

PATHOPHYSIOLOGY

Torticollis may be either congenital or acquired. The etiology of congenital muscular torticollis is unknown. It is believed to be due to intrauterine positioning or trauma to the soft tissues of the neck during delivery, with resulting ischemia of the sternocleidomastoid muscle secondary to venous occlusion. This leads to edema and degeneration of the muscle fibers with eventual fibrosis of the muscle body. Deformities of the face and skull may result if the condition is left untreated. Plagiocephaly (cranial asymmetry), with flattening of the face on the affected side and flattening of the occiput on the contralateral side, is seen most commonly.

Scoliosis is a lateral curvature of the spine, unlike kyphosis and lordosis, which are curves in the antero-posterior plane. Scoliosis can be either functional (nonstructural) or structural. Because no fixed deformity of the spine is associated with functional scoliosis, the apparent curvature disappears on lying down or forward flexion. Structural scoliosis may be idiopathic or caused by various underlying disorders. In structural scoliosis, as the spine curves laterally, it forces the vertebrae to rotate, resulting in deformity of attached structures. For example, a "rib hump" may be produced due to scoliosis in the thoracic spine (see Fig. 77–2B). Pelvic obliquity or flank prominence may be produced when the curvature is in the lumbar spine.

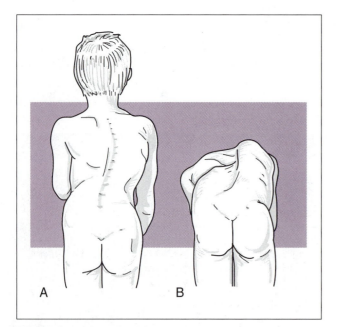

FIGURE 77–2. Scoliosis. A. *Child with scoliosis (rear view).* **B.** *Child with scoliosis performing bend test.*

TABLE 77–1.   Common Causes of Torticollis

Congenital
Congenital muscular torticollis
Pterygium coli (skin web)
Occipitocervical spine anomalies (e.g., Klippel-Feil syndrome)
Acquired
Infectious
   Cervical lymphadenitis
   Retropharyngeal abscess
   Osteomyelitis of cervical vertebrae
Traumatic
   Atlanto-occipital, atlas-axis (C1-C2), or C2-C3 subluxation
   Cervical musculature injury (spastic torticollis)
   Cervical spine fractures
Neurologic
   Tumors (posterior fossa or cervical cord)
   Dystonic drug reactions
   Syringomyelia
   Ocular disturbances (strabismus, nystagmus)
Other
   Sandifer's syndrome (hiatal hernia with gastroesophageal reflux)
   Benign paroxysmal torticollis of infancy
   Rheumatoid arthritis
   Hysteria
   Soft tissue tumors of the neck

DIFFERENTIAL DIAGNOSIS

The differential diagnosis of congenital and acquired **torticollis** is presented in Table 77–1. Congenital muscular torticollis is the most common cause of congenital torticollis. Acquired torticollis is seen primarily in older infants and children. Cervical lymphadenitis is a common cause in children one to five years of age, whereas trauma to the soft tissues or muscles of the neck is seen more frequently in school-age children. Acute episodes (e.g., benign paroxysmal torticollis of infancy) must be differentiated from chronic conditions (e.g., Sandifer's syndrome, rheumatoid arthritis).

Functional or nonstructural **scoliosis** may be secondary to poor posture, leg length discrepancies, or muscle spasm. Structural scoliosis can be classified into idiopathic, congenital, neuromuscular, and miscellaneous forms (Table 77–2). Idiopathic scoliosis, which is by far

TABLE 77–2.   Common Causes of Scoliosis

Functional Scoliosis
Poor posture
Leg length discrepancies
Muscle spasm
   Herniated disk
   Back injury
Structural Scoliosis
Idiopathic
Congenital
Neuromuscular
Miscellaneous
   Trauma (e.g., fractures or dislocations of the vertebrae)
   Intraspinal tumors
   Metabolic disorders (e.g., juvenile osteoporosis, osteogenesis imperfecta, muco-polysaccharidosis)
   Neurocutaneous syndromes (e.g., neurofibromatosis)
   Marfan's syndrome

TABLE 77–3. Common Causes of Back Pain in Children

Infectious
Myalgias (e.g., influenza)
Diskitis (more common in children < 5 years of age)
Vertebral osteomyelitis (pyogenic, tuberculosis [Pott's disease])
Referred pain (pyelonephritis, pneumonia)

Inflammatory
Rheumatologic diseases (juvenile rheumatoid arthritis, ankylosing spondylitis)
Crohn's disease/ulcerative colitis/psoriatic arthritis
Disk space calcification

Neoplastic
Primary vertebral and spinal tumors (e.g., Ewing's sarcoma, osteosarcoma, neuroblastoma)
Metastatic disease (e.g., neuroblastoma)
Benign tumors (e.g., eosinophilic granuloma, osteoid osteoma)

Developmental
Spondylolysis, spondylolisthesis (adolescents)
Scheuermann's syndrome (adolescents)

Traumatic
Herniated nucleus pulposus (disk herniation)
Ligamentous or muscle strain (e.g., overuse syndromes)
Compression fracture of vertebrae

Other
Sickle cell crisis
Osteoporosis (e.g., rickets, osteogenesis imperfecta)
Child abuse
Psychogenic

---

the most common type of structural scoliosis, may be divided into three categories based on age: infantile (0–3 years), juvenile (3–10 years), and adolescent (> 10 years). The adolescent form occurs most frequently.

Congenital scoliosis results from anomalies of the spine such as hemivertebrae or failure of vertebral segmentation. The incidence of cardiac and renal anomalies is increased. Although neuromuscular scoliosis is most often seen in children with spastic cerebral palsy, it may also be apparent in other conditions such as poliomyelitis, meningomyelocele, muscular dystrophy, Friedreich's ataxia, and spinal muscular atrophy.

The miscellaneous causes of scoliosis are uncommon and include trauma, metabolic disorders, and neurocutaneous diseases.

The most common causes of **back pain** in children may be classified into five categories (Table 77–3). Because the spine of children is smaller and has greater flexibility and ligamentous strength, children have a higher tolerance to trauma and injury than adults do. Infection (e.g., diskitis) and neoplasia are perhaps more common in children. Common causes of back pain in adults, such as herniated disks or musculoskeletal low back pain (usually secondary to muscle strain), are uncommon in children. Only about 2% of all herniated disks occur in children. Predisposed individuals often experience their first episode of musculoskeletal low back pain during adolescence or young adulthood.

EVALUATION

History

A careful history may provide clues to diagnosis and etiology (Questions: Torticollis; Questions: Scoliosis; and Questions: Back Pain).

Physical Examination

In children with suspected **torticollis,** a thorough examination with specific attention to the head and neck region should be performed. Limited head rotation toward the affected side with decreased lateral side bending to the opposite side may occur. During the first four to six weeks of life a firm, nontender mobile mass, which gradually regresses by six months of age, may be palpated within the body of the sternocleidomastoid muscle. The hips should be examined for stability because of the association of torticollis with DDH.

In addition, a neurologic examination should also be performed to look for any neurologic deficits that may be signs of an underlying tumor. Fever or signs of inflammation point to infectious causes. Because torticollis may be secondary to visual disturbances such as strabismus, a careful eye examination is warranted.

Questions: Torticollis

- Is there any family history of torticollis?
- What type of delivery did the mother have (e.g., cesarean or vaginal)? Were forceps required?
- When was the head tilt first noticed?
- Does the infant move his or her neck in all directions, or does he or she always prefer to look in one direction?
- Does the infant have any recent history of trauma to the head or neck area?
- Is the head tilt persistent or does it come and go?
- Has the infant been sick or febrile?

Questions: Scoliosis

- Is there a family history of scoliosis?
- Have the parents noticed the curvature of the spine? If so, how old was the child when the condition was first noted?
- Has the curvature increased since it was first noticed?
- Does the child have any back pain?
- Has the child had any previous treatment for the condition?
- (If appropriate) Has the child begun menstruating?

Questions: Back Pain

- How long has the child had the pain?
- Where is the pain localized?
- Is the pain persistent or does it come and go?
- Does the pain radiate anywhere (e.g., down the legs)?
- Is the child limping or having difficulty walking?
- Has the child lost any motor milestones (e.g., skills such as walking or standing that he or she could previously perform)?
- What makes the pain better? What makes it worse?
- Has there been any recent history of trauma or has the child begun participating in a new sport or physical activity?
- Has the child had a fever?
- Has the child had any problems with bowel or bladder function?
- Is the child taking any medication?

Screening for **scoliosis** should be part of the routine health maintenance examination of school-age children and adolescents. Children should be examined with the back fully exposed. The posture should be observed. The presence of any skin lesions such as café-au-lait spots should be noted. Any midline skin defects such as dimples or hair patches should also be noted, because they are often associated with underlying spinal lesions. The spine should be palpated for any signs of tenderness, and a complete neurologic examination should be performed.

The back should be observed for asymmetry of the shoulders, scapulae, or pelvis. Physicians should have children bend forward at the waist to an angle of 90 degrees. This maneuver accentuates the curvature of structural scoliosis and emphasizes the rotational deformity of the spine. For example, in thoracic scoliosis, a characteristic rib hump is apparent on the convex side of the curve.

Scoliosis is described in terms of the primary or major curve, which is predominantly thoracic. The major curve may be single or compensated by a secondary or minor curve, which is predominantly lumbar. The location is defined by the apical vertebra (e.g., T2–T11 = thoracic, T12–L1 = thoracolumbar), the direction of the curvature by the side of convexity, and the severity indicated by the degree of curvature as measured on the spinal radiograph. Curves greater than 15 degrees are abnormal. Mild scoliosis is defined as curvature of less than 20 degrees, moderate as 20 to 40 degrees, and severe as greater than 40 to 45 degrees.

The evaluation of **back pain** begins with observation of children's posture and gait. Any midline skin lesions should be noted. A thorough general physical examination is important because referred pain (e.g., pyelonephritis, nephrolithiasis) may be causing the symptoms in the back. The spine should be palpated for any signs of tenderness. A complete neurologic examination should be performed, and any motor or sensory deficits should be noted. The motor examination should emphasize evaluation of the hips and the lower extremities, including range of motion and strength.

Laboratory Tests

In cases of **congenital torticollis,** laboratory studies are rarely necessary. In acquired torticollis, if any infection is suspected, a CBC and blood and local cultures may aid in the diagnosis.

No specific laboratory tests are required in the evaluation of idiopathic **scoliosis.** Specific laboratory studies may be performed in the evaluation of other forms of scoliosis as indicated by the history and physical examination (e.g., a urine metabolic screen for suspected metabolic disturbances).

Laboratory assessment for **back pain** depends on the history and physical examination. A CBC, blood culture, and ESR may be useful in the evaluation of suspected infectious etiologies. Rheumatologic studies such as a rheumatoid factor or human leukocyte antigen typing may help in the diagnosis of inflammatory conditions.

Imaging Studies

X-rays are generally not useful in children with suspected **torticollis** unless bony anomalies are suspected. MRI of the sternocleidomastoid muscle mass may be considered if an underlying condition (e.g., a branchial cleft cyst) is suspected.

Routine x-rays are not required in the evaluation of all children with mild scoliosis (i.e., minor degrees of curvature noted on physical examination). It may be best to obtain x-rays after orthopedic evaluation is complete. A standing anteroposterior spine x-ray is used to determine the location and direction of the curvature, measure the degree of asymmetry (Cobb's angle), and evaluate the vertebrae. Repeat x-rays of the spine are used to follow the progression of the curvature over time. Because the risk of curve progression before skeletal maturity is a primary concern, hand and wrist x-rays should be taken to assess bone age in prepubertal children with scoliosis.

As with scoliosis, routine x-rays are not indicated in all cases of **back pain.** Various radiologic studies may be ordered depending on the suspected diagnosis. X-rays may be useful in the evaluation of suspected vertebral abnormalities such as spondylolysis and spondylolisthesis. If diskitis is suspected, a bone scan may be more appropriate than x-rays. Similarly, a bone scan or MRI is useful in the evaluation of suspected vertebral tumors.

MANAGEMENT

Treatment of congenital muscular **torticollis** consists of **passive stretching exercises** of the neck. With the neck in a neutral position (i.e., not hyperextended), the head is bent to one side so that the ear on the side opposite to the contracted muscle is brought to the shoulder, or the chin is lowered to touch the shoulder on the affected side. In addition, **changing the placement of the crib** in relation to the nursery door and **repositioning toys and mobiles** in the crib stimulate children to look toward the side opposite the preferred gaze. Torticollis resolves spontaneously in most infants. When the deformity persists beyond the age of one to two years, **surgical release** of the contracted muscle may be indicated.

Management of acquired torticollis depends on etiology. The evaluation and treatment of many of these conditions can be complex and often require consultation with specialists in head and neck surgery, neurology, and orthopedic surgery.

Management of **scoliosis** involves **close follow-up** with careful repeat examinations and radiographic studies. An initial consultation with an orthopedic surgeon is generally advisable, even in minor degrees of curvature. The goal of follow-up is early detection of curvature with implementation of treatment to prevent or reduce curve progression. Children with curves less than 20 to 25 degrees should be monitored for progression. Curves between 25 and 45 degrees do not require bracing in skeletally mature individuals but should be braced (e.g., with Milwaukee brace) in growing children. The goal of **bracing** is not to correct any existing curvature but to prevent further curve progression.

Surgery (e.g., the Harrington rod or posterior spinal fusion) may be indicated for children with curves greater than 45 degrees. These curves have a high likelihood of progression regardless of the patient's age and skeletal maturity.

Although the management of **back pain** is diagnosis-dependent, **rest** and **immobilization** are principles of treatment that apply in many instances. In the management of diskitis, oral antistaphylococcal antibiotics may be necessary in addition to immobilization. If spondylolisthesis and spondylolysis do not respond to rest and immobilization, operative stabilization may be required. In adolescents with low back pain related to muscular injury, conservative treatment including bed rest, heat, and anti-inflammatory medications may be tried for one to two weeks followed by a gradual return to normal activity. It is not advisable to institute such treatment in younger children without pursuing a more extensive evaluation or consultation with an orthopedic surgeon, because the risk of serious disease is significant in this age group.

PROGNOSIS

Congenital muscular **torticollis** responds to conservative management in about 90% of infants. The asymmetry of the face and skull also corrects over time once the contracture of the sternocleidomastoid resolves.

The direction and location of the curvature in **scoliosis** do not change with age, but the degree of curvature may remain stable or progress. Factors associated with a high risk of curve progression include female sex, positive family history for scoliosis, younger age at diagnosis (especially before the adolescent growth spurt), and a larger curve at the time of diagnosis. In addition, a double curve is more likely to progress than a single curve, and a thoracic curve is more likely to progress than a lumbar curve. Left untreated, severe scoliosis can produce cardiopulmonary impairment or cosmetic deformity, which may lead to low self-esteem and poor body image.

The vast majority of cases (80–90%) of low **back pain** in adolescents and young adults resolve spontaneously in two to eight weeks. It is important for patients to learn how to prevent recurrence by improving posture, learning how to lift heavy objects appropriately, and instituting a program of exercises to help strengthen the abdominal and back muscles.

Case Resolution

The history of the infant presented in the opening case scenario is consistent with congenital muscular torticollis. Physical examination helps confirm the diagnosis. The hips should be evaluated thoroughly because of the association of congenital muscular torticollis with congenital hip dysplasia. A program consisting of neck stretching exercises and repositioning of interesting toys and objects in the infant's crib to the side opposite the preferred gaze should be instituted. The infant can be reevaluated in two to three weeks to monitor progress.

Selected Readings

Bunnell, W. P. Back pain in children. Orthop. Clin. North Am. 13: 587–604, 1982.

Bunnell, W. P. Spinal deformity. Pediatr. Clin. North Am. 33:1475–1487, 1986.

Cheng, J. C. Y., and A. W. Y. Au. Infantile torticollis: a review of 624 cases. J. Pediatr. Orthop. 14:802–808, 1994.

Dyment, P. G. Low back pain in adolescents. Pediatr. Ann. 20:170–178, 1991.

Hensinger, R. N. Orthopedic problems of the shoulder and neck. Pediatr. Clin. North Am. 33:1495–1509, 1986.

Kim, G. R. Back pain. *In* R. A. Hoekelman, (ed.). Primary Pediatric Care, 2nd ed. St. Louis, Mosby-Year Book, 1992.

Lonstein, J. E. Natural history and school screening for scoliosis. Orthop. Clin. North Am. 19:227–237, 1988.

Ward, W. T., H. W. Davis, and E. N. Hanley. Orthopedics. *In* Zitelli, B. J., and H. W. Davis (eds.). Atlas of Pediatric Physical Diagnosis, 2nd ed. Philadelphia, J. B. Lippincott, 1992.

GASTROINTESTINAL DISORDERS

VOMITING

Carol D. Berkowitz, M.D.

Hx A six-week-old male infant who has been vomiting after each meal for three days is brought to the office. He is breast-fed, afebrile, and otherwise well. The history of the pregnancy and birth are normal. His birth weight was 3500 grams, and his current weight is 4500 grams.

The physical examination is unremarkable. The mother nurses the infant in the office. Although he feeds hungrily and well, he vomits about five minutes after the feeding. The vomiting is projectile, and the vomitus shoots across the room. The vomitus contains curdled milk. On reexamination of the abdomen, a small mass is felt in the right upper quadrant.

Questions

1. What is the mechanism of vomiting, and how is it different from regurgitation and rumination?
2. What are the common causes of vomiting in infants?
3. What are the common causes of vomiting in older children?
4. What are the unique features of vomiting related to increased ICP?
5. What are some strategies for the management of vomiting in older children?

Vomiting is a common complaint of infants and children, and led Thomas Phaire to write "Many times the stomake of ye child is so feble that it cannot retayne eyther meate or drynke" (The Boke of Chyldren, 1553). **Vomiting** is defined as the forceful ejection of the stomach contents through the mouth. The mechanism involves a series of complex, neurologically coordinated events under the control of the CNS. Projectile vomiting is a distinct condition in which central control does not play a role. Instead, an obstruction blocks the egress of food from the stomach. As a result of this blockage (most commonly seen with pyloric stenosis), reverse peristalsis and ejection of food occur.

In contrast, **regurgitation** is the effortless bringing up of one or two mouthfuls of food without distress or discomfort. This is a frequent symptom of gastroesophageal reflux (GER) (see Chapter 79). **Rumination,** a form

of autostimulation, is the voluntary induction of regurgitation. It is most often noted in infants between the ages of three and six months of age. Rumination occurs in infants with developmental retardation or with a disturbed mother-infant relationship. It is said that affected infants always smell like vomitus, which is on the clothing, but that the vomiting is rarely seen because the presence of another person provides distraction.

Rumination should be considered in infants from deprived environments (e.g., neglectful homes). Cases of rumination have been described in premature infants who were maintained in a neonatal intensive care unit after they no longer needed vigilant care from the nursing staff. Incubators, which were cut off from the outside environment, contributed to the rumination. The condition resolved once the infants were held and nurtured.

EPIDEMIOLOGY

Fifty percent of infants have spitting up or vomiting as an isolated complaint, and fewer than 5% of these infants have significant underlying disease. Vomiting occurs less frequently in older children, who often experience acute, self-limited illnesses such as gastroenteritis.

CLINICAL PRESENTATION

Infants and children may present with vomiting as an isolated complaint or in association with other symptoms, including fever, anorexia, abdominal pain, or diarrhea (D$_x$ Box). When vomiting has persisted over a period of time, weight loss or FTT may occur. Neurologic symptoms, including headache and gait disturbances, may be noted in children with CNS problems.

PATHOPHYSIOLOGY

Vomiting is a reflex reaction that occurs in response to numerous stimuli. The final common pathway involves stasis of food in the stomach, which is related to the rate of gastric emptying. Anything that delays gastric emp-

Dx Vomiting

- Vomiting
- Nausea
- Abdominal pain
- Anorexia
- Diarrhea
- Headache
- Fever

tying may be associated with vomiting. Gastric empty-ing may be retarded by the presence of fat (e.g., a high-fat meal), swallowed mucus (e.g., maternal mucus after birth, nasal mucus with a URI), lax muscle tone, fever, infection, and malnutrition. Vomiting can be divided into three phases: nausea, retching, and emesis.

Nausea, the sensation of the need to vomit, is initiated by afferent fibers in the duodenum that detect stasis in the stomach. Nausea may also be triggered by vestibular or emotional stimuli. Associated autonomic symptoms include faintness, diaphoresis, sweating, pallor, and tachycardia. Anorexia is a key accompanying complaint. The afferent fibers relay the message to the brain to what has classically been referred to as the vomiting center, located in the medulla. Whether the anatomic site is specific and localized or the efferent nuclei are scattered is unclear.

In either case, the response to the stimulus is the discharge of efferent fibers that results in **retching,** the second phase of vomiting. Retching involves the con-traction of abdominal muscles in conjunction with a patterned series of actions of respiratory muscles, including closure of the glottis and depression of the diaphragm. Within the stomach, the fundus remains flaccid, but the antrum and pylorus contract. Relaxation of the lower esophageal sphincter also occurs. The culmination of these reflexes is **emesis** of the gastric contents.

Vomiting related to obstruction does not follow this pattern. With pyloric stenosis, repeated, deep peristal-tic waves reverse direction, leading to projectile vom-iting. No nausea is associated with the vomiting of pyloric stenosis, and affected infants are frequently eager to eat immediately after vomiting. Vomiting related to elevated ICP is also not associated with nausea. In addition, such vomiting, which frequently occurs first thing in the morning on awakening, is unrelated to meals.

Regurgitation, which may be misdiagnosed as vomit-ing, is often related to GER (see Chapter 79 for a more detailed discussion).

DIFFERENTIAL DIAGNOSIS

Vomiting may be related to various different GI or extraintestinal (parenteral) conditions. Some condi-tions respond to medical management, and others mandate surgical intervention (Table 78–1). In acute gastroenteritis, the most common cause of vomiting, the infectious agent may be a virus, such as enterovirus or rotavirus, or a bacterium, such as *Shigella.* Acute gastroenteritis is discussed in greater detail in Chapter 81, Diarrhea. In cases that are not due to gastroenteritis, the differential diagnosis of vomiting is best approached by considering the age of the patient.

Infants

Vomiting in neonates may be associated with the ingestion of irritants such as maternal **blood or mucus.** Either of these substances delays gastric emptying.

Structural anomalies of the GI tract may also cause vomiting in neonates. The higher the structural obstruc-tion, the earlier the onset of symptoms. Lesions of the esophagus, such as esophageal atresia, may be evident in the delivery room, with an unsuccessful attempt to pass a nasogastric tube. Lower GI lesions, such as ileal atresia, may not present for several days. These lesions usually require surgical intervention. Infants with atretic lesions may also have a history of polyhydramnios or a single umbilical artery.

Overfeeding is the most common reason for spitting up in young infants. Frequently, infants who present with vomiting are actually experiencing spitting up or regurgitation. Overfeeding is less likely to occur in breast-fed infants, because they have better control of their satiation. Mothers of bottle-fed infants may feel that the volume of formula consumed by their infants is insufficient. Nursing mothers, on the other hand, cannot "unscrew" their breasts from their bodies to determine how much milk their infants have consumed. Some nonnursing mothers feel the need to reinsert a nipple in the infant's mouth, and infants who are still interested in sucking (nonnutritive sucking) continue to feed, often exceeding the capacity of the stomach. Vomiting then results. The physician should approach breast-fed infants who are vomiting with care and concern.

Food allergies are another eating-related problem. Infants with cow milk formula intolerance may expe-rience vomiting. Associated symptoms such as diar-rhea, rhinorrhea, eczema, and growth failure frequently occur.

TABLE 78–1. Differential Diagnosis of Vomiting in Infancy

Medical Conditions
Gastroenteritis
Ingestion of maternal blood or mucus
Overfeeding
Food allergies
Inborn errors of metabolism
Congenital adrenal hyperplasia
Parenteral infections (e.g., otitis media, urinary tract infection)
Surgical Conditions
Atresia/stenosis of gastrointestinal tract
Pyloric stenosis
Ulcers
Intussusception
Volvulus
Appendicitis

GER is a common cause of regurgitation. Regurgitation may occur with a condition called chalasia, a term that means relaxation. The opposite of this is achalasia, or absence of relaxation. This latter disorder appears to be related to disintegration of the myenteric ganglion. Swallowing may be difficult because of esophageal spasm, and food that is unable to pass into the stomach may be regurgitated. Children with achalasia usually do not present until later in childhood, although they may have a prenatal history of polyhydramnios, a sign suggesting an abnormal swallowing pattern, even in utero.

Metabolic disorders, including inborn errors of metabolism and endocrine problems, may also result with vomiting. For example, children with galactosemia may present with vomiting as well as with jaundice, dehydration, cataracts, and hepatomegaly. Other inborn errors of metabolism include methylmalonic acidemia, disorders of the urea cycle, phenylketonuria, maple syrup urine disease, renal tubular acidosis, hypercalcemia, and diabetes insipidus.

Male infants with **congenital adrenal hyperplasia (CAH)** may present with vomiting and electrolyte disturbance, symptoms indicative of adrenal insufficiency. Affected male infants usually present at about 10 to 14 days of age with vomiting and hyperkalemia (which should not be attributed to hemolysis of the specimen); hyponatremia develops later. In females, CAH is usually detected in the newborn nursery because of ambiguous genitalia. Diagnosis of this potentially lethal condition is critical to ensure the institution of replacement therapy and survival of affected infants.

Vomiting may be symptomatic of **infection** in parts of the body other than the GI tract. Most notably, UTIs of young male infants may cause projectile vomiting, a symptom highly suggestive of pyloric stenosis. These infants are usually febrile, and the diagnosis is considered when the urinalysis or culture is positive. Otitis media may also be associated with vomiting.

Vomiting, especially if unrelated to meals, may occur with **increased ICP**. In young infants, this suggests the possibility of an intracranial hemorrhage as occurs with inflicted, nonaccidental trauma.

Pyloric stenosis, a condition caused by hypertrophy of the muscle surrounding the pyloric channel, is the most common surgical condition associated with vomiting in infancy. The condition affects males much more frequently than females and usually appears in infants between the ages of two weeks and two months. The vomitus is projectile, nonbilious, and frequently contains curdled milk, which reflects delayed gastric emptying, a problem caused by failure of the hypertrophied pylorus to relax.

Affected infants have an intact appetite and are eager to eat. In some infants, starvation leads to few bowel movements and constipation; in others there may be small, frequent, mucus-laden stools (starvation diarrhea) that represent succus entericus. If pyloric stenosis is not diagnosed promptly, infants may fail to gain weight or may exhibit FTT. Symptoms suggestive of pyloric stenosis may result from ulcers in the antrum or the pyloric channel.

Children

Vomiting in children is frequently associated with **gastroenteritis.** Infections elsewhere in the body, particularly UTIs, streptococcal pharyngitis, and otitis media, are also associated with vomiting.

Diabetes mellitus may result in vomiting in older children. Vomiting may also appear in children who are already known to be diabetic. This is particularly true when ketosis is present. Vomiting is also a component of peptic ulcer disease, which is described in more detail in Chapter 83, Abdominal Pain.

Vomiting may be a major symptom of **CNS-related problems,** such as tumors, infections, and other causes of increased intracranial pressure. As previously noted, vomiting in CNS-related conditions is often unrelated to meals and may not be associated with nausea. Autonomic epilepsy and migraine headaches are also associated with vomiting.

Vomiting is one of the hallmarks of **Reye's syndrome,** a disorder that involves an encephalopathy in association with fatty infiltration of the liver. The etiology of the condition is unclear, but the root of the disorder appears to be related to mitochondrial dysfunction. Affected children usually have a history of an antecedent viral illness, most commonly influenza B or chickenpox. Following a period of recovery, they experience altered consciousness with vomiting. Hepatic enzymes and serum ammonia are elevated. Aspirin, which uncouples oxidative phosphorylation, is apparently linked to Reye's syndrome, both epidemiologically as well as theoretically.

Certain **medications,** including theophylline, erythromycin, and digitalis, may also be associated with vomiting.

Familial dysautonomia, a rare condition that affects Jewish individuals, results in vomiting. The disorder is inherited in an autosomal recessive manner and consists of an imbalance in the autonomic nervous system. Children experience intractable vomiting in addition to excess perspiration, inability to produce tears, difficulty swallowing and chewing, and cold hands and feet. They also have hyperpyrexia and hypertension. These children require fluid replacement and management with antiemetics.

Surgical conditions such as appendicitis, gall bladder disease, and twisted ovarian cysts are discussed in Chapter 83, Abdominal Pain.

Adolescents

Vomiting during the adolescent years may be caused by any of the previously mentioned conditions. In addition, adolescents may develop vomiting in association with intentional **ingestion of illicit drugs or alcohol.** Many adolescents have incorrect notions of the sexual activity needed to initiate pregnancy. Teenage girls who have been vomiting, especially for a period of time, should be evaluated for **pregnancy,** regardless of their disclosed sexual activity status.

Adolescents with **eating disorders,** particularly bulimia, vomit but may not disclose their vomiting. They

Questions: Vomiting

- What is the nature of the vomiting (projectile, bilious, nonbilious, regurgitated)?
- How long has the child been vomiting?
- Are any symptoms such as fever or diarrhea associated with the vomiting?
- What is the relationship of the vomiting to meals?
- Does the vomiting occur at night, indicating possible hiatal hernia and gastroesophageal reflux?
- Is there a family history of vomiting?
- Is the child taking any medications?
- Have any measures been taken to relieve the vomiting?

may ingest emetics, such as ipecac, to help control their weight (see Chapter 101, Eating Disorders).

EVALUATION

History

A complete history is essential for correct diagnosis (Questions Box). A positive family history of vomiting may suggest a diagnosis of migraine, peptic ulcer disease, or familial dysautonomia.

Physical Examination

The examination shows the impact of vomiting on children's growth. The weight may provide evidence of the chronicity of the process; weight loss suggests a protracted course. Evidence of other infections, such as otitis media or pneumonia, may also be apparent. The examination of the abdomen may show masses or signs of obstruction and a surgical condition. Distention of the abdomen may be present with an obstruction. Peristaltic waves are an abnormal finding characteristic of pyloric stenosis.

Laboratory Tests

The laboratory assessment is determined by the differential diagnosis. If gastroenteritis is suspected, an examination of the stools for leukocytes and occult blood is appropriate. Specimens for bacterial or viral cultures or viral antigen detection can be submitted. A CBC may support the diagnosis of infection or reveal signs of anemia. In neonates, vomited blood should be evaluated using the Apt test to determine whether it came from the mother or infant.

Electrolytes should be obtained in infants or children with a history of significant vomiting, and may confirm dehydration, acid-base imbalance, or electrolyte disturbance. Infants with pyloric stenosis who vomit stomach contents develop a hypochloremic, hypokalemic alkalosis. A urinalysis also may show evidence of dehydration as well as signs of a UTI. Tests for inborn errors of metabolism, such as urine for amino acid analysis, are appropriate if this is suspected.

Imaging Studies

Radiographic procedures, such as x-rays, ultrasound, and contrast studies, are useful to define obstructive lesions such as pyloric stenosis. A flat plate of the abdomen may show stomach distention, a "double bubble" (air in the stomach and duodenum) or a paucity of intestinal air in cases of high level obstruction. Consultation with a pediatric gastroenterologist may lead to additional diagnostic tests, such as endoscopic evaluation.

MANAGEMENT

The initial step in the management of vomiting infants or children is to ensure adequate hydration and integrity of the cardiovascular bed. This may require the administration of intravenous fluids. **Oral rehydration** is the mainstay of therapy in infants and children whose vomiting is related to gastroenteritis. Small, frequent feedings with clear fluids are better tolerated than large, infrequent feedings, although the latter may be necessary in infants with diarrhea because each feeding may result in a bowel movement. Antiemetics such as phenothiazines are discouraged in children because of the high incidence of side effects, including dystonic posturing.

Further management depends on the diagnosis. Infections should be treated with the appropriate antibiotics. Operative conditions, such as pyloric stenosis or intussusception, should be managed surgically. Inborn errors of metabolism require consultation with a geneticist and dietary manipulation. Congenital adrenal hyperplasia should be managed in consultation with an endocrinologist. This condition necessitates replacement hormonal therapy.

PROGNOSIS

Most cases of acute vomiting resolve spontaneously or are readily managed once the underlying condition is diagnosed. The overall prognosis is therefore quite good.

Protracted vomiting may result in starvation and FTT, however. Severe vomiting may cause tears in the esophagus and lead to hematemesis. Obstructive causes of vomiting in infants respond to surgical intervention. The prognosis for children with Reye's syndrome depends on the severity of the disturbance, with the possibility of death in very sick children.

Case Resolution

The infant in the case history exhibits the signs and symptoms consistent with pyloric stenosis. The boy is a healthy, vigorous breast-fed infant, and his weight gain of 1000 grams in six weeks (average: 25 g/day) is normal. The vomitus is curdled indicating that it has been in the stomach for over three hours. Gastric emptying is delayed. The presence of a mass in the right upper quadrant is also consistent with the diagnosis. An ultrasound would confirm the finding. It would be equally appropriate to keep the infant NPO (nothing by mouth), start intravenous fluids, and obtain surgical consultation.

Selected Readings

Dodge, J. A. Vomiting and regurgitation. *In* Walker, W. A., et al (eds.). Pediatric Gastrointestinal Disease. Philadelphia, B. C. Decker, 1991, pp. 32–39.

Foley, L. C., et al. Evaluation of the vomiting infant. Am. J. Dis. Child. 143:660–661, 1989.

Hebra, A., and M. A. Hoffman. Gastroesophageal reflex in children. Pediatr. Clin. North Am. 40:1233–1251, 1993.

Judd, R. H. *Helicobacter pylori.* Gastritis and ulcers in pediatrics. Adv. Pediatr. 39:283–306, 1992.

Squires, R. H., Jr. Intracranial tumors: vomiting as a presenting sign—a gastroenterologist's perspective. Clin. Pediatr. 28:351, 1989.

CHAPTER 79

GASTROESOPHAGEAL REFLUX

Carlo Di Lorenzo, M.D.

H$_x$ A two-month-old girl has a history of spitting up and vomiting immediately after every meal. Her parents are very anxious and frustrated. The girl's vomiting seems effortless, and the parents have difficulty quantifying the amount of formula that is regurgitated. The child, who has always been in good general health, was the product of a normal pregnancy and delivery and had an uneventful neonatal course. She seems happy, with no apparent abdominal pain, dysphagia, odynophagia, hematemesis, FTT, pneumonia, wheezing, or apnea. The stool is heme-negative, the hematocrit is 40%, and the urinalysis is normal. The physical examination is normal.

Questions

1. How is physiologic gastroesophageal reflux (GER) differentiated from pathologic GER?
2. What groups of children are at risk for GER?
3. What clinical conditions can be caused by GER?
4. How should children with possible pathologic GER be assessed?
5. What management options are available for GER?
6. What is the natural history of GER in children?

Gastroesophageal reflux (GER) is the retrograde movement of gastric contents from the stomach to the esophagus. Such episodes frequently occur physiologically, and the events are brief, asymptomatic, and self-limited. Occasionally, either the overall frequency of reflux or the marked duration of a single episode may cause disease. This is characteristic of pathologic GER. Clinically, pediatric GER takes two forms: infantile and adult. Infantile GER is present during the first months of life and resolves clinically by 18 months of age in at least 80% of affected infants. In contrast, adult GER often manifests initially in children beyond infancy and tends to persist and requires chronic or intermittent therapy.

Understanding of GER in children has been confused by the misuse of terms such as regurgitation, vomiting, and rumination. **Regurgitation** is defined as effortless return of gastric contents to the mouth. **Vomiting** refers to the forceful expulsion of the same material. **Rumination** involves some voluntary effort and contraction of the abdominal muscles, but it is not accompanied by the retching and the retrograde duodenogastric contractions that characterize vomiting.

EPIDEMIOLOGY

The incidence of infantile GER is reported to be 20%, and nearly one-third of affected infants come to medical attention; 80% of these infants (5.4% of all infants) require no workup and only minimal therapy. Of the remaining children who are evaluated, most are successfully treated medically. However, a minority of infants (0.4% of all infants) require antireflux surgery. Boys are somewhat more likely than girls to have pathologic GER in infancy and childhood (ratio: 1.27:1). The cause of this male preponderance is unknown. Some children with particular conditions have a higher risk for developing GER disease.

Neurologic Disease

The incidence of pathologic GER in children with severe neurologic disease is 20 to 70%. Reportedly, the incidence of reflux is inversely proportional to mental age. Neurologic disease associated with hypertonia and spasticity may increase the frequency and duration of reflux episodes by raising intra-abdominal pressure.

In addition, children with spasticity have a higher incidence of sliding hiatal hernia, a predisposing factor for reflux. Hypotonia, supine position, or abnormal postures facilitate GER episodes. Chronic lying in a horizontal position delays the esophageal clearance of refluxate and increases the risk of esophagitis. Children with neurologic diseases often have a decreased gag reflex, which may lead to life-threatening episodes of aspiration of refluxed material.

In particular, children with Down's syndrome are at risk for pathologic GER because they are often hypotonic and have an increased frequency of abnormal esophageal peristalsis. Children with myopathy or systemic sclerosis may also be predisposed to development of esophagitis, because their reflux episodes are poorly cleared by the esophageal peristalsis.

Chronic Respiratory Disease

In children, bronchopulmonary dysplasia (BPD), cystic fibrosis, and asthma are associated with a high prevalence of GER. As many as 20% of premature infants with BPD have abnormal GER, compared with 1 to 2% of preterm infants without BPD. Children with cystic fibrosis have a high incidence of regurgitation, heartburn, and severe esophagitis. The risks for esophagitis are higher in children with severe respiratory disease as compared to those with mild disease. More than 50% of children and adults with asthma have abnormal GER.

Congenital Esophageal Anomalies

Children who have a surgically repaired esophageal atresia have a high incidence of GER disease, which seems to result from an intrinsic abnormality in the esophageal innervation coordinating the esophageal peristalsis. Absence of the intraabdominal segment of the esophagus and damage to the vagus incurred during the surgical repair of the atresia are also believed to contribute to abnormal reflux.

Increased Abdominal Pressure

Increases in intra-abdominal pressure produce higher intragastric pressures that can overcome the opposing pressure of the lower esophageal sphincter (LES). Children who suffer from frequent coughing attacks or are constipated and spend a great amount of time contracting their abdominal muscles in defecatory efforts are at risk for developing GER disease. The chronically increased abdominal pressure in obesity explains the reported 73% prevalence of heartburn in obese adults. The effect of the chronic increase in abdominal pressure during pregnancy is compounded by the effects of progesterone, thus decreasing the LES pressure. Peritoneal dialysis has been shown to increase abdominal pressure and delay gastric emptying, which triggers GER. Placement of a gastrostomy induces abnormal GER by decreasing the LES pressure and length and modifying the gastroesophageal angle. Children with a gastrostomy are also often given rapid bolus feedings that cause a sudden increase in intra-abdominal pressure and induce relaxation of the LES.

CLINICAL PRESENTATION

In infancy, the most common initial symptom is effortless postprandial regurgitation often accompanied by chronic irritability. The loss of regurgitated calories may lead to weight loss or FTT. GI bleeding and pulmonary disorders, including aspiration pneumonia, asthma, and recurrent apnea, are less common. In addition, children with GER may present with signs and symptoms of neurologic disease. Apparent seizures characterized by apnea and stiffening of the body and abnormal posturing of the head and neck have been associated with GER. The main symptoms of GER in older children are heartburn, chest pain, and eructation (belching) (D_x Box). Odynophagia (painful swallowing), dysphagia (difficulty swallowing) secondary to a stricture, and bleeding are less frequent.

PATHOPHYSIOLOGY

GER disease is a multifactorial process in which different abnormalities may predominate in a single patient. The interaction among the multiple factors that results in GER disease is summarized in Figure 79–1. They include competence of antireflux mechanisms, efficiency of esophageal clearance, volume of gastric contents, aggressiveness of refluxed material, and mucosal resistance to injury.

Reflux may occur by one of three general mechanisms: transient LES relaxation, hypotonic LES, or increases in intra-abdominal pressure. For many years, low LES pressure was believed to be the main cause of reflux. It is now evident that most reflux episodes are due to sudden LES relaxations not associated with swallowing. During these episodes, the LES opens completely for 5 to 35 seconds. The main **antireflux mechanism** disappears, and gastric contents move freely from an area with higher resting pressure (stomach) to one with lower resting pressure (esophagus). The transient LES relaxation explains why more than half of the children with GER disease have a normal LES pressure.

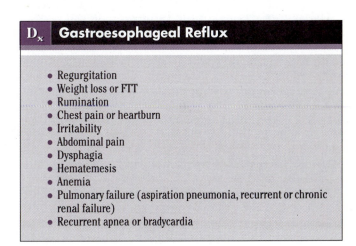

Dx Gastroesophageal Reflux

- Regurgitation
- Weight loss or FTT
- Rumination
- Chest pain or heartburn
- Irritability
- Abdominal pain
- Dysphagia
- Hematemesis
- Anemia
- Pulmonary failure (aspiration pneumonia, recurrent or chronic renal failure)
- Recurrent apnea or bradycardia

FIGURE 79–1. *Pathogenesis of gastroesophageal reflux (GER) disease.*

Spontaneous reflux without LES relaxation occurs only when the basal LES pressure is extremely low (< 5 mm Hg). Most children with very low LES pressure have severe neurodevelopmental delays.

Esophageal clearance determines the duration of esophageal exposure to the injurious effect of refluxate. Esophageal peristaltic contractions rapidly clear fluid volume from the esophagus, and swallowed saliva neutralizes any small amount of residual acid. In the event that peristalsis is abnormal, gravity promotes esophageal clearance when children are upright but not when they are supine. Children who lie supine most of the time or who reflux during sleep have longer esophageal exposure to acid compared to those who are ambulatory or awake. In some children with reflux esophagitis, abnormal esophageal clearance occurs. Esophagitis can cause either abnormal esophageal peristalsis or esophageal stricture. With abnormal peristalsis, swallowing of both liquids and solids is affected; with a stricture, primarily swallowing of solids is altered. The esophageal inflammation may cause further worsening of the peristalsis, triggering a vicious cycle.

Increased **gastric fluid volume** not only makes more volume available for reflux but also increases the frequency of transient LES relaxations. Some children with reflux disease exhibit delayed gastric emptying, which contributes to the development of reflux disease.

The **aggressiveness of the refluxed material** is also important. The degree of esophagitis correlates with the time of hydrochloric acid exposure. Suppression of acid secretion is associated with healing of esophagitis, even when reflux persists. Although acid alone may cause esophageal injury by protein denaturation, pepsin, which becomes an active proteolytic enzyme at pH less than 3.0, contributes substantially to the development of esophagitis. Bile acids and pancreatic enzymes, which may be present in the stomach in patients with duodenogastric reflux, are particularly harmful for the esophageal mucosa.

The mucosal layer, the unstirred water layer, surface bicarbonate, and various aspects of the stratified squamous epithelium affect the **mucosal resistance** to the refluxate. The capacity of the esophageal mucosa to withstand injury and to repair injury appears to be influenced by such factors as age and nutrition.

Children with **hiatal hernias** may exhibit GER. These children lack the intra-abdominal portion of the esophagus, one of the protective mechanisms against reflux. Large, sliding, hiatal hernias may act as fluid traps and promote reflux when the LES opens on swallowing. Although children with large hernias often have severe esophagitis that does not respond to medical treatment, the majority of individuals with hiatal hernias do not have GER. The physician should not equate the presence of a sliding hiatal hernia with the presence of GER disease.

DIFFERENTIAL DIAGNOSIS

The differential diagnosis of reflux symptoms is presented in Table 79–1. **Regurgitation** is a far more frequent symptom in infants than in older children. It is quite easy to diagnose GER as the cause of this symptom. The challenge lies in avoiding inappropriate investigations in children whose only problem is the messiness of regurgitated food. Other causes of vomiting should not be overlooked. Excessive regurgitation causes weight loss, which requires aggressive diagnostic and therapeutic intervention. Poor intake may also contribute to FTT because discomfort due to esophagitis is associated with food intake. In addition, parents may be hesitant to feed infants whose response to eating is regurgitation and irritability. Infantile rumination, which involves regurgitation of previously swallowed food and rechewing and reswallowing of the food, is a particularly ominous presentation of GER disease.

Absence of regurgitation does not rule out GER disease. Esophagitis due to nonregurgitant reflux can present with chest pain or heartburn, abdominal pain, irritability, refusal to feed, dysphagia, hematemesis, and anemia. **Chest pain or heartburn** in response to the acid bathing of the inflamed esophageal mucosa is a common complaint of verbal children. Under the same conditions, infants and younger children are more likely to show irritability or complain of abdominal pain. **Dysphagia** may be a manifestation of esophagitis. **Hema-**

TABLE 79–1.   Differential Diagnosis of Reflux Symptoms

Regurgitation, Vomiting

Stimulation of central vomiting center
Drugs, toxins
Metabolic conditions: diabetic ketoacidosis; diabetes insipidus; lactic acidosis; phenylketonuria; maple syrup urine; methylmalonic acidemia; hereditary fructose intolerance; galactosemia; tyrosinemia; hyperammonemia; fatty-acid oxidation disorders (e.g., medium-chain acyl CoA dehydrogenase deficiency); uremia; renal tubular acidosis

Stimulation of supramedullary receptors
Psychogenic vomiting
Vestibular disease; "motion sickness"
Increased intracerebral pressure: subdural effusion or hematoma; hydrocephalus; cerebral edema or tumor; meningoencephalitis; Reye's syndrome

Stimulation of peripheral receptors
Pharyngeal: gag reflex
Gastric conditions: peptic ulcer disease; dysmotility; obstruction (e.g., bezoar; pyloric stenosis; web)
Intestinal conditions
   Infection; enterotoxin; appendicitis
   Nutrient intolerance (e.g., cow's milk, soy, eosinophilic gastroenteropathy)
   Obstruction (e.g., web; superior mesentric artery syndrome; volvulus; meconium ileus; intussusception; adhesions; meconium plug; Hirschsprung's disease)
Hepatobiliary conditions: hepatitis; cholecystitis
Pancreatic conditions: pancreatitis
Miscellaneous conditions: peritonitis; pyelonephritis; sepsis

Other esophageal diseases
Structural: stricture; ring; etc.
Functional: esophageal body dysmotility, achalasia

Pain, Esophagitis Symptoms
Cardiac pain
Pulmonary or mediastinal pain; chest wall pain (e.g., costrochondritis)
Nonesophagitis upper gastrointestinal inflammation (e.g., peptic ulcer disease)
   Nonesophagitis dysphagia
   Many possible causes of nonspecific irritability in infants (e.g., milk allergy, infantile colic)
   Functional; malingering

Respiratory Symptoms (e.g., Wheeze, Stridor, Cough)
Extrinsic compression (e.g., vascular ring)
Intrinsic obstruction (e.g., malformation, foreign body, cyst, tumor)
Airways reactive to other stimuli (e.g., allergens, infection)
Infection; inflammation; cystic fibrosis; pertussis; asthma
"Central" events (e.g., central apnea)

Neurobehavioral Symptoms (Sandifer's Syndrome, Seizurelike Spells)
Seizures
Dystonic reaction to drugs
Vestibular disorders
Early pertussis

Adapted, with permission, from Orenstein, S.R. Gastroesophageal reflux. *In* Stackman, J.A., III, and R.J. Winter (eds.). Current Problems in Pediatrics 21:223, 1991.

temesis and **anemia** are a consequence of bleeding due to esophagitis.

Some older children with GER disease may develop **Sandifer's syndrome.** They hold their neck in a twisted position, often without realizing they are doing so. This position disappears when reflux is successfully treated and appears to be the children's way of reducing the discomfort associated with reflux.

Certain **respiratory symptoms** in children may actually result from GER disease. Two mechanisms have been suggested to explain respiratory complications of GER disease: (1) pulmonary aspiration of regurgitated gastric contents and (2) bronchoconstriction triggered by refluxate stimulation of an inflamed esophageal mucosa. Pulmonary aspiration of refluxate causes pneumonia, particularly in neurologically abnormal children, whose airway protective mechanisms can be defective. It may be difficult to distinguish aspiration during reflux from aspiration during swallowing in these children. Apnea or bradycardia may occur in neurologically immature infants as a response to various stimuli. Reflux may be an important cause of intrinsic asthma. Children with nocturnal asthma symptoms, including cough, are especially likely to have GER disease. Several studies have shown an improvement in bronchospastic symptoms following medical or surgical treatment of reflux. Stridor, croup, hoarseness, otitis, and sinusitis are other respiratory conditions that have been linked to pathologic GER.

EVALUATION

Diagnostic evaluation of reflux should be undertaken only in children suspected of suffering pathologic effects from reflux. Thus infants with regurgitation but no other sequelae are simply managed with conservative antireflux measures.

History

The diagnostic evaluation begins with a complete history (Questions Box). It is important to inquire about the reflux-associated symptoms even if they are not part of the presenting complaint.

Physical Examination

In most children with GER disease the physical examination is normal. Nevertheless, a complete physical examination should be performed to eliminate conditions discussed in the differential diagnosis (see Table 79–1).

Laboratory Studies

Several diagnostic techniques are available to diagnose different aspects of GER disease (Table 79–2). **Monitoring of intraesophageal pH** for 24 hours is considered the gold standard for diagnosing GER. It allows the physician to correlate symptoms with changes in

Questions: Gastroesophageal Reflux

- Is the emesis effortless, forceful, or projectile?
- When does the infant regurgitate (i.e., how long after a meal; lying supine or prone; during crying, coughing, or diaper change)?
- Has the child ever vomited blood?
- Is the child losing weight or not gaining weight satisfactorily?
- Does the child cry a lot and refuse to eat?
- Does the child have a chronic cough or asthma that is not responsive to conventional therapy?
- Does the child have heartburn exacerbated by citrus juices and relieved by liquid antacids?

TABLE 79–2. Diagnostic Techniques in the Evaluation of Gastroesophageal Reflux

Investigation	Sensitivity	Specificity	Advantages	Disadvantages
Radiology	++	+	Availability; illustrates anatomy	Not physiologic; short duration
Intraesophageal pH monitoring	+++	+++	Accurate; correlates with symptoms	Duration 24 hours; misses postprandial reflux
Endoscopy	++	+++	Detects esophagitis; allows biopsy	Invasive; may be normal when biopsy is abnormal
Scintigraphy	+	++	Noninvasive, physiologic; detects aspiration; measures gastric emptying	Does not detect esophagitis; needs patient cooperation
Esophageal suction biopsy	++	+++	Minimally invasive; detects esophagitis	May be normal in early stages of GER disease
Manometry	+	+	Measures peristalsis and LES pressure	Does not detect esophagitis; may be normal in presence of severe GER disease
Acid perfusion	±	++	Available; easy to perform	Needs patient cooperation; does not detect esophagitis

intraesophageal pH. Although the pH probe can quantify frequency and duration of reflux, it cannot detect reflux for at least one hour following feeding with an infant formula because of the buffering effect of the formula on the intragastric pH. A diagnosis of esophagitis can be obtained either through visualization and biopsy of the esophagus by esophagoscopy or through a blind peroral suction biopsy of the distal esophagus, which provides larger bioptic specimens. Because of the necessarily brief chronology of reflux in infants, children may not have yet developed the pathologic changes diagnostic of esophagitis. Esophageal manometry and intraesophageal acid perfusion have a very limited role in the diagnostic workup of children with GER disease.

TABLE 79–3. Therapy for Gastroesophageal Reflux*

Conservative
Put in prone or completely upright position
Thicken infant feedings (1 Tbsp. rice cereal/oz)
Fast before bed
Avoid large meals, obesity, tight clothing
Avoid provocative foods and medications
    Fatty foods, citrus, tomato, carbonation, coffee, alcohol
    Smoke exposure
    Anticholinergics, adrenergics, xanthines (theophylline, caffeine), calcium channel blockers, prostaglandins
Pharmacologic (Usual Course, 8–12 Weeks)
Prokinetic
    Metoclopramide (0.1 mg/kg/dose qid)
    Bethanechol (0.1–0.3 mg/kg/dose tid or qid)
    Cisapride (0.2–0.3 mg/kg/dose tid)
    Domperidone (not available in the United States)
Antacid
    Cimetidine (5–10 mg/kg/dose qid)
    Ranitidine (2–4 mg/kg/dose tid)
    Famotidine, Nizatidine (adult, 40 mg HS; 300 mg HS)
    Omeprazole (adult, 20 mg HS)
    Antacids (0.5–1 mL/kg/dose, 3–8 times/day: 1–2 hr [PC, HS])
Barrier or miscellaneous mechanism
    Sucralfate slurry (1 g in 5–15 mL solution qid [PC, HS])
    Alginic acid-antacid (2 g 3–8 times/day [PC])
Surgical
Fundoplication
Angelchik prosthesis

*Dosages for children unless otherwise specified.
Adapted, with permission, from Orenstein, S.R. Gastroesophageal reflux. In Stackman, J.A., III, and R.J. Winter, (eds). Curr. Probl. Pediatr. 21:223, 1991.

All children who present with anemia should undergo hemoccult test of the stools. A Hemoccult-positive stool is an important clue that indicates that esophagitis may be causing the anemia.

Imaging Studies

Barium contrast studies of the pharynx, esophagus, and upper GI tract should be performed to rule out anatomic abnormalities such as malrotations, webs, stenoses, and hiatal hernia. The sensitivity of barium fluoroscopy in detecting GER may be poor, and it has a very low specificity; many infants with no clinically significant GER reflux some barium into the esophagus. Scintigraphy measures gastric emptying and diagnoses pulmonary aspiration of gastric contents. This technique involves offering formula containing small amounts of radioactive technetium to children.

MANAGEMENT

A stepwise approach to the treatment of GER disease is summarized in Table 79–3. Most infants with pathologic GER are free of disease within one to two years because of the combined effect of the maturation of the LES function, the introduction of more solid feedings, and the increasing amount of time spent in the upright position.

Optimal positioning for infants with GER disease is prone, with the head of the bed elevated 30 degrees. Although the AAP recommends placing infants in the supine position to decrease the risk of SIDS, this does not apply to infants with GER disease. **Thickening infant formula** with rice cereal decreases the amount of regurgitation, diminishes crying, and increases the caloric density of the formula. When a thickened formula is used, the nipple should be enlarged to allow adequate flow.

Medications are usually added to the regimen when pathologic GER has been demonstrated. **Cisapride,** which has recently been approved for use in GER, is the first-line drug for children with pathologic reflux. Cisapride increases LES pressure, improves esophageal peristalsis, and accelerates gastric emptying. **Acid-**

reducing agents (e.g., H_2-receptor antagonists such as cimetidine, ranitidine, and famotidine; proton pump inhibitors such as omeprazole) should be used when esophagitis is evident.

Infants with rumination may benefit from pharmacologic therapy of GER in combination with any modification of their psychosocial situation, because a problematic parent-infant relationship may play a role in the etiology of infantile rumination.

Surgical therapy is reserved for children who fail to respond to medical treatment or have GER-related, life-threatening events, such as recurrent episodes of apnea or pneumonia. The majority of children who undergo antireflux surgery are neurologically impaired, and 2 to 10% of these infants have Down's syndrome. Nissen fundoplication is the most popular and reliable surgical procedure for treatment of reflux. Success rates of 80 to 90% are reported. Both short- and long-term complications are frequent, however, especially in children with neurologic deficits. These complications include gas bloat, inability to burp and vomit, dysphagia, dumping syndrome (overly rapid gastric emptying), small bowel obstruction due to adhesions, and herniation of the wrap through the hiatus.

PROGNOSIS

The prognosis of infantile reflux is excellent. Most cases resolve in the first year of life. GER that occurs beyond infancy has a less benign course and often requires chronic treatment.

Case Resolution

The girl in the case history has physiologic GER. She requires no diagnostic tests and can be sent home without any pharmacologic intervention. The parents should receive reassurance that the condition is harmless and self-limited. The spitting up will slowly resolve, and the girl should do well.

Selected Readings

Herbst, J. J., S. D. Minton, and L. S. Book. Gastroesophageal reflux causing distress and apnea in newborn infants. J. Pediatr. 95:763–768, 1979.

Orenstein, S. R. Gastroesophageal reflux. *In* Stackman, J. A., III, R. J. Winter (eds.). Curr. Probl. Pediatr. 21:202–241, 1991.

Orenstein, S. R. Prone positioning in infant gastroesophageal reflux: is elevation of the head worth the trouble? J. Pediatr. 117:184–187, 1990.

Orenstein, S. R., P. F. Whitington, and D. M. Orenstein. The infant seat as treatment for gastroesophageal reflux. N. Engl. J. Med. 116:540–543, 1983.

Sondheimer, J. M., and B. A. Morris. Gastroesophageal reflux among severely retarded children. J. Pediatr. 94:710–714, 1979.

Treem, W., P. Davis, and J. Hyams. Gastroesophageal reflux in the older child: presentation, response to treatment and long-term follow-up. Clin. Pediatr. 30:435–440, 1991.

Willinger, M., H. J. Hoffman, and R. B. Hartford. Infant sleep position and risk of sudden infant death syndrome. Report of meeting held January 13 and 14, 1994, National Institutes of Health, Bethesda, MD. Pediatrics 93:814–820, 1994.

CHAPTER 80

GASTROINTESTINAL BLEEDING

Carlo Di Lorenzo, M.D.
Eric Vasiliquskas, M.D.

H_x A four-year-old boy is evaluated for intermittent passing of bright red blood from the rectum for two weeks. Blood either coats the stool or appears as a spot after a bowel movement. The mother reports no vomiting, diarrhea, loss of appetite, weight loss, fever, or abdominal pain. The boy has no history of constipation, straining, or pain with defecation and is taking no medications. The family has no pets and has not traveled recently.

On physical examination, the boy is a well-appearing, energetic, interactive youngster. Weight and height are at the 75th percentile for age. The abdomen is soft, flat, and nontender, and bowel sounds are normally active. No organomegaly or masses are evident. No rashes, bruising, or hemangiomas are present. No tags, fissures, or fistulas are seen on close visual inspection of the perianal area. Digital rectal examination reveals normal sphincter tone, and a small, mobile, pealike mass is palpable in the rectal vault. A film of bright red blood is present on the glove after the examination. A CBC with platelet count and a PT/PTT determination yield normal results.

Questions

1. What is involved in the assessment of children with GI bleeding?

2. How are upper and lower GI tract bleeding differentiated?
3. What conditions usually account for upper and lower GI tract bleeding?
4. What management options are available for GI bleeding?
5. How does the physician decide what type of management is appropriate for each individual patient?

Gastrointestinal bleeding, which is commonly encountered in pediatric practice, is a source of great anxiety for patients and families. GI bleeding ranges in severity, and clinically asymptomatic children with iron deficiency anemia as well as children with acute life-threatening shock from massive hemorrhage may have GI bleeding. Prompt assessment, diagnosis, and treatment are essential. An age-specific differential diagnosis, detailed history, and physical examination indicate the etiology in most patients.

EPIDEMIOLOGY

Children suffering from the stress of major trauma, burns, shock, or sepsis commonly develop multiple superficial erosions of the gastric mucosa. Portal hypertension produces esophageal and gastric varices, which may intermittently bleed briskly, resulting in hematemesis or melena. Patients with coagulopathies from infection, hemophilia, idiopathic thrombocytopenic purpura, poor hepatic synthetic function, vitamin K malabsorption, hypersplenism, giant hemangiomas, platelet dysfunction, platelet inhibitors (aspirin), anticoagulants (Coumadin), or iron intoxication are at high risk as well (see Chapter 58, Bleeding Disorders). GI bleeding may also occur in children with chronic renal failure. Patients taking NSAIDs or corticosteroids and those receiving radiation or chemotherapeutic agents such as Cytoxan, methotrexate, and Adriamycin, which can induce mucositis or neutropenic colitis, may also experience GI bleeding. Opportunistic infections with herpes simplex, CMV, or *Candida* should be considered in immunocompromised children.

Newborns commonly develop gastritis or stress ulcers related to perinatal hypoxia, sepsis, or CNS lesions. Sepsis, vitamin K deficiency, or maternal drugs that crossed the placenta or were passed via the breast milk may result in coagulopathy. Maternal blood swallowed at the time of delivery or ingested from the bleeding nipples of nursing mothers accounts for approximately 30% of blood found in the GI tracts of newborns. Malrotation with midgut volvulus, necrotizing enterocolitis, and Hirschsprung's enterocolitis are life-threatening conditions that require immediate attention. Infants with protein intolerances to cow's milk and soy products may present with hematemesis or rectal bleeding (occult or gross).

DEFINITIONS (D_X BOX)

- **Hematemesis** is the vomiting of blood. Fresh blood is bright red. Once blood is denatured by gastric acid, it assumes a "coffee-ground" appearance. Hematemesis suggests that the source of bleeding lies proximal to the ligament of Treitz.
- **Hematochezia** is the term used for blood passed by the rectum. The discharge may be in the form of pure blood, bloody diarrhea, or blood mixed with stool. Bright red blood almost always originates in the left colon, most commonly in the anorectal region.
- **Melena** refers to black, tarry stools, which usually originate in the upper GI tract and rarely the right colon. The color depends on the volume of blood lost and the transit time; the slower the transit, the darker the color of the stool. Melena results from bacterial degradation of hemoglobin.
- **Occult bleeding** refers to the presence of blood in amounts small enough not to be appreciated visually.
- **Hemodynamic changes** are caused by blood loss. Symptoms include dizziness, dyspnea, tachycardia, and shock. They are the only symptoms that the child with GI bleeding may have on initial presentation.

PATHOPHYSIOLOGY

The body compensates for GI bleeding in a variety of ways depending on the amount of blood lost. When less than 15% of the circulating blood volume is lost, the venous system contracts and extravascular fluid is shifted into the vascular space, thus maintaining both intravascular volume and cardiac output. Very rapid loss of as little as 10% of the blood volume, however, may overwhelm these compensatory mechanisms and lead to shock.

When blood loss exceeds 15%, these homeostatic mechanisms are inadequate. Increased sympathetic output raises the heart rate and force of contraction in an effort to maintain cardiac output. The blood volume is maintained through peripheral vasoconstriction. Oxygen consumption increases. Hyperventilation may result in initial respiratory alkalosis, followed by metabolic acidosis, as blood lactate levels increase secondary to tissue hypoxia.

Blood loss in excess of 30% is associated with hypotension. Decreased cardiac output leads to tissue damage. The resulting metabolic acidosis contributes to the severity of the symptoms. Patients are at risk for acute renal failure, hepatic hypoperfusion, myocardial infarction, and bowel ischemia.

DIFFERENTIAL DIAGNOSIS

Astute clinicians can minimize anxiety and inappropriate diagnostic evaluation by identifying substances that commonly mimic GI blood. Swallowed

---

D_X Gastrointestinal Bleeding

- Bleeding
- Signs of portal hypertension (splenomegaly, caput medusae, jaundice)
- Rash, purpura, hemangioma
- Abdominal mass or distention

blood may come from nongastrointestinal sources such as epistaxis or oropharyngeal lesions. Products that are mistaken for hematemesis include cherry or strawberry candy, red licorice, juice pops, Jello, Kool-Aid, tomatoes, cranberries, beets, antibiotics (ampicillin, amoxicillin), and other medications (Tylenol). Urinary sources of blood or redness in the diaper include hematuria, rifampin, beets, and dyes. *Serratia marcescens* may cause a pink discoloration in the diaper. Chocolate, blueberries, spinach, iron products, and bismuth preparations (Pepto-Bismol) may be mistaken for melena. Menarche should be considered in pubertal females.

The causes of upper and lower GI tract bleeding vary depending on age (Tables 80–1, 80–2, and 80–3).

EVALUATION

To help guide the workup in children with presumed GI hemorrhage, it is important to look for clues in the history and physical examination that quantify the amount and rapidity of the blood loss and help localize the site of bleeding.

History

The physician should first determine whether the blood is actually blood. A thorough history should then be obtained (Questions Box).

Physical Examination

A meticulous examination is important, because the initial signs and symptoms of blood loss such as weakness, dizziness, fatigue, and pain may be nonspe-

TABLE 80–2.   Differential Diagnosis of Lower Gastrointestinal Bleeding

Age Group	Common Causes	Less Common Causes
Neonates (0–30 days)	Anorectal lesions Swallowed maternal blood Milk allergy Necrotizing enterocolitis Midgut volvulus	Hirschsprung's enterocolitis Infectious diarrhea* Coagulopathy Vascular malformations Intestinal duplication
Infants (30 days–1 yr)	Anorectal lesions Midgut volvulus Intussusception Meckel's diverticulum Infectious diarrhea* Milk allergy	Vascular malformations Intestinal duplication Acquired thrombocytopenia
Children (1–12 yr)	Juvenile polyps Meckel's diverticulum Intussusception Infectious diarrhea* Anal fissure Nodular lymphoid hyperplasia	Henoch-Schönlein purpura (HSP) Hemolytic-uremic syndrome Vasculitis (systemic lupus erythematosus) Inflammatory bowel disease
Adolescents (> 12 yr)	Inflammatory bowel disease Polyps Hemorrhoids Anal fissure Infectious diarrhea*	Arteriovascular malformation Adenocarcinomas HSP Pseudomembranous colitis

*Infectious etiologies for lower GI bleeding include *Salmonella, Shigella, Campylobacter jejuni, Yersinia enterocolitica,* enteroinvasive *Escherichia coli,* enterohemorrhagic *E. coli, Clostridium difficile, Entamoeba histolytica,* and *Aeromonas hydrophilia.*

Adapted, with permission, from Olson, A.D., and A.C. Hillemeier. Gastrointestinal hemorrhage. *In* Wyllie R., and J.S. Hyams (eds.). Pediatric Gastrointestinal Disease. Philadelphia, W.B. Saunders, 1993, p. 259.

cific. Most importantly, the physician should determine whether patients are stable or show any signs of shock or impending shock such as tachycardia, pallor, weak pulse, or dyspnea. Vital signs should be measured to help assess volume loss. A decrease of 10 mm Hg during orthostatic blood pressure measurements represents a 10 to 20% intravascular volume loss, and syncope or fainting implies either a larger deficit or a rapid 10% loss. Resting tachycardia and hypotension occur with losses in excess of 30%. A very narrow pulse pressure is an ominous sign, suggesting that the body's compensatory mechanisms are overwhelmed and warning of impending vascular collapse.

The physician should carefully examine the anterior nares and oropharynx. Blood draining into the esophagus and stomach from these areas is the most common nongastrointestinal source of blood in the GI tract. Marked tenderness with or without a palpable mass on abdominal examination raises the possibility of ischemia or intussusception. Bowel sounds may be normal, as expected with a lower GI bleed, or hyperactive, the result of rapid transit of blood through the bowel from the upper GI tract. Signs of obstruction should be noted. Jaundice, hepatomegaly, splenomegaly, ascites, or caput medusae suggests possible hepatic disease and portal hypertension. The practitioner should also inspect the perirectal area, looking for fissures, fistulas,

TABLE 80–1.   Differential Diagnosis of Upper Gastrointestinal Bleeding

Age Group	Common Causes	Less Common Causes
Neonates (0–30 days)	Swallowed maternal blood Gastritis Duodenitis	Coagulopathy Vascular malformations Gastric/esophageal duplication Leiomyoma
Infants (30 days–1 yr)	Gastritis and gastric ulcer Esophagitis Duodenitis	Esophageal varices Foreign body Aortoesophageal fistula
Children (1–12 yr)	Esophagitis Esophageal varices Gastritis and gastric ulcer Duodenal ulcer Mallory-Weiss tear Nasopharyngeal bleeding	Salicylates Henoch-Schönlein purpura (HSP) Vascular malformation Hematobilia Caustic ingestion Foreign body Leiomyoma
Adolescents (> 12 yr)	Duodenal ulcer Esophagitis Esophageal varices Gastritis Mallory-Weiss tear	HSP Thrombocytopenia Dieulafoy's ulcer Hematobilia

Adapted, with permission, from Olson, A.D., and A.C. Hillemeier. Gastrointestinal hemorrhage. *In* Wyllie R., and J.S. Hyams (eds.). Pediatric Gastrointestinal Disease. Philadelphia, W.B. Saunders, 1993, p. 259.

TABLE 80–3. Causes of Occult Gastrointestinal Bleeding

Inflammatory
Peptic esophagitis
Crohn's disease
Ulcerative colitis
Mild enterocolitis
Celiac disease
Eosinophilic gastroenteritis
Meckel's diverticulum
Solitary colon ulcer
Infectious
Helicobacter pylori
Hookworm
Strongyloidiasis
Ascariasis
Tuberculous enterocolitis
Amebiasis
Vascular
Angiodysplasia and vascular ectasias
Gastroesophageal varices
Congestive gastropathy
Hemangiomas
Tumors and Neoplastic
Polyps
Lymphoma
Leiomyoma
Lipoma
Carcinoma
Drugs
Salicylates
Other nonsteroidal anti-inflammatory drugs
Extragastrointestinal
Hemoptysis
Epistaxis
Oropharyngeal bleeding
Artifactual
Hematuria
Menstrual bleeding
Nonspecific Hemoccult test positivity
Miscellaneous
Long-distance running
Coagulopathies
Irritation from nasogastric or gastrostomy tubes
Factitial

Adapted, with permission, from Olson, A.D., and A.C. Hillemeier. Gastrointestinal hemorrhage. *In* Wyllie R., and J.S. Hyams (eds.). Pediatric Gastrointestinal Disease. Philadelphia, W.B. Saunders, 1993, p. 262.

tags, skin breakdown, or evidence of trauma. A digital rectal examination should be performed, and the following questions should be asked: Is a large, hard mass of stool or a polyp palpable? What does the stool look like? Is the blood fresh or denatured? The physician should also check for any evidence of child abuse.

In addition, patients should be examined for any rashes, petechiae, purpura, buccal mucosal discolorations, hemangiomas, telangiectasias, or other vascular lesions that suggest inflammatory bowel disease, Henoch-Schönlein purpura, Peutz-Jeghers polyposis syndrome, or coagulopathy. The presence of scars, which suggest prior surgery, should also be determined.

Laboratory Tests

Depending on the clinical scenario, a type and cross-match, CBC, platelet count, reticulocyte count, Coombs' test, PT, PTT, aspartate aminotransferase, alanine aminotransferase, BUN, and creatinine should be obtained. Gastric contents and stool should be checked for occult blood using the appropriate diagnostic test. Stool may be sent for culture and microscopic examination for leukocytes, ova, and parasites.

Hemoccult and **Hematest** are both used to detect blood in stool. A thin smear of stool is applied to the test pad, and a few drops of developing solution are then added. Hemoglobin and its derivatives (oxyhemoglobin, methemoglobin, reduced hemoglobin, carboxyhemoglobin), when exposed to the hydrogen peroxide developer, catalytically oxidize the guaiac or orthotolidine substrates that are impregnated in pads, producing a color change in the substrate, a positive reaction. **Gastroccult** is based on the same principles and uses guaiac as the substrate, but is more reliable at the low pHs encountered in the stomach.

Blood from the GI tract of newborns should be checked using the **Apt-Downey test,** which detects blood of maternal origin. When 1% sodium hydroxide is added to blood, adult hemoglobin is reduced to a rusty, brownish-yellow color, signifying the presence of maternal blood. Fetal hemoglobin, being much more resistant to denaturization, does not undergo any color change and remains pink or bright red. The substance tested must be grossly bloody (red) and not denatured (e.g., coffee-ground emesis or tarry stools, in which the oxyhemoglobin has already been converted to hematin).

Ingested substances that may produce false-positive results include rare, red meat and peroxidase-containing fruits and vegetables such as broccoli, radishes, cauliflower, cantaloupe, and turnips. Ascorbic acid (vitamin C) and hemoglobin that has been changed to porphyrin by intestinal bacteria may give false-negative results.

Questions: Gastrointestinal Bleeding

- Is the blood loss acute or chronic?
- What is the color and quantity of the blood in the stool or emesis?
- What symptoms preceded the episode of GI bleeding?
- Does the child have a history of vomiting, diarrhea, fever, ill contacts, or travel that may suggest an infectious etiology?
- Has the child experienced abdominal pain?
- Has the child suffered any trauma recently?
- Has the child ingested any substances that might irritate the GI tract such as NSAIDs, steroids, tetracycline, caustic materials, or foreign bodies?
- Does the child have a history of straining with stooling?
- Has there been recurrent retching or forceful emesis, which could cause a Mallory-Weiss tear?
- Does the child have a history of increased stool frequency, weight loss, poor weight gain, or arthritis?
- Do any family members have a history of inflammatory bowel disease?
- Does the child have risk factors for portal hypertension such as a history of umbilical venous catheterization or liver disease?

Diagnostic Studies

If the source of bleeding remains unclear after a complete history and thorough physical examination, a nasogastric (NG) tube should be inserted and the gastric contents aspirated. NG tubes are generally better tolerated than orogastric tubes. The appropriate tube size depends on the size of the child. The largest bore tube that can be tolerated should be used, and the physician should be careful not to induce trauma. Small-bore tubes may suffice for diagnosis, but they obstruct easily and are not useful in removing larger clots. The presence of esophageal varices is not a contraindication to passing an NG tube. Gastric contents are aspirated with a large syringe.

Gastric lavage not only helps localize the site of hemorrhage but also aids in clearing the stomach of blood and clots prior to endoscopic evaluation. In patients with liver disease, it may prevent encephalopathy by avoiding hyperammonemia. Water is as effective as saline for lavage and should be used at room temperature. Cold or iced solutions offer no advantage and may induce hypothermia; large amounts of lavage fluid pass into the intestine and may lower the core temperature. Antacids are not used for lavage, because they interfere with endoscopic evaluation and do not stop bleeding.

If the aspirate does not show blood, the NG tube can be removed. If the aspirate contains bright red blood or coffee-ground material, however, the NG tube may be left in place to monitor ongoing bleeding. Tests of the NG aspirate for the presence of occult blood are rarely useful, because vomiting alone or trauma induced during passage of the NG tube can produce a positive test in the absence of true hemorrhage.

An aspirate showing blood is highly specific for upper tract bleeding. **Esophagogastroduodenoscopy** using flexible endoscopes, if performed within the first 24 hours, identifies the source of bleeding in approximately 90% of cases. Radiologic studies are not sufficiently sensitive for detection of superficial lesions such as esophagitis, gastritis, and Mallory-Weiss tears. When these studies fail to define the site of hemorrhage and the bleeding is massive (> 0.5 mL/min), **arteriography** or an **erythrocyte-labeled technetium-99m (Tc=99m) pertechnetate scan** (tagged RBC scan) should be performed to detect lesions located distal to the ligament of Treitz. These lesions may include hepatic artery aneurysms, hematobilia occurring after trauma, duplication cysts, arteriovenous malformations, and hemangiomas.

A negative aspirate suggests lower GI tract bleeding but does not rule out an upper tract source that is no longer bleeding or a duodenal lesion in which the blood has not refluxed back through the pylorus. **Careful visual inspection** of the anus, **digital examination,** and **proctosigmoidoscopy** reveal the site of lower tract bleeding about 80% of the time.

In the remainder of cases, the diagnosis is made on the basis of **colonoscopy, barium enema,** or **Meckel's scan.** When bright red blood covers the outside of the stool, the source is usually anorectal, such as a fissure, a distal polyp, or proctitis. The cathartic effect of blood on the GI tract can cause rapid transit in children,

however, resulting in bright red blood from an upper GI bleed. Darker blood or blood mixed with the stool suggests a more proximal origin. Melena implies a bleeding site proximal to the ligament of Treitz. Anal fissures, juvenile polyps, and nodular lymphoid hyperplasia are usually associated with minimal bleeding, whereas significant blood loss may be seen with Meckel's diverticulum, a duplication cyst, or an autoamputated polyp. **Plain films** are used to rule out bowel obstruction and perforation. A **barium enema** may be both diagnostic and therapeutic if intussusception is suspected. It can also identify malrotations with secondary intestinal volvulus. In Meckel's scan, intravenously injected Tc-99m pertechnetate loosely binds to plasma proteins and accumulates in functional gastric mucosa, including the ectopic mucosa, which is present in the majority of children with bleeding from Meckel's diverticula. If the diagnosis remains unclear, arteriography or laparotomy may be indicated.

MANAGEMENT

Attention must be focused on stabilizing children prior to initiation of an extensive diagnostic workup. Vigorous cardiovascular resuscitation is essential for orthostatic hypotension, which indicates massive blood loss. Good intravenous access should be established immediately with at least two large-bore lines. Placement of a central venous catheter should be considered. Intravascular volume expansion can be achieved using normal saline, lactated Ringer's solution, whole blood, or a combination of packed red blood cells and fresh-frozen plasma (10–20 mL/kg for 10–20 minutes). In life-threatening circumstances, unmatched blood products are given in an effort to keep patients alive long enough to stop the bleeding.

Once the bleeding has stopped, **packed cells** may be given alone to return oxygen-carrying capacity to normal. Heart rate, blood pressure, and central venous pressure should be carefully monitored to avoid fluid overload. Patients who are at risk for further bleeding should be in a setting where vital signs can be monitored continuously. Coagulopathy should be corrected with **fresh-frozen plasma, platelets,** or **vitamin K** (about 1 mg/yr of age, to a maximum of 10 mg). Hypoxia exacerbates the systemic effects of poor perfusion and resultant metabolic acidosis. All patients suspected of having a massive bleed should receive **supplemental oxygen.** Intubation and ventilator support should be considered. After an acute hemorrhage, equilibration of the hematocrit may take 24 to 72 hours or more, and initial values may not be an accurate reflection of blood volume.

Consultation with the pediatric surgeon and the pediatric gastroenterologist should be sought from the early moments of the evaluation. Although only few conditions require surgery (e.g., Hirschsprung's disease, Meckel's diverticulum), operative procedures should be considered for children who are bleeding severely or for those with undiagnosed, persistent bleeding. The gastroenterologist may assist in diagnosing the condition causing the bleeding by performing endoscopic studies of the upper and lower GI tract. Methods such as injection of sclerosant solutions or use of thermal or electrical coagulation allow the gastroenterologist to stop the bleeding from esophageal varices or peptic ulcers.

PROGNOSIS

Prognosis for infants and children with GI bleeding depends on the condition causing the bleeding. Early, aggressive treatment of the consequences of blood loss is essential to decreasing morbidity and mortality.

Case Resolution

The young child in the case history with episodic, painless rectal bleeding has a juvenile polyp. No associated nausea or vomiting is present. The polyp is palpable on digital rectal examination. Full colonoscopy and therapeu-

tic polypectomy are performed. In addition, the polyp is evaluated for dysplasia, although the majority of polyps found in children are benign. He is referred to a pediatric gastroenterologist.

Selected Readings

Ament, M. E. Diagnosis and management of upper gastrointestinal tract bleeding in the pediatric patient. Pediatr. Rev. 12:107–116, 1990.

Berry, R., and J. Perrault. Gastrointestinal bleeding. *In* Walker and Durie (eds.). Pediatric Gastrointestinal Disease. Philadelphia, B. C. Decker, 1991.

Gonzalez-Peralta, R. P., and J. M. Andres. Polyps and polyposis syndromes. *In* Wyllie, R., and J. S. Hyams (eds.). Pediatric Gastrointestinal Disease. Philadelphia, W. B. Saunders, 1993.

Olson, A. D., and A. C. Hillemeier. Gastrointestinal hemorrhage. *In* Wyllie, R. and J. S. Hyams (eds.). Pediatric Gastrointestinal Disease. Philadelphia, W. B. Saunders, 1993.

Silber, G. Lower gastrointestinal bleeding. Pediatr. Rev. 12:89–93, 1990.

CHAPTER 81

DIARRHEA

Carol D. Berkowitz, M.D.

H$_x$ An eight-month-old male infant is evaluated for a two-day history of fever and blood-streaked, mucus-laden stools. His appetite is reduced, and he is only taking sips of diluted apple juice. He has had a single episode of vomiting. There are no ill contacts. On examination, the patient is irritable with a temperature of 102.2° F (39.0° C), a pulse of 180, a respiratory rate of 58, and a blood pressure of 90/65. The mucous membranes are dry, the fontanelle is depressed, and the skin turgor is reduced. The abdomen is somewhat scaphoid, and bowel sounds are active.

Questions

1. What are the two major categories of diarrhea?
2. What are the common infectious agents that cause diarrhea in infants and children?
3. What are the characteristics of diarrheal stools caused by different etiologies?
4. What conditions lead to prolonged diarrhea in infants and children?
5. How is diarrhea managed in infants and children?

The word "diarrhea" is derived from Greek and means "to flow through." The disorder is characterized by a greater volume of stool, which is associated with a looser consistency and an increased frequency of

stooling. The frequency and consistency of stooling vary from individual to individual. Under normal conditions, stooling frequency is related to genetic factors of muscle function and GI motility. Wide variations in stooling frequency may be seen under certain conditions such as breast-feeding. Some breast-fed infants have a bowel movement every one to two weeks, whereas others may pass stool 12 to 15 times a day.

Diarrhea has several causes, which include infection, inflammation, and exposure to drugs and hormones that affect the absorption of water from the small and large intestines.

EPIDEMIOLOGY

Diarrheal illnesses are very common both throughout the world and in the United States, where diarrhea resulting from acute gastroenteritis is second in frequency only to URIs. An estimated five million children in Latin America, Asia, and Africa die annually from dehydration secondary to diarrhea. In contrast, approximately 500 children die from this condition in the United States each year. These children often come from lower socioeconomic classes.

In the United States, each child experiences an average of 0.9 episodes of diarrhea per year unless enrolled in a daycare facility. In that case, the number increases to up to 4.5 episodes per year, a figure similar to that of children in developing nations. The leading cause of diarrhea in children in developing nations is infection with viruses, bacteria, or parasites. The severity of the infection is influenced by the underlying state of nutrition. An episode of acute gastroenteritis can precipitate severe malnutrition in marginally intact children.

The major route of spread of diarrheal infections is fecal-oral. In developing nations, poor sanitation and contaminated drinking water perpetuate the problem. In the United States, contaminated food supply such as the contamination of eggs and poultry with *Salmonella* is associated with the spread of bacterial gastroenteritis. Puppies have been found to be a reservoir of *Campylobacter* spp.

CLINICAL PRESENTATION

Children with diarrhea present with complaints of frequent, watery stools, which may contain blood or mucus. Affected children may have associated symptoms, including fever, vomiting, bloating, and abdominal pain. Signs and symptoms of dehydration such as decreased skin turgor, dry mucous membranes, depressed fontanelle, diminished tearing, and tachycardia may be present. Persistent diarrhea may be associated with weight loss and failure to gain weight at an appropriate rate (D_x Box).

PATHOPHYSIOLOGY

The consistency of stool depends on the stool's water content. The movement of water into the lumen of the gut is always related to the movement of electrolytes, because no active transport of water occurs. The absorption of water is associated with the active transport of sodium, and the secretion of water is associated with the active transport of potassium. Four different systems influence these processes: (1) the enteric nervous system; (2) the endocrine system; (3) the immune system; and (4) extrinsic factors such as bacterial enterotoxins, drugs, and chemicals. These four systems work by changing the cellular concentration of one or more messengers: cyclic AMP, cyclic GMP, or ionized divalent calcium ion. Medications to counteract diarrhea usually inhibit one of these messengers.

In all cases, diarrhea results when the absorptive capacity of the colon is exceeded. Normal infants

excrete 5 to 10 g/kg of stool per day, of which 60 to 95% is water. Adults pass a total of 100 to 200 g of stool per day. Therefore, the infant colon is already functioning near its absorptive capacity. In cases of certain infections such as rotavirus or enterotoxic *Escherichia coli*, fluid secretion into the lumen of the gut may increase 20-fold.

Diarrhea can be divided into two major categories: osmotic (malabsorptive) and secretory. **Osmotic diarrhea** may be characterized as general or specific. In general osmotic diarrhea, many components of the diet are not absorbed, whereas in specific osmotic diarrhea, certain substances such as lactose are not absorbed. These failures may be related to reduced absorptive surface or absorptive capacity. Infection with certain agents, such as rotaviruses, or bacteria (*Shigella, Salmonella,* or *Campylobacter*) may damage the villous structure of the small intestine and lead to osmotic diarrhea. Simply speaking, stooling stops with the cessation of eating in cases of osmotic diarrhea.

Secretory diarrhea occurs when the bowel continues to secrete water and electrolytes. This type of diarrhea is believed to be related to the presence of intraluminal substances, which are referred to as secretagogues. The best known of these secretagogues are bacterial toxins such as those associated with infection with *E. coli,* one cause of traveler's diarrhea, and *Vibrio comma,* the cause of cholera. In addition, some chemicals, including certain laxatives, dihydroxy bile salts, and long-chain fatty acids, produce secretory diarrhea. Classically, the stooling of secretory diarrhea continues even with cessation of eating.

In reality, both secretory and osmotic components are present in many cases of diarrhea. If the malabsorption of osmotic diarrhea is present, and bile salts or fatty acids remain in the lumen of the gut, their presence may lead to secretory diarrhea. Secretory diarrhea is particularly common in the developing nations of the world, where it is related to infection with organisms such as enterotoxin *E. coli* and *Vibrio comma*. In the United States, vasoactive intestinal peptide-secreting tumors such as ganglioneuroma and neuroblastoma must be considered in the diagnosis.

Steatorrhea refers to the presence of fat in the stools. Approximately 95% of the fat content of food should be absorbed. In infants under the age of 12 months, 10 to 15% of ingested fat may appear in the stool. Fat malabsorption occurs with problems of the small intestine, including giardiasis; liver; and pancreas. Steatorrhea is not related to colonic problems. It may occur in cases of acute gastroenteritis, where the brush border of the small intestine is affected. Fat in the stool is associated with both osmotic diarrhea and secretory diarrhea because the presence of long-chain fatty acids promotes the secretion of chloride and accompanying water.

DIFFERENTIAL DIAGNOSIS

Acute Diarrhea

The major cause of diarrhea in children and infants is related to **acute gastroenteritis,** most commonly with a

D_x Diarrhea

- Liquid stools
- Frequent stools
- Blood in stool
- Mucus in stool
- Fever
- Poor weight gain or weight loss
- Dehydration
- Vomiting
- Abdominal pain

viral infection. The most common virus is rotavirus, which usually occurs during the winter months. This has been referred to as "winter vomiting syndrome." Infants present with an antecedent history of mild upper respiratory symptoms, followed by fever and vomiting. Watery diarrhea, which is usually free of blood or mucus, then occurs. About 10% of infected infants have signs of otitis media. Dehydration may also occur with rotavirus infection. It is typically mildly hypernatremic, with serum sodium values about 150 mEq/L. In the summer months, enteroviral infections may produce similar pathology.

The most common **bacterial agents** associated with gastroenteritis in the United States are *Shigella, Salmonella,* and *Campylobacter.* Both *Shigella* and *Campylobacter* produce signs of colitis, with blood and mucus in the stools. Patients are usually febrile. As a rule, children infected with *Shigella* are sicker, with higher levels of fever and more marked leukocytosis. In addition, they are particularly prone to seizures. Infection with *Salmonella* may also be associated with high fever. Stools may be mucus-laden, and inflammation of the small intestine may be evident. Parasitic infections particularly with *Giardia lamblia, Entamoeba histolytica,* and *Cryptosporidium* may be associated with diarrhea and may follow a more protracted course. Infestation with these organisms does not usually result in fever.

Infectious conditions that do not affect the GI tract may also be associated with diarrhea. **Parenteral or secondary gastroenteritis** occurs with infections of the middle ear and urine. Likewise, infectious hepatitis may be associated with diarrhea and right upper quadrant tenderness.

Other conditions may also result in diarrhea. In newborns, infection with *E. coli* may produce epidemic outbreaks of large, explosive watery, green stools without blood. These outbreaks may result in closure of newborn nurseries. Watery stools may herald the onset of **necrotizing enterocolitis** (NEC); blood is usually present, however. NEC most often affects preterm infants with respiratory distress syndrome. The mechanism of disease production appears to be related to hypoxia of the intestinal mucosa. Enterocolitis may also occur in infants with Hirschsprung's disease. Bloody stools and air in the bowel wall, or pneumatosis intestinales, are the hallmarks of the disorder. Adrenal insufficiency, as well as certain inborn errors of metabolism such as galactosemia may lead to diarrhea. In general, other symptoms such as vomiting occur. Infants may present in shock because of hypovolemia related to dehydration.

Food intolerance may result in diarrhea in infants as well as in older children. Overfeeding or the ingestion of large quantities of fruit juices, dried fruits, or sorbitol-containing products can produce an osmotic diarrhea. Food allergies may also be associated with malabsorption.

In infants, cow protein intolerance can produce diarrhea, steatorrhea, growth retardation, anemia, hypoproteinemia, edema, respiratory symptoms, eczema, eosinophilia, and elevated levels of immunoglobulin E (IgE). Because up to 25% of cow protein-allergic children are also soy protein-allergic, symptoms of diarrhea may not abate when soy formula is offered. However, soy formula does help infants with certain disaccharidase deficiencies, such as lactase deficiency. Although lactose intolerance rarely occurs as a congenital deficiency, it is reported more frequently as a transitory condition following a bout of acute gastroenteritis, when the brush border of the small intestine has been disrupted. Acquired lactase deficiency is fairly common, especially in certain racial groups; it is reported in 10% of Caucasians, 70 to 80% of African Americans, and 90% of Asians. The disorder is associated with diarrhea, cramping, bloating, and abdominal pain after consumption of lactose. The stool has an acid pH, floats because it contains air, and is positive for reducing substances.

Chronic Diarrhea

Chronic diarrhea occurs when symptoms last longer than two weeks. Most cases of acute gastroenteritis resolve within two to five days. Four major conditions are associated with chronic diarrhea without evidence of malabsorption.

Infants and children may have a protracted course of loose stools **following** an episode of **acute gastroenteritis.** In most cases, no cause for the diarrhea can be detected, but infestation with *Cryptosporidium* or *E. coli* may be the source of the problem. The possibility of infection with HIV should be considered in infants and children with protracted diarrhea, especially in geographic areas where disease prevalence is high (see Chapter 106, Pediatric HIV). Certain children with acute diarrhea have such a modified diet (e.g., clear fluids) that they develop starvation stools. These slimy, dark green or golden stools represent succus entericus, the secretion of the small intestine. Starvation stools do not have a fecal odor.

Inflammatory bowel disease, which occurs more commonly in older children and adolescents, is associated with chronic diarrhea. Ulcerative colitis involves inflammation of the mucosa and submucosa with the formation of abscesses. Fever, weight loss, and anorexia are often present. Diarrhea is the hallmark of the disease, and patients experience tenesmus as well as mucus-laden and bloody stools. Evidence of the disease is present on sigmoidoscopy in 95% of affected patients.

Crohn's disease, or regional enteritis, may also lead to chronic diarrhea, although lower abdominal pain relieved by defecation may be a more prominent part of the medical history. Affected individuals frequently experience extraintestinal manifestations of the disease, such as fever, anorexia, weight loss or growth retardation, recurrent stomatitis, uveitis, arthralgia and arthritis, and clubbing. Perianal disease, such as fistulas, may be noted in 70% of patients.

Irritable colon syndrome, which occurs in infants and children between the ages of six months and three years, also results in chronic diarrhea. No stooling during the night, at least a partially formed first stool in the morning, and increased stooling frequency during the day is the classic history. Stooling tends to occur after each meal, suggesting a prominent gastrocolic reflex. Children may have 3 to 10 stools per day, which may be mucus-laden. Alternating periods of constipation may occur. Affected children appear well throughout this illness, and no evidence of weight loss, growth impairment, fever, leukocytosis, steatorrhea, or protein malabsorption is evident. Their appetite remains good. Treatment of this type of chronic diarrhea involves the use of a high-residue diet to add bulk to the stool and thereby prevent small, frequent stools.

Other conditions that lead to chronic diarrhea include intestinal polyposis and the use of certain medications, such as antibiotics, and heavy metals, such as iron. Intestinal polyposis is associated with a history of cramping, and other family members may be affected.

Chronic diarrhea may also be associated with malabsorption. The two most common conditions of malabsorptive chronic diarrhea are cystic fibrosis and celiac disease or gluten enteropathy.

Newborns with **cystic fibrosis** may present with meconium ileus or rarely with acute appendicitis. Children with this disease tend to have voracious appetites because the pylorus fails to contract and food rapidly passes from the stomach into the duodenum. Contraction of the pylorus occurs secondary to the release of enterogastrone, whose secretion depends on the presence of free fatty acids. Children with cystic fibrosis have pancreatic insufficiency and do not produce lipase. Hence, they do not experience a surge in free fatty acids in the serum. Malabsorption occurs because the body fails to digest food effectively. Weight gain is therefore poor. Stools are large, bulky, and foul-smelling secondary to the bacterial overgrowth related to fat and protein malabsorption. Isolated GI complaints are reported in 10 to 15% of patients with cystic fibrosis, but most affected children are also prone to pulmonary infections. Rectal prolapse is another complication.

Celiac disease is related to an allergy to the gliadin portion of the wheat protein, gluten. Characteristically, villous flattening is apparent on small intestinal biopsy. This flattening restricts the absorptive capacity of the intestine and leads to malabsorption. Children with celiac disease have protuberant abdomens, appear bloated, and are frequently irritable because of GI discomfort. Their rate of growth is retarded. Symptoms usually appear when wheat is introduced into the diet, usually between the ages of 6 and 12 months. Stools are mushy, bulky, and foul-smelling. Fat content in the stool may be two to three times the normal level.

EVALUATION

History

A careful history should be obtained (Questions Box).

Physical Examination

Children should be assessed for the presence of dehydration as evidenced by altered vital signs, decreased skin turgor, a sunken fontanelle, dry mucous membranes, and reduced tearing. Evidence of growth retardation should be determined by assessing the growth parameters, particularly weight. Failure to gain weight over a period of months signifies a chronic diarrheal condition with malabsorption.

Laboratory Tests

Stool assessment, a major component of the evaluation, involves four steps. First, the stool is evaluated for its quantity as well as its gross appearance. Undigested pieces of fruits and vegetables in the stool of toddlers are often a sign of poor chewing. Small, threadlike bodies that resemble worms are concretions of bile and are common in the stool of infants. The change in stool volume with fasting can also be checked. Reduced volume in the face of fasting is consistent with osmotic diarrhea.

Second, the stool is subjected to chemical and microscopic analyses to detect the presence of unabsorbed nutrients such as carbohydrates and fats. The presence of carbohydrates may be detected using a small amount of stool liquefied in about one milliliter of water. A Clinitest tablet is added to the sample, and a change in color from blue to green or orange is indicative of the presence of undigested carbohydrate. If the main source of dietary sugar is sucrose, as determined by the history, the specimen must be hydrolyzed by heating with hydrochloric acid. If the specimen sits around for too long a time, the presence of bacteria in the stool may break down the carbohydrate and lead to a false-negative result. The presence of fat can be determined both qualitatively and quantitatively. The stool may be examined under a microscope with just water or using a Sudan or Carmine red stain. If there are 10 or more globules of fat per high-power field, a quantitative fat analysis over a three-day period should be undertaken. Ten percent of children with an abnormal stool fat on microscopic assessment have a normal three-day quantitative stool fat value.

Third, the stool is examined for the presence of blood and leukocytes. Blood may be present in the stool but

---

Questions: Diarrhea

- How long has the diarrhea been present?
- How frequent is the stooling?
- What is the consistency of the stools?
- Is stooling related to eating, which is a sign of osmotic diarrhea, or does it occur even if the child does not eat, which is a sign of secretory diarrhea?
- Do the stools contain any blood or mucus, which suggests a bacterial or parasitic infection?
- Is the child febrile?
- Does the child have any symptoms associated with the stooling problems?
- Does the child have a recent history of travel or exposure to animals?
- Is anyone at home ill?
- Has the child experienced any change in the frequency of urination, which is an important measure of the state of hydration?
- What is the child's diet now? What has it been?

originates from excoriations in the diaper area rather than from the GI tract. To assess for leukocytes in the stool, the mucous component of the stool should be smeared on a glass slide and stained with methylene blue. More than two to four leukocytes per high-power field is abnormal and suggests a bacterial infection. A stool specimen should be submitted for culture and may be evaluated for ova and parasites.

Fourth, the stool is assessed for levels of sodium and potassium and for stool osmolality. These values may be helpful in distinguishing between osmotic and secretory diarrhea.

Additional studies, especially in the face of dehydration or fever, include serum electrolytes, CBC, urinalysis, and urine culture. Sigmoidoscopy or barium enema should be considered after consultation with a gastroenterologist if inflammatory bowel disease or familial polyposis is suspected.

MANAGEMENT

Initial management of children with gastroenteritis involves **adequate hydration and replacement of any fluid or electrolyte deficits.** Bolus therapy may be necessary in children with significant dehydration. Children with significant dehydration may require admission to the hospital and the administration of intravenous fluids. Less severely affected children may be managed as outpatients using oral rehydrating solutions such as Pedialyte or Ricelyte. Alternatively, parents can be advised to make oral rehydrating solutions by using water (1 liter), sugar (4–8 teaspoons), and salt (½ teaspoon).

Dietary manipulation in the treatment of diarrhea is somewhat controversial. Traditionally, affected children have been placed on clear fluids for one or two days, with a gradual return to a more regular diet with time. A **BRAT diet** (**b**ananas, **r**ice or rice cereal, **a**pplesauce, **t**ea or toast) was often recommended because of the intrinsic binding properties of the particular food. Recent studies recommend a full resumption of a normal diet, including dairy products, as the way to ensure adequate nutrition during the acute illness.

Antimicrobial therapy is indicated for infection with certain pathogens such as *Campylobacter*, *E. histolytica*, *G. lamblia*, and *Shigella*. Antimicrobial agents are used to treat *Salmonella* infection in certain populations such as neonates, immunodeficient children, and children with sickle cell anemia. **Antidiarrheal agents** are not usually recommended for the management of diarrhea in children. Diarrhea is believed to be the body's way of eliminating a toxic substance that has been ingested. In addition, the diarrhea often progresses in spite of the medication, which has its most binding effect after the illness has subsided, leading to constipation.

Children with chronic diarrhea secondary to a specific condition should be managed as dictated by the particular disorder.

PROGNOSIS

Most cases of diarrhea in infants and children in the United States are self-limited and resolve without problems. More chronic cases may lead to malnutrition. Enteral feedings or hyperalimentation may be used to ensure a good outcome. Some children require consultation with a pediatric gastroenterologist.

Case Resolution

In the case history, the presence of blood and mucus in the stools suggests a bacterial etiology. The stool should be examined microscopically for the presence of leukocytes using methylene blue. Their presence supports a bacterial etiology. A stool specimen as well as a blood specimen should be sent for culture. Because the infant appears dehydrated (i.e., sunken fontanelle, poor skin turgor, tachycardia), admission to the hospital should be considered to allow for rehydration and the administration of parenteral antibiotics.

Selected Readings

Cohen, M. B. Etiology and mechanisms of acute infectious diarrhea in infants in the United States. J. Pediatr. 118:534–539, 1991.

Huicho, L., and D. Sanchez. Occult blood and fecal leukocytes as screening tests in childhood infectious diarrhea. An old problem revisited. Pediatr. Infect. Dis. J. 12:474–477, 1993.

Murphy, M. S., and W. A. Walker. Celiac disease. Pediatr. Rev. 12:325–330, 1991.

O'Gorman, M., and A. M. Lake. Chronic inflammatory bowel disease in childhood. Pediatr. Rev. 14:475–480, 1993.

Rhodes, J. M., and D. W. Powell. Diarrhea. In Walker, W. A., et al (eds.). Pediatric Gastrointestinal Disease. Philadelphia, B. C. Decker, 1991, pp. 62–76.

Richards, L., M. Claeson, and N. E. Pierce. Management of acute diarrhea in children: lessons learned. Pediatr. Infect. Dis. J. 12:5–9, 1993.

Sondheimer, J. M. Office stool examination: a practical guide. Contemp. Pediatr. (Supplement to Residents):5–14, 1994.

CHAPTER 82

CONSTIPATION

Carol D. Berkowitz, M.D.

Hx   A five-month-old infant is brought to the office for a routine examination by his mother, who complains that her son is constipated. He grunts with each bowel movement, and his face turns bright red. He has soft bowel movements every five days. The infant is breast-feeding and has not yet started other foods. The mother reports that she and her husband are regular and have bowel movements every day.

On examination, the infant's vital signs are normal, and the infant is at the 75th percentile in height and weight. The remainder of the physical examination, including a visual inspection of the anal area, is normal.

Questions

1. What is the definition of constipation?
2. How is the stooling pattern of infants related to their diet?
3. What diseases and medical conditions may be associated with constipation in infants and children?
4. What familial factors relate to constipation?
5. How is routine functional constipation managed?

Constipation refers to the ease of passage of stool. In individuals with constipation, stools are dry, hard, and difficult to pass. Reduced frequency of stooling is sometimes characteristic of constipation, but infrequent passage of soft stool is not considered constipation.

Many factors influence the frequency of stooling in normal children, including familial patterns of intestinal motility and sensitivity, diet, medication, degree of hydration, and disease. In addition, children's reaction to the passage of stool may be misinterpreted as a sign of constipation when in fact it simply represents their physiologic effort to facilitate the passage of stool. Parent-child interactions around the time of toilet training may be associated with resistance on the part of children, resulting in withholding of stool and functional constipation. Assessment of the etiology of constipation requires a careful medical history to determine the age of onset of the symptoms and the presence of contributing factors.

EPIDEMIOLOGY

Complaints related to constipation or fecal soiling account for 3% of all outpatient visits and 10 to 25% of visits to gastroenterologists. The normal frequency of stooling ranges widely. Many people do not have a bowel movement on a daily basis and are not constipated. Ninety-five percent of preschool children have bowel movements every other day, every day, or two or three times a day. The average amount of the stool is 5 to 10 g/kg/day, with most adults excreting about 200 g of stool per day. Transit time increases with age, which means that the frequency of stooling decreases as one gets older (Table 82–1). Longer transit times are associated with harder, drier stools that may lead to bleeding and subsequent withholding of stool.

CLINICAL PRESENTATION

Many infants and children who are constipated present with complaints of infrequent stooling (D$_x$ Box). Some parents are concerned that facial grimacing and grunting during defecation are indicative of constipation in infants. Fecal soiling, which represents overflow incontinence, may also occur in some constipated children. About 60% of constipated children experience recurrent abdominal pain. Poor appetite and poor growth may also be noted secondary to maintenance of a sense of fullness from the feces-filled colon. Some children maintain a withholding posture, where they keep their legs clamped together in an effort to suppress the urge to defecate (Fig. 82–1).

PATHOPHYSIOLOGY

To understand the pathophysiology of constipation, the mechanics of the normal passage of stool must be understood (Fig. 82–2). The rectum is the sensing organ that initiates the process of defecation. As stool moves from the sigmoid colon into the rectum, pressure is exerted on both the walls of the rectum and the rectal valves. This pressure initiates a nervous impulse that triggers relaxation of the internal anal sphincter, which is sensed as urgency and the need to defecate. If it is convenient, defecation occurs. If it is not convenient, the urge to defecate is consciously repressed by voluntary contraction of the external anal sphincter. Subconscious reflex inhibition as well as repression by the contraction of the puborectalis muscle may be involved. Colonic peristalsis may move stool into the

TABLE 82–1. Intestinal Transit Time in Infants and Children

Age	Transit Time
1–3 months	8.5 hours
4–24 months	16 hours
3–13 years	26 hours

Dx   Constipation

- Hard, dry stools
- Infrequent stooling
- Abdominal pain
- Hematochezia (bleeding with stooling)
- Painful defecation
- Anorexia
- Fecal soiling

---

anal canal. Voluntary contraction of the somatic abdominal musculature increases intra-abdominal pressure and facilitates expulsion of stool.

If the urge to defecate has been suppressed, defecation is sometimes difficult. This is an important factor in the pathogenesis of constipation in some school-age children who have an urge to defecate during the school day. These children choose not to go to the restroom for several reasons related to school bathrooms.

A similar phenomenon occurs during toilet training and may lead to chronic functional constipation. In an attempt to maintain independence and a sense of control, children withhold stool. The stool then becomes harder and drier, and attempts to defecate at a later time are associated with pain. This leads to further withholding, and a vicious cycle develops. To accommodate retained stool, the rectum enlarges and loses its propulsive ability. A decrease in sensory sensitivity and subsequent stool retention result.

Other factors may lead to transitory constipation. These include dietary changes; rectal fissures; medications such as aspirin and codeine; intercurrent illness, especially those associated with dehydration such as pharyngitis and URIs; and environmental changes such as vacation travel, a new home or school, birth of a sibling, and family stress. Changes in routine may also contribute to changes in stooling patterns.

Some families are predisposed to constipation. Physiologic factors are believed to be related to stooling difficulties. Absorption of water may be increased, leading to drier, harder stools. In other cases, the bowel is unusually long or poorly motile. In some families, sensitivity to critical rectal volumes appears to be decreased, or particularly large rectal volumes are necessary for initiation of the process of defecation.

Constipation may be related to disorders of innervation of the intestine, thereby not allowing for the normal peristaltic wave. Hirschsprung's disease, a condition reported in 1 in 5000 individuals, involves absence of ganglion cells from the distal rectum and other areas of the more proximal large intestine.

DIFFERENTIAL DIAGNOSIS

The differential diagnosis of constipation is age-related and depends on assessment of the factors that have led to the conclusion that constipation is occurring. For example, infrequent though soft stools are common and normal in breast-fed infants who may have initially experienced frequent, watery stools. This

change in stooling may be misinterpreted as constipation. Similarly, older children may defecate every three to four days and pass soft-formed stools. This is not constipation.

Four conditions should be considered in the differential diagnosis of constipation in infants under the age of six months.

1. **Hirschsprung's disease** may be suspected in young infants in whom the initial passage of meconium has been delayed over 24 hours. Early recognition of this condition may prevent the development of enterocolitis and toxic megacolon, two conditions with high morbidity and mortality. Hirschsprung's disease may not be diagnosed until children are older (age 5–6 years), however.

2. **Hypothyroidism** is also associated with constipation. Infants with hypothyroidism secondary to hypopituitarism are not diagnosed through the newborn screening process because of normal levels of thyroid-stimulating hormone. These children may either appear clinically normal or display some of the features of hypothyroidism (e.g., large anterior and posterior fontanelles; umbilical hernia; coarse facies; large, protruding tongue).

3. **Imperforate anus** can also lead to constipation. Some infants with imperforate anus with perineal fistula may not be recognized immediately in the

FIGURE 82–1. *Child exhibiting retentive posture.*

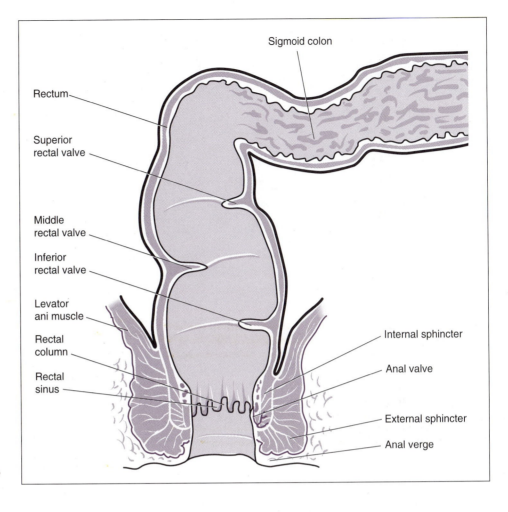

FIGURE 82–2. *Diagram of anus, rectum, and sigmoid colon.*

newborn period because of the subtlety of the condition. These infants may have an anteriorly displaced anus, which does not allow for the easy egress of stool.

4. **Infantile botulism** may result in constipation in infants who are usually between the ages of six weeks and six months. These infants are most often breast-fed or have a history of exposure to honey, corn syrup, or home-grown herbal teas. In addition to constipation, these infants are often febrile, hypotonic, and lethargic. They may be admitted to rule out sepsis. Clinical appearance, with flattened facies and an inability to smile or to gaze away from a light shined directly in the eye, is a clue to diagnosis. Care should be exercised when managing these infants because the administration of gentamicin as part of a rule-out sepsis regimen may potentiate the neuromuscular blockade of the botulinum toxin and precipitate respiratory arrest.

Constipation that begins prior to toilet training indicates possible organic etiology such as **Hirschsprung's disease** or **pseudo-obstruction**. Pseudo-obstruction may also present in older children, who may have a history of abdominal distention, pain, and intestinal paresis. The onset of constipation around the time of toilet training, when stooling has been normal in the past, suggests functional constipation.

Constipation may develop in some children in association with the use of **medications** such as aspirin and codeine, **chemotherapeutic agents** (e.g., vincristine), **heavy metals** (e.g., iron, bismuth [Pepto-Bismol]), and **agents with anticholinergic properties** (e.g., imipramine). A medication history should be obtained in all children with constipation of recent onset. Likewise, **intercurrent illnesses,** particularly those in which children's hydration has been poor (e.g., sore throat, URI), may also be associated with constipation. A diet low in bulk and fiber may be the reason for hard, infrequent stools in some children.

Children with **neurologic disorders** are frequently constipated. This may be secondary to spinal cord dysfunction, as in meningomyelocele, and to the inactivity and low-fiber diet of these children.

EVALUATION

History

The evaluation involves a careful history (Questions Box).

Physical Examination

A complete physical examination should be performed. Although the physical examination is frequently normal, palpation of the abdomen may indicate the

Questions: Constipation

- What is the child's stooling pattern?
- What was the child's age when the problem began?
- What makes up the child's diet?
- Does the child take any medications?
- Does the child have any symptoms associated with constipation, such as recurrent abdominal pain? If so, how long have these been occurring?
- Has the child been sick recently with any illnesses that might cause constipation?
- Has the child recently experienced any changes in routine that could cause constipation?
- Is there a family history of constipation?
- How old was the child when he or she was toilet-trained?
- Is there any bleeding with stooling?
- Have any remedies such as laxatives, enemas, or suppositories been used to relieve the symptoms?

presence of stool-filled intestines. A rectal examination should be performed to assess the location and tone of the anus. In the face of a spinal cord problem, the tone may be decreased. A short anal canal and a dilated rectal segment may be revealed by rectal examination. In other conditions (e.g., Hirschsprung's disease), a tight sphincter or a tight rectal segment may be found. The passage of a large liquid stool after a digital examination is also suggestive of Hirschsprung's disease.

Laboratory Tests

If the history and physical examination suggest hypothyroidism or infantile botulism, appropriate studies should be ordered (e.g., thyroid function studies, stool tests for botulinum toxin). Anorectal manometry may also be carried out by a gastroenterologist. Similar studies that monitor the peristaltic wave can be conducted to diagnose pseudo-obstruction.

Imaging Studies

GI assessment may include the use of radiographic studies, including flat plates of the abdomen. Diagnostic radiographs using contrast material such as barium enemas help establish the diagnosis of imperforate anus and Hirschsprung's disease. It is suggested that the barium enema be attempted without prior cleanout to better document the presence of a dilated, stool-filled rectum.

MANAGEMENT

Most cases of constipation can be evaluated and managed by primary care physicians. The precise management depends on the etiology, with conditions such as Hirschsprung's disease requiring surgical intervention. Children with pseudo-obstruction may show some improvement with cisapride. In the more common cases of familial or functional constipation, the mainstay of management involves **dietary manipulation** and use of **medications** to soften and increase the bulk of the stool.

Many physicians alter the formula of young infants if the formula contains iron. Controlled trials with infant formula have not shown a relationship between iron in the formula and constipation, however. Management of infants with constipation may involve increasing the fluid in their diet or adding fruits or fruit juices, including prune juice. The nonabsorbable carbohydrate Maltsupex may also be effective. The initial dose of one teaspoon per bottle three times a day can be increased to obtain the desired results. Corn syrup should not be given to infants under one year of age because of the risk of infantile botulism.

Management of functional constipation in older children frequently involves dietary manipulation. **Bulk should be added to the diet.** Certain fruits, including papaya and cantaloupe, are very high in fiber. Popcorn is a readily acceptable and effective stool stimulant in children over five years of age. It can be offered as an after-school snack. Some children may need to take **mineral oil.** The dose should be adjusted to produce soft stools without leakage of excess mineral oil from the rectum. Colace adds bulk to the stool. **Laxatives** such as milk of magnesia, which is available over-the-counter, and lactulose (Cephulac), which can be obtained by prescription only, can also be used. Laxatives should not be used on a regular basis, however. They are more appropriate in the management of acute constipation, or briefly, with chronic constipation.

In cases of chronic constipation, management may involve aggressive cleanout, especially if the colon is dilated. **Cleanout** involves the use of **enemas.** Fleet enemas, which are small in volume, may not be as successful as soapsuds enemas, which cause irritation with subsequent peristalsis. Softening the stool using mineral oil enemas is useful. Retraining of the chronically dilated rectum may be accomplished by employing the strategies used in the treatment of encopresis (see Chapter 33, Encopresis). These modalities include the use of stool softeners and laxatives coupled with sitting on the toilet for 15 minutes after meals and assisting with the egress of stool using enemas or suppositories. Behavior modification sometimes is effective. Success is rewarded with positive reinforcement as with the use of star charts or other reward systems.

The symptoms of children with predisposing conditions are more refractory to routine treatment, and they should be managed in consultation with specialists such as pediatric gastroenterologists.

PROGNOSIS

The prognosis varies with the etiology. Functional constipation is usually amenable to routine management. With appropriate surgical treatment, the prognosis for children with Hirschsprung's disease and imperforate anus is excellent.

Case Resolution

The infant in the case scenario has a normal stooling pattern for a breast-fed infant. Stooling frequency is decreased, but the consistency of stools is normal. No diagnostic interventions are warranted at this time.

Selected Readings

Di Lorenzo, C., and A. F. Flores. Use of colonic manometry to differentiate causes of intractable constipation in children. J. Pediatr. 120:690–695, 1992.

Green, M. Constipation and encopresis. *In* Green, M., and R. J. Haggerty (eds.). Ambulatory Pediatrics IV. Philadelphia, W. B. Saunders, 1990, pp. 417–419.

Murphy, M. S. Constipation. *In* Walker, W. A., et al (eds.). Pediatric Gastrointestinal Disease. Philadelphia, B. C. Decker, 1991, pp. 90–110.

Potts, M. J., and J. Sesney. Infant constipation: maternal knowledge and beliefs. Clin. Pediatr. 31:143–148, 1992.

Rosenberg, A. J. Constipation and encopresis. *In* Wyllie, R., and J. S. Hyams (eds.). Pediatric Gastrointestinal Disease. Philadelphia, W. B. Saunders, 1993, pp. 198–208.

C H A P T E R   8 3

ABDOMINAL PAIN

Carol D. Berkowitz, M.D.

H$_x$ An eight-year-old girl has a three-month history of intermittent abdominal pain. The pain is present prior to eating and is intensified by food. Vomiting often follows and relieves the pain. The pain also occurs at night. As a result of her symptoms, the child has missed one to two days of school each week. The family moved to the area six months ago, and initially the child seemed to be adjusting to her new school and environment. In addition, the girl has a history of a five-pound weight loss. She has a positive family history of abdominal pain; her father has been diagnosed with a peptic ulcer.

On physical examination, the vital signs are normal. The weight is at the fifth percentile and the height is at the 25th percentile. There are no abnormal physical findings, and the patient is quiet and cooperative. The rectal examination is normal, and the stool is negative for occult blood.

Questions

1. What are the different types of abdominal pain?
2. What characteristics distinguish functional from organic abdominal pain?
3. What are the common organic causes of recurrent abdominal pain in children?

Abdominal pain is a common pediatric complaint. Pain may be acute or occur on a recurrent basis. Acute abdominal pain in association with vomiting or diarrhea in febrile children is frequently secondary to acute gastroenteritis, whether viral or bacterial. Recurrent or chronic abdominal pain is defined as pain that has occurred on three or more occasions in a three-month period and interferes with the patient's activities.

An organic etiology is found in less than 10% of school-age children with recurrent abdominal pain (RAP). The three leading organic causes of RAP are genitourinary problems such as UTIs and hydronephrosis, peptic ulcer disease, and inflammatory bowel disease. In other cases, constipation is believed to contribute to the symptomatology. When no organic etiology can be established, the term functional abdominal pain is used. This term should not suggest that affected children are malingerers or are confabulating their symptoms. Rather GI function may be disturbed or children may have increased sensitivity to the normal degree of gastric discomfort and distention that all individuals experience.

EPIDEMIOLOGY

Abdominal pain, one of the most common symptoms of childhood, is often fleeting and therefore not brought to medical attention. Acute pain may be related to multiple etiologies, which occur with variable frequency in different age groups. RAP, also a common problem, is reported in 10 to 25% of school-age children.

CLINICAL PRESENTATION

Children who experience abdominal pain may present with pain that may be characterized as persistent or intermittent, waxing and waning or steady and unrelenting, sharp or dull, and worsened or unaffected by movement. They may have associated complaints, including vomiting, diarrhea, constipation, fever, weight loss, headache, and anorexia (D$_x$ Box).

PATHOPHYSIOLOGY

Abdominal pain has two major causes: **inflammation** and **smooth muscle distention.** Pain from inflammation

---

Dx   Abdominal Pain

- Abdominal pain
- Abdominal wall rigidity
- Abdominal tenderness
- Vomiting
- Alterations in bowel sounds
- Diarrhea or constipation
- Anorexia
- Fever

---

results from inflammation of the mucosa, serosa, and peritoneal lining. Guarding and rigidity are distinguishing features. Inflammatory pain is characteristically well-localized and constant. Motion makes the pain worse. The pain of acute appendicitis, which is localized to McBurney's point and intensified by movement (e.g., hopping on one foot), is classic inflammatory pain.

Inflammation of the peritoneal lining may result in two different types of pain. Pain from inflammation of the parietal peritoneum is referred to the dermatome with the same innervation, because the parietal peritoneum has the same innervation as the abdominal musculature. Inflammation of the visceral peritoneum (i.e., that surrounding the viscera) is innervated by the autonomic nervous system. Pain that results from inflammation of the visceral peritoneum produces symptoms similar to those of distention of the viscera. The pain is vague and poorly localized, waxes and wanes, and is usually felt in the midepigastrium.

Pain from distention of smooth muscle also waxes and wanes, is poorly localized, and is unaffected by motion. Distention of any hollow viscus, including the stomach, intestines, biliary tree, fallopian tubes, or ureters, can result in such symptomatology. A classic example of such pain is renal colic, where the patient is writhing because of the discomfort.

DIFFERENTIAL DIAGNOSIS

In assessing the possible disease entities that may account for abdominal pain, patient age and duration of symptoms are the key differential components. As previously mentioned, acute gastroenteritis is a major diagnostic category when children have abdominal pain and fever, particularly if vomiting or diarrhea is associated with the pain.

The location of the pain may provide a clue to the etiology. Disease affecting the stomach is usually appreciated in the epigastrium. Duodenal problems are noted between the xiphoid and the umbilicus, small intestinal pathology is appreciated in the periumbilical area, and cecal inflammation may be felt from the epigastrium to McBurney's point. Disease in the colon is less specifically noted but is usually felt in the hypogastrium. Bladder and colon problems may be suprapubic or sacral. Pain may also be referred to the back. Classically, biliary colic is noted in the high midback, and pancreatic inflammation noted in the lower midback. Renal colic is

also noted in the back, but more in a lateral or costovertebral angle (CVA tenderness) site.

Acute and Recurrent Abdominal Pain

Young Infants: Medical Conditions

A unique disorder of infants, **colic** has been referred to as paroxysmal fussiness of infancy (see Chapter 26, Crying and Colic). The onset of symptoms is usually between two and four weeks of age, with resolution by three to four months. Although recurrent abdominal pain appears to be present, abdominal pain has never been established as the cause of colic. Colic is characterized by fussiness and crying. Symptoms usually appear after feeding, particularly late in the day around dinner time. Infants cry, clench their fists, and flex their legs. A gas-cry–air swallowing cycle seems to occur. The symptoms may respond to a number of measures, including rhythmic motion and antigas medications. Infants with colic usually appear well otherwise and often have accelerated weight gain secondary to repeated feeding made in efforts to quiet them.

Abdominal pain may also occur with **food allergy,** particularly cow's milk protein allergy. Generally, symptoms such as vomiting, diarrhea, Hematest-positive stools, FTT, rhinitis, eczema, pallor, irritability, and a positive family history of allergies are associated with food allergies. Congenital disaccharidase deficiency may result in abdominal pain, but diarrhea is also usually present.

Young Infants: Surgical Conditions

Intussusception occurs in infants between the ages of 6 and 24 months. Children may have been previously well or have experienced a recent bout of diarrhea. Vomiting is reported in about 50% of patients, and pallor is frequently present. An etiology is noted in less than 2.5% of affected infants, although a lead point (lymphoma or Meckel's diverticulum) may be found in 5 to 10% of older children. The intussusception most often involves the area around the ileocecal valve. Compression of the vessels within the bowel wall may lead to necrosis and gangrene. The presence of blood and mucus in the stools gives a "currant jelly" appearance, although the initial stool is often normal, having been the stool that was present in the rectum prior to the intussusception.

The abdominal examination of affected children may be benign except for pain over the area of the intussusception or may reveal the presence of a mass. Bowel sounds may be increased secondary to the obstruction. The rectal examination may reveal blood and the presence of a mass. Fever and leukocytosis may also be noted. A flat plate of the abdomen may show an obstructive pattern, with distended loops of bowel and air fluid levels. Intussusception is both diagnosed and managed by a barium enema, which reduces the intussusception using hydrostatic pressure. In some countries, such as

China and Canada, air rather than barium may be used to reduce the risk of barium peritonitis should gangrene of the bowel be present.

School-Age Children: Medical Conditions

Peptic ulcers may develop in children in three situations. One, acute infantile ulcers may occur in newborns secondary to stress and hypoxia. Two, stress ulcers may occur in children who are the victims of trauma, including burns and hypoxia (e.g., after submersion). Third, adult or chronic ulcers may develop in children with no apparent precipitating factors. A positive family history of peptic ulcer disease is reported in 25% of children. Unlike the classic ulcer symptoms of adults, in which pain occurs on an empty stomach and is relieved by eating, younger children may find that ulcer-related pain is exacerbated by eating and relieved by vomiting. Hematemesis and Hematest-positive stools are clues to the diagnosis. Recent evidence suggests an association between ulcer disease and infection with *Helicobacter pylori*.

Primary peritonitis is secondary to infection with *Streptococcus pneumoniae* and is seen in children with nephrotic syndrome and sickle cell disease, and in young girls with fever, abdominal pain, and vaginal discharge.

Mesenteric adenitis may produce symptoms indistinguishable from appendicitis (see below), although children may not be so ill-appearing. Nausea and vomiting and a history of an antecedent URI are often present.

Parenteral infections such as tonsillitis or pneumonia may present with fever and abdominal pain. In addition, hepatitis may result in pain and tenderness localized to the right upper quadrant in association with anorexia. Hepatitis in children is usually due to hepatitis A, and many infected children are anicteric (see Chapter 85, Hepatitis).

Pancreatitis produces abdominal pain that is often referred to the back. In the past, mumps was the most common cause of pancreatitis. At present, certain medications (e.g., steroids, chemotherapeutic agents) induce pancreatitis as a side effect. Familial and recurrent forms of pancreatitis are also reported. Trauma, particularly from injuries sustained as a result of impact against handle bars of bicycles, is a common cause. In children with pancreatitis and no apparent etiology, trauma related to child abuse should be considered.

Parasitic infestations, particularly with *Giardia lamblia,* may produce abdominal pain, often with bloating and diarrhea.

Genitourinary problems may result in abdominal pain. An abnormal urinalysis provides clues to the etiology. Renal stones occur infrequently in children, and boys are more often affected than girls. In two-thirds of affected children, stones are detected incidentally or in association with a urinary tract infection. Stones may be composed of calcium phosphate or oxalate, magnesium, uric acid, cystine, or xanthine. In addition to flank or abdominal pain, patients may also experience hematuria, fever, recurrent UTI, and persistent pyuria.

Hematologic and vascular disorders such as sickle cell disease, rheumatic fever, and Henoch-Schönlein purpura (HSP) may also present with abdominal pain. Sickle cell anemia should be considered in African-American children with abdominal pain. HSP, which is also referred to as anaphylactoid purpura, is characterized by a hemorrhagic skin rash, joint pain, and renal abnormalities in addition to abdominal pain. This pain may result from a number of processes, including vasculitis and ischemia of the bowel wall, edema of the bowel wall, and intussusception of the small intestine. The intussusception may be difficult to diagnose because the colon is unaffected and a barium enema is normal.

Diabetes mellitus may lead to abdominal pain secondary to cramping of accessory muscles of respiration.

Acute intermittent porphyria is an uncommon cause of abdominal pain in children. The pain is often colicky and may be associated with constipation, nausea, and vomiting. Neurologic symptoms such as pain or paresthesia in the extremities may be present. Often symptoms are precipitated by the ingestion of medications (e.g., barbiturates, sulfa drugs). Some antispasmodic medications such as Donnatal elixir contain phenobarbital and can precipitate an attack. The diagnosis is made by evaluating the urine for the presence of protoporphyrins.

School-Age Children: Surgical Conditions

Appendicitis is the most common surgical condition that produces abdominal pain in school-age children. Appendicitis may even occur in newborns, where it is seen in association with conditions such as cystic fibrosis and Hirschsprung's disease that lead to diminished passage of stool. The condition is frequently difficult to diagnose in children under the age of three or four years for two reasons: (1) examination of such young children for pain is difficult and (2) symptoms are similar to those of acute gastroenteritis (i.e., fever, abdominal pain, anorexia). Classically, patients complain of periumbilical pain that localizes to the right lower quadrant in one to five hours. They often have a low-grade fever, with a temperature of 100.4° F (38° C). Vomiting and increased urinary frequency may occur. Stooling is variable.

The physical examination may reveal guarding and localized pain as well as rebound tenderness. A positive psoas or obturator sign may be present, indicating inflammation of these muscles. Tenderness may also be noted on rectal examination. Leukocytosis over 10,000/µL is also noted. An x-ray of the abdomen may reveal one of four signs: a fecalith in the appendix (appendicolith), air in the cecum (sentinel loop), blurring of the shadow of the psoas muscle, or edema of the abdominal wall on the right side. A chest x-ray is also useful to rule out the presence of pneumonia, which may produce symptoms that mimic appendicitis.

Meckel's diverticulum may be responsible for abdominal pain in a number of ways. It may serve as the lead point for an intussusception, may cause symptoms of ulcer disease (pain or hemorrhage) secondary to the presence of ectopic gastric mucosa, or may become acutely inflamed as in appendicitis. Meckel's diverticulum follows the rule of twos: it affects 2% of the population, is two feet from the ileocecal valve, is two inches in length, and is two times more common in males than in females.

Adolescents

In female adolescents, **gynecologic problems** such as torsion of the ovary, mittelschmerz, dysmenorrhea, and pelvic inflammatory disease must be considered as causes of abdominal pain (see Chapter 70, Menstrual Disorders). In addition, pain may result from gall bladder disease secondary to cholelithiasis or cholecystitis. Cholelithiasis is also a consideration in previously pregnant adolescent patients with abdominal pain and fatty food intolerance.

Recurrent Abdominal Pain

As noted previously, most children with RAP do not have a diagnosable condition that accounts for their pain. Much has been written about the family dynamics of these children and the reactions of families to children's pain. Although many children seem to outgrow the pain, some investigators believe that a percentage of these children experience irritable bowel syndrome as adults. Other children with abdominal pain may have nonulcer dyspepsia. The association of nonulcer dyspepsia with infection with *H. pylori* is speculative. Lactose intolerance may account for abdominal pain in another subset of children.

EVALUATION

History

A thorough history should be obtained (Questions Box). Pain made worse by eating is characteristic of both peptic ulcer disease in children and cholecystitis. Pain relieved by defecation is suggestive of inflamma-

---

Questions: Abdominal Pain

- What is the nature of the pain? Is it sharp or dull, well or poorly localized, intermittent or relentless, worsened or unaffected by movement?
- How often does the pain occur?
- How long has the pain been present?
- Do any maneuvers, such as eating or lying down, reduce the symptomatology?
- Is the pain related to meals in any way? Is it worse after eating?
- Are any symptoms such as fever, weight loss, anorexia, vomiting, diarrhea, constipation, dysuria, or headache associated with the pain?
- Does any one else in the family have similar symptoms?
- Does the pain occur at night and on weekends?

---

tory bowel disease. An organic etiology is suggested by pain that awakens children at night and is lateral rather than periumbilical. Associated symptoms such as fever, weight loss, anorexia, vomiting, diarrhea, leukocytosis, and an elevated sedimentation rate also suggest an organic etiology.

Physical Examination

The physical examination should include an assessment of the severity of the pain. Children should be observed when they do not suspect that they are being watched. For example, a child who stands up and hops around when the physician leaves the room may have pain with a psychosomatic basis. Detection of abdominal tenderness may be ascertained during auscultation of the abdomen by pressing down with the stethoscope. In young children suspected of having an acute abdomen, sedation with a non–pain killer may be necessary to assess the presence of tenderness. Sedated children with an acute abdomen awaken with palpation of the abdomen.

A rectal examination is also an integral part of the evaluation. In prepubescent girls with genitourinary symptoms or adolescent females, a genital assessment should be included.

Abnormal findings such as abdominal masses or perianal skin tags are clues to an organic etiology. Children who appear vigilant and keep their eyes open during the examination often have organic problems.

Laboratory Tests

The laboratory assessment is determined by the differential diagnosis. In general, laboratory tests include a CBC, a urinalysis, and an ESR (in recurrent cases). In children with suspected lactose intolerance, a hydrogen breath test is recommended by some physicians, although a trial of dietary manipulation or use of exogenous lactase (e.g., Lactaid) may be more cost-effective. Other laboratory tests, such as serum amylase or liver function studies, are appropriate if pancreatitis or hepatitis is suspected. Stool evaluation for occult blood and parasites is also helpful. Consultation with a gastroenterologist should be considered in patients suspected of having ulcer disease or inflammatory bowel disease. Specialists may order diagnostic procedures such as endoscopy to arrive at the diagnosis.

Imaging Studies

In general, a flat plate of the abdomen should be obtained, especially if an acute surgical condition is suspected. A chest x-ray may also be ordered in children with acute symptoms consistent with appendicitis. Barium enema is indicated to diagnose intussusception. Technetium scans help detect Meckel's diverticulum if ectopic gastric mucosa is present. Ultrasonography is useful in suspected cases of cholelithiasis and cholecystitis.

MANAGEMENT

Management depends on the suspected cause of the abdominal pain. Medical conditions warrant treatment with **pharmacologic agents.** Peptic ulcer disease requires H_2-blockers such as cimetidine. Infection with *H. pylori* is managed with amoxicillin and Pepto-Bismol. Urinary tract infections should be treated with antibiotics. Conditions such as appendicitis mandate **surgical intervention.**

The management of children with RAP is challenging. A three-tiered empiric trial has been suggested. First, a high-fiber diet should be implemented. This helps alleviate the abdominal pain symptoms of children with irritable bowel syndrome. Second, antacids or H_2-blockers are used empirically to see if symptoms respond to decreased acid levels. The use of H_2-blockers is currently very popular for the treatment of adults with abdominal pain. Third, a trial of Lactaid or a lactose-free period may also be implemented. Psychological referral has been suggested, but it is more appropriate for the primary care physician to explore and address some of the psychosocial concerns that may be contributing to children's symptoms.

PROGNOSIS

In general, the prognosis for children with acute abdominal pain is good, although it varies depending on the condition. In 30 to 50% of children with RAP, the symptoms resolve within two to six weeks of diagnosis. Thirty to 50% of affected children experience abdominal pain as adults, however, although the pain does not limit their activities. As adults, these individuals may experience irritable bowel syndrome or other chronic nonspecific complaints, such as headache, backache, and chronic pelvic pain.

Case Resolution

In the case history, the girl has the classic symptoms of peptic ulcer disease. Her symptoms are exacerbated by eating and relieved by vomiting. In addition, the family history is positive. Further evaluation may include an upper GI series or consultation with a gastroenterologist. Management involves the institution of H_2-blockers.

Selected Readings

Boyle, J. T. Chronic abdominal pain. *In* Walker, W. A., et al (eds.). Pediatric Gastrointestinal Disease. Philadelphia, B. C. Decker, 1991, pp. 45–53.

Gartner, J. C. Recurrent abdominal pain: who needs a workup? Contemp. Pediatr. (Supplement to Residents)11:28–34, June 1994.

Gryboski, J. D. Peptic ulcer disease in children. Pediatr. Rev. 12:15–21, 1990.

Hamilton, A. B., and L. K. Zeltzer. Visceral pain in infants. J. Pediatr. 125:S95–S102, 1994.

Hirsch, B. Z. Recurrent abdominal pain. *In* Snyder, J. D., and W. A. Walker (eds.). Common Problems in Pediatric Gastroenterology and Nutrition. Chicago, Year Book Medical Publishers, 1989.

Oberlander, T. F., and L. A. Rappaport. Recurrent abdominal pain during childhood. Pediatr. Rev. 14:313–319, 1993.

Ross, A. J. Acute abdominal pain. *In* Walker, W. A., et al (eds.). Pediatric Gastrointestinal Disease. Philadelphia, B. C. Decker, 1991, pp. 42–44.

Silverberg, M. Chronic abdominal pain in adolescents. Pediatr. Ann. 20:179–185, 1991.

Stevenson, R. J., and M. M. Ziegler. Abdominal pain unrelated to trauma. Pediatr. Rev. 14:302–311, 1993.

CHAPTER 84

JAUNDICE

Carol D. Berkowitz, M.D.

H$_x$ A 2-month-old male infant is brought to the office for a routine well child checkup. He was the product of a full-term, normal, spontaneous, vaginal delivery, with a birth weight of 3600 g. He has been feeding well, exclusively at the breast. Loose stools follow each nursing.

On physical examination, the infant weighs 4900 g. The examination is normal except that the boy appears jaundiced. On further questioning, the mother states that her son has been jaundiced since shortly after birth, and she feels that his appearance has not changed. The color of the stool is yellow.

Questions

1. What are the common causes of unconjugated hyperbilirubinemia in young infants?
2. What are the common causes of conjugated hyperbilirubinemia in young infants?

3. What are the usual causes of jaundice in older children and adolescents?
4. What is the appropriate management of hyperbilirubinemia in breast-fed infants?

Jaundice is a condition that occurs when bilirubin reaches a level in the blood that makes it visibly apparent. In newborn infants, this level is 5 mg/dL. In older children and adolescents, jaundice becomes apparent at serum bilirubin levels of 2 mg/dL. The term **physiologic jaundice** is used to denote the jaundice that normally occurs following birth. In full-term infants, bilirubin reaches its peak of about 6 mg/dL between the second and fourth days of life. Levels above 10 mg/dL are probably not physiologic. Bilirubin generally returns to a normal level (< 1 mg/dL) by 12 days of age. Premature infants experience their peak level of bilirubin, which may be up to 10–12 mg/dL, between the fifth and seventh days of life. Levels over 14 mg/dL are probably not physiologic. Levels may be elevated in premature infants for up to two months.

Although physiologic jaundice, a benign finding, affects all infants, other more serious disorders may present with similar symptomatology. The physician must be able to differentiate between these conditions to ensure appropriate intervention and management. New-onset jaundice in older children and adolescents is caused by other disorders.

EPIDEMIOLOGY

Jaundice is nearly universal in neonates because of the rapid turnover of red blood cells and the relative immaturity of the liver. Breast milk jaundice affects about 1% of breast-fed infants. Various illnesses, particularly bacterial infections, also may precipitate jaundice in newborns. Neonatal cholestasis (conjugated hyperbilirubinemia), which is seen in a small number of cases of neonatal jaundice, is due to neonatal hepatitis or extrahepatic biliary atresia 70 to 80% of the time. Jaundice occurs much less frequently in the postneonatal period and is most often secondary to viral hepatitis (see Chapter 85, Hepatitis).

CLINICAL PRESENTATION

Children with jaundice have yellow skin, conjunctiva, and mucous membranes. In newborns, the coloration may not be appreciated by parents because of its gradual onset and the parents' inexperience. The finding may be apparent in otherwise asymptomatic infants during routine health maintenance visits.

Aside from the yellow color, children with jaundice may also present with symptoms related to the cause of the jaundice, including vomiting, anorexia, FTT, acholic (white) stools, dark urine, fatigue, and abdominal pain or fullness (D_x Box).

D_x Jaundice

- Yellow skin, mucous membranes, and conjunctiva
- Tenderness in the right upper quadrant of the abdomen
- Hepatomegaly
- Anorexia
- Acholic stools
- Vomiting
- Pruritus

PATHOPHYSIOLOGY

Bilirubin, a yellow pigment found primarily in bile, forms from the breakdown of hemoglobin. Blockage along any point in the physiologic or anatomic pathway may result in increased levels of bilirubin and the appearance of jaundice (Fig. 84–1). After the breakdown of hemoglobin, unconjugated bilirubin is taken up by intracellular proteins (Y proteins) in the liver. Uptake depends on hepatic blood flow and the presence of the necessary binding proteins. Once in the liver, unconjugated bilirubin is conjugated by the enzyme glucuronyl transferase. Conjugated bilirubin, which is water-soluble, can be eliminated through the kidneys. Follow-

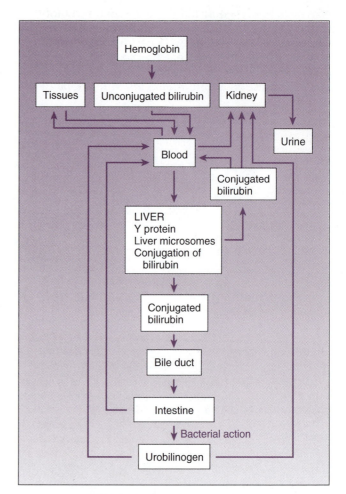

FIGURE 84–1. *The bilirubin pathway.*

ing conjugation, bilirubin passes into the bile through the bile canaliculi. It then moves to the GI tract, where some of it may be reabsorbed (enterohepatic circulation), or be acted on by bacteria to form urobilinogen, which may appear in the urine or stool.

In neonates, a number of factors contribute to physiologic jaundice. Increased destruction of red blood cells occurs, because the red blood cell survival in infants is only 70 to 90 days, as opposed to 120 days in older children. Hepatic uptake is lower, perhaps as a result of decreased levels of hepatic proteins as well as decreased hepatic blood flow. Levels of glucuronyl transferase do not reach adult values until the second week of life. These decreased levels of glucuronyl transferase mean that conjugation of bilirubin occurs at a slower rate. In some infants, glucuronyl transferase levels remain low; these individuals remain prone to jaundice at times of illness, stress, and starvation (Gilbert's syndrome). Some breast-fed infants also experience prolonged jaundice. It is believed that some unknown substance in the mother's milk, perhaps pregnanetriol, blocks glucuronyl transferase. Reabsorption of bilirubin is increased through the enterohepatic circulation because of the diminished number of bacteria in the GI tract in young infants.

In older children, similar mechanisms may act to cause an increase in the bilirubin level. Hemolytic anemias (e.g., glucose-6-phosphatase or pyruvate kinase deficiencies) may lead to increased red blood cell destruction. Inflammatory or infectious processes involving the liver, such as hepatitis, may impair the ability of the liver to excrete bilirubin. Pharmaceutical and toxicologic agents may also interfere with the ability of the liver to metabolize bilirubin.

DIFFERENTIAL DIAGNOSIS

The differential diagnosis of jaundice in children involves three criteria: (1) age, (2) the type of hyperbilirubinemia (conjugated or unconjugated), and (3) if the hyperbilirubinemia is conjugated, the nature of the obstruction (intrahepatic or extrahepatic). The latter two factors are particularly important in determining the etiology of jaundice in young infants. A diagrammatic representation of the differential diagnosis of jaundice in children is shown in Figures 84–2, 84–3, and 84–4.

Infants Under Eight Weeks of Age
Unconjugated Hyperbilirubinemia

Jaundice occurs universally in all newborns, but marked elevation of bilirubin levels or persistence of jaundice beyond 2 weeks of age warrants assessment. When less than 15% of the total bilirubin is direct, unconjugated hyperbilirubinemia is present. This is best determined by measuring the levels of total and direct bilirubin in the blood. **Physiologic jaundice** is associated with unconjugated hyperbilirubinemia. The hematologic workup of affected infants is normal. Jaundice related to breast-feeding may resemble physiologic jaundice, but bilirubin levels rise during the

second week of life when physiologic jaundice is improving. In breast-fed infants, levels may reach as high as 25–30 mg/dL. Breast milk jaundice usually peaks by the age of 4 weeks and decreases by 10 weeks.

Conditions associated with slow intestinal transit time and increased enterohepatic circulation, such as hypothyroidism, also may result in jaundice. As with physiologic and breast milk jaundice, the hematologic workup is normal. High intestinal obstructions, such as pyloric stenosis, duodenal atresia, annular pancreas, and jejunal atresia may lead to jaundice, perhaps because of starvation and decreased levels of glucuronyl transferase.

Crigler-Najjar syndrome type I, which involves a deficiency in glucuronyl transferase, is associated with neonatal jaundice. Because of very high bilirubin levels, type I disease may lead to kernicterus unless managed with exchange transfusion.

Hematologic problems may also produce jaundice in the neonatal period. Such problems are most often associated with blood group (usually Rh or ABO) incompatibility between mothers and infants, but some minor blood group determinants can precipitate similar problems. Jaundice occurs in affected infants because of the rapid destruction of red blood cells. Other infants may have a hemolytic anemia such as spherocytosis.

Jaundice may also occur if excess blood is present in the infant's system. Situations in which elevated hemoglobin is associated with jaundice include maternal-infant or twin-twin transfusions, infants who are small for gestational age, delayed clamping of the umbilical cord, infants of diabetic mothers, and infants with hyperviscosity syndrome.

Conjugated Hyperbilirubinemia

When over 15% of the total bilirubin is direct, the jaundice is categorized as conjugated hyperbilirubinemia. Total parenteral nutrition is the most common cause of conjugated hyperbilirubinemia in the neonatal intensive care unit but does not usually present a diagnostic dilemma. In other cases, determination of whether the problem is intrahepatic or extrahepatic is the major consideration. Some conditions of intrahepatic involvement represent a spectrum involving progression from inflammation of bile canaliculi (hepatitis) to their destruction (biliary atresia).

Inflammation of the hepatocytes is hepatitis. This disease may be caused by an infection in the liver or elsewhere in the body (e.g., sepsis and UTIs in young infants). UTIs are usually caused by *Escherichia coli.* Three mechanisms of action for jaundice in bacterial infections have been postulated: (1) increased hemolysis, with an increased reticulocyte count; (2) toxic hepatitis, with inflammation and lymphocytic infiltration in the liver; and (3) poor nutrition secondary to fever and illness. The common pathway seems to be some degree of hepatocellular necrosis, with pericholangitis, bile duct proliferation, and mild amounts of portal fibrosis. The hepatic involvement resolves with appropriate antibiotic therapy of the primary infection.

Primary liver infection may be due to hepatitis A, B,

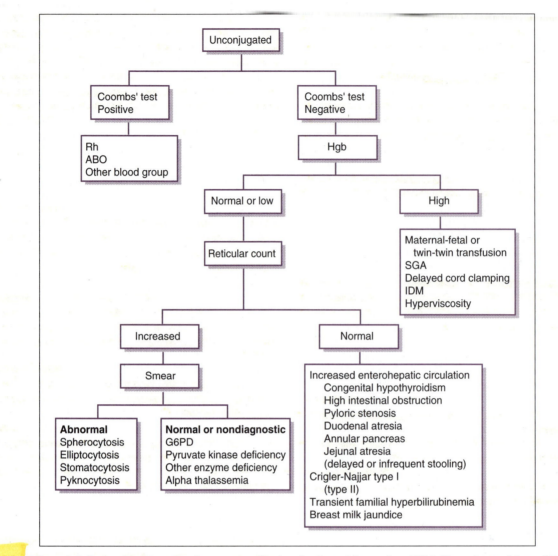

FIGURE 84–2. *Differential diagnosis of jaundice in neonates (during the first eight weeks of life). Unconjugated hyperbilirubinemia.*

or C, or other so-called **TORCH** agents (**t**oxoplasma, **r**ubella, **c**ytomegalovirus, **h**erpesvirus). Infants infected prenatally often have low birth weights, hepatosplenomegaly, petechial rashes, and ocular findings such as cataracts and chorioretinitis. **Other infectious causes include syphilis, coxsackie B virus, echovirus II, adenovirus 2,** *Listeria monocytogenes,* **and tuberculosis.**

Differentiating among these conditions is usually done on the basis of culture or serology. Certain physical and epidemiologic findings may help to distinguish these entities, however. Syphilis is more common in the developing nations of the world. Jaundice may appear within the first 24 hours of life or be of later onset. Infection with *L. monocytogenes* infection may be associated with the presence of focal granulomas on the posterior pharynx. Similar granulomas in the liver are evident.

Metabolic diseases and **inborn errors of metabolism** may also lead to hepatitis. Most of these conditions are inherited in an autosomal recessive manner. In addition to jaundice, infants may present with vomiting, irritability, lethargy, anorexia, hepatomegaly, hypoglycemia,

FTT, bleeding, or cataracts. Galactosemia may be detected through neonatal screening. Infants with hereditary fructose intolerance present after exposure to fructose, sucrose, or sorbitol. Alpha-1 antitrypsin deficiency may account for 20 to 30% of cases of idiopathic neonatal liver disease.

Other metabolic conditions that lead to jaundice in newborns include hereditary tyrosinemia, infantile Gaucher's disease, Niemann-Pick disease, and Wolman's disease. Cystic fibrosis may also cause cholestatic jaundice because of the presence of inspissated bile in the bile canaliculi. Fifty percent of these infants have meconium ileus, meconium peritonitis, or intestinal atresia. "Plugged" bile ducts may be seen with severe hemolytic anemia where bilirubin production is markedly elevated. Drugs may also induce intrahepatic cholestasis.

A number of syndromes are associated with persistent intrahepatic cholestasis. Alagille's syndrome (arteriohepatic dysplasia) is characterized by unusual facies, cardiovascular anomalies, and a paucity of intralobular bile ducts.

Extrahepatic biliary atresia accounts for about 30%

of cases of cholestasis in newborns. Obliteration of the biliary tree is apparent. Infants are often well until 3 to 6 weeks of age, when they develop conjugated hyperbilirubinemia. Choledochal cysts appear as dilatations of the biliary tree and obstruct the passage of bile.

Older Infants, Children, and Adolescents

The approach to the differential diagnosis of jaundice in older infants and children is similar to the process in young infants. In cases of unconjugated hyperbilirubinemia, the level of indirect bilirubin helps clarify the differential diagnosis. Patients whose indirect bilirubin is greater than 6 mg/dL may have **Crigler-Najjar syndrome type II** and respond favorably to phenobarbital. Patients with levels under 6 mg/dL may have hemolytic anemia. **Congestive heart failure** and **hyperthyroidism** may also produce unconjugated hyperbilirubinemia. **Gilbert's disease,** a benign condition in which the bilirubin rises in response to stress and starvation, may result in jaundice. **Drugs,** including rifampin and birth control pills, may also be associated with unconjugated hyperbilirubinemia.

Conjugated hyperbilirubinemia may result from two different processes: (1) cholestasis and (2) hepatocellular inflammation or injury. Signs of cholestasis are high levels of alkaline phosphatase (three times normal), increased 5′ nucleotidase, and increased gamma glutamyl transpeptidase. Cholestatic jaundice, related to drugs (estrogens) and alcohol, may occur on an intrahepatic basis. **Byler's syndrome** is a familial disorder characterized by intrahepatic cholestasis. Extrahepatic cholestasis is seen with cholelithiasis or other obstructions of the biliary tree. Cholelithiasis may occur in individuals with hemolytic anemia and in female adolescents who have been pregnant. Hepatocellular injury most often results from hepatitis (discussed in Chapter 85, Hepatitis), including infectious, alcoholic, and drug-induced hepatitis. Rarer disorders include Dubin-Johnson syndrome and Rotor's syndrome.

EVALUATION

History

A careful history must be obtained (Questions Box).

Physical Examination

Patients should be evaluated for evidence of organomegaly, ocular anomalies, rashes, hearing deficits, and unusual facial features. The unique facial features are

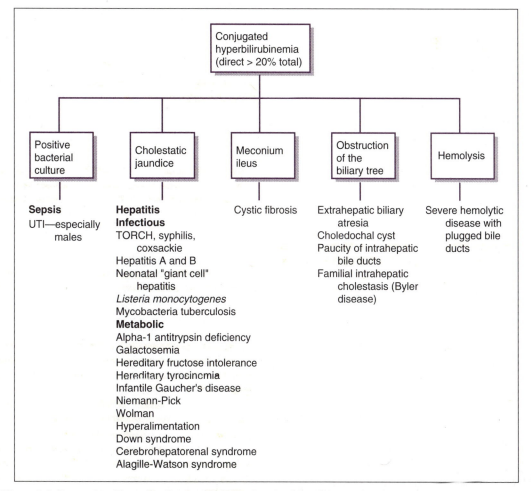

FIGURE 84–3. *Differential diagnosis of jaundice in neonates (during the first eight weeks of life). Conjugated hyperbilirubinemia.*

FIGURE 84–4. *Differential diagnosis of jaundice in older infants, children, and adolescents.*

pathognomic for certain genetic disorders such as Byler's or Alagille's syndromes. Rashes and lymphadenopathy are associated with certain infectious conditions, including congenital infections (TORCH) in newborns and infectious mononucleosis in adolescents. Patients should also be checked for the presence of any cardiac anomaly, which may suggest a genetic syndrome or congestive heart failure.

Laboratory Tests

The aim of the laboratory assessment is to discover where the bilirubin metabolism is abnormal. The total bilirubin as well as the fractionated bilirubin levels should be determined. The presence of elevated levels of direct-reacting bilirubin represents conjugated hyperbilirubinemia. The demonstration of a yellow color to the foam of a shaken specimen of urine is a rapid test for conjugated hyperbilirubinemia.

In children with unconjugated hyperbilirubinemia, a CBC with reticulocyte count and evaluation of the peripheral smear confirm hemolytic anemia. In neonates, the Coombs test should be performed, and infant and maternal blood types should be determined. The hemoglobin should also be obtained. A normal or low hemoglobin may be seen in the face of hemolytic anemia. An elevated reticulocyte count or an abnormal peripheral blood smear indicates hemolysis. Hemolytic anemias with abnormal peripheral smears include spherocytosis, elliptocytosis, stomatocytosis, and pyknocytosis.

In children with conjugated hyperbilirubinemia, tests should be performed to determine if infections such as bacteremia, UTI, congenital infection, or hepatitis are present. Evaluation for metabolic diseases should also be obtained by assessing the urine for the presence of reducing substances (e.g., Clinitest tablet) or amino acids. The status of liver function can be determined by evaluating aspartate aminotransferase, serum glutamic pyruvic transaminase (SGPT), and serum glutamic oxaloacetic transaminase (SGOT), alkaline phosphatase, or 5′ nucleotidase.

Questions: Jaundice

- What associated symptoms are present?
- How long have the symptoms been present?
- Does the child have a fever, which may suggest the presence of an infection?
- What is the color of the stools (acholic stools suggest obstruction)?
- Does the child have a family history of jaundice or consanguinity?
- What makes up the child's diet? If the child is an infant, is he or she breast-fed or bottle-fed?
- When did the parents first notice the jaundice?
- Has the child been jaundiced previously?
- Has the child been vaccinated against hepatitis B?
- Is there a history of foreign travel or shellfish ingestion?

Imaging Studies

The anatomy of the biliary tree can be evaluated using ultrasound. Choledochal cysts may be visualized using this modality. Other imaging tests, including excretion studies (radioisotope scans), can be used to help differentiate hepatitis from biliary atresia. Consultation with a pediatric gastroenterologist may be appropriate.

MANAGEMENT

The management of jaundice depends on the cause of the condition. Physiologic jaundice and jaundice secondary to breast-feeding frequently require no intervention. Some practitioners use **bilirubin-reducing lights,** but other clinicians believe that breast-fed infants can tolerate bilirubin levels as high as 25–30 mg/dL without danger of kernicterus. Infants who are preterm, ill, or have jaundice as a result of hemolysis may be at a greater risk from elevated bilirubin levels. **Exchange transfusion** may be indicated in addition to placement under bilirubin-reducing lights. A rule of thumb: Preterm infants should receive exchange transfusions when the bilirubin reaches the infant's weight (e.g., 11 mg/dL in an 1100-g infant).

Medications play a limited role in the management of jaundice. **Phenobarbital** may speed up the liver's excretion of bilirubin, even in cases of hemolytic anemia. This drug is also useful in the management of jaundice due to certain genetic conditions such as Crigler-Najjar syndrome type II. The appropriate **antibiotics** should be used to combat infections associated with jaundice.

Infants with biliary atresia may require **surgery.** Surgery links the surface of the liver to the intestinal tract, allowing for passage of bilirubin directly into the lumen of the small intestine. Adolescents with gallbladder disease may also require surgical intervention (i.e., a cholecystectomy).

PROGNOSIS

The majority of infants with elevated bilirubin levels have physiologic jaundice or jaundice related to breast feeding. The prognosis is excellent in these children. Other conditions may be less amenable to therapy and may require ongoing medical or surgical intervention. Children with metabolic abnormalities usually require lifelong nutritional intervention, those with hepatic disease may succumb to their hepatic dysfunction, and those treated with surgical correction of biliary atresia may have recurrent episodes of cholangitis leading to cirrhosis and the eventual need for liver transplantation.

In contrast, older infants, children, and adolescents with jaundice often have self-limited conditions that spontaneously resolve.

Case Resolution

In the case history, the infant is breast-fed, which raises the possibility of breast milk jaundice. Bilirubin and hemoglobin determination are appropriate to assess the bilirubin level and confirm the absence of hemolysis. One approach to the diagnosis of breast-feeding as the etiology of the jaundice is to stop breast-feeding for a day or two to see if the bilirubin level decreases. (Sometimes an infant may not resume breast-feeding.) Biliary atresia or metabolic or infectious hepatitis should be also be considered because of the infant's age.

The presence of normal-colored stools is reassuring, however, and excludes biliary atresia. The urine should be checked for the presence of reducing substances, which is a noninvasive way of evaluating the infant for galactosemia. The birth record should be obtained. Knowledge of the maternal and infant blood types would allow evaluation for mother-infant blood group incompatibility.

Selected Readings

Balistreri, W. F., and J. T. Stocker. Pediatric Hepatology. New York, Hemisphere Publishing, 1990.

Gartner, L. M. Neonatal jaundice. Pediatr. Rev. 15:422–432, 1994.

Heubi, J. E., and C. C. Daugherty. Neonatal cholestasis: an approach for the practicing pediatrician. Curr. Probl. Pediatr. 20:239–295, 1990.

Mews, C., and F. R. Sinatra. Cholestasis in infancy. Pediatr. Rev. 15:233–240, 1994.

Mowat, A. P. Liver Disorders in Children, 2nd ed. London, Butterworth, 1987.

Newman, T. B., and M. J. Maisels. Evaluation and treatment of jaundice in a term newborn: a kinder, gentler approach. Pediatrics 89:809–818, 1992.

HEPATITIS

Monica Sifuentes, M.D.

H$_x$ A 7-year-old boy is brought to the office with a one-week history of intermittent fever, vomiting, diarrhea, and diffuse abdominal pain. His mother reports the appearance of "yellow eyes and skin" on the day before the visit. Her son was previously in good health. He is taking no medications and has no ill contacts. The boy came to the United States five years ago. The pregnancy and delivery in El Salvador were normal. He has no history of recent travel outside of the United States.

The physical examination is significant for a temperature of 100.4° F (38.0° C), a pulse of 100, and a blood pressure of 110/63. The child is a well-developed, well-nourished male with yellow skin and sclera. The abdomen is soft, with minimal diffuse tenderness and normal bowel sounds. The liver edge is palpated 5 cm below the right costal margin, and no splenomegaly is present. The rectal examination is normal, with guaiac-negative stool.

Questions

1. What conditions could account for symptoms of jaundice and GI upset?
2. What is the appropriate evaluation for children with suspected hepatitis?
3. What are the most common causes of hepatitis in children?
4. What complications are associated with viral hepatitis?
5. What treatments are currently available for viral hepatitis, and how does treatment differ depending on the specific etiology?

Hepatitis is an inflammation of the liver that can occur as the result of an exposure to a toxin, such as a chemical or drug, or an infectious agent. Viruses are the most common cause in children, and a majority of cases are the result of hepatitis A or B infection. Other common viruses that can cause hepatitis in children are EBV, varicella-zoster virus, and herpes simplex virus. However, their contribution to the overall morbidity and mortality associated with infectious hepatitis is minimal. Recent public health efforts have been aimed at immunizing infants, adolescents, and other high-risk individuals against hepatitis B, thus reducing the incidence of this illness as well as its long-term consequences.

EPIDEMIOLOGY

Approximately 60,000 cases of viral hepatitis are reported each year in the United States, the majority of which are hepatitis A and hepatitis B. Other etiologies include hepatitis C (formerly called non-A, non-B hepatitis) and unidentified causes. The total number of hepatitis cases is probably underestimated as a result of underreporting.

Certain situations are associated with increased risk for infection with hepatitis A. These include crowded living conditions, chronic care facilities, military institutions, prisons, day care centers, and homosexuality. Poor personal hygiene and sanitation are also risk factors. Hepatitis A is found worldwide, but specific locations are associated with an increased incidence of the disease: Central and South America, Africa, the Mediterranean region, and Asia. Children less than 15 years of age have the highest incidence of the disease, and both sexes are equally affected.

Groups at high risk for hepatitis B include illicit parenteral drug users, homosexuals, heterosexuals with multiple sexual partners, health care workers, recipients of hemodialysis, household contacts of carriers of hepatitis B virus (HBV), and immigrants from HBV-endemic areas. Individuals who live in crowded environments with poor hygienic standards, such as institutions for the developmentally disabled or correctional facilities, are at risk for hepatitis B. Areas with the highest incidence of hepatitis B include Southeast Asia, most of Africa, the Pacific Islands, China, and parts of the Middle East.

Approximately 10 to 15% of primary infections with HBV result in a chronic carrier state. The younger children are when they are infected with HBV, the more likely they are to become chronic carriers. Between 70 and 90% of infants born to infected mothers become carriers, and at least 50% of children infected before the age of five years become carriers. Boys have a greater risk of becoming carriers than girls.

Hepatitis C accounts for 20 to 40% of all viral hepatitis. High-risk individuals are recipients of transfusions of blood or blood products, intravenous drug users, health care workers with blood exposure, and, rarely, sexual or household contacts of infected persons. No identifiable source can be found in at least 35% of cases. In the pediatric population, recipients of blood and blood products (e.g., hemophiliacs), dialysis patients, institutionalized children, and "high-risk" infants (e.g., maternal history of intravenous drug abuse, STDs, HIV coinfection) are most likely to have hepatitis C.

Because hepatitis D only occurs as a coinfection with hepatitis B, high-risk groups are the same, with the exclusion of health care workers and homosexual males. High prevalence rates occur in eastern Europe, Central Africa, southern Italy, and the Middle East.

No cases of hepatitis E acquired in the United States have been reported, although the disease has been epidemic in other countries such as Mexico, Asia, North Africa, and India. Young and middle-aged adults are most commonly affected.

CLINICAL PRESENTATION

Children with hepatitis have diffuse abdominal pain, decreased appetite, nausea, and vomiting. Additional symptoms may include fever and malaise. Unlike in adults, jaundice is not always present, especially not in infants and young children. Hepatomegaly is universally not found on physical examination, along with varying degrees of right upper quadrant discomfort (D$_x$ Box). A nonspecific macular rash and arthralgias can also occur early in the course of hepatitis B.

PATHOPHYSIOLOGY

Hepatitis A

Hepatitis A, formerly called infectious hepatitis, is caused by a picornavirus composed of single-stranded RNA. The most common modes of transmission are through close personal contact and contaminated food and water. This generally occurs by fecal contamination and oral ingestion. Shellfish, such as raw oysters, clams and mussels, are a frequent source of infection. Infected food handlers may also transmit the disease.

The average incubation period for hepatitis A is 28 to 30 days (range: 15–50 days). Peak viral secretion occurs before the onset of jaundice. The virus is shed in the stool two to three weeks before the onset of jaundice and up to one week after its appearance. Most young children, however, are anicteric, and so infections often go unnoticed during this highly contagious period (Fig. 85–1).

A chronic carrier state for hepatitis A does not exist, although fulminant infections can occur. Lifelong immunity is conferred after a single infection.

Hepatitis B

Hepatitis B, formerly called serum hepatitis, is caused by a double-shelled DNA virus. The disease is usually spread by contact with infected blood or blood products, but it can also occur through close interpersonal contact. Although hepatitis B surface antigen (HBsAg) is

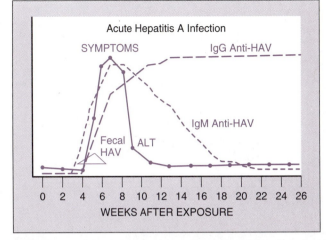

FIGURE 85–1. *Course of acute hepatitis A infection.* *(Reproduced, with permission, from Tabor, E. Etiology, diagnosis and treatment of viral hepatitis in children. In Aronoff, S.C., et al. [eds.].* Advances in Pediatric Infectious Diseases. *Chicago, Year Book Medical Publishers, 1988.)*

found in numerous body secretions such as blood and blood products, feces, urine, tears, saliva, semen, breast milk, vaginal secretions, cerebrospinal and synovial fluid, only serum, semen, vaginal secretions, and saliva are contagious. No fecal-oral transmission occurs. Transmission is facilitated through percutaneous inoculation (e.g., tattooing, intravenous drug use) and exposure of cuts in the skin and mucous membranes to contaminated fluids on objects such as razors and utensils. Sexual transmission occurs via semen, vaginal secretions, and saliva. Perinatal vertical transmission occurs in mothers who are acutely infected or chronic carriers. Although the exact mode of transmission is unclear for household contacts, postnatal infection from household exposure is reported.

The average incubation period for hepatitis B is three to four months (range: 1–6 months). Figure 85–2 depicts the typical course of acute hepatitis B, along with the course of the chronic carrier state.

Hepatitis C

Hepatitis C results from infection with a single-stranded RNA virus. Like HBV, the hepatitis C virus (HCV) can be spread through contact with contaminated blood or, rarely, through household or sexual contact with infected individuals. Studies indicate that perinatal transmission does occur but is relatively uncommon.

The incubation period is variable, ranging from approximately 4 to 12 weeks. Most affected children are anicteric.

Hepatitis D

Acute delta hepatitis, or hepatitis D, is caused by a distinct single-stranded RNA virus that requires HBsAg for replication. Both the virus and a delta antigen are enclosed in an envelope of HBsAg. Transmission is simi-

D$_x$	**Hepatitis**

- Diffuse abdominal pain
- Nonspecific symptoms (fever, malaise, anorexia, nausea, and vomiting)
- Jaundice (not necessarily in all cases)
- Dark urine and light-colored stool
- Pain or tenderness over the liver area
- Hepatomegaly

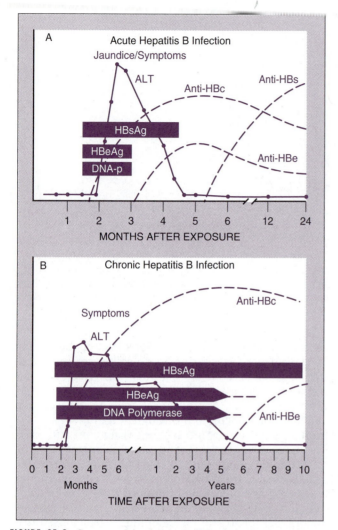

FIGURE 85–2. *Course of hepatitis B infection.* (*Reproduced, with permission, from Tabor, E. Etiology, diagnosis and treatment of viral hepatitis in children. In Aronoff, S.C., et al. [eds.].* Advances in Pediatric Infectious Diseases. *Chicago, Year Book Medical Publishers, 1988.*) A. *Acute hepatitis B infection.* B. *Chronic hepatitis B infection.*

lar to hepatitis B, but vertical transmission is uncommon.

Hepatitis D occurs either as a coinfection with HBV or a superinfection in a chronic carrier of HBV. The disease is usually more severe than hepatitis B.

DIFFERENTIAL DIAGNOSIS

The differential diagnosis of hepatitis depends on patient age. Possible causes in neonates include congenital infections such as toxoplasmosis, CMV, and syphilis, in addition to hepatitis B. Anatomical abnormalities causing biliary obstruction (e.g., biliary atresia) should also be considered (see Chapter 84, Jaundice).

In infants and children, viral etiologies include EBV, CMV, herpes simplex, varicella-zoster, rubella, rubeola, coxsackie B, adenovirus, and HIV. Acute or chronic anemias such as sickle cell disease can also cause hepatomegaly and jaundice. Other rarer conditions to consider include cystic fibrosis, α_1-antitrypsin defi-

ciency, drug-induced hepatitis (e.g., treatment with isoniazid, phenytoin), and congenital disorders such as Caroli's disease (intrahepatic dilation of the bile ducts).

In adolescents, specific drugs that cause liver toxicity include oral contraceptives, alcohol, acetaminophen, and tetracycline. Viral etiologies to consider in this age group are the same as those listed for children.

EVALUATION

History

A comprehensive history should be obtained in children of all ages (Questions Box). A dietary history may also be helpful when considering hepatitis A.

A complete maternal and obstetrical history, which includes the following questions, should be taken. Does the mother have any history of intravenous drug use? Does the mother come from an area where hepatitis is highly endemic, such as Southeast Asia? Did the mother receive prenatal care? Was hepatitis B screening performed prenatally or at delivery? Did the mother have any known sexual contacts with hepatitis B, or did she have multiple sexual partners?

The physician should ask adolescents about sexual activity, STDs, and the number of sexual partners. In addition, it is important to inquire about parenteral drug use and tattoos.

Physical Examination

Because most children with viral hepatitis are asymptomatic, and all forms of the disease are clinically indistinguishable, a complete physical examination should be performed to rule out other etiologies. Growth parameters, particularly weight, should be obtained and compared to previous measurements. The temperature should be recorded, especially if children have a recent history of fever. In children who are vomiting, signs of dehydration (e.g., tachycardia, evidence of orthostatic hypotension, dry mucous membranes, tenting of the skin, sunken eyes, lethargy) should be noted.

Questions: Hepatitis

- Does the child have any history of fever, malaise, anorexia, or weight loss?
- Has the child experienced any vomiting or diarrhea?
- Is any abdominal pain or discomfort present? If so, in what location?
- Are yellow eyes or any changes in skin color apparent? If so, for how long?
- Is the color of the urine dark and the stool light?
- What is the child's recent travel history?
- Has the child ingested any shellfish in the previous one to two months?
- Has the child been in contact with any individuals with hepatitis or jaundice (including sexual contacts)?
- Does the child have a history of transfusion with blood or blood products?
- Does the adolescent have a history of intravenous drug use?
- Does the mother have a history of hepatitis, intravenous drug use, STDs, or multiple sexual partners?

In addition, the skin should be examined for jaundice, evidence of pruritus (e.g., excoriations), or a nonspecific rash. Icterus of the sclera, tympanic membranes, and palate should also be noted. The abdomen should be palpated for tenderness and organomegaly, particularly hepatomegaly. The liver span should also be measured because it will help monitor the patient's progress. Splenomegaly, which is not typically found in hepatitis, indicates a different diagnosis, such as leukemia, or another infectious cause, such as CMV. A rectal examination should also be performed to look for masses or blood in the stool.

A neurologic examination is important to document any signs of encephalopathy from hyperammonemia, which occurs more commonly in chronic liver disease or fulminant hepatic failure.

Laboratory Tests

A limited number of laboratory studies are initially needed. These include liver function tests (LFTs) (alanine aminotransferase [ALT], aspartate aminotransferase [AST], gammaglutamyl transferase [GGT], and total bilirubin) and coagulation studies (PT/PTT). A PT is particularly useful because of its rapid turnaround time and predictive utility; if the value is greater than three seconds above the upper limit of normal (INR>1.5), the prognosis is poor. A urinalysis for bilirubin should be done. Serologies for hepatitis A (HAV-IgM and HAV-IgG) and hepatitis B (HBsAg, anti-HBs, HBeAg, anti-HBe, and anti-HBc) should also be performed.

In patients at high risk for hepatitis C, serum antibodies to HCV (anti-HCV) should be sent. A confirmatory test such as a polymerase chain reaction or recombinant immunoblot assay, which measures antibody to various regions of the HCV genome, can also be considered. Serologic markers for hepatitis D (IgM and IgG anti-HDV) can be sent when concurrent HBV infection is evident. Isolation of the hepatitis D antigen (HDAg) in the liver, however, is the "gold standard" test for diagnosis of hepatitis D.

MANAGEMENT

For most cases of hepatitis A, B, C, and D, therapy consists of general **supportive care.** No specific therapy is available, and disease is usually self-limited. Adequate nutrition and hydration are of primary importance. Therefore, the **intake of sufficient food and fluids** should be ensured. A low-protein diet during the acute phase of the illness may be considered as well. The use of **antipyretics** such as acetaminophen or ibuprofen for fever usually does not pose a problem in patients with acutely elevated LFTs and mild disease. Physical activity should be limited until patients feel better and LFTs return to normal. Children and adolescents can return to school when they are no longer jaundiced; they can resume a normal diet at that time.

In children with more severe symptoms, intravenous hydration and an antiemetic, such as phenergan, are indicated. Hospitalization is required for children who are moderately to severely dehydrated, are unable to keep fluids down, or have evidence of fulminant liver failure. Treatment is aimed at correcting any metabolic abnormalities or electrolyte disturbances, including hypoglycemia. Coagulopathies should be corrected with vitamin K, fresh-frozen plasma, and cryoprecipitate. Total parenteral nutrition may be required to maintain caloric needs. Consultation with a pediatric gastroenterologist is important for children with acute fulminant liver failure or chronic, active hepatitis.

Treatment of chronic, active hepatitis B and C with recombinant alpha interferon has been effective in adults. Approximately 30 to 50% of patients have responded with normalization of LFTs, particularly ALT, and histologic improvement. Fifty percent of patients, however, relapse when treatment is discontinued. Corticosteroids and acyclovir have also been used without benefit. There has been limited experience and success with these treatments in the pediatric population.

PREVENTION

Hepatitis A

Handwashing by food handlers, medical personnel, and day care workers is a primary method for prevention of the spread of hepatitis A. **Enteric precautions** should be used for infected patients. **Immune globulin** is recommended for postexposure prophylaxis for all people who have had intimate exposure to infected individuals. It is indicated for all household and day care contacts but not for contacts at school or work. The dose is 0.02 mL/kg within 48 hours of exposure, given no later than two weeks after exposure. Preexposure prophylaxis is recommended for travelers to endemic areas. If the stay is less than three months, the dose is the same as for postexposure prophylaxis, and for longer stays, the dose is 0.06 mL/kg every five months. An inactivated hepatitis A vaccine has been recently licensed for use in the United States. The benefit of routine immunization of all individuals versus only those at risk (e.g., postexposure) has yet to be determined.

Hepatitis B

Preventive strategies for hepatitis B include preexposure and postexposure prophylaxis and universal immunization of all infants beginning shortly after birth. In addition, the vaccination of high-risk adolescents and other selected individuals is recommended.

Hepatitis B immune globulin (passive immunization) is recommended for infants born to known HBsAg-positive mothers or mothers considered at risk for the disease (history of intravenous drug use, STDs, or multiple sexual partners). Passive immunization is also recommended for sexual partners of persons with acute hepatitis B infections, household contacts (especially children less than one year of age) of persons with acute infection, and mucosal or percutaneous exposure to HBsAg-positive blood. Simultaneous active immunization with the hepatitis B vaccine is recommended in these cases.

Immunization with the hepatitis B vaccine (active immunization) is currently recommended for all infants, sexually active adolescents, intravenous drug users, homosexual males, children receiving blood or blood products regularly (e.g., hemophiliacs), children in chronic care facilities, household contacts of chronic carriers, and health care professionals. The schedule consists of three doses. Infants should receive the first dose before discharge from the nursery or shortly thereafter, the second dose one to two months later, and the third dose at 6 to 18 months of age. Intervals for other individuals should be similar.

Perinatal vertical transmission of hepatitis B can be prevented by giving newborns hepatitis B immune globulin (0.5 mL intramuscularly) within 12 hours after birth and hepatitis B vaccine concurrently (at a different site) prior to discharge. This practice prevents approximately 90% of chronic infections in infants born to mothers with HBsAg and hepatitis Be antigen (HBeAG).

PROGNOSIS

The prognosis for children with viral hepatitis depends on etiology as well as age. With hepatitis A the prognosis is generally good, with an uneventful recovery. Infants and children infected with hepatitis B, on the other hand, are at high risk of becoming chronic carriers. Approximately 25% of carriers develop chronic, active hepatitis, which often progresses to cirrhosis. In addition, the risk of developing hepatocellular carcinoma is 12 to 300 times higher in these patients compared to the rest of the population.

Chronic hepatitis also occurs with hepatitis C, but fortunately this does not occur commonly in children. Approximately 50% of patients with acute disease later develop chronic, active hepatitis, and 10 to 20% progress to cirrhosis and hepatic failure.

Likewise, complications of hepatitis D, such as cirrhosis and portal hypertension, are not uncommon. They occur more frequently than with hepatitis B, however, and progress more rapidly. Infection with hepatitis E does not result in a chronic condition.

Fatal hepatitis A is a rare occurrence. The overall mortality associated with hepatitis B, C, and E is also low (approximately 1–2%). For hepatitis D, however, it is more variable, ranging from 2 to 20%. Figures increase to 30% for hepatitis B with coinfection with hepatitis D. In addition, hepatitis E can be fatal in 20% of infected pregnant women.

Case Resolution

In the case history, the boy has a classic presentation of viral hepatitis despite no history of travel to an endemic area. Because he does not appear to be dehydrated or seriously ill, he can be managed as an outpatient. Statistics point to a probable infection with hepatitis A. Serologies for both hepatitis A and B should be performed, however, in addition to LFTs and coagulation studies. The parents should be informed of the probable diagnosis and receive prophylaxis with immune globulin. They should also be educated regarding the infectivity of the disease and counseled about supportive therapy. The boy should be scheduled for a follow-up visit in a few days for repeat LFTs and coagulation tests. The prognosis is good.

Selected Readings

American Academy of Pediatrics, Committee on School Health. Prevention of hepatitis B virus infection in school settings. Pediatrics 91:848–850, 1993.

American Medical Association. Prevention, Diagnosis, and Management of Viral Hepatitis. Chicago, American Medical Association, 1995.

A-Kader, H. H., and W. F. Balistreri. Hepatitis C virus: implications to pediatric practice. Pediatr. Infect. Dis. J. 12:853–866, 1993.

Centers for Disease Control and Prevention. Protection against viral hepatitis: recommendations of the Immunization Practices Advisory Committee (ACIP). M.M.W.R. 39(S–2):1–26, 1990.

Frymoyer, C. L. Preventing the spread of viral hepatitis. Am. Fam. Physician 48:1479–1486, 1993.

Krugman, S. Viral hepatitis: A, B, C, D, and E—infection. Pediatr. Rev. 13:203–212, 1992.

Krugman, S. Viral hepatitis: A, B, C, D, and E—prevention. Pediatr. Rev. 13:245–247, 1992.

Lee, M. A., and H. C. Meissner. Hepatitis in adolescents. Adol. Med. State Art Rev. 2:499–507, 1991.

Nowicki, M. J., and W. F. Balistreri. The Cs, Ds, and Es of viral hepatitis. Contemp. Pediatr. 9:23–42, 1992.

Shapiro, C. N. Epidemiology of hepatitis B. Pediatr. Infect. Dis. J. 12:433–437, 1993.

Shapiro, C. N., and S. C. Hadler. Hepatitis A and hepatitis B virus infection in day-care settings. Pediatr. Ann. 20:435–441, 1991.

Stevens, C. E., et al. Prospects for control of hepatitis B virus infection: implications of childhood vaccination and long-term protection. Pediatrics 90:170–173, 1992.

NEUROLOGIC DISORDERS

C H A P T E R   8 6

HYPOTONIA

Kenneth R. Huff, M.D.

Hₓ   A 6-month-old girl is brought to the office because she does not reach for her toys anymore. The pregnancy was full term, but the mother remembers that the fetal kicking was less than with an older brother. Delivery was uncomplicated, and the infant fed well. The girl began to show visual attention at two to three weeks, smiled socially at one month, and pushed up while prone at two months. Although she turned over at four months, she has not done this in the last month. She no longer reaches up to the mobile over her crib.

On examination, the girl lies quietly on the table and watches the examiner intently. Her growth parameters, including head circumference, are normal. After she has been undressed, it is apparent that she "see-saw" breathes (i.e., abdomen rises with inspiration) and has a "frog leg" posture. Her cranial nerve examination is normal except for head turning strength. When she is pulled to a sitting position, her head lags far behind and her arms are straight at the elbows. She cannot raise her arms off the table. When a rattle is placed in her hands, she manipulates the toy, which she regards from the corner of her eye. Her deep tendon reflexes are absent, but her pain sensation is intact.

Questions

1. How is the level of nervous system involvement determined in infants with hypotonia?
2. What is the significance of the loss of developmental milestones or abilities?
3. What are the related clinical management issues?
4. When is genetic counseling appropriate for children with hypotonia?

cell, peripheral nerve components, myoneural junction, muscle fibers in the motor unit) is most important in determining the etiology of hypotonia in infants and children.

EPIDEMIOLOGY

In infants, hypotonia is not an uncommon finding, and nonneuromuscular causes of hypotonia are more common than neuromuscular conditions. These include hypoxic ischemic encephalopathy and brain lesions related to premature birth. Duchenne's muscular dystrophy is the most common neuromuscular condition of childhood. The incidence of Duchenne's muscular dystrophy is 1:1700–3500 male births. Spinal muscular atrophy is the next most common condition, with an incidence close to that of cystic fibrosis. Both disorders are due to gene mutations.

CLINICAL PRESENTATION

Hypotonic infants have delayed motor milestones, decreased movements, and poor head and trunk control (Fig. 86–1). Older children may have decreased ability to resist with strength testing of individual muscle groups as well as impaired functional strength in walking, sitting, or running (Dₓ Box).

PATHOPHYSIOLOGY

Tone is a product of connective tissue structural elements, including ligaments, tendons, and joint cap-

Infants with decreased tone are referred to as hypotonic, or "floppy." Hypotonia is most simply defined as lower than normal resistance to passive motion across a joint. Although this resistance has other components, muscle strength is a key component of this resistance. In infants who cannot cooperate with testing, tone can be effectively used as a measure of strength. Identification of the level of the nervous system affected (e.g., upper motor neurons, spinal cord, anterior horn

---

Dₓ   Hypotonia

- Decreased resistance to passive movement of a joint
- Muscular weakness in older children
- Etiologic diagnosis related to the nervous system level of the lesion

FIGURE 86–1. *Hypotonic infant being pulled into sitting position. Arms are completely extended, head control is poor, and legs are abducted at the hip.*

sules; muscle fiber number and integrity, leading to strength; and nerve fiber input to muscle. The control of tone through the anterior horn cell is complex and involves more than just corticospinal tract influences. Tone may be most directly decreased by lesions of the neuromuscular apparatus, but lesions in any of these elements at any level can affect tone.

The nature of the lesions can be quite varied. Structural abnormalities of muscle fibers can result from congenital myopathies, genetically induced degenerative death of anterior horn cells in spinal atrophy, and birth asphyxia in ischemic encephalopathy. All of these conditions produce hypotonia.

DIFFERENTIAL DIAGNOSIS

Any of the numerous causes of **static encephalopathy**, including hypoxia, ischemia at birth, cerebral dysgenesis, or intracranial hemorrhage, may result in hypotonia in infants. Common neuromuscular causes are **spinal muscular atrophy, congenital myopathy,** and **myotonic dystrophy.** In older children, postinfectious neuritis, hereditary neuropathy, and muscular dystrophy frequently lead to hypotonia with weakness (Table 86–1).

It is often useful to distinguish **CNS causes** from peripheral nervous system or neuromuscular causes. Children with a CNS problem may have a below-normal level of attention or range of awareness and may lack age-appropriate social skills. Fine motor coordination, quality and repertoire of movements, and language may be affected in older children. The deep tendon reflexes may be brisk or easily elicited. In contrast, children with hypotonia caused by neuromuscular lesions may have an interested and visually attentive facial appearance in the presence of severe weakness that allows only sparse

or nearly absent limb movements. Deep tendon reflexes may be difficult to elicit or absent in many children with such lesions.

Older children may display a pattern of weakness that gives a clue to the level of involvement. If the weakness is preferentially in upper extremity extensor and lower extremity knee flexor, ankle dorsiflexor, and ankle everter muscle groups, the disturbance may involve upper motor neurons or CNS causes. This differential weakness may be present and contribute to hypotonia for a long period before spasticity intervenes and affects tone. If the weakness involves agonist and antagonist equally, however, it may represent a neuromuscular process.

EVALUATION

A methodical assessment of clinical and laboratory features in children can help narrow a very wide differential diagnosis by localizing the lesion to a level of the nervous system (Table 86–2).

History

Past history is useful for correct diagnosis (Questions Box). Information about the pregnancy and birth is important. For example, relatively decreased fetal movements may signify an early degenerative condition. Birth events should be investigated for sources of possible trauma to the neonatal nervous system, such as prematurity or birth asphyxia. The physician should determine whether or not any skills have been lost. Any associated loss of tone or strength could signify a progressive condition, rather than a static problem as would occur with a birth injury. The acuteness of the developing weakness is an important clue in the differential diagnosis.

TABLE 86–1. Differential Diagnosis of Infantile Hypotonia

Level	Specific Lesion
Cerebral hemisphere	Static encephalopathy related to perinatal or prenatal insults
	Dysgenesis (e.g., Down's syndrome)
	Degenerative conditions (e.g., storage disease)
Spinal cord	Traumatic transection
	Dysraphism or other malformation
Anterior horn cell	Spinal muscular atrophy
	Poliomyelitis
Peripheral nerve	Leukodystrophy
	Type III hereditary sensory-motor neuropathy
	Acute polyneuritis (rarely occurs in infancy)
Myoneural junction	Myasthenia gravis
	Toxin (botulism or "mycin" antibiotic)
Muscle	Congenital structural myopathy
	Congenital myotonic dystrophy
	Congenital muscular dystrophy
	Mitochondrial myopathy
Systemic	Amino and organic acidopathies, hypercalcemia, renal acidosis, rickets, scurvy, celiac disease, hypothyroidism, collagen disease, congenital heart disease

TABLE 86–2. Approach to the Diagnosis of Hypotonia

Clinical Feature	Anatomic Site				
	Cerebrum	Spinal Cord	Anterior Horn Cell	Neuromuscular Junction	Muscle
Alertness	Decreased	Normal	Normal	Normal	Normal
Cry	Decreased	Normal	Normal/weak	Weak	Normal/weak
Eye movements	Sometimes abnormal	Normal	Normal	Abnormal	Normal
Tongue fasciculations	Absent	Absent	Present	Absent	Absent
Muscle bulk	Normal	Normal	Decreased	Normal	Decreased
Deep tendon reflexes	Normal/increased	Decreased/increased	Absent	Normal	Normal/decreased

In addition, the family history should be determined. It may indicate a genetic explanation for the hypotonia or a maternal basis for the perinatal weakness.

Physical Examination

Dysmorphic features should be noted in developmentally delayed children because they may suggest possible cerebral dysgenesis. Some dysmorphic features (e.g., hypoplastic mandible; high, arched palate) may suggest a congenital neuromuscular condition. Age-appropriate cognitive abilities should be assessed as a measure of cerebral function. This evaluation may range from primarily observation of visual attention in very young infants to assessment of language and academic skills in older children. Cranial nerve examination with regard to eye movements, facial strength, and presence of tongue fasciculations is important, especially in the differential diagnosis of many neuromuscular conditions (e.g., spinal muscular atrophy, congenital myopathies).

Tone and strength should be examined carefully in both trunk and limbs. Individual joint movements should be observed, and agonist-antagonist strengths should be tested bilaterally to check for asymmetries and focal discrepancies. The presence of deep tendon reflexes should also be carefully noted. Sensory testing is important in suspected neuropathies, radiculopathies, and myelopathies.

Observation rather than formal neuromuscular testing is often easier and more revealing, particularly in infants and preschool-age children. Useful activities to observe include walking, running, climbing stairs or stepping onto a stool, lying on the floor and rising to a standing position unassisted, smiling, tightly closing eyes, and speaking. In the case of hypotonic neonates, the mother may also need to be examined for the presence of signs of myotonic dystrophy or myasthenia gravis.

Laboratory Tests

The purpose of laboratory tests is to confirm the suspected level of involvement (Table 86–3). Serum **creatine phosphokinase (CPK),** a screen for muscle fiber necrosis, should be requested when the history suggests a degenerative condition or the examination indicates the cause of the hypotonia is in the neuromuscular unit. CPK is one to two orders of magnitude higher than normal in children with muscular dystrophy, and it may also be mildly elevated in female carriers of the mutant dystrophin gene early in life. The serum CPK level may be less markedly elevated in children with inflammatory myopathies such as dermatomyositis and polymyositis and to some extent following muscle trauma, including EMG.

Useful information about the presence of neuropathic, primary myopathic, and neuromuscular junction disorders can be obtained from the **nerve conduction velocity** and **EMG.** Demyelinating neuropathies slow nerve conduction or produce signs of a segmental block. If the hypotonia is the result of motor neuropathy, an axonal neuropathy may have depressed amplitude of the nerve action potential or fibrillation potentials on EMG. In some myopathies, bizarre or small amplitude potentials and myotonia may be seen on EMG. Decremental response to stimulation and other abnormalities are evident with myasthenia gravis and neuromuscular junction blockade caused by the botulinus toxin. An intravenous edrophonium (Tensilon) test can confirm a diagnosis of myasthenia gravis in patients with easy fatigability on history or examination.

When properly handled, a **muscle biopsy** gives useful diagnostic information about neuromuscular disorders that may cause hypotonia. A large section of tissue should be frozen for histochemical studies, and part of the muscle should be fixed in glutaraldehyde for electron microscopy to determine if ultrastructural abnormalities such as those seen in specific congenital or mitochondrial myopathies are present. Histochemical studies can differentiate neuropathic changes from

---

Questions: Hypotonia

- Were the fetal movements of the child abnormal or less than those of previous pregnancies?
- Was the pregnancy full term? Was the delivery complicated?
- Do the mother, any siblings, or other family members suffer from a similar weakness?
- Has the child lost any developmental skills? Is the problem getting worse?
- If the weakness is worsening, how rapidly is it progressing?

TABLE 86–3 Laboratory Tests Useful in the Diagnosis of Hypotonia Caused by Neuromuscular Lesions

	Anatomic Site		
Test	Anterior Horn Cell	Neuromuscular Junction	Muscle
Muscle enzymes	Normal	Normal	Normal/increased
Tensilon test	Normal	Abnormal	Normal
Electromyography (EMG)	Neuropathic abnormal	Decremental	Myopathic
Muscle biopsy	Group atrophy	Normal	Myopathic

myopathic changes related to fiber type specificities, as well as convey structural abnormalities pointing to dystrophy or congenital myopathy. Various special stains can also give information about metabolic myopathic disorders.

When myopathy is suspected on the basis of clinical evidence, biopsy tissue samples can be subjected to specific analyses such as dystrophin protein levels, glycolytic enzyme activity analysis, respiratory chain enzyme complex assays, carnitine levels, or fatty acid transport assays to confirm the diagnosis. Various molecular techniques, including specific nucleic acid probes, restriction fragment length polymorphism analysis, and linkage analysis can be used in blood or tissue studies to help diagnose particular genetic disorders (e.g., Duchenne's or other X-linked muscular dystrophies, myotonic dystrophies, mitochondrial cytopathies). Cytogenetic analysis may be useful when Down's or Prader-Willi syndromes are suspected as causes of nonparalytic hypotonia.

Imaging Studies

A CT or MRI scan is indicated in two situations: (1) when deficits in mental status, cognitive function, or attention are apparent in children with hypotonia and (2) when neurologic examination suggests an upper motor neuron component, such as active deep tendon reflexes or persistent ankle clonus, to the weakness or hypotonia. Imaging studies should also be performed in children who have hypotonia as part of a multiorgan system dysgenesis, such as with a chromosomal aberration, because of the relatively higher likelihood of a CNS component to the dysgenesis.

MANAGEMENT

The management of hypotonic infants frequently depends on the underlying diagnosis. For example, an infant with a congenital myopathy that is expected to improve with time should receive total supportive care, including long-term ventilatory support and gastrostomy feeding. In contrast, an infant with the severe infantile type of spinal muscular atrophy would not be supported as aggressively because of the degenerative nature of the diagnosis and the terminal prognosis.

It should be remembered that children with profound weakness easily succumb to respiratory infections and have difficulty with recovery from anesthesia; therefore, they require vigilance, **early intervention,** and **intensive respiratory support.** In nonprogressive or slowly progressive conditions, **orthopedic surgery** can help through procedures that improve joint function by equalizing or stabilizing muscles of different strengths. If children have rehabilitative potential, **physical and occupational therapy** can accelerate recovery or maximize function.

In older children with acquired acute hypotonic weaknesses, such as those listed in Table 86–4, more directed therapies are indicated. Acute postinfectious polyneuritis requires careful frequent monitoring of respiratory status and artificial ventilation when significant loss of vital capacity has occurred. Children should be considered for **plasmapheresis** when their condition rapidly worsens early in the course of the disorder. **Immunoglobulin therapy** is still somewhat controversial, but it may be considered in children who are too small for the venous access required for pheresis. Specific antisera are available for botulinus toxin. Dysimmune myasthenia can be treated with anticholinesterase medication, immunoglobulin therapy, and thymectomy when resistant to medication. Chronic relapsing polyneuritis and myositis can be treated effectively with anti-inflammatory agents such as prednisone and immunoglobin therapy.

Treatment and care of children with muscular dystrophy is presently directed toward maintaining mobility and preventing contractures through physical therapy, bivalved casts, and braces. Inactivity increases disability. Adjunctive steroid therapy is useful in children with Duchenne's dystrophy, but beneficial effects are temporary and must be weighed against steroid toxicity. Many new hardware technologies (e.g., long leg braces, electric wheelchairs, battery-operated ventilators) have allowed affected children to overcome previously insurmountable handicaps.

TABLE 86–4. Specific Etiologies of Hypotonia Caused by Acute Generalized Weaknesses

Acute postinfectious polyradiculoneuritis (Landry-Guillain-Barré syndrome)
Postinfectious myositis
Enteroviral poliomyelitis
Acute myasthenia gravis
Infantile botulism
Tick paralysis
Periodic paralysis (hyperkalemic, hypokalemic, and normokalemic)

PROGNOSIS

Genetic conditions may progress to a terminal outcome. The course can be quite variable, however. The variability may relate to different alleles at the same locus, as in the case of spinal muscular atrophy, or different mutations of the same locus, as in the case of Duchenne's and Becker's muscular dystrophy. Weakness in infants with congenital myopathy or infantile botulism frequently improves with time. The immunologic neuromuscular disorders frequently have a relapsing, remitting course, but they may respond to appropriate treatment.

Case Resolution

The 6-month-old girl in the case history is judged to have hypotonia with a neuromuscular cause, in part because of her alert appearance and absent deep tendon reflexes. Neuropathic abnormalities on EMG and muscle biopsy confirm the diagnosis of spinal muscular atrophy suggested by her rapidly progressive course. The family receive

genetic couseling, become involved in a support group, and eventually reach a decision to forego intubation with eventual respiratory failure in their daughter. The physician coordinates hospice services for the family.

Selected Readings

Brooke, M. H. A Clinician's View of Neuromuscular Diseases, 2nd ed. Baltimore, Williams & Wilkins, 1986.

Buist, N. R. M., and B. R. Powell. Approaches to the evaluation of muscle diseases. Int. Pediatr. 7:320–326, 1992.

Dubowitz, V. Muscle Disorders in Childhood, 2nd ed. (1995) Philadelphia, W. B. Saunders, 1995.

Engle, A. G. Myasthenic syndromes. In Engel, A. G., and B. Q. Banker (eds.). Myology. New York, McGraw-Hill, 1986, p. 1955–1990.

Epstein, M., and Sladky, J. The role of plasmapheresis in childhood Guillain-Barré syndrome. Ann. Neurol. 28:65–69, 1990.

Fenichel, G. M. Clinical Pediatric Neurology, 2nd ed. Philadelphia, W. B. Saunders, 1993, pp. 169–195.

Menkes, J. H. Textbook of Child Neurology, 4th ed. Philadelphia, Lea & Febiger, 1990, pp. 601–635.

Shapira, Y. Clinical aspects of mitochondrial encephalomyopathies. Int. Pediatr. 8:225–232, 1993.

Wessel, H. B. Dystrophin: a clinical perspective. Pediatr. Neurol. 6:3–12, 1990.

CHAPTER 87

HEADACHES

Kenneth R. Huff, M.D.

H$_x$ A 12-year-old girl complains of headaches. She has been sent home from school twice in the last six weeks and has experienced headaches for at least a year. The headache begins as a dull feeling over both eyes, radiating up to the top of the head and eventually developing a pounding character. The girl has no preliminary visual symptoms or other warning prior to the head pain.

The last episode began in an afternoon class after the girl had been outside on a hot sunny day for physical education. The headache worsened as she walked home from school. She went to her room, closed the curtains, and lay down. Because of nausea and loss of appetite, she skipped dinner, but she did not vomit. She reportedly had no diplopia, vertigo, ataxia, or limb weakness; her speech was observed to be articulate and coherent. She took 160 mg of acetaminophen without obtaining significant relief, but she eventually fell asleep. The following morning she felt fine.

Between headaches, the girl's behavior is unchanged, and she continues to earn above-average grades. She has not experienced any major changes in her home environment. The girl's mother initially denies having "migraines,"

but she admits to needing to lie down because of headaches about once a month. A detailed neurologic examination of the girl is completely normal.

Questions

1. What are the major causes of headache?
2. How do the symptoms help differentiate the causes?
3. How does family history influence the etiology of headache?
4. What is the appropriate treatment for the problem headache?

Headaches, which are very common in adolescents and older children, frequently prompt parents to bring their children to the physician's attention. The physician must differentiate headaches that are symptomatic of a progressive intracranial process from those that may possibly be intermittently disabling but do not necessitate surgery. The cornerstone of this determination is obtaining key historical information and noting abnormalities on examination of the nervous system. Decisions about management strategies are most influenced by etiology and the impact the headaches are having on the child's life.

EPIDEMIOLOGY

Chronic, recurrent headaches in children that are not related to a self-limited condition are frequently lumped together as "migraine," which includes classic and common migraine. Numerous potential triggering factors are involved, and it is presumed that the cranial vessels play a pathogenic role. The prevalence of migraines is about 3% for all children. Headaches are also commonly associated with trauma, acute intercurrent infection, or systemic illness. The contribution of symptomatic headaches (for example those due to tumors, vascular abnormalities, or meningitis) to the overall prevalence of headache is relatively small. Initial symptoms usually begin between 6 and 12 years of age, but many adolescents may present with headache problems for the first time.

A multigenerational family history of "sick headaches" is found in the majority of children with migraine. This history must be specifically elicited by the physician, however, because its significance is often discounted by parents.

CLINICAL PRESENTATION

Younger children may complain of head pain or present with nausea or vomiting. Adolescents may report persistent, dull, aching or pounding head pain. The pain may be episodic, stable in frequency, and similar to that experienced by other family members to some degree (D_x Box). Alternatively, it may be increasing in intensity or frequency and be associated with neurologic signs, suggesting an intracranial mass lesion. Classic migraine, which is relatively unusual in children, is distinguished from common migraine by the presence of an aura and sensory symptoms that precede the headache. Both types of headache may be associated with lethargy, slowness of movement and response, intolerance of intense sound or light, and loss of appetite.

PATHOPHYSIOLOGY

Pain fibers are carried in the trigeminal nerves from the scalp, skull, meninges, and vessel walls within the

TABLE 87–1. Triggers of Migraine

Glare, dazzle, bright sunlight, or fluorescent lighting
Physical exertion, fatigue, lack of sleep, hunger
Change in ambient temperature or humidity
Allergic reactions, pungent odors
Certain foods, alcoholic beverages, and cold foods or beverages
Anxiety, stress, and worry
Head trauma
Menstruation and oral contraceptives
Refractive errors (rare)

brain. Traction on these fibers or inflammation at the endings produces the pain that is associated with blood clots, other mass lesions, or meningeal inflammation. Traditionally, migraine and tension headaches in adults have been viewed as etiologically distinct. This distinction is less valid with younger children. However, a number of different pathogenic mechanisms may lead to different headache syndromes within the framework of childhood migraine. Several different mechanisms that involve one or many environmental factors may "trigger" headache in genetically predisposed individuals (Table 87–1). The relevant neurotransmitter at the nerve endings may be serotonin (perhaps emanating from platelet stores), but release may be precipitated by a cascade of local cytokines in and around vessel walls due to these triggers. The role of genetic susceptibility and environmental agents is currently being investigated.

DIFFERENTIAL DIAGNOSIS

Acute Headaches

Emergent causes should be considered if headaches have an abrupt onset, develop rapidly, are especially severe, or if children describe them as "the worst of my life." **Intracranial hemorrhage** from a ruptured aneurysm, an arterial-venous malformation, or rarely, as a secondary effect from hypertension is foremost on the list of such causes. If children have a condition that may potentially lead to stroke, such as coagulopathy, hemoglobinopathy, or heart disease, the stroke may become hemorrhagic and produce acute, severe headache.

Nonhemorrhagic meningeal irritation, such as the inflammation produced by bacterial or viral meningitis, may also cause acute headaches. These conditions may render patients confused and lethargic while still conscious and are often associated with fever. Both types of meningitis produce signs of meningeal irritation: nuchal rigidity (stiff neck) and Kernig's and Brudzinski's signs.

Tumor-related Headaches

Children with brain tumors may also present with headaches that increase in frequency or severity and generally are not localized. Some children with brain tumors experience vomiting without complaining of headaches. If headaches occur, they may awaken children from sleep because of the relative shift in intracranial traction forces due to gravity and the horizontal position.

Chronic or Recurrent Headaches

Sinus infection may be a cause of either chronically recurring headaches or acute headaches, especially if children relate that the pain is more facial than cranial. Symptoms of chronic nasal congestion, allergies, and postnasal drip may be associated with **sinus headaches**.

Other types of headaches may recur. **Tension headaches** may produce the feeling of a tightening band around the head, occur later in the day, and be associated with a stressful environment. **Posttraumatic headaches** may recur with decreasing severity up to several months following head trauma. **Cluster headaches** are associated with lancinating pain, unilateral tearing, and nasal stuffiness. The pain of **migraine headaches** is dull in character, and if headaches are severe, patients shun other intense sensory stimuli.

EVALUATION

History

Information should be obtained from patients, parents, and other caregivers concerning the quality, intensity, and location of the headache as well as associated symptoms before and during the headache (Questions Box). The duration, clinical course, and conditions that evoke, intensify, or alleviate the pain are also important. It is useful to have children describe a typical episode (perhaps the most recent), including the circumstances of when and where the headache began and how it affected activities at the time. The degree to which the headache problem affects the child's life-style influences the management plan.

Questions: Headaches

- Where is the child, what time of day is it, and what is the child doing when a typical headache begins?
- Where is the pain located? How severe is the pain? How long does the pain last?
- Is nausea, vomiting, or photophobia associated with the headache?
- What does the child do after getting the headache? Does the episode require cessation of activities?
- Does the child take any medication for the pain? Does this or anything else make the child feel better?
- How long ago did the first headache occur? Are the headaches becoming more frequent or severe?
- Have headaches ever awakened the child at night?
- Have there been any changes in speech, vision, gait, or personality, or any loss of skills or abilities between headaches?
- Does the child have any warning symptoms before the pain? Does unilateral visual loss, weakness or numbness, diplopia, confusion, or loss of consciousness occur with the headache?
- How often does the child miss school because of a headache?
- Do other members of the family have headaches? Do they ever need to lie down with these headaches?

Physical Examination

A thorough examination is needed to determine if neurologic findings suggest an emergent problem or potential neurosurgical condition such as meningitis, intracranial hemorrhage, or brain tumor. The examination should assess for the presence of sinus tenderness by palpation, nuchal rigidity, funduscopic pathology, and any focal neurologic signs. Signs are referable to the part of the brain involved by a neoplasm or other space-occupying lesion (e.g., ataxia and cranial nerve dysfunction for posterior fossa tumors; constricted visual fields or hypothalamic dysfunction [endocrine abnormalities] for suprasellar tumors; hemiparesis, hemisensory deficits, or language dysfunction for cerebral hemispheric tumors). Increased ICP may lead to papilledema, general hypertonicity, positive Babinski signs, spastic gait, loss of continence, or confusion or stupor due to blockage of CSF by the tumor.

Rarely, children in the midst of a migraine headache may display confusion, aphasia, unilateral numbness, or less commonly, weakness, hemianopsia, or ophthalmoplegia. In these circumstances, the diagnosis of migraine is reached only after other diagnostic tests have eliminated more emergent conditions.

Laboratory Tests

If stiff neck is present and focal or lateralized neurologic signs are absent, an immediate CSF examination is indicated to diagnose the cause of meningeal inflammation. When hemorrhagic fluid is encountered, it is often useful to centrifuge a specimen to check for xanthochromia and to count cells in a subsequent sample to differentiate a traumatic spinal tap from subarachnoid hemorrhage.

Imaging Studies

If signs or symptoms of increased ICP are apparent, a CT or MRI scan must be obtained to diagnose the etiology of the headaches correctly. Focal neurologic signs also suggest the need for a CT or MRI scan. Radiologic studies, including CT or plain films, are helpful with the diagnosis of chronic or recurrent sinus headaches. Cerebral angiography may be necessary to locate a focal source of subarachnoid hemorrhage.

MANAGEMENT

After a careful assessment has shown no structural abnormalities, the appropriate management is often just **reassurance.** Families should be told that the problem will not progress and is not caused by a surgical lesion. Sometimes pointing out the familial basis of a child's headaches (and their similarities to parents' headaches) may help parents understand the benign nature of the condition and find effective strategies for helping a child deal with the problem.

However, it may be apparent from the historical information that children are suffering significantly from the headaches or are so debilitated or handicapped by

TABLE 87–2. Drugs Useful in Childhood Headaches

Abortive (Symptomatic)

Acetaminophen	325–975 mg q4h (15 mg/kg/dose) (max: 5 doses/24 hr)
Ibuprofen	200–800 mg q6h (10 mg/kg/dose) (max: 40 mg/kg/24 hr)
Butalbital (Fioricet)	50 mg q4h (1.5 mg/kg/dose) (max: 9 mg/kg/24 hr)
Ergotamine, SL	2–4 mg, then 2 mg q30min prn (max: 6–12 mg [older children and adolescents])
Sumatriptan, SC	6 mg (may repeat after 1 hr) (max: 2 doses/24 hr [older children and adolescents])
Dihydroergotamine, IV	0.25–1 mg at onset and 1 mg/h × 2 (max: 6 mg/wk [older children and adolescents])
Dexamethasone, IV	4–16 mg single dose (0.25 mg/kg) or rapidly tapering q6h

Prophylactic

Diphenylhydantoin	5 mg/kg, divided bid (max: 7 mg/kg [follow serum level])
Propranolol	10–40 mg bid to qid (max: 40–80 mg/24 hr if ≤ 35 kg; 120–160 mg/24 hr if > 35 kg; no more than 320 mg/24 hr)
Cyproheptadine	1–4 mg bid–qid (0.25–0.5 mg/kg/24 hr) (max: 16 mg/24 hr)
Amitriptyline	25–75 mg qhs (max: 150 mg/24 hr [older children and adolescents])

the frequency of the occurrences that their life-style is adversely affected. In such cases, symptomatic or prophylactic treatment, or a combination of both types, is warranted (Table 87–2). **Symptomatic treatment** often begins with a trial of an adequate dose of **acetaminophen**. If this is not effective, **NSAIDs** may be beneficial. If severe headaches resolve with sleep, then a short-acting **barbiturate** such as butalbital may be effective. For severe, recurrent headaches, **sumatriptan** has proved beneficial and has relatively mild side effects, but it must be given by injection. Refractory headaches may require intravenous **dihydroergotamine** under medical observation.

The decision to begin a **prophylactic medication** should be based on a combination of frequency and severity of the headaches. The virtues of potentially controlling headache-related symptoms must be weighed against the risk of side effects. In younger children, anticonvulsants such as **diphenylhydantoin** have been found to be successful antimigraine agents.

Propranolol and **nadolol,** unlike other beta-blocking drugs, have demonstrated efficacy as prophylactic agents. **Amitriptyline** is also an effective preventive treatment in older children and adolescents; a single bedtime dose should be used at first. A one-to-two-week trial is necessary before concluding the initial treatment has been ineffective. Amitriptyline can also be combined with propranolol if necessary.

PROGNOSIS

Many children with headaches have a good prognosis and do not require ongoing intervention after families are reassured of the benign nature of the problem. For the remainder of children, symptomatic medications are frequently effective. Prophylactic medication is necessary in a few cases. If headaches are controlled expeditiously, children frequently experience remission, and early withdrawal of the prophylactic medications is often possible without exacerbation.

Case Resolution

In the case history, the child's symptoms and the circumstances of the headache suggest a diagnosis of migraine. No laboratory tests or imaging studies are necessary. The girl is begun on amitriptyline and instructed to keep a calendar of headache occurrences. She has two headaches in the first two weeks, which are aborted effectively with ibuprofen. Following these episodes, she has no further recurrences, and the amitriptyline is withdrawn successfully after three months.

Selected Readings

Barlow, C. F. Headaches and Migraine in Childhood. Clinics in Developmental Medicine No. 91, Spastics International Medical Publications. Oxford, U.K., Blackwell Scientific Publications, and Philadelphia, J. B. Lippincott, 1984.

Fenichel, G. M. Migraine in children. *In* Pediatric Neurology. Neurol. Clin. North Am. 3:77–94, 1985.

Moskowitz, M. A. The neurobiology of vascular head pain. Ann. Neurol. 16:157–168, 1984.

Prensky, A. L. Diagnosis and treatment of migraine in children. Neurology 29:506–510, 1979.

Rothner, A. D. Diagnosis and management of headache in children and adolescents. *In* Neurol. Clin. North Am. 1:511–526, 1979.

TICS

Kenneth R. Huff, M.D.

Hx An eight-year-old boy has unusual recurring behaviors that began two to three months ago. He stretches his neck or raises his eyebrows several times a day. Sometimes he is able to suppress these actions. The boy's parents report that in the last two years he has displayed repetitive behaviors, including blinking, grimacing, rubbing his chin on his left shoulder, making a "gulping" sound, and sniffing. Originally they thought the sniffing was related to hay fever, but the boy has no other allergic symptoms. He does not use profane words. In conversations, he sometimes repeats the last phrase of a sentence that was just used whether by himself or someone else. In addition, he must touch each light switch in the hallway every time he leaves his room, and he must retie his shoelaces several times until they are exactly the same length. Although his schoolwork has not deteriorated, he has always had trouble completing tasks and finishing homework. Both his teacher and his best friend have asked about his strange behavior. His mother has a psychological problem with her son's gulping sounds (i.e., they recur in her own mind), and she recalls that her father had a habit of frequently looking over one shoulder for no apparent reason.

Although during examination the boy does not exhibit any unusual behaviors, he raises his eyebrows twice and places his hand over his crotch several times while his parents are interviewed. Except for mild fine motor dyscoordination, the neurologic examination is normal.

Questions

1. What are the characteristics of tics?
2. What are the social implications of tics?
3. Should pharmacologic treatments be part of the management of tics?
4. What other problems are associated with movement disorders?

EPIDEMIOLOGY

Tics are relatively common in children but often go unrecognized as movement disorders. The onset of tics is generally between 6 and 12 years of age but can be as late as 21. Many cases of Gilles de la Tourette's syndrome, a common cause of tics in children, are familial, although other family members may have symptoms so mild that they never seek medical attention. The only manifestation in some family members may be obsessive-compulsive symptoms. Symptoms occur in multiple generations and in both sexes. The prevalence of tics is higher in males than in females.

CLINICAL PRESENTATION

Children with tics display sudden, repetitive movements of the face, neck, or shoulders in the context of normal behaviors. These actions can be suppressed for periods of time, however. The involuntary movements include the vocal apparatus, and different movements may appear over a period of weeks or months. Often children have associated problems of learning difficulties and obsessive behaviors (D$_x$ Box).

PATHOPHYSIOLOGY

Tics are a movement disorder, and therefore are thought to be related to an abnormality in deep structures within the cerebral hemispheres. So far no lesion visible on brain imaging studies has been correlated with the symptoms. It is hypothesized that abnormal neural function is related to an abnormality in dopamine neurotransmitter mechanisms of action, and evidence in patients shows this to be the case. This evidence has led to a "hypersensitive receptor" for dopamine theory in the patients.

In patients with Tourette's syndrome, the cerebrospinal fluid contains low levels of homovanillic acid, a dopamine metabolite. In addition, amphetamines and

Tics are brief, abrupt, nonpurposeful movements or utterances. They occur in a background of normal activity and are repetitive and involuntary but can be suppressed. Movements usually involve the face, neck, or shoulders and sometimes muscles in the limbs or other parts of the body. Tics may either mimic normal, sometimes complex movements or involve a series of orchestrated simple movements. In contrast, habits are complex, voluntary, purposeful, repetitive behaviors that involve several movements and suggest more directed actions.

D$_x$ Tics

- Sudden, brief uncontrolled movements
- Repetitive sounds from the vocal apparatus
- Variable manifestations historically
- Associated behavior problems

methylphenidate increase dopamine release, and in some instances, these agents precipitate tic symptoms. Haloperidol blocks the dopamine receptor and therefore may block some of the negative feedback from a potentially hypersensitive receptor for dopamine. This then allows for more dopamine release and subsequently higher levels of homovanillic acid. The observations of clinical response and side effects with low amounts of haloperidol and the finding of homovanillic acid levels remaining high long after disappearance of the neuroleptic drug both support this hypothesis.

DIFFERENTIAL DIAGNOSIS

The duration, frequency, and appearance of the movement, and circumstances of occurrence of tics help distinguish them from several other episodic movement disorders. Myoclonus is a lightninglike, nonsuppressible jerk of a small group of muscles, and chorea involves nearly constant, small amplitude movements of the fingers, hands, and feet that are often accompanied by grimacing movements of the face. Tremor is an oscillatory movement of an extremity or the head. Hemiballismus is an uncontrollable episodic throwing movement of an extremity. Hyperexplexia is a hyperactive startle response provoked by touch or sudden noise. Torticollis, or neck writhing, may be paroxysmal. Paroxysmal kinesiogenic choreoathetosis, an unusual episodic condition precipitated by a sudden movement, is characterized by a twisted trunk and limb posture lasting a few seconds and not accompanied by loss of consciousness. Hypnogogic jerks and bruxism are persistent normal variant behaviors that occur in sleep.

Tic disorders are sometimes divided into three groups: (1) **simple transient tics,** which are monomorphic (always the same appearance over a period of months), last less than 12 months, and may be caused by particular environmental situations or psychological states; (2) **chronic tics,** which last longer than 12 months but are a single type; and (3) the **tics of Tourette's syndrome** (Table 88–1). However, all three types of tic disorders are sometimes found in the same family.

Tourette's syndrome is a common cause of tics in children. It is defined by multiple different tics displayed over time. These include motor tics and vocal tics produced by some sudden movement of air or saliva within the larynx, nasopharynx, or oropharynx, causing a perceptible sound.

A number of different types of tics have been described as part of Tourette's syndrome (Table 88–2). Many affected children describe a "sensory tic," which is an indescribable, uncomfortable feeling that is relieved by a motor tic. In addition to tics, patients may have other unusual behaviors including echopraxia (repetitive gestures), copropraxia (obscene gestures), and coprographia (obscene writing). Unusual speech patterns include repetitive, irrelevant, or nonsense words, pallilalia (repeating one's own words), echolalia (repeating another's words), and coprolalia (obscene speech). Diagnosis is often delayed because of misunderstandings about the manifestations (Table 88–3). Other psychobehavioral problems, including ADHDs and obsessive-compulsive behaviors, may be associated with Tourette's syndrome, although all affected children do not have these problems.

EVALUATION

History

A thorough history should be taken when evaluating children with potential tic disorders. The physician should find out as much as possible about the duration, circumstances of occurrence, and frequency of the movements (Questions Box). Parents may imitate the behavior or, if possible, bring in a videotape of the child's behavior. This may give the physician important information.

TABLE 88–2.   Types of Tics Seen in Children With Gilles de la Tourette's Syndrome

Simple Tics

Clonic
Dystonic

Complex Tics

Series of different or similar simple tics
More complicated coordinated movement
Copropraxia and coprographia

Vocal Tics

Oropharyngeal, nasopharyngeal, or laryngeal sounds
Consonants or syllables
Meaningful or nonsense words or phrases
Coprolalia
Pallilalia and echolalia

Sensory Tics

TABLE 88–3.   Misconceptions in Diagnosing Gilles de la Tourette's Syndrome

Attributing the unusual tic symptom to attention-getting or emotionally based behavior
Diagnosing the episodic behavior as a seizure on the basis of inadequate historical information
Attributing a vocal tic to an upper airway, sinus, or allergic condition
Attributing an ocular tic to an ophthalmologic problem
Requiring tics to be observed in the office before making the diagnosis
Waiting for coprolalia to be present before making the diagnosis
Assuming severe tics are necessary for the diagnosis or assuming tics are a normal developmental phase

---

TABLE 88–1.   Conditions Necessary for Diagnosis of Gilles de la Tourette's Syndrome

Multiple motor and vocal tics variably manifested over time
Tics present for at least one year
Onset of tics before 21 years of age
Tics not due to another known condition or substance

Questions: Tics

- How long and how often has the child been displaying the unusual behaviors?
- In what circumstances do the unusual behaviors occur? For example, do the behaviors occur when the child is eating or sleeping, engrossed in an activity, or excited? Or do they occur when attention is on the child or after a startle or other triggering behavior?
- Can the parents or other caregivers imitate the child's unusual behavior?
- Is the child having difficulty at school (cognitively or socially)?

Physical Examination

The physician should observe children for abnormal behaviors during the course of the parent interview and physical examination, although very frequently tics are not seen. A screen of cognitive abilities and fine motor coordination should be included in the examination.

Laboratory Tests

Children with suspected movement disorders should be screened for potential metabolic abnormalities. The evaluation should include routine determinations of calcium, magnesium, glucose, liver function enzymes, and ceruloplasmin levels. Thyroid function tests should also be requested. Endocrine hormone problems may produce low calcium, magnesium, or glucose as well as abnormal thyroid functions. They may also cause movement disorders that are difficult to distinguish from tics. Wilson's disease affects liver enzymes and ceruloplasmin levels and is associated with many movement problems, including tics.

Imaging Studies

MRI of the brain should be performed to determine whether anatomic abnormalities in the basal ganglia such as congenital lesions or evidence of metabolic abnormalities such as calcium deposition are present.

MANAGEMENT

Goals of management should include (1) reduction in the frequency of tics during critical circumstances with a minimum of medication side effects and (2) attention to other learning or behavioral handicaps that may coexist. Before physicians prescribe drug treatment, they must consider the severity of the tic disorder and the potential for possible psychosocial handicapping. Some children do not need medication for the movement disorder, and they and their families can be reassured with an understanding of the problem. Other children may experience remission for weeks or months with medication, and can then reduce or discontinue the drug.

Several drugs are useful in the treatment of tic disorders. **Haloperidol** has proved effective in doses ranging from 0.5–6 mg/day in divided doses. Children should begin with a low dose that is then titrated up to maximum efficacy or development of intolerable side effects. The primary disadvantage of this medication is cognitive sedation. **Clonidine,** in the form of the Catapres transdermal skin patch, is also useful. **Pimozide** (Orap) is also effective. An ECG is recommended before beginning this drug because it has been associated with electrocardiographic abnormalities.

Treatment for children with Tourette's syndrome should be multimodal and address all problematic aspects of the syndrome (Table 88–4). Children with Tourette's syndrome should be assessed for learning disabilities and ADHD. Interventions may include individualized instruction, education, **pharmacotherapy,** and **psychotherapy.** Methylphenidate is not necessarily contraindicated in children with Tourette's syndrome; recent reports indicate that the drug does not worsen tics in all patients.

Children with Tourette's syndrome and their families also frequently benefit from lay **educational materials** about the disorder. **Support groups** composed of other families with children with the syndrome and local chapters of the Tourette Syndrome Association may help. Referral for psychologic or psychiatric counseling for patients and their families may be necessary, because in its severe form, Tourette's syndrome may be socially devastating and may provoke secondary emotional problems as well as primary handicapping psychobehavioral aberrations.

PROGNOSIS

The prognosis in the majority of children with tics is good, and these children can have a productive educational experience and appropriate peer relationships. The physician must often individualize and optimize the management strategy to realize this prognosis in more difficult cases, however. Because the movements may remit for long periods of time, the psychologic adjustments allowed by appropriate therapy become very important in the long-term prognosis.

TABLE 88–4. Therapies Useful in Gilles de la Tourette's Syndrome

Tics
Clonidine (Catapres transdermal patch): alpha-adrenergic agonist
Haloperidol (Haldol) (low dose): dopamine receptor blocker
Pimozide (Orap): dopamine receptor blocker
Attention Deficit/Hyperactivity Disorder and Learning Disability
Clonidine (Catapres transdermal patch): alpha-adrenergic agonist
Methylphenidate (Ritalin): if tics are not worsened
Desipramine: tricyclic antidepressant
Education interventions: individualized or small-group instruction
Obsessive-Compulsive Disorder
Fluoxetine (Prozac): Serotonin uptake inhibitor (nontricyclic)
Clomipramine (Anafranil): tricyclic antidepressant
Depression and Adjustment Problems
Psychotherapy (individual and family)
Imipramine: tricyclic antidepressant
Support group

Case Resolution

The boy in the case history is diagnosed as having Tourette's syndrome. After a discussion with his family about the disorder, he is treated with Catapres patches. A questionnaire is sent to his teacher concerning attention deficit symptoms at school. At a six-week follow-up visit, he has fewer tics and is doing better in school (classroom situation of 15 students for most of the day).

Selected Readings

Comings, D. E., and B. G. Comings. A controlled family history study of Tourette syndrome. I. Attention deficit hyperactivity disorder, learning disorders and dyslexia. J. Clin. Psychiatry 51:275–280, 1990.

Cantwell, D. P. Tics and Tourette's disorders. Int. Pediatr. 6:170–175, 1991.

Shapiro, A., et al. Gilles de la Tourette Syndrome, 2nd ed. New York, Raven Press, 1988.

Singer, H. S., I. H. Hahn, and T. H. Moran. Abnormal dopamine uptake sites in postmortem striatum from patients with Tourette's syndrome. Ann. Neurol. 30:558–562, 1991.

C H A P T E R   8 9

ACNE

Monica Sifuentes, M.D.

Hx A 15-year-old adolescent male seeks a preparticipation sports physical. He is healthy, and he has no questions, complaints, or concerns.

The adolescent is well developed and well nourished, with normal vital signs, including blood pressure. The physical examination is entirely normal except for the skin. Erythematous pustules are present across the hairline, and cystic lesions are evident over both cheeks. Scattered blackheads are located over the nose and cheeks as well. The chest and back are clear, with no lesions.

Questions

1. What is the pathogenesis of acne vulgaris?
2. What are some contributing factors in the development of acne?
3. What are the different types of acne lesions?
4. What management options are available for the treatment of mild, moderate, and severe acne in adolescents?
5. What are the indications for the use of isotretinoin (Accutane)?
6. What is the prognosis for adolescent patients with acne?

Acne vulgaris is a common condition that most frequently occurs in adolescents. The spectrum of disease varies from individual to individual and may be caused by a variety of factors. Regardless of the etiology and extent of acne, the disease can be devastating to adolescents both physically and psychologically. Primary care physicians should therefore acknowledge acne as a medical problem even when patients do not mention it and should treat the condition accordingly.

EPIDEMIOLOGY

Most cases of acne that require treatment occur in individuals 9 to 19 years of age, although the condition can also affect young infants. Boys and girls are equally affected, but the condition is usually more severe in boys. Certain individuals may be genetically susceptible to acne. No ethnic groups are predisposed to acne, but certain cultural practices, such as the use of oily grooming agents by some African Americans, can lead to a specific pattern of lesions. Estimates indicate that more than 85% of adolescents in the United States are affected with acne and that more than $124 million dollars is spent annually on acne treatments.

Several factors contribute to the development of acnelike eruptions. Internal agents include endogenous hormones (e.g., androgens, progesterone) and specific drugs (e.g., oral contraceptives, isoniazid, phenytoin, corticosteroids, lithium-containing compounds). External agents include skin bacteria, especially *Propionibacterium acnes;* industrial chemicals (e.g., petroleum, animal and vegetable oils); oil- or wax-containing cosmetics; greasy sunscreen or suntan preparations; and local pressure from objects such as headbands, shoulder pads, or helmets. Excessive perspiration and emotional stress can also aggravate acne. Specific foods such as chocolate, soda, and french fries have not been shown to cause or worsen acne.

CLINICAL PRESENTATION

The lesions of acne vulgaris primarily affect the face, chest, back, and shoulders, and can be noninflamed or inflamed (Dx Box). Noninflamed lesions, or comedones, can be opened or closed to the environment. Closed comedones ("whiteheads") are small, flesh-colored bumps, and open comedones ("blackheads") contain central, dark material. Inflamed lesions are

---

Dx **Acne**

- Occurrence predominantly during puberty
- Lesions more severe in males
- Location on face, chest, back, and shoulders
- Open comedones ("blackheads") or closed comedones ("whiteheads")
- Inflamed papules or pustules
- Nodules or cysts may be present
- Possible exacerbation around menses

typically erythematous papules or pustules and may be more cystic in appearance.

PATHOPHYSIOLOGY

Although the exact etiology of acne remains unclear, the pathogenesis of acne involves certain processes.

1. **Abnormal follicular keratinization.** The earliest change in the formation of acne occurs in the horny cells that line the sebaceous follicle. A disturbance in the differentiation of these cells leads to excessive shedding of the cells into the lumen. Impaction of the follicle occurs as these horny cells stick together.

2. **Overproduction of sebum.** The sebaceous gland is highly responsive to hormonal stimulation, namely androgens. With the rise in androgens during puberty, hypertrophy of the sebaceous gland occurs, and the production of sebum is increased. The flow of sebum is obstructed by the above follicular hyperkeratosis, resulting in retention of all material.

3. **Proliferation of _P. acnes._** The overproduction of sebum in acne provides a ripe environment for the proliferation of _P. acnes,_ an anaerobic diphtheroid that, along with _Staphylococcus epidermidis_ and _Pityrosporum ovale_, is part of the microflora of the sebaceous follicle. In addition, _P. acnes_ possesses a lipase that hydrolyzes sebum triglycerides into free fatty acids. These acids irritate the follicular wall and cause inflammation.

4. **Inflammation.** The expulsion of sebum into the dermal layer of the skin occurs as a result of the rupture of the pilosebaceous follicle. This initiates an inflammatory process and the formation of inflammatory lesions such as pustules and cysts. In addition, _P. acnes_ produces biologically active extracellular materials, which increase the permeability of the follicular epithelium. The bacterium also produces chemotactic factors that are responsible for the migration of inflammatory cells to the area.

5. **Comedones.** The above processes can lead to a number of noninflammatory and inflammatory lesions (Table 89–1). Comedones are early noninflammatory lesions made up of sebum, horny cells, and bacteria. They can be closed or open. A **closed comedo,** or "whitehead," is a dilated plugged sebaceous follicle that is closed to the surface of the skin. An **open comedo,** or "blackhead," occurs as a result of dilatation of the follicular orifice at the surface of the skin and open communication with the outside environment. The dark color at the surface of the skin is believed to result from melanin in the horny cells, not dirt.

Questions: Acne

Medical Aspects
- How long has the adolescent had acne?
- Has the adolescent ever received treatment for acne?
  - How long did treatment continue?
  - What treatment methods were used?
  - For what reasons was the therapy discontinued?
- Is the adolescent currently using any treatment products?
  - Do the lesions seem to be getting better or worse?
- If the acne has never been treated, is treatment desired?
- Do any activities, medications, or environmental agents seem to exacerbate the lesions?
- Does the adolescent have a family history of acne?
- Is the adolescent taking any oral medications?

Psychological Aspects
- Is the adolescent bothered by the lesions?
- Is the adolescent embarrassed about his or her appearance? If so, does this embarrassment prevent the adolescent from participating in certain activities?
- Is the adolescent ever ridiculed by his or her peers because of the acne?

6. **Pustules** and **papules** are inflammatory lesions. Pustules lie in the superficial epidermal layer of the skin, and papules occur in the lower dermal layer. Because of their deeper location, they are often accompanied by a more severe inflammatory reaction, and scarring may result. **Nodules** or **cysts** are suppurative inflammatory lesions located deep within the dermis. Associated with the most severe form of acne, nodules are the result of deep pustules that rupture and then become lined with epithelium. When nodules are present, significant scarring is a major problem.

EVALUATION

History

The primary historical issues to explore in patients with acne vulgaris are both medical and psychological (Questions Box). From a medical standpoint, practitioners should determine how long the acne has been present and if the condition has ever been treated. Psychological aspects should include questions to assess the patient's overall self-esteem. Expectations regarding treatment and recovery should also be assessed at the initial visit before therapy is begun.

Physical Examination

The physical examination should focus on the primary sites of acne: face, chest, back, and shoulders. The entire skin should be inspected closely at the first visit, however. Individual lesions should be checked for signs of inflammation and infection at each follow-up visit. Their distribution should also be recorded along with their response to treatment. The presence or absence of scarring should also be assessed as a measure of the severity of acne and a predictor of outcome.

TABLE 89–1.   Classification of Acne

Grade one	Noninflammatory acne → open and closed comedones
	Closed comedones then lead to any of the next three levels of inflammatory acne
Grade two	Early inflammatory acne → presence of either comedones or papules (obstructed follicles)
Grade three	Moderate, localized inflammatory acne → pustules or larger, more inflamed papules
Grade four	Severe, more generalized inflammatory acne → cystic, nodular lesions

Laboratory Tests

No laboratory studies are needed either at the time of the initial evaluation or during the treatment of mild to moderate acne. In the case of severe acne, however, when isotretinoin is indicated, several pretreatment studies are necessary. A CBC, liver function tests, and a fasting lipid profile are recommended. In addition, a pregnancy test must be performed within two weeks of starting isotretinoin in sexually active female adolescents. These studies should be obtained in consultation with a dermatologist, who is generally responsible for prescribing isotretinoin.

MANAGEMENT

The general management of acne should include patient education regarding the pathophysiology of the condition to dispel any myths regarding its etiology and treatment. In addition, the patient's motivation should be assessed to better individualize therapy. Parental involvement is optimal in cases of severe acne.

All adolescents with acne should follow these general recommendations:

1. Wash skin with mild soap and water once or twice daily.
2. Use cosmetics sparingly or switch to oil-free products.
3. Avoid picking and excessive scrubbing.
4. Note that dietary modifications are not indicated.
5. Follow the prescribed regimen carefully (Table 89–2).

The specific therapies prescribed depend on the severity of the acne and patients' ability to comply with the proposed treatment. The most effective regimens include topical products such as benzoyl peroxide, retinoic acid, and antibiotics; systemic antimicrobials; hormonal agents; and isotretinoin. Most often, however, combination therapy is used and later modified according to patients' responses. Physicians should remember that the acne often looks worse before it gets better. Noticeable improvement usually takes four to six weeks.

Topical Therapy

Several topical products are available for the treatment of acne. **Benzoyl peroxide** is bactericidal for

TABLE 89–2. Treatment of Acne

Classification	Recommended Treatment Regimen
Grade one	Benzoyl peroxide 5% or 10% every other day or once a day. May increase to twice a day, if tolerated
Grade two	Benzoyl peroxide as above *plus* topical antibiotics twice a day. Retinoic acid in resistant cases
Grade three	Benzoyl peroxide 10% twice a day (may alternate with retinoic acid once a day) *plus* oral antibiotics
Grade four	Above treatment for grade three acne, *plus* referral to a dermatologist for possible treatment with isotretinoin

Modified from Greydanus, D.E. Acne vulgaris: pathway to the adolescent. Adolesc. Health Update 2:1989, p. 5.

P. acnes and acts as a comedolytic agent as well. Although over-the-counter lotions are available, the more effective gel preparations are preferable. The lowest concentration possible should be used initially. Higher concentrations should be used in cases in which the trunk or back are involved.

Therapy should be initiated gradually, especially if used in combination with retinoic acid, because benzoyl peroxide is inherently irritating and drying. Initially, a thin application should be made once a day every other day, and the frequency should be increased as tolerated. Allergic contact dermatitis rarely develops, but if it does, treatment must be discontinued.

Tretinoin or retinoic acid (Retin-A) is the mainstay of therapy for noninflammatory acne. This vitamin A derivative reduces microcomedo formation by normalizing follicular keratinization and decreasing the adhesiveness of horny cells shed into the follicular lumen. It is available by prescription as a gel, cream, or liquid in several different concentrations.

Like benzoyl peroxide, retinoic acid can be very irritating and may cause some peeling. Therefore therapy should be initiated cautiously with a cream or gel, which is less potent and drying than the liquid preparation. To further reduce irritation, patients should be instructed to wash with a mild soap no more than two times a day and to wait at least 20 to 30 minutes for the skin to dry completely before applying the product. Physicians often recommend that patients apply retinoic acid before bedtime rather than in the mornings, which tend to be more hectic. Patients should also be cautioned against excessive sun exposure while using retinoic acid, because this agent lowers the sunburn threshold. Alternate daily treatment with benzoyl peroxide is warranted in cases of inflammatory acne.

Antibiotic Therapy

Both topical as well as systemic antibiotics can be used in the treatment of inflammatory acne. **Topical antibiotics** are often useful in patients with inflammatory lesions that are unresponsive to benzoyl peroxide or retinoic acid alone. Such antibiotics act by inhibiting the growth of *P. acnes* and reducing the number of comedones, papules, and pustules. Erythromycin, tetracycline, clindamycin, and meclocycline are available as topical preparations. The **erythromycin gel** is most popular; the recommended dosage is twice daily. Allergic reactions from topical formulations rarely occur. Compared to systemic antibiotics, topical preparations have fewer systemic side effects because of decreased absorption.

Systemic antibiotics are the mainstay of therapy in patients with nodular or cystic inflammatory acne and in patients who have not responded to topical antibiotics. However, systemic agents have not been shown to be effective with comedonal acne. The success of oral antimicrobial therapy relates to the suppression of *P. acnes* and the inhibition of bacterial lipases. As a result free fatty acids and other byproducts are reduced, thereby decreasing inflammation.

Tetracycline and **erythromycin** are probably the most frequently prescribed oral antibiotics. Other systemic antibiotics that can be used to control inflammatory acne include clindamycin, doxycycline, and minocycline. These agents are particularly beneficial when lesions fail to respond to tetracycline. Tetracycline and doxycycline are not recommended in children less than eight years of age or in pregnant females. The most common side effects include candidal vaginitis, especially in females who also take oral contraceptives, and GI disturbances. The ultimate goal of oral antibiotic therapy is use of the minimum dose to control lesions and minimize side effects.

Hormonal Therapy

Hormonal therapy is indicated in females over 16 years of age who are unresponsive to other forms of treatment and who are not candidates for isotretinoin. **High-dose estrogen** (> 50 mg of ethinyl estradiol or mestranol) suppresses sebum production. It cannot be used in males because of its feminizing effects. Estrogen is usually prescribed in the form of oral contraceptives and administered for 21 days. A trial for no more than one year is recommended because of possible thromboembolic events.

Low-dose glucocorticoids (dexamethasone) are indicated in females with acne accompanied by virilization or any other evidence of excessive androgens. These agents work by decreasing adrenal androgen production. Low-dose glucocorticoids in combination with oral contraceptives can also be extremely effective.

Isotretinoin Therapy

Isotretinoin (Accutane), a systemic oral analog of vitamin A, is currently the most effective treatment available for severe pustulocystic acne that is resistant to conventional therapy. This agent is also useful in patients with a propensity for scarring. It influences all aspects of acne formation: sebum secretion, skin microflora, and inflammatory responses.

Because isotretinoin has numerous potentially serious side effects, referral to a dermatologist is recommended for patients who require isotretinoin therapy.

The most significant of these side effects is teratogenicity. Therefore, isotretinoin should be used cautiously in women of childbearing age, and the drug should not be prescribed in pregnant or nursing women. Compliance with effective contraception must be established before the initiation of treatment. Isotretinoin can also elevate triglyceride levels, particularly in patients with diabetes mellitus, obesity, alcohol abuse, and familial hyperlipidemia. To ensure informed consent as well as avoid potential complications, patients must receive careful instructions prior to the initiation of therapy and must be followed closely during the course of their treatment.

PROGNOSIS

Fortunately, the large majority of uncomplicated cases of acne (approximately 90%) resolve in the third decade of life. For those individuals with pustulocystic lesions, however, acne and significant scarring can continue to be a problem. Therefore, aggressive treatment is imperative.

Case Resolution

In the case history, the adolescent should be offered treatment for his acne. This may include benzoyl peroxide, retinoic acid (Retin-A), and oral antibiotics. The common side effects of the medications (e.g., dry skin, peeling) should be reviewed. A follow-up appointment should be arranged after three to four weeks to assess compliance with and tolerance of the treatment regimen.

Selected Readings

Greydanus, D. E. Acne vulgaris: pathway to the adolescent. Adolesc. Health Update 2:1–6, 1989.

Hurwitz, S. Acne vulgaris: pathogenesis and management. Pediatr. Rev. 15:47–52, 1994.

Hurwitz, S. Clinical Pediatric Dermatology: A Textbook of Skin Disorders of Childhood and Adolescence, 2nd ed. Philadelphia, W. B. Saunders, 1993.

Lucky, A. W. Update on acne vulgaris. Pediatr. Ann. 16:29–38, 1987.

Winston, M. H., and A. R. Shalita. Acne vulgaris: pathogenesis and treatment. Pediatr. Clin. North Am. 38:889–903, 1991.

CHAPTER 90

DISORDERS OF THE HAIR AND SCALP

Geeta Grover, M.D.

H$_x$ A six-year-old child presents with a one-week history of a swelling on the right side of her scalp that is associated with hair loss. She has previously been in good health, and she has no history of fever. On examination, she is afebrile, has normal vital signs, and appears well. An area of nontender, boggy swelling 2 × 2 cm with associated alopecia is apparent over the scalp in the right temporal area. Small pustular lesions are scattered over the involved area. Generalized scaling of the scalp and occipital adenopathy are evident.

Questions

1. What are the common causes of circumscribed hair loss in children?
2. What are the common causes of diffuse hair loss in children?
3. What features distinguish tinea capitis from alopecia areata?
4. What is the treatment for tinea capitis? Is there a role for topical antifungal agents?

Disorders of the scalp may be either congenital or acquired during childhood or adolescence. Conditions may be further classified according to the presence or absence of hair loss (alopecia) and whether the hair loss is diffuse or circumscribed.

EPIDEMIOLOGY

Acquired circumscribed hair loss is more commonly seen than diffuse hair loss. The vast majority of cases of acquired circumscribed hair loss result from tinea capitis, alopecia areata, or trauma.

Tinea capitis is a fungal infection of the scalp most often caused by the dermatophytes *Microsporum canis* or *Trichophyton tonsurans*. *T. tonsurans* accounts for about 90 to 95% of all cases. Tinea capitis, which is rare in infants and postpubertal adolescents, is seen primarily in prepubertal children between the ages of two and ten years. Boys are affected more often than girls.

Human-to-human transmission is rare with *M. canis* but does occur with *T. tonsurans*. Children who handle dogs or cats, which harbor *M. canis*, are susceptible to infection. Asymptomatic carriers of *T. tonsurans* make up about 4% of the general population.

Alopecia areata is an idiopathic disorder with an incidence of about 17/100,000 population. The cause is unknown, but an autoimmune mechanism has been suggested. Family history is positive in 10 to 20% of affected patients. Although alopecia areata may develop at any age, it generally begins before the age of 25.

Trichotillomania may be seen in association with other compulsive disorders such as thumb sucking and nail biting (see Chapter 31, Thumb Sucking and Other Habits). Usually the scalp hair is involved, but eyebrows or eyelash hair may also be affected. Although trichotillomania may be seen at any age, it primarily occurs in adolescents and children who are 4 to 10 years of age.

CLINICAL PRESENTATION

Children may present with specific complaints, including localized baldness, pruritus, scaling, or inflammation (D$_x$ Box). Occasionally, lymphadenopathy, particularly in the occipital area, is the major presenting symptom.

PATHOPHYSIOLOGY

An understanding of the physiology of the normal hair growth cycle helps in the evaluation of hair and scalp disorders. The scalp of an average human being contains about 100,000 hairs. Average healthy terminal hair grows at about 2.5 mm per week or approximately 1 cm per month.

The hair follicle is responsible for the majority of disturbances of hair growth because the hair shaft itself is a nonliving structure. Normal hair growth is a cyclical process composed of three stages. The anagen phase, the period of active hair growth, lasts for an average of three years (range: 2–6 years). Normally, about 85 to 90% of scalp hair is in this phase at any one time. The catagen phase, the transition period, lasts for about 10 to 14 days. The telogen phase, the final resting phase, lasts for about three to four months. The average individual loses about 50 to 100 telogen hairs per day.

Infection begins when the dermatophytes *M. canis* and *T. tonsurans* invade the hair follicle. The initial stage of infection with either organism is noninflammatory and may last two to eight weeks. *M. canis* spores remain

---

D$_x$ **Disorders of the Hair and Scalp**

- Circumscribed or generalized hair loss (alopecia)
- Scaling
- Pruritus
- Erythema of the scalp
- Localized or generalized swelling of the scalp

on the hair surface (ectothrix). In contrast, *T. tonsurans* spores are located inside the hair shaft (endothrix) and may cause the involved hairs to break easily. The noninflammatory stage may be followed by the inflammatory stage, or kerion, which represents a delayed hypersensitivity reaction to the organism. Histologically, the kerion consists of a mononuclear cell infiltrate.

In alopecia areata, histologic examination of a scalp biopsy reveals a dense, lymphocytic infiltrate around the hair follicle in areas of alopecia. The hairs at the margins of alopecia are easily plucked. They have clubbed or attenuated ends when examined under a low-power microscope. This appearance is pathognomonic, and these hairs are often referred to as "exclamation mark" hairs.

DIFFERENTIAL DIAGNOSIS

Scalp Disorders Without Associated Hair Loss

These conditions are divided into those disorders seen most often in neonates and young infants and those seen more frequently in children and adolescents (Table 90–1). **Caput succedaneum,** a generalized edema involving the soft tissues of the scalp, and **cephalhematoma,** a subperiosteal hematoma, are two of the most common lesions of the scalp that occur during the neonatal period. A cephalhematoma does not extend beyond the suture lines of the affected bone, which distinguishes it from caput succedaneum. Both conditions result from birth trauma and generally resolve spontaneously within a few weeks to months without further complications.

Other common neonatal scalp infections include **scalp abscess** and **herpes simplex infection.** When fetal scalp electrode monitors are used, a scalp abscess at the site of the monitor is seen in about 1 in 200 births. The most commonly implicated pathogens are staphylococci, gram-negative enteric bacteria, and gonococci. Management depends on the severity of the infection (i.e., associated cellulitis or signs of systemic involvement). Herpes simplex infections of the scalp are not uncommon in neonates, because the scalp usually has the longest contact with the cervix, the site of infection transmission. Herpes lesions are typically vesicular, but petechial, purpuric, or bullous lesions may also be apparent. Although skin lesions may be present at birth, they typically develop between five and ten days of life.

TABLE 90–1. Common Disorders of the Scalp Without Associated Hair Loss

Neonatal Period and Early Infancy
Birth trauma to the scalp (e.g., caput succedaneum, cephalhematoma)
Scalp abscess (at fetal scalp electrode site)
Herpes simplex infection
Cradle cap/seborrheic dermatitis

Childhood and Adolescence
Seborrheic dermatitis*
Head lice (pediculosis capitis)
Psoriasis*

*May occur with or without associated hair loss.

Seborrheic dermatitis is an erythematous, greasy, scaly eruption that occurs mainly on the scalp, face, and postauricular and intertriginous areas (see Chapter 92, Papulosquamous Eruptions). This condition is seen primarily in infants under the age of six months and in adolescents. Seborrheic dermatitis that involves the scalp of neonates is known as cradle cap. This noninflammatory, diffuse, greasy scaling of the scalp usually develops during the first several months of life.

Unlike atopic dermatitis, seborrheic dermatitis is generally nonpruritic. Occasionally the inflammatory process is severe enough to result in diffuse hair loss. Psoriatic lesions of the scalp can mimic seborrhea, and skin biopsy may be required for definitive diagnosis.

Head lice (pediculosis capitis) are an extremely common childhood infestation that affects girls more often than boys. Lice are spread by direct contact with infected individuals or infested clothing, combs, or brushes. Pruritus is the primary symptom. The ova or nits may be visible as small, oval, whitish specks found most commonly in the hair above the ears and the occipital region. They are difficult to remove. Unlike nonspecific scales, nits fluoresce under Wood's light examination.

Scalp Disorders Associated With Hair Loss

Table 90–2 lists the common scalp disorders associated with hair loss. When evaluating hair loss in children, it is important to determine whether the loss is diffuse or circumscribed.

Nevus sebaceus is a common cause of congenital circumscribed hair loss. Lesions are solitary, well-circumscribed plaques on the scalp that may be yellow or tan and round or oval. They can sometimes occur on the face as well. Nevus sebaceus should be differentiated from epidermal nevi. Epidermal nevi tend to occur more on the extremities but may develop anywhere on the body, including the scalp. They range in appearance from oval, hyperpigmented wartlike lesions to linear lesions that consist of a series of confluent papules.

Aplasia cutis congenita is a congenital skin defect with localized areas of epidermal, dermal, and subcutaneous tissue loss. Lesions can occur anywhere on the body, but the majority are found along the midline of the scalp. At birth, the lesions usually appear as small, depressed, hairless areas with associated ulceration or erosion of the skin. Etiology is unknown, and other developmental defects such as cleft lip or palate and syndactyly may be seen. Small defects generally heal well, whereas larger defects may require surgical excision and eventual skin grafting.

Tinea capitis, a fungal infection of the scalp, is one of the most common causes of acquired hair loss in children. This condition is characterized by patchy alopecia with broken-off hairs and scaling of the scalp. *T. tonsurans* infection sometimes appears as a series of black dots within the affected area due to the presence of fragmented hairs. Occasionally, an intense hypersensitivity response may result in a boggy swelling of the scalp known as a **kerion.** The surface of the kerion may

**TABLE 90–2. Common Disorders of the Scalp
With Associated Hair Loss**

Circumscribed Hair Loss

Congenital
  Aplasia cutis congenita
  Nevus sebaceus
  Epidermal nevus
Acquired
  Tinea capitis
  Alopecia areata
  Traction alopecia
  Trichotillomania
  Discoid lupus erythematosus
  Secondary syphilis

Diffuse Alopecia

Congenital
  Congenital hypothyroidism
  Hair shaft defects (e.g., Menkes' kinky hair syndrome)
  Ectodermal dysplasias
Acquired
  Seborrheic dermatitis
  Psoriasis
  Telogen effluvium
  Anagen effluvium (secondary to toxins or chemicals)
  Endocrine
    Hypothyroidism-hypoparathyroidism-hypopituitarism
    Diabetes mellitus
    Androgenic alopecia (e.g., male pattern baldness)
  Other
    Nutritional (e.g., acrodermatitis enteropathica)
    Systemic lupus erythematosus

be smooth or covered with small pustules, mimicking a bacterial infection. Uncomplicated tinea capitis leaves no scars, but kerions may result in permanent hair loss.

Alopecia areata, which frequently leads to hair loss, is characterized by well-defined areas of complete hair loss without associated scaling, irritation, or inflammation of the scalp. Hairs at the periphery of bald patches can usually be easily plucked. Associated nail defects, including nail pitting and ridging, may be seen in about 20% of affected individuals. Occasionally, alopecia totalis (loss of all scalp hair) or alopecia universalis (loss of all body and scalp hair) may result. Onset at younger age and more extensive involvement are poor prognostic signs.

Common traumatic causes of alopecia are traction alopecia and trichotillomania. **Traction alopecia** often occurs along the margins of the hairline secondary to having the hair pulled back in tight ponytails or braids. **Trichotillomania** is a self-induced form of traction alopecia in which children twist or pull out their hair either consciously or subconsciously (see Chapter 31, Thumb Sucking and Other Habits). The frontal and temporoparietal areas, which are most accessible to children's hands, are most commonly involved. Trichotillomania may mimic other types of alopecia, but the diagnosis can usually be made on the basis of the bizarre patterns of hair loss with hairs broken at differing lengths. Children occasionally eat the hairs as they are pulled out, resulting in the formation of a **trichobezoar** (hair ball) in the stomach.

Discoid lupus erythematosus and **secondary syphilis** are uncommon causes of localized hair loss from the scalp in children. The patches of alopecia in discoid lupus erythematosus often have hypopigmentation with erythematous margins, whereas those of secondary syphilis are numerous and small in size, with distinct margins.

A variety of structural defects, endocrine and metabolic disorders, and toxins may be associated with diffuse loss of scalp hair (see Table 90–2). **Intrinsic structural defects of the hair** may cause hairs to break, thus resulting in failure of hair growth. In some forms of **ectodermal dysplasia,** the number of hair follicles is reduced or they are altogether absent, giving the appearance of sparse or thinning hair.

Telogen effluvium is a common cause of diffuse hair loss that may occur two to four months after a variety of events, including pregnancy, discontinuation of oral contraceptives, severe febrile illness, or severe emotional stress. Hair loss results from the abrupt conversion of numerous scalp hairs from the anagen (growth) phase to the telogen (resting) phase. Loss of more than 100 hairs per day is considered abnormal. Patients may complain of losing several hundred hairs a day, but the occurrence of clinically significant baldness is rare. Estimates indicate that individuals must lose about 25% of their hair before thinning becomes clinically apparent. The hair loss may continue for several weeks, but complete regrowth usually occurs within 6 to 12 months.

Anagen effluvium results in the loss of growing hairs due to a sudden cessation of the growing phase. It occurs most commonly after systemic chemotherapy.

EVALUATION

History

The age of the child guides the differential diagnosis, because some lesions are more common at one age than another (Questions Box).

Physical Examination

The scalp should be examined to see if the hair loss is diffuse or circumscribed and whether scalp hairs can

---

Questions: Disorders of the Hair and Scalp

- Is the child losing any hair?
  - If so, is the child losing hair from all over the scalp or only from localized areas on the scalp?
  - Has the child lost any body hair (e.g., eyebrows, eyelashes) in addition to the scalp hair?
  - How long has the child been losing hair?
- Is the scalp pruritic or scaling?
- Have the parents noticed the child twisting or pulling the hair?
- Is the child's hair often in ponytails or braids?
- Has there recently been any significant stress in the child's life?
- Do any pets live in the home?
- Is the child taking any medications?
- Is anyone else in the home or anyone in close contact with the child having similar symptoms?

be plucked easily. Signs of irritation, inflammation, or scaling of the scalp should also be noted, as well as the presence of adenopathy, nail changes, or hair loss elsewhere on the body.

Wood's light examination of the scalp for fungus is helpful if positive. A negative examination does not rule out the possibility of fungal infection, however, because *T. tonsurans*, the most common cause of tinea capitis, does not fluoresce. *M. canis,* which causes about 5 to 10% of cases, fluoresces yellow-green under the Wood's light.

Laboratory Tests

Laboratory assessment is useful in some cases. If fungal infection is suspected, a KOH examination should be performed by the primary care physician. The scalp in the involved areas should be scraped with a No. 15 blade. The scrapings should be placed on a glass slide, dissolved in KOH solution, and examined under the microscope. Hyphae and spores within the hair shaft (e.g., *T. tonsurans* infection) or surrounding the hair shaft (e.g., *M. canis* infection) should be noted.

In addition to microscopic examination, many dermatologists recommend routine fungal cultures in all cases of suspected tinea capitis. Hair or scalp scrapings are inoculated onto Sabouraud's agar or Dermatophyte Test Medium (DTM). Within 5 to 14 days, a distinctive growth seen on the Sabouraud's agar or a color change from yellow to red in the DTM confirms the diagnosis. A negative KOH examination in addition to a lack of inflammation and scaling may be required for differentiating trichotillomania or alopecia areata from tinea capitis.

The diagnosis of telogen effluvium is usually suggested by the history and counting the number of hairs lost each day. If the diagnosis is in question, the patient may be referred to a dermatologist for examination of the involved hair roots and determination of the anagen-telogen ratio, which is usually about 85:15. A telogen count of more than 25% is considered to be diagnostic of telogen effluvium. The ratio of anagen to telogen hairs is normal in trichotillomania.

A more extensive laboratory workup may be required if the hair loss is persistent or the history or physical examination are suggestive of systemic disease (see Table 90–2). Studies that may be considered include liver function tests, thyroid function studies, a serum Venereal Disease Research Laboratory (VDRL) test or antinuclear antibodies (ANA), and serum electrolytes.

MANAGEMENT

Management depends on the diagnosis. Herpetic infection requires immediate attention and systemic antiviral therapy, because the risk of systemic infection is significant.

Children suspected of nevus sebaceus should be referred to a dermatologist. Early identification and excision are important, because 10 to 15% of lesions undergo secondary neoplastic changes during puberty or adulthood.

Infantile **seborrheic dermatitis** usually resolves spontaneously by the age of six to eight months. **Mineral oil** can be massaged into the scalp to soften the scale in children with thick scaling of the scalp due to seborrheic dermatitis or cradle cap. A soft brush may be used to loosen the scale before shampooing. An **antiseborrheic shampoo or a topical corticosteroid solution** may be required for more severe cases. In adolescents, seborrhea of the scalp may be treated with **shampoos containing zinc or selenium** such as Head & Shoulders or Selsun, respectively. **Tar shampoos** or topical corticosteroid solutions can be used if pruritus is significant.

Head lice may be treated with **pyrethrin products** such as permethrin 1% cream rinse (Nix). A fine-toothed comb or tweezers may be required after rinsing to remove the ova or nits of head lice. An application of vinegar after shampooing may also facilitate removal of nits. Heat, such as that associated with blow-drying the hair, also kills the lice.

Oral griseofulvin administered for at least six to eight weeks is given for **tinea capitis.** Although griseofulvin can have many side effects, including GI disturbances, hepatotoxicity, and leukopenia, it is generally well tolerated by children. Hematologic, renal, and liver function studies can be monitored in children on high doses or prolonged treatment. Topical antifungal agents are not effective on the scalp. A course of oral **prednisone** may be required in conjunction with the griseofulvin if a kerion is present. Children with kerion are often misdiagnosed as having a bacterial infection of the scalp and treated with oral antibiotics. However, the pustules in kerion are sterile, and antibiotics are not required.

Children believed to have alopecia areata should be referred to a dermatologist immediately. Therapy for **alopecia areata** consists of **both topical and intralesional corticosteroids.** Many psychosocial factors should be considered when treating children with this condition. Children with severe forms of the disease may benefit psychologically from wearing a wig. The National Alopecia Areata Foundation is available as a support group for affected children and their families.

PROGNOSIS

Common disorders of the scalp such as seborrheic dermatitis, head lice, and tinea capitis generally respond well to treatment and result in no long-term sequelae. The course and prognosis of alopecia areata is quite variable and may be difficult to predict. Generally, the prognosis for regrowth is good if hair loss has occurred in only a few patches. The prognosis for complete regrowth of hair is usually poorer with younger age at onset and more widespread involvement.

Case Resolution

The child presented in the case scenario exhibits physical findings of a kerion. Diagnosis can be made clinically on the basis of the appearance of the lesion. The diagnosis is established by microscopic evidence of hyphae and culture confirmation. Treatment with griseofulvin should be initiated. The child should be examined in two weeks to ascertain the response to therapy and check for any adverse reactions.

Selected Readings

Atton, A. V., and W. W. Tunnessen. Alopecia in children: the most common causes. Pediatr. Rev. 12:25–30, 1990.

Goldgeier, M. H. Fungal infections of the skin, hair and nails. Pediatr. Ann. 22:253–259, 1993.

Honig, P. J. Skin conditions: misdiagnosed and just plain missed. Contemp. Pediatr. 7:96–113, August 1990.

Hurwitz, S. Disorders of hair and nails. *In* Hurwitz, S. Clinical Pediatric Dermatology, 2nd ed. Philadelphia, W. B. Saunders, 1993. pp. 481–514.

Levy, M. L. Disorders of the hair and scalp in children. Pediatr. Clin. North Am. 38:905–919, 1991.

Rasmussen, J. E. Cutaneous fungus infections in children. Pediatr. Rev. 13:152–156, 1992.

CHAPTER 91

DIAPER DERMATITIS

Geeta Grover, M.D.

H$_x$ A 6-month-old infant has a three-day history of a rash in the diaper area. The mother has been applying cornstarch, but the rash has gotten worse and has spread to the inner thighs and the abdomen. The infant has no history of fever, upper respiratory tract symptoms, vomiting, or diarrhea. He was seen in the emergency room one week ago for acute gastroenteritis, which has since resolved.

On examination, a poorly demarcated, shiny, erythematous rash is noted over the convex surface of the buttocks, lower abdomen, and genitalia, with relative sparing of the intertriginous creases. The rest of the physical examination is within normal limits.

Questions

1. What are the common causes of rashes in the diaper area (diaper dermatitis)?
2. What are the features that distinguish one type of diaper dermatitis from another?
3. What systemic diseases may present with diaper dermatitis?
4. What are some common treatments for diaper dermatitis?

Diaper dermatitis is used to describe a wide variety of skin disorders that present with a rash in the area covered by the diaper. The most familiar form of diaper rash, irritant contact diaper dermatitis, is one of the most common skin disorders of infants and young children. Successful management requires making the correct diagnosis and identifying the etiology and associated factors.

EPIDEMIOLOGY

Diaper dermatitis occurs in infants and young children between birth and two years of age, with a peak incidence at seven to nine months. Its estimated prevalence is approximately 10% in children under two years of age.

CLINICAL PRESENTATION

The lesions of diaper dermatitis primarily affect the skin of the buttocks, lower abdomen, perineal area, and proximal thighs. Most commonly, a poorly demarcated, glistening erythema is apparent over the convex surfaces, with relative sparing of the intertriginous folds (Fig. 91–1A). Candidal infection is characterized by a beefy red, sharply demarcated eruption with small, satellite papules and pustules along the margins. The eruption is primarily concentrated within the skin folds (D$_x$ Box) (Fig. 91–1B).

PATHOPHYSIOLOGY

Many factors are involved in the pathophysiology of diaper dermatitis. Prolonged contact with urine, feces,

---

D$_x$ Diaper Dermatitis

- Age less than two years
- Erythematous rash over anogenital region
- Associated gastroenteritis, antibiotic therapy, or oral thrush

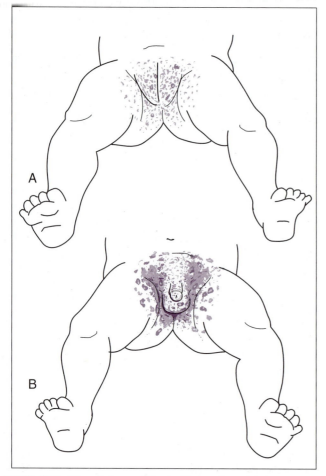

FIGURE 91–1. *Diaper dermatitis. A. Diaper dermatitis secondary to contact. Surface areas are affected. Diaper dermatitis secondary to Candida. B. Intertriginous areas are affected, and satellite lesions are present.*

or irritating chemicals plays an important role in the initiation of these disorders. Friction generated as the infant tries to move around may further aggravate the condition and lead to maceration of the skin. Secondary infection, most often with *Candida albicans,* may be seen in many cases.

For many years it was believed that ammonia produced by bacterial breakdown of urea was the causative factor in the majority of cases of diaper dermatitis. Recent studies have refuted this finding. Currently it is thought that wetness increases the skin's permeability to irritants such as fecal proteases and lipases, which are the major irritants responsible for diaper dermatitis. Although ammonia in the urine is not enough to initiate the dermatitis, it may aggravate existing inflammation.

Whether diaper type (i.e., cloth or disposable) plays any role is controversial. Experts agree that leaving wet diapers on infants for prolonged periods may increase skin damage.

DIFFERENTIAL DIAGNOSIS

Technically, any rash that occurs in the area covered by the diaper can be called diaper dermatitis, but certain rashes occur primarily in this area in infants and young children. The differential diagnosis of diaper dermatitis is presented in Table 91–1.

Irritant contact dermatitis, the most common cause of diaper dermatitis, is most prominent on the skin of the buttocks, perineal area, lower abdomen, and inner thighs. The skin of the creases is relatively unaffected. Exposure to proteolytic enzymes and irritant chemicals in the face of excessive heat or moisture is believed to lead to this condition. Friction with the diaper at sites of contact may aggravate it. Such a rash is poorly demarcated and gives the skin a glistening, red appearance.

Candidal diaper dermatitis, due to infection with *C. albicans,* typically begins in the creases (intertriginous areas) and then spreads to other surfaces. Sometimes associated with oral thrush, it is also a common sequelae to systemic antibiotic therapy. The rash appears bright, beefy red with sharp, raised borders and small satellite papules, vesicles, and pustules along its margins. Scales may also be noted along the edge. *C. albicans* can be a cause of secondary infection of already inflamed skin as well as a primary causative factor in some cases of diaper dermatitis.

Seborrheic diaper dermatitis, like candidal diaper dermatitis, also primarily affects the intertriginous areas of the groin. The lack of pruritus distinguishes it from atopic dermatitis. The rash has a characteristic salmon-colored, greasy appearance with a yellowish scale. Satellite lesions are not evident. Seborrheic dermatitis of the face, scalp, neck, and postauricular areas are usually seen in association with the seborrheic dermatitis of the diaper area.

Less common causes of diaper dermatitis are **allergic dermatitis, impetigo,** and **perianal streptococcal disease.** True **allergic contact dermatitis** in the diaper area is rare in the first two years of life, but irritation caused by harsh soaps or cleansing agents may be commonly seen.

Impetigo, especially bullous impetigo, is a not uncommon eruption in the diaper area. Bullous impetigo is usually caused by *Staphylococcus aureus.* The rash presents as bullae 1 to 2 cm in diameter within the diaper area. Characteristically, the bullae rupture, leaving superficial erosions with thick, honey-colored crusts. The lesions may spread outside the diaper area, and fever and regional lymphadenopathy may be noted later in the course of the disease.

TABLE 91–1. Differential Diagnosis of Diaper Dermatitis

Most Common Causes
Irritant contact dermatitis
Candidiasis
Seborrheic dermatitis
Less Common Causes
Allergic dermatitis
Impetigo
Perianal streptococcal disease
Atopic dermatitis
Psoriasis
Acrodermatitis enteropathica
Histiocytosis X

Perianal streptococcal disease due to group A beta-hemolytic streptococcus manifests as a well-demarcated, erythematous, pruritic, and usually tender perianal rash. Rectal bleeding and painful defecation may also be noted.

Systemic diseases that may present as rashes in the diaper area include psoriasis, atopic dermatitis, acrodermatitis enteropathica, and histiocytosis X. **Psoriasis** may occur anywhere on the body, but lesions typically occur on the scalp, face, elbows, and knees. In infants psoriasis may involve the diaper area. Unlike lesions elsewhere on the body, which are typically well-circumscribed, erythematous plaques with a thick, silvery scale, psoriatic lesions in the diaper area may be difficult to differentiate from seborrheic dermatitis or candidal infection. Psoriasis should be considered in the differential diagnosis of a diaper rash that persists despite seemingly adequate therapy. Skin biopsy, family history of psoriasis, or nail involvement may help confirm the diagnosis.

Atopic dermatitis is rare in the diaper area, even in infants who have lesions elsewhere on the body. The relative sparing of the diaper area is perhaps a result of the increased moisture of the skin in this area (see Chapter 92, Papulosquamous Eruptions, for a discussion of atopic dermatitis).

Acrodermatitis enteropathica is a rare, inherited disorder of zinc metabolism that presents in early infancy with diarrhea, failure to thrive, and skin lesions involving the distal extremities, perioral, and perineal areas. Erythematous, moist, vesicular, pustular, and eczematoid skin lesions may be apparent. Lesions in the diaper area are often mistaken for candidiasis. The etiology appears to be impaired gastrointestinal zinc absorption. Treatment consists of oral zinc supplementation.

Histiocytosis X, another rare cause of diaper dermatitis, refers to a group of disorders characterized by proliferation of histiocytes within the bone, liver, spleen, lungs, lymph nodes, and skin. Skin lesions may involve the diaper area but more commonly affect the scalp and neck. The lesions appear as small, reddish-brown, scaling papules and pustules; ulceration may be apparent in the inguinal and perineal areas. Diagnosis can be confirmed by skin biopsy.

EVALUATION

History

A thorough history should be obtained (Questions Box). Candidal diaper dermatitis should be suspected if oral antibiotic therapy has recently been used.

Physical Examination

On physical examination, the presence of skin lesions elsewhere on the body should be noted. This is particularly important in the case of a persistent, resistant, or recurrent diaper rash, where systemic diseases such as psoriasis must be considered. The distribution of the rash within the diaper area itself may

Questions: Diaper Dermatitis

- When did the rash begin?
- Does the rash resolve and then recur?
- Is the rash pruritic?
- Have any home remedies or previous treatments been used? Which ones?
- Does the child have a family history of atopic dermatitis or psoriasis?
- Is the child taking antibiotics now or been using them recently?
- What type of diapers are used?
- How frequently are the diapers changed?

provide clues to the diagnosis. Candidal dermatitis occurs primarily in the creases, whereas irritant contact dermatitis usually affects the convex areas of the skin with relative sparing of the intertriginous areas. Streptococcal disease manifests primarily as marked perianal erythema.

Laboratory Tests

Although the diagnosis of candidal diaper dermatitis is usually evident clinically, microscopic examination of skin scrapings with KOH may be performed to establish the diagnosis. Typically, budding yeast with hyphae and pseudohyphae is seen. The diagnosis of perianal streptococcal disease or bullous impetigo may be confirmed by bacterial cultures from the perianal area or bullous lesions, respectively.

MANAGEMENT

The mainstay of therapy and the key to prevention is **good hygiene**, which involves keeping the diaper area clean and dry. Gentle but thorough cleansing of the diaper area with water alone or water and a mild soap is usually sufficient. The area should then be patted dry and allowed to air dry completely if possible. Too frequent cleansing with harsh soaps or scrubbing too vigorously can actually aggravate skin that is already damaged and inflamed.

In addition, the diaper should be **changed frequently**. The diaper area should be exposed to as much air as possible (e.g., by allowing the infant to sleep without a diaper). In the absence of any inflammation, **dusting powders,** such as cornstarch powder, may be used to minimize friction and moisture. **Moisture-resistant barrier ointments or creams** such as zinc oxide or petrolatum are usually not needed if the above hygiene measures are carried out routinely. The role of hygiene in all forms of diaper dermatitis cannot be over-emphasized. Topical application of medicated creams and ointments is not effective in the presence of poor hygiene.

Irritant contact dermatitis usually responds to hygienic measures and the application of barrier ointments and low-potency **topical corticosteroids** such as 0.5% or 1% hydrocortisone cream. Seborrheic dermatitis usually resolves spontaneously but can also be treated with low-potency topical corticosteroids. Candidal diaper dermatitis responds to **topical antifungal creams** such as nystatin, miconazole, or clotrimazole. In addition, a low-potency corticosteroid may be required if inflammation is severe. Oral penicillin usually clears perianal streptococcal disease, but the relapse rate is high. The topical antibiotic mupirocin may be used to treat bullous impetigo only if the lesions are few and isolated. Oral antibiotics (e.g., erythromycin, cephalexin) may be required for more extensive disease. Combination creams containing both a corticosteroid and an antifungal should not be recommended routinely because they usually contain high-potency corticosteroids.

PROGNOSIS

Although recurrence of diaper dermatitis is common, the usual varieties respond well to measures aimed at keeping the diaper area clean and dry and to medicated creams.

Case Resolution

The infant presented in the case scenario has irritant contact dermatitis. He has a recent history of gastroenteritis, and stool is known to be particularly irritating to the skin. Treatment includes keeping the diaper area clean and dry and topical application of a low-potency corticosteroid cream.

Selected Readings

Honig, P. J. The great masqueraders: skin disorders that fool the eye. Contemp. Pediatr. 8:98–109, 1991.

Hurwitz, S. Skin lesions in the first year of life. Contemp. Pediatr. 10:110–128, 1993.

Hurwitz, S. Clinical Pediatric Dermatology, 2nd ed. Philadelphia, W.B. Saunders, 1993, pp. 34–39.

Leyden, J. J. Diaper dermatitis. Dermatol. Clin. 4:23–28, 1986.

CHAPTER 92

PAPULOSQUAMOUS ERUPTIONS

Carol D. Berkowitz, M.D.

Hx A six-month-old female infant presents with an erythematous, confluent, and scaly rash on the cheeks. The extremities are also covered with a fine papular rash. The infant has had some scaling behind the ears and on the scalp since birth, but the symptoms have recently increased. The mother has been applying baby oil to the scalp to relieve the scaliness. Except for some intermittent rhinorrhea, the infant has otherwise been well. Immunizations are deficient; she received only the first set when she was two months old. The family history is positive for bronchitis. The infant's weight is at the 75th percentile, and the height is at the 50th percentile. Vital signs are normal. The physical examination is normal except for the presence of the rash.

Questions

1. What are the characteristics of papulosquamous eruptions?
2. What are the common conditions associated with papulosquamous eruptions in children?
3. What are the appropriate treatments for the common papulosquamous eruptions?

approach. First, rashes are assessed in terms of appearance, whether macular (flat), papular (raised), squamous (scaly), vesicular (fluid-filled), or bullous (large, fluid-filled). Next, the extent of the rash is determined. Rashes may be described as generalized or localized. Location is also important. The site of a localized rash may be consistent with certain diagnoses, for instance, diaper dermatitis.

Alternatively, rashes that are associated with fever can be differentiated from those that are not. Rashes seen in febrile children are called exanthems. Exanthems may be associated with enanthems, or lesions in the oral cavity (see Chapter 93, Maculopapular Rashes).

Papulosquamous eruptions, the subject of this chapter, are raised, scaly lesions. They are often localized to certain parts of the body, but the site may vary according to the age of the child. The rashes are frequently pruritic, but children are usually afebrile. The presence of a secondary infection may lead to fever, however.

EPIDEMIOLOGY

Although a large number of conditions may cause papulosquamous eruptions in children, a select number of diagnoses account for the majority of problems. Two of the most common causes of papulosquamous erup-

Rashes, a common problem in children, can be classified in ways that help to establish a diagnostic tions in children are atopic dermatitis and scabies. Atopic dermatitis affects about 3 to 5% of children under age five years and accounts for about 4% of pediatric emergency department visits. The itching associated with atopic dermatitis and other pruritic rashes is worse at night, which is one reason for the frequent visits.

Scabies is believed to affect 300 million persons worldwide, making it a frequent complaint of children seen in general pediatric practices. Although the existence of epidemics and pandemics of scabies has been suggested, the disorder does not appear to occur in regular cycles. Reports of infestations rise when populations are forced into close proximity (e.g., during wars). Increased reporting of scabies is related to increased physician recognition of the disorder. When one family member is affected, scabies is noted in another family member in about two-thirds of cases. When the infection is absent in household contacts, physicians should not be dissuaded from diagnosing scabies, however.

CLINICAL PRESENTATION

Papulosquamous eruptions consist of erythematous raised, scaly lesions that may involve the face, trunk, or extremities. The lesions are often highly pruritic, and scratching may lead to excoriation or secondary infection. Sometimes multiple family members are affected (D_x Box). Chronicity may lead to thickening or lichenification of involved skin.

PATHOPHYSIOLOGY

The pathophysiology of atopic dermatitis has not been definitively established. The disorder, which is attributed to immune dysfunction, is characterized by IgE overproduction and diminished cell-mediated immunity. Inflammatory hyperactivity of the skin and other sites, including the lungs and nasal tissues, results.

The inflammatory response in scabies is triggered by an infestation with a mite, *Sarcoptes scabiei*. The adult female burrows under the skin and lays her eggs. After two weeks, the eggs become adults. Affected individuals may be asymptomatic on first exposure. With time, usually 10 to 30 days after infestation, signs and symptoms including pruritus and rash become apparent. This reaction relates to the development of cellular or humoral immunity to the mite, feces, or eggs. In infants, rashes may develop in areas away from the site of infestation as a sign of an allergic reaction to foreign material.

D_x Papulosquamous Eruptions

- Raised, scaly papules
- Pruritus
- Afebrile, unless secondary infection is present
- Allergic personal or family history
- Intertriginous rash

DIFFERENTIAL DIAGNOSIS

The major conditions that are associated with papulosquamous eruptions in children are atopic dermatitis, seborrheic dermatitis, allergic contact dermatitis, scabies, xerosis, lichen planus, psoriasis, papular urticaria, flea bites, fungal infections of the skin, and infantile acropustulosis dermatosis.

Eczema is a general term that is used to denote a papulosquamous eruption. The two most common eczematous conditions seen in children are atopic eczema or dermatitis and seborrheic dermatitis. **Atopic dermatitis** is a disorder of infancy and childhood. Sixty percent of affected individuals become symptomatic with a pruritic rash during the first year of life, and 85% develop symptoms during the first five years. The area of involvement changes with age. In infancy and childhood, the face and extensor surfaces are involved, and the diaper area is often spared (Fig. 92–1A). By adolescence, the flexor surfaces show the characteristic changes of chronic inflammation with lichenification and accentuation of the flexure folds. Clinically, erythema and a pruritic papular eruption are apparent. Scratching and rubbing leads to excoriation, weeping, and eventually lichenification. Changes in coloring, including hypo- and hyperpigmentation, may also occur. Xeroderma, or dry skin, is a frequent coexisting condition. Lesions around mucosa (Dennie-Morgan infraorbital fold under the eye and cheilitis around the mouth) may also be seen. Symptoms of other allergic conditions, such as rhinorrhea, wheezing, or food-related allergies, may occur.

Seborrheic dermatitis, which develops during the first three months of life, is characterized by scaliness, particularly of the scalp. Scalp eruptions are referred to as cradle cap. In addition, seborrheic dermatitis has a predilection for intertriginous areas, including the folds in the diaper region and the area behind the ears (Fig. 92–1B). A scaly eruption involving the eyebrows and around the nose may also be apparent. The reddish or pinkish rash may have a greasy quality. Use of baby oil often exacerbates the condition, and secondary infections may occur either with *Candida*, particularly in the intertriginous areas, or with *Pityrosporum*, in the scalp. Seborrheic dermatitis is less pruritic than atopic dermatitis, and this feature can be used to distinguish between the two conditions. The intertriginous involvement and the onset shortly after birth also differentiate these two types of dermatitis.

Allergic contact dermatitis occurs when individuals come into physical contact with an irritant or a specific allergen. The disorder is more commonly observed in individuals with atopic dermatitis. Hands and exposed areas are frequently affected. Although the rash is papulosquamous, it is often also oozing and subsequently lichenified.

Scabies may resemble atopic or seborrheic dermatitis in infants and young children. The lesions may be papules, pustules, or vesicles. The characteristic burrow, which is only about 1 cm long, is often difficult to appreciate unless certain diagnostic maneuvers are undertaken. The lesions are most often noted on the skin of the hands and feet, including the palms and soles

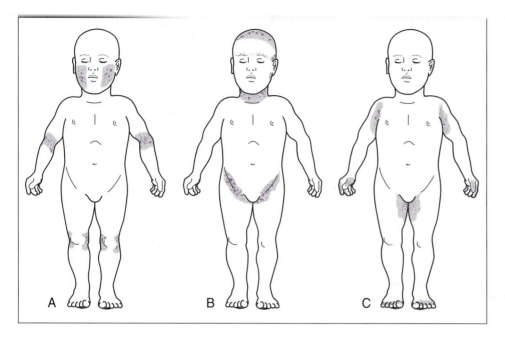

FIGURE 92–1. *Typical distribution of papulosquamous eruptions in children.* A. *Atopic dermatitis: usually located on cheeks, creases of elbows, and knees.* B. *Seborrheic dermatitis: usually located on scalp, behind ears, thigh creases, and eyebrows.* C. *Scabies: usually located on axillae, webs of fingers and toes, and intragluteal area.*

in infants and young children. Intertriginous areas such as the intragluteal region, groin, and fingerwebs are commonly infected (Fig. 92–1C). In infants, the face and head may be involved. Scratching and secondary infection may alter the appearance of the rash. Reddish-brown nodules may be characteristic of chronic infection. These nodules are believed to be an immune reaction to the dead mite. In institutionalized or immunosuppressed individuals, the rash may become covered with thick crusts, a condition referred to as "Norwegian scabies."

Xerosis, or xeroderma, refers to dry skin. This condition is frequently noted in patients prone to atopic dermatitis, but it may be seen in other individuals under drying conditions, such as low humidity and frequent bathing with drying soaps. The skin may be scaly and pruritic, and scratching may result in excoriations. A papular eruption is usually absent.

Lichen planus is an uncommon papulosquamous eruption. The polygonal, brownish-pink, scaly lesions are located on flexor surfaces.

Psoriasis, although a papulosquamous eruption, is more plaquelike. In older children the face and scalp are affected, but in infants the eruption is frequently noted in the diaper area, where it is very erythematous. The white, silvery scale, usually noted when the eruption affects the extensor surfaces, is milder because of the hydrating effect of occlusive diapers. Like seborrheic dermatitis, psoriasis may become secondarily infected by *Candida.* In general, psoriasis is only mildly itchy.

Papular urticaria is noted in children between the ages of three and ten years. The eruption may be triggered by the presence of insect bites, particularly **flea bites**. The papular, extremely pruritic lesions are usually confined to the extremities.

Fungal infections (tinea corporis and tinea pedis) may also appear as papulosquamous eruptions. Sometimes the lesions assume a characteristic distribution, with the papules grouped in a circle, and central clearing of the scaliness.

Infantile acropustulosis consists of very pruritic papules and vesicles on the sides of the hands and the feet. The lesions may be mistaken for scabies. African-American and Native American children under the age of three years have a predilection for this condition.

EVALUATION

History

A thorough history should be obtained (Questions Box). The presence of a rash in other family members suggests a contagious condition such as scabies or a familial disorder such as atopic dermatitis or psoriasis. An onset in the first few weeks of life is consistent with seborrheic dermatitis. It is important to determine if any medications have been used, because these may modify the appearance of the rash.

PHYSICAL EXAMINATION

The physical examination helps define the exact nature of the eruption and its distribution, which is

---

Questions: Papulosquamous Eruptions

- How long has the child had the rash?
- What did the rash look like when it first appeared?
- Are other family members affected?
- Have any medications been used to treat the rash?
- Is pruritus present?
- Does the child have any other symptoms such as wheezing or rhinorrhea?
- Does the child have a history of any contact between the affected skin and any irritating substance?
- Has the child been febrile?

often the clue to its etiology. The entire body should be examined, and particular attention should be paid to the intragluteal region and web spaces between fingers and toes. Certain rashes have characteristic appearances. For example, a circular cluster of scaly papules with central clearing signifies tinea corporis, and the presence of burrows characterizes scabies.

Laboratory Tests

Certain diagnostic tests may help clarify the etiology. The burrow of the mite that causes scabies may not be readily apparent, but a number of studies make it more easily detectable. The ink test helps visualize the burrow. A washable felt tip marker is rubbed across the web spaces, and excess ink is removed with water or alcohol. The ink penetrates through the stratum corneum, thus outlining the burrow. Scrapings should also be taken to identify the mite, eggs, or feces. The yield is reported to be as high as 90 to 95% if proper technique is followed. Alternatively, mineral oil may be placed on the web space or on a No. 15 scalpel blade. Multiple burrows or web spaces are scraped. The material is then spread on a glass slide and viewed under low power.

Scrapings of skin also assist in diagnosing candidal or tinea infections. These scrapings should be mixed with KOH, which facilitates the dissolution of epithelial debris, and allows for identification of the yeast or fungus.

If a secondary bacterial infection is suspected, cultures of the skin are indicated. No other specific diagnostic tests, short of a skin biopsy, assist in the diagnosis.

MANAGEMENT

The management is determined by the diagnosis. **Topical steroids** are used to treat various papulosquamous eruptions. These drugs are the mainstay of therapy designed to minimize inflammation. The agents usually prescribed in cases of atopic as well as seborrheic dermatitis are triamcinolone 0.1% and hydrocortisone 1% (cream or ointment). Sometimes brief courses of systemic steroids (4–5 days of prednisone) may be needed during more severe exacerbations. Psoriasis does not usually respond to hydrocortisone 1% alone and may require a combination tar-hydrocortisone preparation.

Management of atopic dermatitis involves the **reduction of dryness and irritation.** Children may bathe, but they should avoid using drying soaps. Within three minutes of leaving the bath tub they should apply moisturizers to ensure that the skin is hydrated. Seborrheic dermatitis may respond to topical steroids, but additional scalp treatment may be necessary. Baby oil may be applied to help loosen the scales. Parents should be told to massage the child's scalp gently. The scalp should then be washed using either a mild baby shampoo or an over-the-counter antiseborrheic shampoo (usually containing sulfur and sialic acid). The scalp may be brushed with a soft-bristle tooth brush

to loosen scales further while the shampoo is on the scalp.

Antibiotics are indicated if secondary infection is present. The most common pathogen involved is *Staphylococcus aureus*. A five-day course of erythromycin may be adequate to treat the infection. Some children are colonized with erythromycin-resistant organisms, however, and they should therefore be treated with a cephalosporin, dicloxacillin, or amoxicillin-clavulanate.

If children with atopic dermatitis develop infection with **herpes simplex** (eczema herpeticum), they should be treated with **acyclovir**. Atopic children are also prone to infection with warts and molluscum contagiosa. These conditions should be appropriately managed. Other measures in the management of atopic dermatitis include the use of tars and sunlight.

Coinfection with **_Candida,_** which occurs with seborrheic dermatitis and psoriasis, requires the use of **topical medications** such as nystatin, clotrimazole, or miconazole. Antifungal shampoos may also help in reducing the scaling due to fungal agents such as *Pityrosporum*.

Three major medications are used to treat scabies. They all work by killing the mites causing the infestation. **Lindane (Kwell),** which has been used for over 50 years, is a 1% cream. It is generally applied from the neck down and left in place for 8 to 12 hours. At the end of this time it should be removed by bathing. Because of concern about the absorption of lindane and its potential neurotoxicity, the drug should not be used in young infants or patients with a seizure disorder. It is recommended that a repeat application of the drug be administered in seven days in all symptomatic patients. A mild topical steroid, such as hydrocortisone 1% cream, may be used in between applications to decrease the inflammatory response to the mites.

Crotamiton 10%, an antiscabies medication, lacks the neurotoxic effects of lindane. However, the efficacy of crotamiton is low—reportedly only 40 to 50% after two daily applications. Five days of daily applications are therefore recommended, which is both less convenient and more costly for patients. **Permethrin** (Elimite), a newer product, requires only a single application and is safe for individuals of all ages. An over-the-counter treatment for lice, permethrin is currently the drug of choice for the treatment of scabies.

Antihistamines may play a role in reducing the pruritus, especially during the night. Hydroxyzine seems to have the best effect.

PROGNOSIS

In general, the prognosis for children with papulosquamous eruptions is excellent with appropriate management, which is contingent on accurate diagnosis. Both atopic dermatitis and seborrheic dermatitis tend to improve as children get older. Children with atopic dermatitis frequently face remissions and exacerbations, particularly associated with seasonal changes. Scabies also improves with appropriate management. Psoriasis may have a more prolonged course, and children with this condition often require medical intervention into adulthood.

Case Resolution

The infant's presentation in the case history is characteristic of seborrheic dermatitis. The infant experienced the onset of symptoms shortly after birth, and the involvement of the scalp with scaling and crusting supports the diagnosis of seborrheic dermatitis. The mother should be advised that although she may use the baby oil to loosen the scale on the scalp, she should shampoo immediately afterwards using an antiseborrheic or antifungal shampoo. A mild topical steroid, such as hydrocortisone 1%, may also be recommended. If skin scrapings reveal secondary infection with *Candida*, an antifungal cream should be added to the regimen.

Selected Readings

Birmhall, C. L., and N. B. Esterly. Summertime, and the critters are biting. Contemp. Pediatr. 11:62–77, 1994.

Cohen, B. Atopic dermatitis: breaking the itch-scratch cycle. Contemp. Pediatr. 9:64–81, 1992.

Hanifin, J. M. Atopic dermatitis in infants and children. Pediatr. Clin. North Am. 38:763–789, 1991.

Hogan, D. J., L. Schachner, and C. Tanglertsampan. Diagnosis and treatment of childhood scabies and pediculosis. Pediatr. Clin. North Am. 38:941–957, 1991.

Hurwitz, S. Skin lesions in the first year of life. Contemp. Pediatr. 10:110–128, 1993.

Mallory, S. B. Neonatal skin disorders. Pediatr. Clin. North Am. 38:745–761, 1991.

Nigro, J. F., and N. B. Esterly. Psoriasis—chronic but controllable. Contemp. Pediatr. 10:114–130, 1993.

Rabinowitz, L. G., and N. B. Esterly. Atopic dermatitis and ichthyosis vulgaris. Pediatr. Rev. 15:220–226, 1994.

Rasmussen, J. E. Scabies. Pediatr. Rev. 15:110–114, 1994.

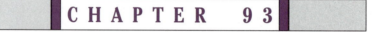

CHAPTER 93

MACULOPAPULAR RASHES

Carol D. Berkowitz, M.D.

H*x* A 10-month-old infant girl is brought to the office with a history of rhinorrhea, cough, and fever for three days prior to the onset of a confluent, erythematous rash. The rash started on her face. She has been irritable, and her eyes are red and teary. Her immunizations include three sets of diphtheria-pertussis-tetanus (DPT), oral polio, *Haemophilus influenzae* type B and hepatitis B vaccines. No one at home is ill. The girl was seen in the emergency department two weeks before because she caught her finger in a car door.

On physical examination, the girl's temperature is 39° C (102° F). A confluent maculopapular rash is evident on the face, trunk, and extremities, with prominent bilateral posterior cervical nodes. Rhinorrhea and conjunctivitis are also present.

Questions

1. What are the common causes of febrile maculopapular rashes in children?
2. What features distinguish one disease from another?
3. What are the public health considerations concerning viral exanthems in children?

More than 50 different viruses in addition to bacteria and rickettsia cause childhood exanthems. These exanthems may be macular, papular, or vesicular. In most cases, these rashes are seen in conjunction with fever, and sometimes other symptoms, including rhinorrhea, conjunctivitis, and lymphadenopathy. Although many of the common childhood illnesses of the past are now prevented by immunizations, not all segments of the population are adequately immunized. In addition, some children are not eligible for immunization because of their young age. Allergic reactions to medications, particularly antibiotics, may also result in eruptions, although these often have no associated symptoms. Differentiating viral exanthems from allergic reactions may be difficult in febrile children who have empirically been started on antimicrobial agents.

EPIDEMIOLOGY

In most children, the viruses that cause maculopapular exanthems produce mild disease without significant morbidity or long-term sequelae. Of greater concern is that some diseases are a public health risk because of potential spread through the population. Maculopapular eruptions are a common presenting complaint, particularly in certain age groups and at certain times of the year.

Measles, a viral disease, had been virtually eliminated in the United States. Periodic resurgences have occurred, particularly among unimmunized preschoolers and 15–19-year-old adolescents. In addition, young infants are also at risk because of decreased levels of passively transferred maternal immunity related to lack of maternal natural infection or immunization. Vaccine-related immunity apparently wanes more rapidly in mothers than does naturally acquired immunity. In a recent outbreak of measles in the Los Angeles area, Hispanic children of poorer immigrant parents were 12.6 times more likely to develop measles than nonimmigrant children. The incubation period of measles is about one week. Individuals are infectious during the second half of this week, before the rash erupts, and then for several days following its appearance.

Rubella now rarely occurs, but sporadic outbreaks are reported, particularly during the springtime. Adolescents and young adults are at greatest risk for the disease. Congenital rubella syndrome may develop in the offspring of pregnant women who have rubella. The incubation period is 15 to 21 days.

Erythema infectiosum, also called fifth disease, is most commonly seen in children aged 5 to 15 years. The disease is caused by parvovirus B19 and spread through respiratory secretions. The incubation period is generally 4 to 14 days but may be up to 20 days.

Roseola may affect children from 6 months to 3 years of age, although the majority are under the age of 1 year. The illness is due to infection with human herpesvirus 6 or 7, and the virus is shed in the saliva, even among healthy, previously infected infants. The incubation period is 5 to 15 days.

Enteroviruses are the most common cause of exanthems during August, September, and October and account for two thirds of all exanthems that occur during the summer. Thirty different types of enteroviruses are recognized. Previously these viruses were categorized as coxsackievirus, echovirus, or poliovirus, but now newly identified strains are grouped under picornavirus. Infection is spread through the fecal-oral route. Exanthems are more common in young children, and infection of the central nervous system is more common in older children. The incubation period is three to seven days, with an absent or brief prodrome.

Kawasaki disease is of uncertain etiology, although recent evidence suggests that the disorder may be related to a new strain of *Staphylococcus aureus,* producing a toxic shock syndrome–like toxin (TSST). Most patients are under the age of 2 years, and 80% are below the age of 5 years. Males outnumber females by a ratio of 1.5 to 1. The incidence of the disorder among Asians is higher. Caucasians and African Americans in the United States are also affected. The incubation period is unknown.

Scarlet fever is a bacterially transmitted illness that can produce a maculopapular eruption. The rash and illness are due to an exotoxin produced by group A beta-hemolytic streptococcus. A resurgence of disease related to exotoxin A, which causes more severe cases, has occurred. These cases may be associated with a toxic shock–like picture, with the classic rash of scarlet fever. Scarlet fever is usually seen in young children with pharyngitis. The incubation period is two to five days.

Dx Maculopapular Rashes

- Macular, papular, or maculopapular rash
- Fever
- Enanthems (lesions in the mouth)
- Lymphadenopathy
- Respiratory symptoms

CLINICAL PRESENTATION

Maculopapular eruptions may involve the face, trunk, or extremities. The rash is usually erythematous, and the lesions are flat or slightly raised. Occasionally, lesions within the mouth, referred to as enanthems, are evident. Most children are febrile (D_x Box).

PATHOPHYSIOLOGY

The mechanism for development of a rash is variable. In some cases, the rash is the reaction of the body to infection or to the presence of a toxin. In general, the sequence involves exposure to an infectious agent and then acquisition of the agent either through droplet infection or fecal-oral contamination. The agent, usually a virus, then replicates, perhaps in the reticuloendothelial system. Lymph nodes enlarge, reflecting the involvement of the reticuloendothelial system. Associated viremia may be present.

In a toxin-mediated rash (e.g., scarlet fever), previous exposure to the toxin is believed to sensitize the individual. An antibiotic-related rash may represent an allergy to the antibiotic itself, or not infrequently, a reaction to one of the ingredients in the antibiotic preparation. Reactions to ampicillin and amoxicillin are especially common in patients infected with EBV.

DIFFERENTIAL DIAGNOSIS

Maculopapular rashes are associated with several diseases, such as measles, rubella, erythema infectiosum, roseola, enterovirus-caused diseases, Kawasaki disease, and scarlet fever.

The rash associated with **measles** is preceded by rhinorrhea, conjunctivitis, cough, and fever (temperature: 39.4° C [103° F]), which last for several days before the eruption of the exanthem. Lesions within the oral cavity, called Koplik's spots, are well-circumscribed white lesions (Fig. 93–1) that usually resolve after about two to three days, with the appearance of the rash. Other oral lesions, referred to as Forschheimer spots, are pinpoint, rose-colored, petechial spots on the soft palate. The conjunctivitis associated with measles is purulent, which distinguishes it from Kawasaki disease.

The measles rash itself usually begins on the head, particularly behind the ears and around the margin of the scalp and then spreads over the rest of the body. Initially the lesions are discrete papules that coalesce and become pruritic. As the rash resolves the lesions become brawny, and desquamation occurs.

FIGURE 93–1. *Koplik's spots.*

As with other viral exanthems, the measles rash is associated with lymphadenopathy, particularly in the posterior cervical region. The major complications of measles in children in developed nations are pneumonia, encephalitis, and secondary bacterial infections. In developing nations, children with marginal nutritional status are at high risk of dying from measles or its complications. Arthritis has been reported as a complication in adults. In individuals who were initially immunized with killed measles vaccine (1963–1967), acquisition of measles results in atypical measles, which is characterized by a papular or vesicular eruption that may be hemorrhagic. Pneumonia is always present, and associated findings include hepatosplenomegaly and weakness.

Rubella produces a relatively minor illness in children, although adults, particularly women, may experience a painful arthritis. The rash consists of fine macules and papules, starting on the face and progressing caudally. Lymphadenopathy, particularly of the postauricular nodes, is characteristic of the disease.

Erythema infectiosum is characterized by a sudden onset of the rash. Prodromal symptoms are mild, and may include low-grade fever, headache, and malaise. The rash is variable, and the classic pattern of the markedly erythematous "slapped cheek" appearance is present in only 50% of cases. If involved, the extremities may initially have a discrete maculopapular eruption, which then assumes a fine, lacy quality. The rash on the extremities usually appears one to four days after the malar eruption but may last for weeks, waxing and waning. Most children are only mildly ill, but children with underlying hematologic disorders may experience aplastic crises because of the affinity of parvovirus B19 for developing red blood cells.

Roseola is another viral exanthem that usually causes a mild illness in children. Defervescence usually accompanies the rash, which consists of fine pink macules or papules on the neck and trunk. On average, the rash lasts about four days, although it may be very evanescent, lasting from a few hours to one to two days. Infants may appear sickest during the prodromal phase, when the fever is high (temperature: often 39° C [102.2° F] or above) and infants are irritable. Workups to rule out sepsis are often warranted. During the prodromal phase, as well as following the eruption of the rash, lymphadenopathy is seen in the occipital, cervical, and postauricular nodes.

The rashes associated with **enterovirus infections** are highly variable. They may resemble measles or rubella or may be distinct and characteristic, such as hand-foot-and-mouth disease, usually seen with coxsackievirus A16. The rash of hand-foot-and-mouth disease may be vesicular or maculopapular. Lesions may be anywhere in the mouth and progress from vesicles to sharply demarcated ulcers. Often low-grade fever, anorexia, sore throat, and malaise are present. Other enteroviral infections may have similar systemic symptoms, and some may cause gastroenteritis or aseptic meningitis.

The rash of **Kawasaki disease** is also highly variable; it may be morbilliform, urticarial, scarlatiniform, or resemble erythema multiforme. The rash is often intensified in the perineal area, where it peels, like the rash of scarlet fever. Other signs and symptoms in addition to the rash characterize Kawasaki disease. Temperature over 39.4° C (103° F) occurs for at least five days. A nonpurulent conjunctivitis is present, and erythema of the mucous membranes of the mouth, fissuring of the lips, and hypertrophy of the papilla of the tongue are also evident. Cervical lymphadenopathy is present. The distal extremities are also involved; erythema or edema of the palms and soles and desquamation of the tips of the fingers or toes, often around the nails, is apparent. The presence of this symptom complex should suggest the diagnosis. The major complication of Kawasaki disease is coronary artery aneurysms, which are reported in 15 to 20% of affected children. This problem can be averted with appropriate management, but the diagnosis must be considered before the necessary therapy is instituted.

Scarlet fever is the most common bacterially caused exanthem. Symptoms of fever (temperature: 39.4° C [103° F]), headache, vomiting, malaise, and sore throat appear suddenly. The tonsils are covered with a white exudate, and palatal petechiae are seen. The tongue initially has a white coating. Edema of the papillae make them appear prominent, and the finding is referred to as strawberry tongue (Fig. 93–2). The face is flushed, except around the mouth (circumoral pallor), but a discrete facial rash is absent. The fine rash is concentrated on the trunk and it is intensified in flexor folds. The bright red lines noted in the antecubital fossa are called Pastia's lines. As the scarlet fever rash resolves, desquamation begins in four to five days.

Adenoviruses account for 2 to 4% of rashes and occur more commonly in winter and spring. This usually mild rash has nonspecific characteristics. Conjunctivitis, rhinitis, pharyngitis, lymphadenopathy and, occasionally, pneumonia accompany the rash.

Infection with EBV is associated with rash in young children and in adolescents on antibiotics. The eruption is morbilliform, and the lesions may be erythematous or copper-colored. Fever, upper respiratory symptoms, lymphadenopathy, hepatosplenomegaly, and facial and peripheral edema, including unilateral periorbital edema may be noted.

EVALUATION

History

A thorough history should be obtained (Questions Box).

Physical Examination

The focus of the physical examination is to help define the characteristics of the eruption such as location, extent, and degree of coalescence. The presence of any associated physical findings such as fever, lymphadenopathy, enanthem, desquamation, rhinorrhea, conjunctivitis, organomegaly, or CNS symptomatology should be determined.

Laboratory Tests

Laboratory assessment may be helpful in certain conditions. Serologic testing is most valuable for defining a community outbreak of a specific disease such as measles. In most viral exanthems, the results of serologic studies are not available until the condition has resolved and the patient has recovered. Tests may include acute and convalescent titers for specific viruses. Alternatively, IgM levels of antibodies against certain infections may be used to document that the infection was recent. Because neutropenia and lymphocytosis

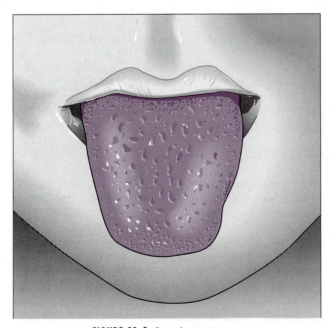

FIGURE 93–2. *Strawberry tongue.*

> **Questions: Maculopapular Rashes**
>
> - What does the rash look like?
> - What symptoms, if any, are associated with the rash?
> - How long has the child had these symptoms?
> - Is the child taking any antibiotics?
> - Does the child have any ill contacts?
> - What is the child's immunization status?

characterize many viral illnesses, such findings are not helpful in differentiating specific causal agents. Lymphocytosis with characteristically atypical lymphocytosis, distinguishes EBV infection. Although a mononucleosis spot test is usually positive in older children and adolescents, it may be nonreactive in young children, where infection is documented by specific EBV serology.

Scarlet fever is characterized by leukocytosis. In addition, a throat culture or antigen assay reveals the presence of group A beta-hemolytic streptococci. If the pharyngitis has resolved, serologic studies such as antistreptolysin O or anti-DNAase provide evidence of the recent infection.

Kawasaki disease is associated with specific laboratory abnormalities, including an elevated platelet count and IgE. A slit lamp examination of the eye may show uveitis.

Imaging Studies

Ultrasound, if performed in children with suspected Kawasaki disease, may reveal hydrops of the gallbladder. An echocardiogram to check for evidence of coronary artery aneurysm is a mandated part of the evaluation in this disorder.

MANAGEMENT

The management of most viral exanthems is supportive and symptomatic. In cases where complications such as encephalitis or pneumonia develop, hospitalization is indicated. Antibiotic therapy should be initiated if bacterial coinfection is suspected. Antibiotics in the form of penicillin should be given when patients have scarlet fever.

The management of Kawasaki disease includes the administration of intravenous immune globulin (IVIG), which should be started within 10 days of onset. IVIG may work by binding to the toxin that is suspected of precipitating the illness. Low-dose aspirin to prevent coronary thrombosis is also recommended.

PROGNOSIS

The prognosis for most maculopapular rashes of childhood is excellent, with full resolution of symptoms unless children are very young or have some underlying condition. In some young infants, viruses that cause exanthems may produce severe complications such as pneumonia and encephalitis.

Selected Readings

Beutner, K. R. Cutaneous viral infections. Pediatr. Ann. 22:247–252, 1993.

Committee on Infectious Disease, American Academy of Pediatrics. 1994 Redbook: Report of the Committee on Infectious Disease. Elk Grove Village, IL, American Academy of Pediatrics, 1994.

Farrar, W. E., et al. Infectious Disease. Text and Color Atlas. London, Gower Medical Publishing, 1992.

Frieden, I. J., and S. D. Resnick. Childhood exanthems, old and new. Pediatr. Clin. North Am. 38:859–885, 1991.

Leung, D. Y. M., et al. Toxic shock syndrome toxin-secreting *Staphylococcus aureus* in Kawasaki syndrome. Lancet 342:1385–1388, 1993.

McMillan, J. A. HHV-6 and roseola: a "new" virus explains an old disease. Contemp. Pediatr. 9:89–98, 1992.

Makhene, M. K., and P. S. Diaz. Clinical presentations and complications of suspected measles in hospitalized children. Pediatr. Infect. Dis. J. 12:836–840, 1993.

Rowley, A. H., F. Gonzalez-Crussi, and S. T. Shulman. Kawasaki syndrome. Adv. Pediatr. 38:51–74, 1991.

CHAPTER 94

VESICULAR EXANTHEMS

Monica Sifuentes, M.D.

H$_x$ A 2-year-old toddler is evaluated for a two-day history of fever (temperature: 39.5° C [103° F]), runny nose, decreased appetite, and a rash over the abdomen. The boy has had no previous known exposures to chickenpox (varicella). He attends day care daily. No one at home is ill. The boy is currently taking no medications except for acetaminophen for fever, and he has no past history of dermatologic problems.

On physical examination, the heart rate is 120 beats/min, the respiratory rate is 20 breaths/min, and the temperature is 38.0° C. The toddler's overall appearance is nontoxic. The skin examination is significant for a few scattered erythematous vesicular lesions over the abdomen and one papule on the back. The rest of the examination is normal.

Questions

1. What are the most likely causes of vesicular exanthems in febrile children?
2. How can types of vesicular rashes be differentiated on the basis of patient history?
3. What are the key historical questions to ask?
4. What is the natural course of varicella?
5. What treatment options are available for children with varicella? What options are available for other vesicular exanthems?

Exanthems are generalized, erythematous rashes that often accompany viral or bacterial illnesses. These eruptions have different physical appearances and can be macular, papular, vesicular, or petechial. Vesicles are elevated, fluid-filled lesions that measure 0.5 cm or less in diameter. Bullae are quite similar but are more than 0.5 cm in diameter. Vesicles may be grouped, generalized, or linear depending on their etiology, and their specific distribution is often helpful in formulating a differential diagnosis. This chapter will focus on common vesicular exanthems in children.

EPIDEMIOLOGY

Epidemiologic factors help differentiate infectious from noninfectious etiologies. Patient age, season of the year, presence or absence of similar cases in the community, regular attendance at day care or school, and lower socioeconomic class, which may contribute to exposure, should all be considered. Gender and ethnicity, on the other hand, are not usually helpful from an epidemiologic standpoint.

CLINICAL PRESENTATION

Vesicular exanthems are distinctive lesions that are raised and fluid-filled (D$_x$ Box). They may be located anywhere on the child's body and, depending upon the etiology, may or may not be pruritic. Other symptoms that may accompany such rashes include fever, upper respiratory symptoms, and decreased appetite.

PATHOPHYSIOLOGY

Numerous infectious conditions cause vesicular eruptions (Table 94–1). Parasites such as the tiny itch mite,

Dx Vesicular Exanthems

- Raised, fluid-filled vesicles on the skin
- Lesions may be pruritic
- Possible associated fever, URI symptoms, myalgias
- History of affected contacts
- Lesions on mucous membranes

Sarcoptes scabiei, can cause an intensely pruritic vesicular eruption in combination with papules and linear burrows (see Chapter 92, Papulosquamous Eruptions). Fungal pathogens that cause vesiculopustular lesions that appear on the feet and toes include *Trichophyton rubrum, T. mentagrophytes,* and less commonly, *Epidermophyton floccosum.* A delayed hypersensitivity reaction secondary to contact with an oleoresin of the poison ivy or poison oak plant causes the classic linear vesicular lesions of *Rhus* dermatitis. Contact with other allergenic substances may also produce a vesicular rash. The etiology of dyshidrotic eczema, a vesicular eruption involving mainly the hands and feet, is unknown.

DIFFERENTIAL DIAGNOSIS

The differential diagnosis of acute vesicular exanthems can be organized according to the distribution of the lesions. Distinctive locations as well as specific patterns are important to consider in each individual case. The presence or absence of fever (a temperature ≥ 38.3° C [101° F]) can also be key to developing the appropriate differential (Figure 94–1). Epidemiologic, as well as historic, information may suggest the diagnosis. For example, known exposure to varicella (chickenpox)

TABLE 94–1. Common Causes of Acute Vesicular Exanthems

Infectious
Viral
Varicella-zoster virus
Herpes simplex virus
Enterovirus: coxsackievirus A16
Bacterial
Staphylococcus aureus
Parasitic
Sarcoptes scabiei
Fungal
Trichophyton rubrum
T. mentagrophytes
Noninfectious
Contact dermatitis
Rhus (plant) dermatitis
Dyshidrotic eczema

10–21 days prior to a vesicular eruption facilitates diagnosis of this disease. A history of hiking or camping suggests possible contact with poison ivy or poison oak. In addition, the presence of a specific prodrome can often be elicited with primary or recurrent herpes simplex. Pain on swallowing often occurs with coxsackie virus infection. A past history of similar lesions lessens the likelihood of acute primary infection and suggests a chronic condition such as the recurrent disorder pompholyx (dyshidrotic eczema).

EVALUATION

History

A thorough history should be obtained (Questions Box). Practitioners must inquire about the current state of general health, as well as the specific details about the eruption.

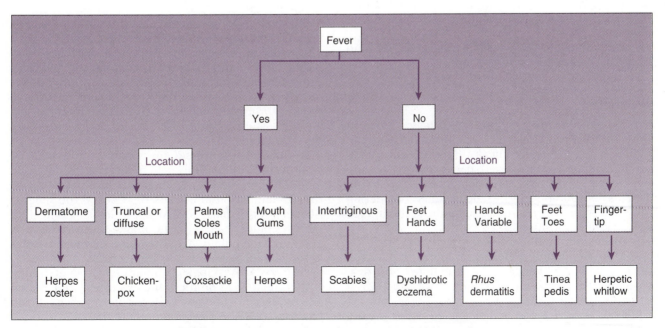

FIGURE 94–1. *Approach to the evaluation of vesicular eruptions.*

Physical Examination

Although the physical examination focuses on the skin, other aspects of the examination are helpful diagnostically. Vital signs should be taken to verify the presence or absence of fever. The oropharynx should be examined closely for vesicular or ulcerative lesions on the tongue, gingiva, buccal mucosa, anterior tonsillar pillars, and posterior pharynx. The lips should also be examined for any evidence of vesicular lesions that may occur with a primary or recurrent herpes simplex infection.

Patients should be completely unclothed to permit a thorough examination of the skin. The distribution of the lesions should be noted. Physicians should determine whether the vesicles are grouped in a particular dermatomal distribution, as with zoster (shingles), or more generally distributed and in various stages of development, as with varicella. A linear distribution may suggest contact with poison ivy or poison oak. Physicians should also ask the following questions: Do the lesions include or exclude the palms and soles? Are the buttocks involved? Are the lesions concentrated on one specific part of the body, such as the feet and toes or the hands? Are the sizes of the lesions uniform? If not, are other larger bullous-like lesions present in addition to vesicles?

It is also helpful, if at all possible, to examine the skin of family members for similar lesions.

Laboratory Tests

Few, if any, laboratory studies are usually needed in healthy children with vesicular eruptions because the diagnosis is often made clinically. Serologies are indicated in immunocompromised patients with an unknown history of varicella and a definite exposure to the virus. This information may be helpful when considering prophylaxis with varicella-zoster immune globulin (see Chapter 17, Immunizations).

Definitive confirmation of scabies can be made by microscopic examination of skin scrapings from suspicious lesions. The presence of the adult mite or the ova, larva, or feces is diagnostic. For children with suspected tinea pedis, a skin scraping mixed with potassium hydroxide can be performed and examined under the microscope. Fungal cultures can also be taken. A Tzanck smear showing multinucleated giant cells that contain intranuclear viral inclusions may be useful in making a preliminary diagnosis of a herpesvirus, but commercially available monoclonal antibody tests are more accurate. A culture for herpes simplex can also be done in specific cases that pose diagnostic dilemmas.

MANAGEMENT

The mainstay of treatment for most vesicular eruptions is parent and child education as well as reassurance. Conditions are usually self-limited and require only **supportive therapy.** For example, hand-foot-and-mouth disease is self-limited and no treatment except parental reassurance and education regarding adequate hydration is necessary. Special circumstances exist in immunocompromised children such as those with HIV or AIDS and patients who are receiving chemotherapeutic agents or systemic corticosteroids.

Topical agents such as calamine lotion, oatmeal soaks, or Aveeno baths should be used in children with intense pruritus or multiple lesions. Topical products, which are potentially sensitizing (e.g., diphenhydramine-containing agents) should not be used. Cool wet compresses with plain water or Burow's solution can be quite soothing in cases of *Rhus* dermatitis. Wet compresses may also be helpful with open, macerated lesions of dyshidrotic eczema.

Antipyretics (acetaminophen, ibuprofen) may be used to treat otherwise healthy children with varicella. Aspirin-containing medications should be avoided in children with varicella because of the association with Reye syndrome. Herpetic whitlow is often treated aggressively with antipyretics and topical pain medications to decrease the pain of the accompanying gingivostomatitis.

Oral antihistamines (diphenhydramine or hydroxyzine) may be used in children with varicella for treatment of pruritus. These drugs are also helpful in *Rhus* dermatitis.

Steroids may be effective in the control of some vesicular rashes. Topical steroids can be used for outbreaks of vesicles of dyshidrotic eczema on the palms, soles, and lateral aspects of the hands. Although these agents are used by many practitioners to treat *Rhus* dermatitis, their role is minimal. In severe cases of *Rhus* dermatitis, a short course of systemic steroids, such as prednisone, 1 to 2 mg/kg/day, may be warranted.

Oral acyclovir should be considered in otherwise healthy individuals only when the risk of developing moderate to severe varicella is increased. According to the Committee on Infectious Diseases of the American Academy of Pediatrics (AAP), acyclovir is indicated in patients older than 12 years of age, those with chronic cutaneous or pulmonary disorders, or those receiving chronic salicylates or corticosteroids (systemic or aerosolized). Acyclovir is most effective if initiated within the first 24 hours of the exanthem, and it should not be used to prevent varicella in otherwise healthy children. (See the 1994 *Red Book* of the AAP for further details and specific recommendations regarding immunocompromised children and the role of varicella-zoster immune globulin.) A live attenuated varicella vaccine is now licensed for use in the United States and is available for all nonimmune individuals.

Additional recommendations for children with varicella include keeping fingernails short in young children to prevent superinfection of lesions from scratching. Children should drink plenty of fluids to avoid dehydration. Patients are considered contagious from one to two days prior to the onset of the rash until the lesions are all scabbed over (usually five to seven days after the rash develops), at which time, children may return to school. In children with persistent or recurrent fever, secondary complications should be considered.

Treatment for zoster, or shingles, is primarily symptomatic and should consist of pain medications. Acyclovir can be considered if the eruption becomes generalized or affects immunocompromised patients. Herpetic whitlow and herpes gladiatorum do not require treatment with antiviral agents such as acyclovir.

Bullous impetigo requires **oral antistaphylococcal therapy** with agents such as amoxicillin and clavulanate (Augmentin), erythromycin, or cefalexin (Keflex). Augmentin should be given three times a day for a total dose of 20–40 mg/kg/day. Diarrhea is the most common side effect and is dose dependent. The dose of either erythromycin or Keflex is 40 mg/kg/day and should be given four times daily. Erythromycin should be taken with meals or milk because gastrointestinal upset is not uncommon.

For the treatment of tinea pedis, topical **antifungal agents,** such as 2% miconazole (Micatin), 1% tolnaftate (Tinactin), and undecylenate (Desenex), are available over the counter in powder form and can be applied twice daily. Antifungal creams (clotrimazole, ketoconazole), also available over the counter, can be used twice daily for four to six weeks. Vesicular lesions should be treated with wet compresses of Burow's solution, 1:80. The recommended application is 10 to 15 minutes three to four times a day for three to five days. In severe cases, an oral antifungal preparation, griseofulvin, may be prescribed for an extended period.

Tinea pedis can be difficult to control. Its treatment is centered around meticulous foot hygiene. Because careful foot care is often not a priority for most patients, complete eradication is not realistic. Patients should be instructed to wash and change their socks when they return from school, dry their feet completely, avoid occlusive shoes, and wear open-air shoes or sandals whenever possible. Cotton socks are recommended.

PROGNOSIS

Overall, the prognosis for vesicular exanthems is good, with most children recovering in 1–2 weeks, depending on the etiology. Secondary infections can occur with varicella, however, and should be suspected in children with persistent or recurrent fever. These complications include cellulitis, otitis media, pneumonia, and meningoencephalitis. Long-term sequelae associated with these secondary infections are rare. Reye syndrome, another complication of chickenpox, has an excellent prognosis when diagnosed early.

Case Resolution

In the case presented at the beginning of the chapter, the toddler has a classic presentation of primary varicella (chickenpox). Management should include symptomatic treatment with acetaminophen and antihistamines, along with topical preparations such as calamine lotion and oatmeal or Aveeno baths. The parent should be instructed regarding the natural course of this infection and be informed that the infection is highly contagious. In addition, symptoms indicating possible complications, such as persistent or recurrent fever, circumferential redness or swelling of the lesions, and shortness of breath, should be reviewed with the parents.

Selected Readings

Calvelli, F., and A. A. Gaspari. When the vesicles aren't chickenpox. Contemp. Pediatr. 10:48–62, 1993.

Eichenfield, L. F., and P. J. Honig. Blistering disorders in childhood. Pediatr. Clin. North Am. 38:959–976, 1991.

Feder, H. M., and S. Long. Herpetic whitlow: epidemiology, clinical characteristics, diagnosis, and treatment. Am. J. Dis. Child. 137:861–863, 1983.

Freiden I. J., and S. D. Resnick. Childhood exanthems. Pediatr. Clin. North Am. 38:859–887, 1991.

Hurwitz, S. Clinical Pediatric Dermatology, 2nd ed. Philadelphia, W. B. Saunders, 1993.

Schachner, L., and S. Press. Vesicular, bullous and pustular disorders in infancy and childhood. Pediatr. Clin. North Am. 30:609–629, 1983.

THE NEW MORBIDITY

CHAPTER 95

ATTENTION DEFICIT/HYPERACTIVITY DISORDER

Iris Wagman Borowsky, M.D., Ph.D.

Hx A 9-year-old boy is seen in the emergency department after nearly colliding with a car while riding his bicycle. He sustained only minor abrasions from a fall. The boy's mother states that her son is impulsive and frequently engages in risky behaviors. She reports that he is extremely active and has a short attention span. He is in the fourth grade and an average student, but he has a hard time following directions and is easily distracted in class. In addition, he tends to have trouble keeping friends.

In the examining room, the boy is quiet but answers questions appropriately. Except for a few scrapes, his physical examination is entirely normal.

Questions

1. What are the primary symptoms of attention deficit/ hyperactivity disorder (ADHD)? What other conditions should be considered in the differential diagnosis of ADHD?
2. What other psychiatric disorders or neurodevelopmental disabilities commonly coexist with ADHD?
3. What is the appropriate evaluation of children with suspected ADHD?
4. What treatment modalities are useful in the management of ADHD?

Three major symptoms—inattention, impulsivity, and hyperactivity—are characteristic of ADHD. The *Diagnostic and Statistic Manual of Mental Disorders* (4th ed.) identifies three diagnostic subtypes of ADHD: (1) predominantly inattentive type, (2) predominantly hyperactive-impulsive type, and (3) combined type. Most children and adolescents with the disorder have the combined type, exhibiting symptoms of both inattention and hyperactivity-impulsivity.

Symptoms of ADHD must appear before seven years of age and persist for at least six months before the disorder can be diagnosed. The behaviors are more frequent and severe than those typically seen in normal children at the same level of development and interfere with functioning in at least two settings (e.g., home and school).

EPIDEMIOLOGY

An estimated 3 to 5% of school-age children have ADHD. Boys are affected approximately six times as often as girls.

CLINICAL PRESENTATION

Children with ADHD have problems with selective attention. They may make careless mistakes or fail to pay attention to details. In addition, they are easily distracted and have difficulty concentrating on tasks long enough to complete them (D_x Box). Difficulties following instructions and organizing tasks and activities are also characteristic of ADHD. Poor impulse control manifests as difficulty awaiting one's turn, frequently blurting out answers, and interrupting or intruding on others. Symptoms of hyperactivity include fidgetiness, difficulty remaining seated or playing quietly, and subjective feelings of restlessness in adolescents. Difficulties with social relationships and low frustration tolerance are also commonly seen in children with ADHD.

PATHOPHYSIOLOGY

The etiology of ADHD is unknown. Genetic, neurologic, and dietary factors may play a role.

D_x Attention Deficit/Hyperactivity Disorder (Core Symptoms)

- Inattention
- Impulsivity
- Hyperactivity

TABLE 95–1.   Differential Diagnosis of Attention Deficit/Hyperactivity Disorder

Developmental delay
Learning disability
Language disorder
Sensory deficiencies (especially hearing impairment)
Autism
Seizure disorder
Iron deficiency
Environmental toxins (lead)
Side effects of medication (phenobarbital)
Hyperthyroidism
Congenital infection
In utero exposure to drugs or alcohol
Previous brain insult (trauma, infection)
Family stresses
Ineffective parenting
Psychiatric disorders
   Conduct disorder
   Oppositional disorder
   Anxiety disorders
   Affective disorders (depression, bipolar illness)
   Personality disorders (aggression, antisocial behavior)
   Substance abuse

Family studies indicate that **genetic factors** influence the development of ADHD. First-degree relatives of children with ADHD have a 25% risk of similar problems. In addition, behavioral ratings and measures of attention are more alike in monozygotic twins than in same-sex dizygotic twins.

ADHD may be the result of **neurologic factors.** Patients with frontal lobe disorders exhibit inattention, impulsivity, and hyperactivity. The frontal and prefrontal regions of the brain appear to be involved in selective attention, distractibility, inhibition, planning, and organization. ADHD may be the result of neuroanatomic factors. Psychostimulants, the most effective pharmacologic therapy for ADHD, alter dopamine and catecholamine metabolism. Thus ADHD may have a neurochemical basis.

Various **dietary ingredients,** such as sugar, aspartame, food coloring, and food additives, have been implicated as a cause of hyperactivity and other behavioral problems in children. Many parents have put their children on special diets with no additives. Well-controlled studies have now shown that sugar and food additives have no adverse effects on behavior or cognitive function in children. Nevertheless, many parents believe that certain foods have negative effects on their children's behavior.

DIFFERENTIAL DIAGNOSIS

The symptoms of ADHD can be seen in a variety of conditions (Table 95–1). Developmental delay is frequently confused with ADHD. Sensory deficiencies, especially hearing impairment, can also imitate attention deficits. Inattention is often a component of autism, also called pervasive developmental disorder, but autistic children exhibit stereotyped behaviors and markedly impaired speech and social interactions. Iron deficiency anemia and low-level lead poisoning also may have detrimental effects on behavior and development.

Seizure disorders, such as petit mal (absence) or partial complex seizures, may be misdiagnosed as ADHD. Possible side effects of certain medications, such as phenobarbital or theophylline, may mimic ADHD. Hyperthyroidism can cause the symptoms of ADHD, but other signs of increased metabolism, such as elevated heart rate, tremors, or weight loss, should be apparent. Exposure to alcohol or drugs in utero has been associated with subtle difficulties with learning and attention at a later time. Congenital infections, CNS infections in early childhood, and traumatic brain injuries may produce behaviors similar to those seen in ADHD.

In addition, psychosocial problems, such as family stresses (e.g., marital discord, unemployment, poverty, substance abuse) or ineffective parenting (e.g., inconsistent discipline) must be considered in the differential diagnosis of ADHD. Comorbidity is extremely common in children with ADHD. Up to 44% of these children carry another psychiatric diagnosis, 32% carry two other diagnoses, and 11% carry three other diagnoses. Learning or language disabilities, conduct disorder, oppositional disorder, anxiety, depression, and bipolar illness commonly coexist with ADHD in children. In adolescents and young adults, personality disorders such as aggression and antisocial behavior and substance abuse are often seen together with attention deficits. These conditions can magnify the symptoms of children with ADHD or may explain the symptoms entirely.

EVALUATION

History

The diagnostic evaluation of ADHD should begin with a description by caregivers of the child's problem behaviors, including examples of situations in which the behaviors occur. A thorough history should be obtained (Questions Box). The physician should find out how parents handle their child's behavioral problems; this provides insight into their parenting style. Family stresses should be evaluated. Interviewing the child alone provides an opportunity for the child to describe

---

Questions: Attention Deficit/Hyperactivity Disorder

- What are the problem behaviors?
- How old was the child when the behaviors began?
- Where do the behaviors occur (at home, at school, or in both settings)?
- Did the child's mother develop any infections during the pregnancy?
- Did the child's mother use alcohol, marijuana, or any other drugs during the pregnancy?
- Were there any perinatal complications?
- At what age did the child attain various developmental milestones?
- Does the child take any medications?
- Does the child have any history of trauma, seizures, meningitis, or recurrent OM?
- What is the child's temperament and personality?
- Does the family have a history of ADHD, learning disability, or substance abuse, or other psychiatric disorders?

his or her thoughts and feelings. The physician should ask what problems the child is having at home and at school and find out how the child is coping with these difficulties.

Copies of report cards and teachers' descriptions of children's behavior are extremely helpful in obtaining the school history. Speaking to children's current teachers directly may also be useful. In addition, many rating scales (e.g., Conners scales, child behavior checklist) have been developed to allow parents and teachers to report children's behavior in various domains (e.g., inattention, hyperactivity, anxiety, aggression). These scales are used to aid in the diagnosis of ADHD as well as to evaluate the effects of treatment.

Physical Examination

The physical examination should include an assessment of growth parameters and any minor congenital anomalies as well as a careful neurologic examination. The child's weight, height, and head circumference should be plotted on a growth curve and the pattern of growth evaluated. Children should be examined for dysmorphic features such as the facies associated with fetal alcohol syndrome. A neurologic examination should include an assessment of the child's affect, speech, hearing, and vision. Some children with ADHD exhibit indicators of neuromaturational delays, the so-called soft neurologic signs, such as choreiform movements, involuntary movements, and motor slowness.

Observing the child's behavior during the office visit is important, but most children with ADHD do not display hyperactivity in the office. Interaction between the child and his or her parents should be observed. The physician should note whether the child listens to parental instructions and how parents deal with any misbehavior. Does the child cooperate with the examination? How well does the child relate to adults? The physician should watch the child play (e.g., draw, play with toys) and note the child's organization of activities, attention span, distractibility, and motor activity.

Laboratory Tests

The history and physical examination should direct the laboratory evaluation. Referral for further evaluation of speech, hearing, and vision should be done if indicated. A hematocrit and lead level are useful to rule out iron deficiency anemia and lead intoxication. Thyroid function tests are appropriate if signs or symptoms of hyperthyroidism are present (e.g., increased appetite, hyperactive precordium).

Psychometric tests of intelligence (IQ) and academic achievement help identify learning disabilities. Tests designed specifically to measure attention and impulsivity can be helpful, particularly in assessing response to medication.

Diagnostic Studies

An EEG is indicated if absence or partial complex seizures are suspected.

MANAGEMENT

Treatment of ADHD must be multifaceted and long-term to be successful. Family education is essential, and counseling about ADHD should provide factual information about the disorder, emphasize the strengths of children and families, and address parental concerns. The physician can ease parents' guilt by telling them that their children's problems are not the result of insufficient parenting. Children who discover that their problems are not their fault may feel that a heavy burden has been lifted from their shoulders. Both parents and children may find it difficult to accept that the child has a chronic disorder, however. The pediatrician can help by supporting families' efforts to seek treatment. Support groups for parents of children with ADHD can also provide assistance.

Behavior Management

The goals of behavior management include helping children learn to follow rules and complete important tasks, increasing children's self-control, and reducing stress within families. Management of overactive children who have difficulty focusing attention, following rules, and controlling impulses can be challenging for both parents and teachers. As often as possible, parents should give children positive feedback for good behavior and should set a good example for children. Parents should focus on one behavior at a time, such as doing homework, putting toys away, or completing chores.

Behavioral techniques include rewards for positive behaviors (e.g., verbal praise, hugs, points or stars on a chart that can be traded for material objects, special time with a parent or friend) and punishments for unacceptable behaviors (e.g., time out, loss of a privilege, extra chores, reduction in allowance). Acceptable and unacceptable behaviors should be clearly defined, and rewards and punishments should be spelled out in a contract drawn up with children. Because children with ADHD tend to lose interest in these behavioral programs over time, parents must be creative in periodically varying the rewards and penalties.

Educational Interventions

The pediatric practitioner can play an important role in optimizing each child's educational experience by keeping in contact with the child's teachers and attending school conferences where specific educational alternatives for the child with ADHD are discussed. Most children with ADHD can be managed in the regular classroom. If they are having behavioral or academic difficulties in the regular classroom, special educational placement in a smaller, more focused setting for part or all of the day may be indicated.

Teachers can help children with ADHD focus their attention and follow directions in the classroom in several ways (Table 95–2). In addition, they should focus on and nurture children's strengths and provide children with many opportunities to experience success in the classroom. In addition, teachers should be supportive and try not to embarrass children. Positive rein-

---

TABLE 95–2. Strategies for Managing Children With ADHD in the Classroom

Seat children in the front of the classroom, where distractions can be minimized and teachers can see whether children are paying attention

Cue children secretly to remind them to refocus their attention

Give clear instructions and repeat them frequently

Shorten work periods by allowing children to get up and move around (e.g., handing out papers, cleaning chalkboard)

---

forcement for good behavior as well as negative consequences for misbehavior should be addressed. immediately. This can be achieved through a system in which points are gained or lost for specific behaviors. Accumulated points can be "cashed in" at the end of the day for a desired activity (e.g., playing a game). Teachers who are most successful in working with children with ADHD are able to set firm limits and discipline children without anger or frustration, while at the same time remaining flexible enough to recognize when a change in tactics is necessary.

Because children with ADHD are easily provoked into misbehavior and are prone to clashes with peers, they can also benefit from closer supervision in unstructured school areas such as the playground, cafeteria, halls, and bus. Programs designed to improve social competence and peer relationships (e.g., group social skills training, therapeutic recreational activities) may also be helpful.

Pharmacotherapy

Research has shown that medications produce short-term benefits for children with ADHDs, including longer attention span, better impulse control, and lower activity levels. Significant long-term effects such as improved social adjustment and school achievement have not been demonstrated. When used in combination with other treatment approaches, medications usually help school-age children. Children below five years of age are less likely to respond to drug therapy and are at greater risk of experiencing adverse effects.

Psychostimulants, the most commonly used agents for ADHDs, have an estimated response rate of 80%. The most commonly prescribed psychostimulants are methylphenidate (Ritalin), dextroamphetamine (Dexedrine), and pemoline (Cylert). Some children suffer adverse effects such as decreased appetite, insomnia, tics, headaches, and stomach aches. Methylphenidate, the most widely used and best studied of the psychostimulants, is usually prescribed first because it has minimal side effects. The usual effective dose is 0.3–0.7 mg/kg. An initial dose of 5 to 10 mg is typically given in the morning. If teachers report an improvement in morning classroom behavior, this dose can be continued; otherwise, it should be increased in increments of 2.5 or 5.0 mg per week until an effective level is reached. This dose can then be given two or three times a day. The third dose is given to help children complete homework assignments in the late afternoon. Weekend dosing is optional, depending on children's behavior and scheduled activities. Sustained-release methylphenidate is available to

simplify dosing, but this form of the drug may not be as effective as the tablets.

A poor response to one stimulant does not predict a poor response to another. Dextroamphetamine and pemoline, which are both longer-acting than methylphenidate, may be appropriate if frequent dosing is a problem.

The physician should maintain close contact with children's teachers to monitor effects of medication, both positive and negative. Children who are doing well should have a brief examination approximately every two months, with particular attention to weight, height, and blood pressure. For children who are beginning to lose weight, the dose and schedule of medication can be changed to improve appetite at mealtimes. Growth delay warrants stopping medication for several weeks to allow catch-up growth to occur.

If psychostimulants are not effective or produce unacceptable side effects, clonidine or antidepressants (e.g., TCAs, monoamine oxidase inhibitors) may be introduced. These agents have some positive effects on the behavior of children with ADHDs.

PROGNOSIS

ADHD is a chronic condition, and over 50% of affected children continue to exhibit symptoms of ADHD into adulthood. Adults have an increased incidence of anxiety, low self-esteem, antisocial behavior, alcohol and drug abuse, interpersonal difficulties, and job changes. Poor outcomes are associated with lower intelligence, lower economic status, conduct problems, and family psychopathology (e.g., alcohol or drug abuse). Individual outcomes can be very good, however.

Case Resolution

In the case history presented at the beginning of this chapter, the boy's mother expresses concerns about her son's behavior. She describes symptoms of ADHD. The boy is referred to his primary care physician for diagnostic evaluation, which should include a full history, physical examination, and an assessment from his school.

Selected Readings

American Psychiatric Association: Diagnostic and Statistical Manual of Mental Disorders, 4th ed. Washington, D.C., American Psychiatric Association, 1994.

Culbert, T. P., G. A. Banez, and M. I. Reiff: Children who have attentional disorders: Interventions. Pediatr. Rev. 15:5–14, 1994.

Kelly, D. P., and G. P. Aylward: Attention deficits in school-aged children and adolescents: current issues and practice. Pediatr. Clin. North Am. 39:487–512, 1992.

Reiff, M. I., G. A. Banez, and T. P. Culbert: Children who have attentional disorders: diagnosis and evaluation. Pediatr. Rev. 14:455–464, 1993.

Rostain, A. L. Attention deficit disorders in children and adolescents. Pediatr. Clin. North Am. 38:607–635, 1991.

Wolraich, M. L., et al. Effects of diet high in sucrose or aspartame on the behavior and cognitive performance of children. N. Engl. J. Med. 330:301–307, 1994.

CHAPTER 96

PHYSICAL ABUSE

Carol D. Berkowitz, M.D.

Hx A 6-month-old male infant arrives at the emergency department after becoming limp and nonresponsive at home. The mother states that her son was fine when she left him in the care of her boyfriend before going to the store for cigarettes. When she returned one hour later, he was asleep, but then he seized and stopped breathing. The infant is being ventilated by a bag.

On examination, the infant is pale and limp. The heart rate is 100 beats/min, and the blood pressure is 90/30. The only abnormality is the presence of bilateral retinal hemorrhages.

Questions

1. What are the major lethal injuries associated with physical abuse of children?
2. What are the types of injuries seen in physically abused children?
3. What are the presenting complaints of children with head injuries?
4. What are the legal obligations of physicians in the area of child abuse?

Physical child abuse was first described in the pediatric literature in 1962 by Kempe and Silverman in their classic paper on the battered child syndrome. Child abuse or maltreatment takes many forms, including physical abuse, FTT, sexual abuse, emotional abuse, prenatal exposure to substances such as drugs and alcohol, and Munchausen syndrome by proxy, a complex disorder in which parents confabulate or create a medical condition in their children.

The nature and extent of inflicted injuries is variable and includes bruises, burns, fractures, lacerations, internal hemorrhage, and ruptures. Physicians must be aware of the legal obligations related to the suspicion of child abuse. They must assess the nature of the injuries, initiate appropriate medical therapy, and determine if the history offered is consistent with the medical findings.

EPIDEMIOLOGY

Over two million cases of child abuse are reported annually in the United States. Certain factors are associated with physical abuse. Most victims are young children; two-thirds are under the age of 3 years, and one-third are under the age of 6 months. These young children are frequently demanding. Crying infants and toilet-training toddlers are particularly at risk for abuse. Factors such as lower socioeconomic class and domestic violence, including spousal abuse, substance abuse, and poor parenting skills, place children at risk for abuse.

CLINICAL PRESENTATION

Children who have been physically abused present with injuries that range from nonsevere to lethal (D_x Box). Visible bruises, bites, and burns may be noted. Children may also have symptoms related to fractures, such as crying or refusal to walk or move an extremity. More severely injured children may present with seizures, apnea, shock, or cardiopulmonary arrest.

PATHOPHYSIOLOGY

Injuries in children who experience physical abuse are the result of direct trauma inflicted on the children. Head injuries, the most deadly form of abuse, may result from either a direct blow to the head or shaking. Classically, a crying infant is vigorously shaken and suffers acute axonal brain injury. This leads to "shaken baby syndrome" or "shaken impact syndrome." The infant stops crying and falls asleep. Subdural bleeding occurs as bridging blood vessels are disrupted. In addition, brain swelling, apnea, and seizures result. The child may exhibit retinal hemorrhages as well as skeletal trauma. Such injuries are frequently associated with a fatal outcome or long-term damage to the CNS.

Circumstances surrounding other inflicted injuries is similar. Abusive parents often have unrealistic expectations of their children, especially around the time of toilet training. These parents have often been victims of abuse themselves. Corporal punishment is the only disciplinary modality they know. These parents also exhibit poor impulse control. Frequently they do not intend to harm their children but desire to alter

Dx **Physical Abuse**

- Bruises
- Bites
- Burns
- Fractures
- Intracranial hemorrhage
- Intraabdominal hemorrhage
- Retinal hemorrhage
- History that changes
- Injuries not explained by history

TABLE 96–1.   Causes of Retinal Hemorrhages

Inflicted head trauma
Nonintentional head trauma (rare)
Birth trauma
Blood dyscrasias
Meningitis
Papilledema
Hypertension
Cytomegalovirus retinitis
High-altitude illness
Lead toxicity
Carbon monoxide toxicity
Methanol intoxication

Questions: Physical Abuse

- What caused the injury?
- Was the child healthy until the injury occurred?
- Has the child sustained similar injuries in the past?
- Is there a family history of any conditions that would account for easy bruisability or fragility of the bones (e.g., von Willebrand's disease, osteogenesis imperfecta)?
- Is the child developmentally normal? Are the child's motor skills normal?
- Who was with the child when the injury occurred?
- What was done immediately after the injury? Was medical care sought?

---

children's behavior, and sometimes the outcome is unexpected.

DIFFERENTIAL DIAGNOSIS

When evaluating children with physical injuries, the major differentiation involves distinguishing between injuries that are intentional from those that are nonintentional. Practitioners should be suspicious of stories that change or are inconsistent with the injuries that children have sustained. Unwitnessed injuries in young children, particularly if they are preambulatory, should also be suspect.

Bruises, burns, and fractures may be intentional or nonintentional. Normal ambulatory children sustain bruises over bony prominences such as the shins with nonintentional trauma. Bruises over soft areas such as the thighs and cheeks or the pinnae of the ear suggest inflicted trauma. Injuries to the oral mucosa may result from efforts at forced feeding or occlusion of the mouth in an effort to silence crying. Retinal hemorrhages in infants most often result from intentional head trauma, such as shaking. They may also be due to other medical conditions (Table 96–1).

Children may be intentionally burned by being immersed in hot water or having hot objects such as irons or cigarettes held against them. Children who are immersed in hot water develop burns that may envelop an entire extremity, usually in a glove or stocking pattern, or form a doughnut pattern on the buttocks. These burns are distinct from splash or spill burns, which take on a drip pattern.

Long bone (especially humerus and femur) fractures should be suspect, particularly in preambulatory infants. Most falls do not result in fractures. Certain fractures, such as metaphysical chip fractures and rib, sternum, and scapula fractures, are suggestive of inflicted trauma.

Numerous medical conditions may mimic abuse. Bullous impetigo may resemble burns. A coagulopathy may lead to multiple bruises. Leukemia, thrombocytopenia, and aplastic anemia are also associated with bruises. Osteogenesis imperfecta may result in multiple fractures. Osteoporosis may be associated with meningomyelocele, and pathologic fractures of the long bones may occur as a result. Bone cysts may also lead to pathologic fractures.

EVALUATION

Children who present with injuries need to be evaluated with a careful history and complete physical examination. Infants with altered mental status should be evaluated in a similar manner, because their symptoms may be secondary to intracranial injury.

History

The history should focus on an explanation for the medical findings (Questions Box). Children should be interviewed alone if they are of an appropriate age. Physicians should determine if other risk factors, such as domestic violence or substance abuse, are present.

Physical Examination

Children's state of hygiene and growth should be noted. The physical examination should be comprehensive. The location and color of bruises should be carefully recorded. Bruises tend to heal in distinctive patterns (Table 96–2). Large, blue spots, which are frequently apparent over the lower back in African-American, Hispanic, and Asian children, are referred to as Mongolian spots. These should not be mistaken for bruises.

Physicians should check for burns or other injuries, including pinch marks in the genital area, which may be inflicted on toddlers who have had a toilet-training accident.

In addition, physicians should look for any characteristic patterns that may have resulted from inflicted injuries, such as slap marks to the face or gag marks

TABLE 96–2.   Discoloration Caused by Healing Bruises

Color	Healing Period
Swelling without discoloration	< 1 day
Purple color	1–5 days
Green color	5–7 days
Yellow color	7–10 days
Brown color	10–14 days

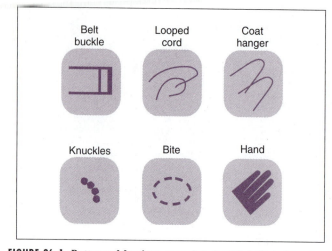

FIGURE 96–1. *Patterned bruises associated with inflicted trauma.*

around the mouth. Belts, cords, and blunt instruments may also produce particular marks, such as repetitive loop marks (Fig. 96–1). Bite marks leave indentations of teeth that are unique to the perpetrator. Inflicted burns may also assume a characteristic pattern, such as a glove-stocking distribution (Fig. 96–2).

Practitioners should be aware that infants with injuries of the head and abdomen may present with no external signs of trauma but have seizures, apnea, or altered mental status, often with no explanation. The retina should be evaluated for hemorrhages.

Children with abdominal injuries may be in shock or have gastrointestinal symptoms such as vomiting, abdominal pain, or distention. Injuries may include hematomas of the bowel wall, perforations of the bowel, or trauma to solid organs such as the liver, spleen, pancreas, or kidneys. On physical examination, children may have signs of a surgical abdomen with rigidity, guarding, and diminished bowel sounds.

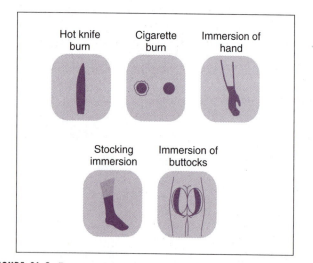

FIGURE 96–2. *Patterned burns associated with inflicted trauma.*

Laboratory Tests

Children who present with bruises should have a hematologic assessment, with a CBC and differential, including a platelet count, a PT, and a PTT. Cultures from lesions may help differentiate infection from burn injury.

Children with suspected abdominal trauma should be evaluated with a CBC, urinalysis, liver function studies, and amylase. These studies may demonstrate anemia secondary to hemorrhage, hematuria from renal injury, and elevated amylase from pancreatic trauma (see Chapter 40, Abdominal Trauma).

Imaging Studies

Children with bruises should be evaluated with a skeletal survey to determine the existence of additional injuries or evidence of skeletal dysplasia.

Children with symptoms of head injury should be evaluated with CT scans and MRI studies. The combination of these two modalities is particularly useful in dating intracranial bleeding (see Chapter 41, Head Trauma).

Abdominal x-rays may demonstrate a disordered motility pattern with air-fluid levels or distended loops of bowel. Other imaging studies may show organ disruption or hemorrhage. Free air may be present under the diaphragm if there has been bowel perforation.

MANAGEMENT

The management of children who are suspected victims of abuse focuses on medical stabilization and psychosocial investigation. Injuries should be treated in the appropriate manner. Children with extensive internal injuries frequently require admission to an intensive care unit. Consultation with appropriate surgical specialists in neurosurgery, orthopedics, or general surgery should be obtained.

The psychosocial assessment of the family often requires the expertise of a social worker. Further assessment may require an in-home evaluation such as that conducted by law enforcement or child protective services. States require that physicians who suspect child abuse report these suspicions to appropriate agencies. Physicians do not have to be certain of the abuse.

These mandated agencies pursue the evaluation. Children may be removed from their homes and placed in foster homes to ensure their safety. Cases of suspected abuse are usually evaluated in court to determine the safety of children's environment, the ability of parents to care for their children, and the criminal culpability of suspected perpetrators. Physicians may be expected to offer evidence in such hearings.

PROGNOSIS

The prognosis is variable. Some children succumb to inflicted injuries before coming to medical attention, and others sustain permanent neurologic damage. Even in cases in which the physical well-being of children is assured, their self-esteem has often been irreparably damaged.

Case Resolution

The opening vignette describes a classic case of shaken baby syndrome. The infant was left alone with an individual with limited parenting skills. Most likely, the crying infant was vigorously shaken, resulting in axonal injury, subdural hemorrhage, loss of consciousness, altered mental status, and seizures. The infant is intubated, given anticonvulsants, and admitted to a pediatric intensive care unit. Consultation with neurosurgery, ophthalmology, and social service is obtained. Appropriate imaging studies and skeletal surveys are performed when the infant is sufficiently stabilized.

Selected Readings

Chadwick, D. L. The diagnosis of inflicted injury in infants and young children. Pediatr. Ann. 21:477–483, 1992.

Davis, H. W., and B. J. Zitelli. Childhood injuries: accidental or inflicted? Contemp. Pediatr. 12:94–112, 1995.

Duhaime, A. C., et al. Head injury in very young children: mechanisms, injury types, and ophthalmologic findings in 100 hospitalized patients younger than 2 years of age. Pediatrics 90:179–185. 1992.

Johnson, C. F. Inflicted injury versus accidental injury. Pediatr. Clin. North Am. 37:791–814. 1990.

Kempe, C. H., et al: The battered child syndrome. J.A.M.A. 181:17–24, 1962.

Leventhal, J. M., et al. Fractures in young children: distinguishing child abuse from unintentional injuries. Am. J. Dis. Child. 147:87–92, 1993.

Reece, R. M. (ed.). Child Abuse: Medical Diagnosis and Management. Philadelphia, Lea & Febiger, 1994.

Sirontnak, A. P., and R. D. Krugman. Physical abuse of children: an update. Pediatr. Rev. 15:394–399, 1994.

CHAPTER 97

CHILD SEXUAL ABUSE

Carol D. Berkowitz, M.D.

Hx A four-year-old girl is brought to the emergency department with the complaint of vaginal itching and discharge. Her past health has been good, and she has no medical problems. She lives with her biologic parents and her two-year-old brother.

On physical examination, the vital signs are normal, and the child is well except that the genital area is swollen and erythematous and a green vaginal discharge is present. The girl is interviewed briefly but denies that anyone has touched her. The mother states that she has never left her daughter unattended and is angered by the questions.

Questions

1. What are the anogenital findings in prepubescent and postpubescent children who may have experienced sexual abuse?
2. What behavioral problems are common in children who have been sexually abused?
3. What are the pitfalls in disclosure interviews of children who have been sexually abused?
4. What is the significance of sexually transmitted diseases in children who have been sexually abused?

Child sexual abuse is the involvement of children and adolescents in sexual activity that they cannot consent to because of their age and developmental level. An age disparity exists between the victims, who are younger, and the perpetrators, who are older. The intent of the abuse is the sexual gratification of the older individuals.

Sexual abuse has been recognized with increasing frequency since the 1980s, in part because medical knowledge about the anogenital anatomy in both normal and molested prepubescent children has expanded. Technical advances have altered the manner in which these children are evaluated. In particular, the colposcope, with its potential for magnification, and photographic or videotape documentation has been valuable. Parental awareness and school-based programs have led to increased disclosures about abuse as well as greater willingness on the part of adults to believe these disclosures.

Patient interviews are another key component of the assessment process. Nonleading, open-ended questions are asked by experts as few times as possible.

EPIDEMIOLOGY

Over two million cases of child abuse are reported annually in the United States. Between 20 and 40% of these cases involve allegations of child sexual abuse. Exact figures on the prevalence of child sexual abuse are not readily available, because they depend on reports of a condition that may not come to medical attention for many years. Anonymous surveys indicate that about

20% of women and 10 to 15% of men have been sexually abused before reaching adulthood.

Victims of sexual abuse come from all socioeconomic and ethnic groups. Approximately 75% of victims who come to medical attention are girls and 25% are boys. Some investigators believe that the statistics for boys are falsely low because boys are generally reluctant to disclose their abuse. Girls are often victimized by male family members, such as fathers (biologic fathers and stepfathers), mothers' boyfriends, uncles, and grandfathers. Boys are more likely to be molested out of the home by nonrelatives, including coaches and teachers. Boys are more likely than girls to be abused by female perpetrators.

Frequently, the sexual abuse has been occurring for several years. The mean time from onset of abuse to disclosure is three years. Sometimes children are not ready to disclose but the abuse is discovered accidentally because the victims develop symptoms, such as vaginal discharge, or functional complaints. A routine or comprehensive physical examination may reveal anogenital abnormalities.

STDs, which vary in frequency in different geographic locations, are reported in between 2 and 28% of children who have been sexually abused (average estimated range: 10–15%). The incidence is higher in older children, particularly in adolescents.

CLINICAL PRESENTATION

Children may present with complaints related to the anogenital region such as bleeding, pain, swelling, dysuria, vaginal discharge, or difficulty stooling. More often, children have no specific anogenital symptoms. Instead, they have nonspecific complaints such as headache, abdominal pain, or vague systemic symptoms (e.g., fatigue). Behavioral changes may also be noted. These include sleep disturbances, hyperactivity, enuresis, encopresis, decreased appetite, depression, and so on. Some children may present with a history of sexually abusive experiences (D$_x$ Box).

PSYCHOPHYSIOLOGY

Children suffer sexual abuse after becoming entrapped. Children may be enticed with promises of rewards or presents. They may be made to feel special or grown-up by being allowed to engage in adult behavior. Some children do not regard the sexual experiences as threatening but rather a means by which

D$_x$ Child Sexual Abuse

- Anogenital erythema
- Anogenital bleeding
- Genital discharge
- Anogenital scarring
- Behavioral symptoms
- Disclosure of abuse

TABLE 97–1. Child Abuse Accommodation Syndrome

Secrecy
Helplessness
Entrapment and accommodation
Delayed, unconvincing disclosure
Retraction

they can obtain the love they crave. Only when they grow older do they realize that these sexual relationships were not normal or appropriate.

Other children are coerced into sexual activity with threats of physical harm. Once they have acquiesced, they are maintained in the relationship with threats of reprisal if they disclose the abuse. Children feel both guilty and responsible for what has happened. This sense of responsibility is often perpetuated by the legal system, which may remove the children from their families and place them in a foster home or juvenile facility.

Lastly, some children enter into sexual relationships out of curiosity. They too become entrapped, particularly because they were so willing to participate.

Children who disclose the abuse often experience what has been referred to as the child abuse accommodation syndrome (Table 97–1). This syndrome attempts to explain how children adjust to abuse. A key component of the syndrome is the need for secrecy. Disclosures are often partial or incomplete, and they are frequently recanted as children are made to feel responsible for any resulting disruption of families.

DIFFERENTIAL DIAGNOSIS

A number of medical conditions that involve the anogenital area may be mistaken for sexual abuse (Table 97–2).

Children may sustain accidental injuries to the genital area, usually straddle injuries that follow falls. Most often the labia majora, labia minora, or periurethral areas are affected. Bleeding and pain are presenting complaints; the hymen is unaffected.

Bleeding is also a frequent complaint in girls with urethral prolapse, a condition reported most often in prepubescent African-American girls between the ages of four and eight years. These girls have a protuberant mass extruding from the urethra. The condition is of uncertain etiology but it is not related to abuse.

TABLE 97–2. Conditions Mistaken for Sexual Abuse

Genital
Accidental trauma
Lichen sclerosus et atrophicus
Urethral prolapse
Congenital malformations
Hemangioma
Anal
Inflammatory bowel disease
Hemorrhoids
Anal abscess associated with neutropenia
Perirectal abscess
Perianal streptococcal infection

TABLE 97–3.   Conditions Associated With Vaginal Discharge

Sexually Transmitted Diseases
Gonorrhea
Chlamydial
Trichomonas
Bacterial vaginosis
Conditions That Are Not Transmitted Sexually
Candidiasis
Shigellosis
Group A beta-hemolytic streptococcus infection
Vaginal foreign body

TABLE 97–4.   Problems Reported in Sexually Abused Children

Enuresis
Encopresis
Sexualized behavior
Pseudomaturity
Recurrent urinary tract infections
Vaginal discharge
Sleep disturbances
Suicide

Lichen sclerosus et atrophicus, which is less common, is a dermatologic condition that may produce macules, papules, or hemorrhagic blisters in the anogenital area. The affected skin becomes atrophic, hypopigmented, and easily traumatized. The key to differentiating this condition from injuries related to sexual abuse is that the hymen is unaffected in lichen sclerosus et atrophicus.

Congenital malformations may also affect the anogenital area, particularly if tissues fail to fuse along the median raphe, which appears denuded as a consequence. Other congenital malformations include hemangiomas that may bleed and be mistaken for traumatized tissue. These tumors are most often noted in infants under two to three years of age, and they usually regress with time.

Medical conditions may also affect the perianal area and be mistaken for abuse. Crohn's disease may lead to fissures, fistulas, perirectal abscesses, or tags. In general, Crohn's disease affects older children and produces other symptoms such as fever, weight loss, and stooling problems, or extraintestinal symptomatology. Perirectal abscesses may occur in patients with neutropenia, sometimes as the presenting complaint of leukemia. Hemorrhoids occur rarely in children, and their presence should raise concern about intra-abdominal venous congestion, as seen in portal vein thrombosis.

Vaginal discharges (Table 97–3) may be related to sexual abuse, particularly if they are secondary to STDs such as gonorrhea or *Chlamydia* infection. Other agents may produce similar symptoms, yet not be sexually related, including *Candida, Shigella,* and group A beta hemolytic streptococci. The streptococci may produce a painful erythematous rash in the perianal area, which is frequently misdiagnosed as secondary to trauma or sexual abuse.

EVALUATION

The extent and urgency of the evaluation is in part dependent on whether the allegations involve an acute abusive episode or one that occurred in the past.

History

In all cases, a careful, comprehensive medical history should be obtained, including allegations related to the abuse. A general medical history should be taken as well, with particular attention to prior trauma or operative procedures involving the anogenital area. A psychological history should also be obtained; certain behavioral problems may occur more frequently in children who have been abused (Table 97–4).

Children must also be interviewed. The interview is best accomplished by someone with professional expertise in the areas of interviewing and child sexual abuse. This individual may be the physician, or a social worker, psychologist, or rape counselor. The interview should be structured to include open-ended questions, such as "Tell me what happened" (Questions Box). Ancillary methods, such as drawings or anatomically detailed dolls, may be used but are best left to experts with experience in these controversial modalities. Statements that children make should be recorded in the medical record as close to verbatim as possible. At some facilities interviews are videotaped or recorded on an audiotape. In addition, legal experts, such as individuals from the district attorney's office or law enforcement agency, may observe interviews through a one-way mirror.

Physical Examination

It is helpful for the examiner to be familiar with the normal anogenital anatomy of prepubescent children. The anatomy of boys remains constant throughout childhood, except for the increase in size of the penis and testes and the appearance of pubic hair during adolescence. Figure 97–1 shows the normal anogenital anatomy of girls, which changes from infancy through adolescence. All girls are born with a hymen, which is thick and full and covers the hymenal orifice in newborns. As maternal hormones regress, the hymen becomes thinner and more translucent, frequently taking on a crescentic configuration. When puberty begins, the

Questions: Child Sexual Abuse

- What happened?
- Has anything like this happened before? If so, what happened the first time?
- Who did this to you?
- Has anyone else done this to you?
- How often has this happened?
- Where were other people (e.g., mother) when this happened?
- Did you tell anyone what happened?
  - Who?
  - What did they do?

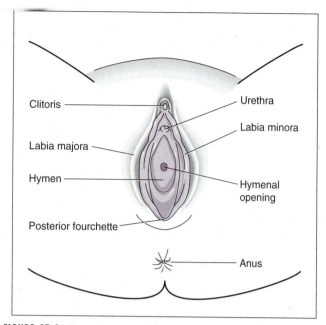

FIGURE 97–1. *Normal anogenital anatomy of prepubescent girls.*

hymen once again becomes thickened, scalloped, and full. Penetration of the hymen in postpubescent adolescents may result in stretching without tearing of the tissue. In prepubescent children, transections may heal with little residual evidence. The physician must realize that a normal anogenital examination does not preclude sexual abuse. Many types of abuse (such as orogenital contact and fondling) are not expected to lead to any apparent changes.

In cases of acute molestation evidence of injury may be readily apparent, particularly if the examination is performed with the assistance of magnification such as colposcopy. Injuries related to penile penetration usually involve the hymen in the six o'clock position and the area of the posterior fourchette (see Fig. 97–1).

The evaluation of children who have been molested in the past or on a chronic basis is more problematic. Many injuries heal with little residual scarring. Scarring that does occur may appear as disruptions in the hymenal contour, with notches or concavities. The pattern of blood vessels may also be interrupted, and areas of increased or decreased vascularity may be apparent. Sometimes marked reduction or attenuation in the hymenal tissue is present.

Male genitalia are less often injured by sexual abuse. More often the injuries seen in prepubescent boys, as well as some girls, involve changes in the perianal area. The incidence of these changes in all children who have been sodomized is unknown but is believed to be low. When changes do occur, they may appear as scars, tags, or irregularities in anal contour and anal tone.

Laboratory Tests

When the molestation has occurred within 72 hours of the examination, forensic evidence should be collected, as required by law enforcement. This evidence usually involves samples of vaginal washings and dried secre-

tions, which are evaluated for the presence of sperm or semen. In addition to confirming that sexual assault has occurred, presence of semen may help establish or eliminate an individual as a suspect. Forensic packages, which are referred to as rape kits, have specific instructions concerning the appropriate collection of samples.

A laboratory evaluation of any vaginal discharge is necessary. It is impossible to determine the etiology of the discharge accurately simply by its characteristics. In general, cultures of the vagina or urethra, rectum, and throat of children who have suffered sexual abuse should be assessed for the presence of *Neisseria gonorrhoeae*. These cultures should be evaluated in a reliable laboratory because of the legal implications of venereal infections in young children. Children who acquire these infections outside of the neonatal period are deemed to be victims of sexual abuse. Cultures to test for the presence of *Chlamydia* should be obtained. Rapid diagnostic studies, such as direct fluorescent antibodies, are not reliable in prepubescent children. Assessment for other STDs, such as herpes genitalis and condyloma acuminatum, should be based on clinical findings. Testing for syphilis should be performed if children have symptoms consistent with the diagnosis (e.g., condyloma latum, alopecia, rashes), if they have another STD, or if they live in a high prevalence area. Recommendations for testing for HIV are similar. The presence of disease in perpetrators also suggests the need for testing victims.

Other laboratory tests may be indicated if conditions other than sexual abuse are suspected. These include a CBC for leukemia or a barium enema for Crohn's disease.

MANAGEMENT

The management of children who have been sexually abused has three major components.

One, any medical problem sustained as a result of the abuse, such as traumatic injuries, must be addressed. In addition, STDs should be managed. The appropriate treatment of these conditions in pediatric patients is presented in Table 97–5. (See Chapter 69, Sexually

TABLE 97–5. Management of Sexually Transmitted Diseases in Children

Infection	Medication	Dose
Neisseria gonorrhoeae	Ceftriaxone	125 mg IM (< 45 lb) 250 mg IM (> 45 lb)
Chlamydia	Erythromycin	30–40 mg/kg/day for 7 days
	Doxycycline (> age 8 yr)	100 mg bid for 7 days
Herpes genitalis	Acyclovir	200 mg q4h for 10 days
Trichomonas	Metronidazole	30–50 mg/kg/day, divided (max: 250 mg tid)
Bacterial vaginosis	Metronidazole	15 mg/kg/day for 7 days (max: 500 mg bid)
Syphilis	Benzathine penicillin	50,000 units/kg, single IM dose (max: 2.4 million units)

Transmitted Diseases, for a more extensive discussion of STDs in adolescents.) Adolescents who have been the victims of an acute assault should be offered pregnancy counseling and STD prophylaxis.

Two, the emotional well-being of patients must be ensured. In cases of acute assault, crisis intervention is mandatory. If children have been the victims of chronic or prior sexual abuse, referral to appropriate counseling services should be implemented.

Three, the physician must report the incident of sexual assault or abuse to the appropriate agencies, as mandated by the laws of the locality in which the physician practices. The physician may be required to testify in court about particular findings and whether abuse occurred. Testifying may be intimidating. It is helpful for the physician to review the medical records ahead of time and to discuss this information with the attorney who subpoenas the physician.

PROGNOSIS

Several factors influence the prognosis in cases of child sexual abuse, including relationship of the perpetrator to the child, chronicity of the abuse, support following the disclosure, and preexisting psychosocial conditions. Physical injuries are usually nonexistent or minor, and healing occurs with minimal residual evidence. In most cases, psychologic counseling is indicated. Such counseling is beneficial, and emotional recovery is not only possible but likely to occur in a supportive environment.

Case Resolution

In the case history presented at the beginning of this chapter, the mother claims that no one has access to her child, but the girl's symptoms strongly suggest an infection with *N. gonorrhoeae*. Secrecy about abuse is very common. Both the child and the mother should be interviewed by a skilled person. Cultures for gonorrhea should be carefully collected and sent to the most reliable laboratory. Antibiotic therapy may be initiated if the child is symptomatic. The case may be referred immediately to social service and law enforcement agencies if there is a disclosure. Alternatively, if the child denies the abuse, the referral may be deferred pending laboratory confirmation of the diagnosis.

Selected Readings

Behrman, R. E. (ed.). The Future of Children: Sexual Abuse of Children. Palo Alto, CA, Center for the Future of Children, The David and Lucile Packard Foundation, 1994.

Berkowitz, C. D. Child sexual abuse. Pediatr. Rev. 13:443–452, 1992.

Chadwick, D. L., et al. Color Atlas of Child Sexual Abuse. Chicago, Year Book Medical Publishers, 1989.

DeJong, A. R., and M. A. Finkel. Sexual abuse of children. Curr. Prob. Pediatr. 20:489–567, 1990.

Finkel, M. A., and A. R. DeJong. Medical findings in child sexual abuse. *In* R. M. Reece (ed.). Child Abuse: Medical Diagnosis and Management. Philadelphia, Lea & Febiger, 1994, pp. 185–247.

Krugman, R. D., and J. M. Leventhal (eds.). Child Sexual Abuse. Report of the Twenty-Second Ross Roundtable on Critical Approaches to Common Pediatric Problems. Columbus, OH, Ross Laboratories, 1991, pp. 1–101.

CHAPTER 98

FAILURE TO THRIVE

Carol D. Berkowitz, M.D.

H_x   A 2-year-old girl is brought to the office because of her small size. She was born at term but weighed only 2200 grams (less than fifth percentile) and measured 43 centimeters (less than fifth percentile). The mother is a 30-year-old gravida V para IV aborta I who smoked during pregnancy but denies using alcohol or drugs. She received prenatal care for only two weeks prior to delivery, and she claims to have felt well.

The child's physical health has been good. She is reported to be normal developmentally but speaks only four to five single words. She has not yet started toilet-training.

The family history for medical problems, including allergies, diabetes, and cardiac and renal disease, is negative. The mother is 5 feet (152 cm) tall, and the father is 5 feet, 4 inches (163 cm) tall. The girl has three siblings, aged five years, four years, and three years, who are all normal. The father is no longer in the household. The mother is not employed outside of the home, and she receives public assistance. She states that frequently there is not enough food in the home, although she receives food stamps.

On physical examination, the girl is less than the fifth percentile in height and weight. Although she is very active, she does not use any understandable words. The rest of the examination is normal.

Questions

1. What are the key prenatal factors that affect the growth of children?
2. How can caloric adequacy of a diet be assessed?
3. How do parental measurements affect their children's stature?
4. What are the behavioral characteristics of infants with environmental failure to thrive?
5. What are some strategies to increase caloric intake of infants and children?

Failure to thrive (FTT) can be defined as the failure of children to grow and develop at an appropriate rate. The term FTT first appeared in the pediatric literature in 1933. Previously, the condition was referred to as "cease to thrive." The term "growth deficiency" is sometimes used. FTT is one way of consolidating two common pediatric problems, growth retardation and short stature, together.

Historically, FTT has been divided into two distinct categories, organic and nonorganic. In organic FTT, an underlying medical problem, such as cystic fibrosis or congenital heart disease, is believed to contribute to the failure to grow at an appropriate rate. In nonorganic FTT, also referred to as environmental deprivation, inadequate growth is attributed to lack of nourishment and a nonnurturing home environment. It is important to recognize that many children have growth problems with both organic and environmental components.

The diagnosis of FTT is made when the growth parameters of children as plotted on a standardized curve are below the fifth percentile in height or weight. Children who are above the fifth percentile may also be diagnosed with FTT if the rate of growth has decelerated and two major percentiles (e.g., decreased from the 75th percentile down to the 10th percentile) have been crossed within six months (D$_x$ Box).

The challenge for the physician caring for the child with FTT is to determine the etiology of the problem, which may not be readily apparent. Nonspecific, nondirected laboratory tests are not helpful because their yield is low and their cost is high. The evaluation of small, underweight children requires a careful history and physical examination as well as an assessment of mother-infant interactions. A home visit helps because it permits evaluation of the mother-infant relationship in a more natural setting and an assessment of the family's economic and food resources.

D$_x$ Failure to Thrive

- Weight below fifth percentile
- Height below fifth percentile
- Weight for height below fifth percentile
- Rate of growth too slow
- Delayed developmental milestones

EPIDEMIOLOGY

The prevalence of FTT varies in different segments of the population. Poverty puts children at risk for undernutrition, and 12% of Medicaid recipients are less than the third percentile in weight. Child neglect can lead to FTT but is not a necessary component; approximately 60% of cases of child abuse are reported for child neglect. Several other factors may contribute to variations in growth. All of these are not the result of a pathologic process but may reflect variations in individual genetic potential.

Environmental FTT occurs in three different family settings. In the type 1 family, an acute depressive episode in the mother is the key component. Family living conditions are good, and the educational background of the mother is adequate. The depressive episode is most commonly related to a loss that occurred during the pregnancy or shortly after delivery. The mother is too depressed to interact appropriately with her children. The type 2 family has marginal financial resources. The mother may be chronically depressed and the father involved in alcohol or substance abuse. Domestic violence frequently occurs. Spacing between children is less than 18 months, and the number of children is often the same as the age of the oldest child. The mother is too overwhelmed to meet the needs of the children. The type 3 family also involves a mother who is depressed and has experienced losses, usually of a chronic nature. Her financial and educational background are adequate, but she views one of her children (the one who now presents with FTT) as bad or evil and the source of all her problems. As a result, an individual child is singled out, and the neglect is intentional.

CLINICAL PRESENTATION

Children with FTT present with low weight, short stature, or poor appetite. Sometimes parents may express concern, and at other times teachers may detect children's growth problems. Some children with FTT are diagnosed during a health maintenance visit or when they are being evaluated for another medical problem, such as a febrile illness.

PATHOPHYSIOLOGY

The common pathway for the development of FTT in both organic and nonorganic cases is insufficient calories to sustain growth. Caloric intake may be inadequate for several reasons. Some factors are societal, specifically poverty and inadequate access to food. Other factors may involve increased caloric needs. Certain chronic conditions are characterized by increased caloric expenditure (e.g., some forms of chronic lung disease) or increased loss of ingested food (e.g., diarrhea).

In environmental FTT a disturbed mother-infant interaction is believed to contribute to reduced caloric intake and any associated GI symptoms (i.e., vomiting). Although various disturbances in mother-FTT infant dyads have been described, maternal depression is the most common maternal feature noted in environmental FTT. Infants withdraw after unsuccessful attempts to interact with nonresponsive mothers, and infants become apathetic and disinterested in food. Alternatively, overactive mothers, some of whom have a bipolar (manic-depressive) disorder, are out of synchrony with their infants. The infants become agitated, especially during feedings, and cannot feed and frequently vomit. These infants, who may interact with persons other than their mothers, usually do well in other environments.

Older children with FTT have disturbed hypothalamic-pituitary functioning. The etiology of this dysfunction is uncertain but has been attributed to sleep disturbances.

DIFFERENTIAL DIAGNOSIS

The growth of children with FTT may be impaired with regard to weight, height, head circumference, or any combination of growth parameters. If weight is the only abnormal parameter, inadequate caloric intake is probably the major problem. If height is reduced and the weight is appropriate or high for height, the diagnosis may be short stature rather than FTT. Small head circumference in the face of low growth parameters suggests a central nervous system basis for the growth delay. It is important to determine if children's skills are developmentally appropriate when determining the etiology of FTT. Affect and interactional skills should also be noted. Environmentally deprived infants are apathetic and noninteractive. They may appear to have cerebral palsy or infantile autism, but their symptoms resolve with a change in surroundings.

The most common causes of short stature include familial short stature and constitutional delay. Children with short stature are short because the parents are short. Except for a deceleration in growth, which usually occurs between the ages of 6 and 18 months, children with constitutional delay appear healthy. They have a delayed bone age that is comparable to their height age (the age when their height is at the 50th percentile), however. In children with either familial short stature or constitutional delay, growth parameters at birth are usually normal.

Children with low growth parameters at birth may have been premature or have suffered from intrauterine growth retardation (IUGR). Most studies support the notion that well premature infants exhibit catch-up growth (head circumference by 18 months, weight by 24 months, and height by 40 months). Ill preterm infants may not demonstrate such catch-up growth either because of increased caloric needs related to residual medical problems (e.g., bronchopulmonary dysplasia) or impaired nutritional intake resulting from certain conditions (e.g., cerebral palsy).

Children who are small for gestational age may have suffered any of several in utero insults that affect postnatal growth, including exposure to cigarettes, alcohol, and illicit drugs. In addition, maternal infection with such diseases as rubella may result in a congenital infection in infants with subsequent growth impairment.

> ### Questions: Failure to Thrive (Pregnancy and Delivery)
>
> - Was the pregnancy planned?
> - How did the mother feel when she learned that she was pregnant? Was the infant wanted?
> - Was prenatal care obtained?
> - How many times has the mother been pregnant?
> - Is there a history of abortions, either spontaneous or therapeutic?
> - How much did the mother drink during the pregnancy, if at all?
> - How much did the mother smoke during the pregnancy, if at all?
> - How much did the mother use drugs during the pregnancy, if at all? Which drugs did she use?
> - Did the mother take any medications during the pregnancy?
> - Did the mother have any rashes or illnesses during the pregnancy?
> - Was the infant term or premature?
> - How much did the infant weigh?

A number of other conditions may lead to disturbed growth, including endocrine disorders, skeletal dysplasias, food allergies, and malabsorption. These conditions occur less frequently and are usually more readily apparent as children undergo the evaluation for the growth problem.

EVALUATION

History

Careful questioning about certain topics provides clues to diagnosis in about 95% of cases. The physician should learn about the pregnancy and delivery, children's medical and dietary history, and the family history.

It is important to obtain a history of the pregnancy and delivery (Questions: Pregnancy and Delivery). Recurrent spontaneous abortions suggests that mothers may have an underlying problem such as a balanced chromosomal translocation that leads to fetal wastage. Mothers who have experienced repeated losses may have difficulty bonding with subsequent infants. The physician should determine whether mothers used cigarettes, alcohol, or drugs during the pregnancy by asking mothers questions beginning with the phrase "How much?" Any medications taken by the mother may affect the subsequent growth of their infants.

A review of children's medical history may also provide a clue to the etiology of FTT (Questions: Medical and Family History). It is essential that the physician obtain as many of the previous growth parameters as

> ### Questions: Failure to Thrive (Medical and Family History)
>
> - Is the child's growth rate normal or slow?
> - Has the child had any previous illnesses (e.g., gastroenteritis, recurrent pneumonia)?
> - Does the child tire easily?
> - How tall are the parents?

possible to determine whether children are small but growing at a normal rate or if their rate of growth is too slow. Previous illnesses should be assessed because these events may interrupt growth temporarily. Certain complaints may indicate underlying organic disorders, and recurrent infection raises the possibility of infection with HIV. A history of easy fatigability may be a clue to congenital heart disease. Although most children with congenital heart disease grow normally, growth problems may occur with congestive heart failure, some forms of cyanotic heart disease, and complex atrial septal defects. Children with urinary incontinence may have renal disease that interferes with their growth. The presence of seizures may be a sign of a CNS problem that makes it difficult to obtain adequate nutrition. Some children with seizures are heavily medicated and are too sleepy to eat.

A family history as well as a social history is important to obtain. Determination of parental heights, which is best accomplished by measuring the parents, is critical. This is particularly important in children with short stature. Specific mid-parental height curves allow the physician to determine if children's height is appropriate given the parental stature.

A nutritional assessment is an essential part of the history. The physician or another member of the health care team, such as a dietician, can perform this assessment. The dietary history can be determined either by using a 24-hour recall of children's intake during the previous day or a prospective three-day diary, in which parents record the kinds and quantities of foods their children eat. This nutritional information can be used to find ways to alter children's diet to ensure adequate and balanced meals.

Physical Examination

The essential component of the physical examination is determination of growth parameters. Calculation of the body mass index (BMI = weight [kg] divided by height [m]^2) is useful. Children with a low BMI are suffering from undernutrition. Short children with a normal BMI are not. Children should also be evaluated for dysmorphic features. It is important to remember that children with Down's syndrome grow at different rates than other children, and separate standardized curves for assessing these children are available (see Chapter 18, Well Child Care for Children with Trisomy 21). The presence of one major congenital anomaly or two minor anomalies suggests the existence of other anomalies. The incidence of growth hormone deficiency is reportedly higher in children with cleft lip and palate. Children with heart murmurs may have FTT related to congenital heart disease.

Infants with environmental FTT exhibit behavioral characteristics that are easy to recognize. They refrain from making eye contact and exhibit gaze avoidance. Infants are not cuddly and do not like being held. When held, they may arch their back in an effort to avoid the holder. Their muscles seem tense, and they are often considered to be hypertonic.

Psychosocial Assessment

The evaluation of children with FTT and their families entails a detailed psychosocial assessment to determine what environmental factors may be affecting children's growth. Such an assessment is helpful even if the FTT has an organic basis, because chronic disease has an effect on family functioning. This evaluation can be carried out by a primary care physician, social worker, or psychologist. The key is to query the caretaker about living conditions, adequacy of food supply, and economic resources.

Laboratory Tests

Routine laboratory tests appropriate for any pediatric health maintenance visit should be obtained in children with FTT if these studies have not been performed recently. Such tests include hematocrit, lead level (screening at some time between age six months and six years), and urinalysis. Other laboratory tests should be determined by the findings on history and physical examination. Evaluation for endocrinopathies, such as hypothyroidism or growth hormone deficiency, should be carried out in children whose bone age is less than their height age. Genetic consultation or chromosomal assessment should be performed in children with dysmorphic features or in families with a history of fetal wastage.

Imaging Studies

X-rays to determine bone age are useful in children with short stature that is not related to parental heights. Children with constitutional delay have a bone age that is consistent with their height age.

MANAGEMENT

Adequate Caloric Intake

Ensuring that children receive appropriate caloric intake is essential. The caloric intake, which averages 120–150 cal/kg/day for most infants, should be based on children's ideal rather than actual weight (see Chapter 11, Nutritional Needs). For infants on formula, the physician should review the exact preparation of formula with the mother. Overly diluted formula results in an unusually large intake volume with a lack of weight gain. For infants who are breast-fed, the physician should observe a feeding session to be certain that mothers have an adequate milk supply and infants are able to suck and swallow appropriately. Infants should be weighed before and after feeding. Some infants with FTT have neurologic problems that prevent them from sucking and swallowing consistently without becoming fatigued.

Children who are slow feeders may require formula concentration (Table 98–1). These infants may also receive added calories in the form of Polycose (glucose polymer) or oil such as medium-chain triglycerides mixed in the milk. Older children may be placed on supplemental feedings such as Pediasure or instant

TABLE 98–1. Concentration of Infant Formula to Increase Caloric Intake

Concentrated Infant Formula (13 oz can)		
Formula (oz)	*Water (oz)*	*Calories (cal/oz)*
13	13	20
13	10	23
13	8	25
Powdered Formula		
Formula (scoops)	*Water (oz)*	*Calories (cal/oz)*
1	2	20
5	8	25

breakfast drinks. These drinks are a less expensive form of nutritional supplementation than Pediasure and are well tolerated. Up to 24 oz per day of the breakfast drinks can be consumed. They should be mixed with whole milk and given in addition to, not in place of, a balanced diet.

Mothers should be advised that many children preferentially tolerate six small meals a day rather than three large ones. In addition, parents should be told that access to nonnutritional foods such as cookies adversely affects children's appetites. The physician should inform parents regarding foods that can be added to children's diets to increase caloric intake. These foods include powdered milk, cheese, sour cream, avocado, and peanut butter.

Parenting Issues

Some parents need more help about appropriate child-rearing practices than the physician can provide. They should be enrolled in parenting programs that address multiple aspects of the parenting process. Mothers with substance abuse problems may need to participate in drug treatment programs. Other caregivers may need individual counseling for depression or emotional problems.

In some middle-class families, meal time has evolved into a battle of control. Some children find that food is supplied in a manner more conducive to its consumption at school rather than at home. Parents should be counseled about avoiding conflicts about meals with children, because the children win simply by closing their mouths. Parents should be encouraged to allow toddlers independence around meal time.

Families may also require supplementary services to ensure that food supplies are adequate and financial resources are sufficient. Such services include food stamps, Supplemental Food Program for Women, Infants, and Children (WIC), and Aid to Families with Dependent Children (AFDC).

Home Visitation

Home visitation services provide useful diagnostic information and help parents implement advice. Such information may include lack of access to running water, overcrowding, and inadequate food resources. Home visitation may be available in the community through the use of public health nurses or private visiting nurse

agencies. These nurses should interact with the primary care physician so that families' compliance with treatment recommendations can be determined.

Child Protective Services

Child protective services (CPS) may be necessary if parents are unable to comply with medical recommendations, if children do not grow, or if there is intentional neglect on the part of families. In some families with children with FTT, the home environment is not safe for the children, and they require placement elsewhere. Type 3 families need immediate referral to CPS, and some type 2 families also need such a referral (see Epidemiology).

Hospitalization

Hospitalization is occasionally necessary if infants with FTT are severely malnourished and food must be given in a controlled environment. These infants may also have intercurrent illnesses that require inpatient care. In addition, health care professionals may determine that the home environment is unsafe and that no other placement, such as foster care, is available.

Children with both organic and nonorganic FTT usually gain weight in the hospital. Thus the hospitalization of children with FTT simply to demonstrate appropriate weight gain in a different environment is considered neither appropriate nor cost-effective. Some children with environmental FTT do not gain weight in the hospital, however, because they are subjected to many diagnostic tests that interfere with nutritional intake (e.g., being NPO).

PROGNOSIS

Many children with FTT respond dramatically to change in diet or in environment. Improvement in affect and cognitive functioning frequently follows nutritional improvement. These children grow and achieve and maintain normal stature. With early intervention, cognitive abilities also can be fully realized. Even when intervention has been delayed, catch-up growth and development are expected.

Case Resolution

In the case scenario presented, the full-term infant had a low birth weight, which suggests IUGR. Although the mother reports using no alcohol or drugs, such denial is not uncommon. The child's growth pattern should be determined to see if the rate of growth has changed recently, and the BMI should be calculated to check for both undernutrition and short stature. A mid-parental height curve should be used to determine if the child's short stature is related to the parents' short stature. Intervention should involve mobilizing resources for the child and family to ensure adequate food and financial and emotional support.

Selected Readings

Bithoney, W. G., H. Dubowitz, and H. Egan. Failure to thrive/growth deficiency. Pediatr. Rev. 13:453–459, 1992.

Drotar, D. (ed.). New Direction in Failure to Thrive: Research and Clinical Practice. New York, Plenum Press, 1985.

Frank, D. A., and D. Drotar. Failure to thrive in child abuse: medical diagnosis and management. *In* Reece, R. M. (ed.). Child Abuse: Medical Diagnosis and Management. Philadelphia, Lea & Febiger, 1994, pp. 298–324.

Frank, D. A., M. Silva, and R. Needlman. Failure to thrive: mystery, myth, and method. Contemp. Pediatr. 10:114–133, 1993.

Helfer, R. E. The neglect of our children. Pediatr. Clin. North Am. 37:923–942, 1990.

LaFranchi, S., C. E. Hanna, and S. H. Mandel. Constitutional delay of growth: expected versus final adult height. Pediatrics 87:82–87, 1991.

McHugh, M. Child abuse in a sea of neglect: the inner-city child. Pediatr. Ann 21:504–507, 1992.

CHAPTER   99

INFANTS OF SUBSTANCE-ABUSING MOTHERS

Carol D. Berkowitz, M.D.

H$_x$ An infant is born by emergency cesarean section because of abruptio placentae. The mother is a 29-year-old gravida VI para IV aborta II with a history of crack cocaine and heroin abuse during pregnancy. The infant is 36 weeks' gestation. The birth weight is 2400 grams, and the length is 43 centimeters. The physical examination is normal.

The infant does well for the first 10 hours but then develops jitteriness, with irritability, diarrhea, sweating, and poor feeding. A urine toxicology test on the infant and mother are positive for cocaine.

Questions

1. What complications affect infants secondary to maternal substance abuse during pregnancy?
2. What withdrawal symptoms do newborn infants experience as a result of maternal substance abuse during pregnancy?
3. What typical behavioral and learning problems are found in infants and children whose mothers abused illicit substances during pregnancy?
4. What are the appropriate management strategies for infants who have experienced in utero drug exposure?

Maternal substance abuse during pregnancy places infants at risk for a number of medical as well as psychosocial and developmental problems. The particular problems experienced by infants depend on the drug (or drugs) to which they have been exposed. Many infants have been exposed to several drugs in addition to cigarettes and alcohol. The long-lasting effects of alcohol exposure are well-established, but the effect of newer drugs is less well-defined. Illicit drugs change in their popularity and availability at different points in time.

The environment into which children are born also affects their health and and eventual development. Environments in which substance abuse is common are frequently suboptimal for normal growth and development for several reasons: (1) the impact of substance abuse on parenting; (2) fragmentation of families; (3) domestic violence; (4) incarceration of significant family members; (5) illnesses, including HIV infection, and (6) limited financial resources. Because of these environmental problems, many drug-exposed infants are cared for by foster parents or nonparental family members. All these factors compound the assessment of problems related to drug exposure versus the accompanying environmental conditions. This differentiation is of less significance to the practitioner, who must anticipate and care for the multiple problems that drug-exposed children manifest, than to the researcher or epidemiologist.

EPIDEMIOLOGY

About 15% of the 56 million women between the ages of 15 and 44 years are substance abusers. An estimated 15% of infants who are born have been exposed to drugs or alcohol. Figures for inner city hospitals are different from those of small community hospitals in rural areas. In one high prevalence area, 70% of infants screened were positive for cocaine. A study in a suburban hospital revealed that 12% of infants tested positive for cocaine. Screening may be done by the use of questionnaires, by testing urine, or both. Hair or meconium is sampled less commonly.

CLINICAL PRESENTATION

Neonates who have been exposed to drugs such as heroin and methadone may present with symptoms of drug withdrawal, such as tremors, sneezing, sweating, vomiting, diarrhea, poor appetite, irritability, and seizures. Some cocaine-exposed infants have birth defects (e.g., absent limbs). Pre- and postnatal growth failure and microcephaly are associated with maternal alcohol abuse. Learning disabilities and ADHD are noted in older children who have been exposed in utero to alcohol and drugs. Oppositional and impulsive behavior may also be a presenting complaint.

PATHOPHYSIOLOGY

Drugs used by pregnant women may affect infants in three different ways. One, the drugs may be addictive and result in symptoms of withdrawal during the neonatal period; two, they may be toxic and lead to impaired functioning and neurodevelopmental problems; and three, they may be teratogenic and cause congenital anomalies and a dysmorphic appearance. The mechanism of action of the various substances on the developing fetus can be understood in terms of their biochemical properties.

In utero exposure to heroin and methadone results in physiologic addiction. These drugs are opiates that bind to opiate receptor sites in the brain and in the gut. When the opiates are no longer present, individuals experience withdrawal. In utero exposure is also believed to affect the respiratory center and may predispose infants to disturbed ventilatory control, and subsequent SIDS (see Chapter 38).

Cocaine is addictive, toxic, and teratogenic. It interacts with three receptor sites in the brain. One, cocaine blocks the reuptake of norepinephrine. Higher levels of norepinephrine are associated with an increased incidence of preterm labor. Heart rate and blood pressure rise, and vasoconstriction, diaphoresis, and tremors occur. Vasoconstriction may affect the placenta and lead to anomalies of placentation, such as placental infarcts or abruptio placentae. The fetus, who may also be affected by periods of vasospasm, hypoperfusion, and ischemia, may develop anomalies such as atresia of the GI tract, stroke, and absent limbs. In addition, cocaine-exposed infants have a higher incidence of cutaneous hemangiomas.

Two, cocaine decreases the reuptake of dopamine. This effect is apparent in cocaine-using mothers, who have decreased appetite, which affects maternal nutrition during pregnancy. Stereotypic behavior, hyperactivity, and sexual excitement may be associated with sexual promiscuity and the risk of HIV and STDs.

Three, cocaine decreases serotonin reuptake, leading to decreased sleep. The sleep cycle of cocaine-exposed infants is often disrupted.

Phencyclidine (PCP) has sympathomimetic effects, including increases in blood pressure, heart rate, respiratory rate, deep tendon reflexes, and tone. In addition, PCP has cholinergic effects, causing sweating, flushing, drooling, and pupillary constriction. Infants exposed to PCP in utero do not exhibit these symptoms, however, but display neurologic and developmental disorganization.

Alcohol has multiple teratogenic effects, including

Dₓ Infants of Substance-Abusing Mothers

- Symptoms of withdrawal (see Table 99–1)
- Growth retardation
- Developmental delay
- Sexually transmitted diseases
- Congenital anomalies

---

impairment of growth of the brain and the body. The impact on growth may be apparent at birth and continue after the newborn period. The disturbed neurologic development is also evidenced by microcephaly, microphthalmia, ptosis, mental retardation, and ADHD.

DIFFERENTIAL DIAGNOSIS

The major differential diagnoses relate to the symptomatology produced by the abused substance or substances (Dₓ Box). Infants exposed to addictive substances may present in the neonatal period with symptoms of withdrawal. Exposure to heroin and methadone is most commonly associated with this symptom pattern (Table 99–1). The irritability and jitteriness characteristic of in utero drug exposure may also be seen with hypoglycemia, hypocalcemia, and hypomagnesemia. These biochemical disturbances are often found in infants of diabetic mothers.

Sometimes the neurologic instability associated with drug withdrawal may progress to the point that infants experience a seizure. Other causes of seizures, such as intraventricular hemorrhage or pyridoxine dependency, must be considered in the differential diagnosis. Sepsis, with or without fever, may also be associated with irritability. In addition, GI disturbances such as poor feeding, vomiting, or diarrhea in the newborn period are associated with drug withdrawal. Infectious gastroenteritis and formula intolerance are part of the differential diagnosis.

Specific syndromes of dysmorphic appearance may also be the result of alcohol or drug exposure. Fetal alcohol syndrome is the most comprehensive syndrome of dysmorphic appearance related to maternal substance abuse during pregnancy. Other causes of dysmorphic syndromes, such as gene and chromosome problems, must be ruled out.

TABLE 99–1.   Symptoms of Neonatal Withdrawal Syndrome

Irritability
Jitteriness
Tremors
Seizures
Sneezing
Hiccups
Vomiting
Diarrhea
Sweating
Poor feeding

In older children, presenting symptoms related to maternal substance abuse may take the form of neurobehavioral problems, such as impulsive behavior, antisocial behavior, and ADHD. It may not be readily apparent that the origin of children's difficulties lies in maternal substance abuse during pregnancy. Diagnosis is often difficult because of maternal denial and the many environmental factors that may be contributing to children's neurodevelopmental problems. A specific neurodevelopmental problem associated with maternal cocaine abuse involves a hearing impairment and a disorder in which the processing of speech are affected. Delayed speech development may be noted.

FTT may also be a presenting complaint in infants or children who have been exposed to drugs or alcohol (see Chapter 98, Failure to Thrive, for a discussion of the differential diagnosis of FTT). It is important to consider maternal substance abuse in all patients who have been diagnosed with FTT, particularly if the affected children were small for gestational age.

Maternal substance abuse should be considered in all infants who present with certain infections such as STDs (most commonly hepatitis B, HIV, and syphilis).

EVALUATION

History

The possibility of maternal substance abuse should be considered in the face of certain maternal risk factors. These factors include the absence of prenatal care, evidence of poor maternal nutrition, poor maternal weight gain, presence of STDs, maternal hypertension and tachycardia, abruptio placentae, precipitous delivery, and a history of domestic violence.

Infants who manifest symptoms of withdrawal should be evaluated for the possibility of maternal substance abuse. This assessment involves an appropriate history as well as a toxicologic evaluation. Mothers disclose their drug history to varying extents, depending on the circumstances of the interview. If mothers are concerned about the health and well-being of their infants and do not fear legal repercussions, they are more likely to discuss their drug use. An appropriate drug history should be obtained in a nonjudgmental manner (Questions Box).

Questions: Infants of Substance-Abusing Mothers

- Did the mother use any substances such as alcohol, cigarettes, marijuana, or prescription and illicit drugs during the pregnancy?
- Has she ever used these substances? Is she currently using these substances?
- If so, how much? How frequently? By what route? To what extent is she trying to abstain?
- Is the mother at risk for sexually transmitted diseases? Has she ever been tested?
- Did the mother have prenatal care? When did the care start?
- What is the status of other children in the family?
- Does the father abuse alcohol or drugs?

Physical Examination

Infants should be assessed for the common complications related to maternal substance abuse. They should undergo a full physical examination to check for the presence of any anomalies. Growth measurements should be noted, and physicians should determine if intrauterine growth retardation or microcephaly is evident. Premature infants should be monitored for all the problems related to prematurity, such as intraventricular hemorrhage and necrotizing enterocolitis. Signs of neonatal withdrawal syndrome should be assessed (see Table 99–1).

Laboratory Tests

In addition to obtaining a toxicologic history, screening for drugs should also be performed. The legal guidelines for screening mothers for drugs vary in different localities. In general, infants can be screened on medical grounds without parental consent because the information obtained is important in the care of the infant. Screening of the mother's urine without her consent is more problematic, however, because of the potential legal implications of a positive test.

Some centers have drug panels, which screen for the most commonly used substances, such as cocaine metabolites, opiates, amphetamines, barbiturates, and marijuana metabolites. Most of these tests, which utilize immunoassays, require 1–2 mL of infant urine. These tests are inexpensive and sensitive but not very specific. For example, antihistamines cross-react with amphetamines, and morphine (used during delivery) cannot be distinguished from heroin. Other tests using mass spectroscopy or gas chromatography are more expensive and require larger samples of urine.

Newer methods check for the presence of illicit drugs, particularly cocaine, in infant hair or meconium. These tests are able to document the presence of drugs in the time prior to delivery and may be positive even if urine screening is negative at the time of birth.

Further evaluation in the neonatal period should include an evaluation for the presence of STDs, particularly HIV, hepatitis B, and syphilis.

Imaging Studies

Some investigators recommend that cocaine-exposed infants be routinely evaluated with ultrasound for the presence of CNS hemorrhages. Other neuroimaging techniques should be used if infants appear lethargic in the nursery.

MANAGEMENT

In the neonatal period, the management of drug-exposed infants requires attention to medical condition, such as prematurity, that may accompany drug exposure. Likewise, STDs such as congenital syphilis should be treated. Hepatitis B vaccine and hepatitis B immunoglobulin should be administered if appropriate.

**TABLE 99–2. Pharmacologic Management
of Neonatal Drug Withdrawal**

Medication	Dosage
Tincture of paregoric	1–4 drops/kg/dose PO q4–6h
Phenobarbital	1–3 mg/kg/dose PO or IM q6h
Methadone	0.1 mg/kg/dose PO q12h

Symptoms of neonatal substance withdrawal may also require treatment. Infants may respond to **swaddling** as a means of decreasing their increased irritability. In addition, they may require **medication.** Table 99–2 lists the substances commonly used to manage the symptoms of neonatal drug withdrawal. In general, these agents should be used in infants with vomiting, diarrhea, and marked irritability. Medications should be tapered over time, allowing infants to outgrow the dosage.

Social service is a key component of management. In many jurisdictions, child protective services must be notified about positive toxicologic tests on newborn infants or their mothers. Likewise, infants who display symptoms of neonatal drug withdrawal may also have to be reported to these agencies. These agencies are generally responsible for performing a home assessment and determining the adequacy of the environment. In some cases, infants may be assigned to foster homes. Parents may be ordered to participate in drug treatment programs and parenting classes.

After the newborn period the focus of management is provision of **well child care.** Infants who have been exposed to cocaine in utero should have BAER testing in early infancy to detect hearing impairment. Attention should be paid to physical growth and administration of immunizations. Monitoring of neurodevelopmental status should be carried out. If a sensory impairment or neurodevelopmental delay is apparent, children should be referred to appropriate community agencies.

Symptoms of ADHD in older children may require similar intervention, with recommendation for specific school programs as well as pharmacologic treatment. Regular assessments of school performance should be obtained from children's teachers. Standardized neurodevelopment tests should be administered at periodic intervals to ensure appropriate progress.

PROGNOSIS

Many infants, particularly those exposed to alcohol in utero, suffer long-term sequelae such as neurodevelopmental disabilities. Remedial educational programs help, but do not cure, such disabilities. Initial reports suggested that the effects of in utero cocaine exposure were equally devastating. More recent studies show that a key factor determining the outcome in cocaine-exposed infants is the environment in which they are raised. A stable, nurturing environment minimizes the many adverse effects of drug exposure and promotes normal neurodevelopment by enforcing the acquisition of skills and knowledge.

Case Resolution

The case history presented highlights the typical features of the drug-exposed infant. Management includes testing for hepatitis B, syphilis, and HIV and administering medication such as phenobarbital if the irritability does not respond to swaddling or other measures. The situation should be reported to child protective services to ensure an assessment of the infant's home environment.

Selected Readings

Berlin, C. M. Effects of drugs on the fetus. Pediatr. Rev. 12:282–287, 1991.

Callahan, C. M., et al. Measurement of gestational cocaine exposure: sensitivity of infants' hair, meconium, and urine. J. Pediatr. 120:763–768, 1992.

Dixon, S. D., K. Bresnahan, and B. Zuckerman. Cocaine babies. Meeting the challenge of management. Contemp. Pediatr. 7:70–92, 1990.

Fulroth, R., B. Phillips, and D.J. Durand. Neurologic manifestations of cocaine exposure in childhood. Pediatrics 93:557–560, 1994.

Ostrea, E. M., et al. Drug screening of newborns by meconium analysis: a large-scale, prospective, epidemiologic study. Pediatrics 89:107–113, 1992.

Siddiqi, T. A., and R. C. Tsang. Babies of substance-abusing mothers: an overview. Pediatr. Ann. 20:527–530, 1991.

Singer, L. T., R. Garber, and R. Kliegman. Neurobehavioral sequelae of fetal cocaine exposure. J. Pediatr. 119:667–672, 1991.

Volpe, J. Effect of cocaine use on the fetus. N. Engl. J. Med. 326:399–407, 1992.

Zuckerman, B., and K. Bresnahan. Developmental and behavioral consequences of prenatal drug and alcohol exposure. Pediatr. Clin. North Am. 38:1387–1406, 1991.

CHAPTER 100

SUBSTANCE ABUSE

Monica Sifuentes, M.D.

A 17-year-old adolescent male is brought to your office by his father with a chief complaint of chronic cough. You have followed this patient and his siblings for several years and know the family quite well. The father appears very concerned about "this cough that just won't go away." The adolescent is not concerned about the cough, however, and reports no associated symptoms such as fever, sore throat, chest pain, or sinus pain. You ask the father to step out of the room for the rest of the interview and the physical examination.

On further questioning, the patient reports that he smokes a few cigarettes a day and has tried marijuana as well as cocaine. He denies regular use of these substances, but reports exposure to these drugs at parties and when he hangs out with "certain friends." The adolescent is now in the eleventh grade, attends school regularly, and thinks school is "OK." His grades are average to above average, but he thinks he might fail history this semester. Although he used to play baseball, he dropped out last year. He hopes to get a part-time job at a local fast food restaurant this summer if his parents let him. Currently he is sexually active and uses condoms occasionally. He denies suicidal ideation and exposure to any firearms.

On physical examination, he appears well developed and well nourished with an occasional dry cough. He is afebrile, and his respiratory rate, heart rate, and blood pressure are normal. Pertinent findings on examination include slight conjunctival injection bilaterally and mild erythema of the posterior pharynx. No tonsillar hypertrophy is apparent. The rest of the examination is within normal limits.

Questions

1. What are the most common manifestations of substance use and abuse in adolescents?
2. What are the risk factors associated with substance abuse in adolescents?
3. What other conditions must be considered when evaluating adolescents with a history of chronic substance abuse?
4. What laboratory evaluation, if any, should be considered in adolescents with suspected substance use or abuse?
5. What are the specific consequences, if any, of short-term and long-term use or abuse of substances such as alcohol, marijuana, cocaine, opiates, and hallucinogens?

Primary care practitioners can become involved in adolescent substance abuse either through prevention and anticipatory guidance or through the identification and treatment of a substance abuse problem in their patients. Ideally, all adolescent patients should be questioned and counseled about the use of illicit drugs, alcohol, and tobacco at each health maintenance visit (see Chapter 7, Screening in Adolescents, and Chapter 4, Talking to Adolescents). Unfortunately, this rarely occurs because most health care professionals often feel uncomfortable opening this "Pandora's box." Primary care practitioners thus lose a valuable opportunity to adequately assess adolescents for substance abuse.

Substance use can be defined as the use of or experimentation with illicit drugs, alcohol, or tobacco. Illicit drugs include marijuana; cocaine; amphetamines; hallucinogens such as lysergic acid diethylamide (LSD), mescaline, and psilocybin, which is found in *Psilocybe mexicana* mushrooms; opiates; and phencyclidine (PCP). **Substance abuse** refers to the chronic use of mind-altering drugs in spite of adverse affects. **Addiction** is the term applied to compulsive and continued use of a substance in the face of these adverse consequences. The substance may produce physical dependence or symptoms of withdrawal when it is discontinued.

EPIDEMIOLOGY

Current Trends and Prevalence Rates

A wide range of substances are currently being used by young adolescents in the United States. Alcohol, tobacco, and marijuana are clearly the more common and most popular substances.

In a recent survey of graduating high school seniors, approximately 90% admitted to **alcohol** use at some time. Two-thirds of students reported drinking alcohol during the month preceding the survey, and 3 to 5% admitted that they used alcohol daily. Binge drinking has probably contributed most to the overall morbidity and mortality associated with alcohol use in adolescents. Among high school seniors in the class of 1991, 30% reported having five or more drinks in a row at least once during the previous two weeks.

Although **tobacco** use among adolescents decreased from 1975 to 1991, approximately 20% of teenagers still report smoking one or more cigarettes per day in the past month. Eleven percent of adolescents smoked a half a pack or more cigarettes per day in 1991 compared to 19% in 1977. Three to four percent of 12- and 13-year-olds smoke regularly.

In 1991, 29% of high school seniors admitted to using an illicit drug during the previous 12 months. The overall lifetime prevalence was 44%, indicating that nearly two out of five graduating seniors admitted to using an illicit substance at some time in the past. It is important to remember that these statistics do not include the estimated 15 to 20% of students who drop out of school before their senior year.

Marijuana is the most commonly used illicit psychoactive substance. In 1986, 50% of high school seniors reported ever having used marijuana, and in 1991, nearly 25% admitted to having used it in the previous 12 months. Daily use of marijuana has declined over the years to approximately 2% of high school students. However, 9% of students still report a history of daily smoking for at least one month in their lifetimes.

The use of other substances amongst adolescents has generally taken a downward trend since 1986, although figures continue to be disturbing. Reportedly, approximately 9% of high school graduates in 1990 tried cocaine, with approximately 2% having used it in the previous month. The overall annual prevalence rate for cocaine usage was 4%. The 1991 prevalence rate for LSD usage was slightly higher at 5%, and its use has shown no appreciable decline in the past 10 years. Some authors report an even higher incidence of LSD usage among adolescents in treatment programs. Amphetamine prevalence rates have decreased to an annual rate of 8% in 1991, compared to a peak of 26% in 1981.

Concurrently, the reported use of over-the-counter nonprescription stimulants that contain caffeine or phenylpropanolamine has increased. Other substances used to "get high," such as inhalants, are often used by younger students (preteens). Usage in 1991 was reportedly 6.6%, which showed an upward trend from previous years.

Although not considered an illicit substance, anabolic steroids are abused by some adolescents, mostly males, to increase muscle size and strength. In 1991, approximately 2% admitted to using them at some time in their lives. Other studies indicate as many as 5.5% of high school students participating in sports use anabolic steroids (6.6% males, 3.9% females).

Demographics

Although adolescents now begin using most illicit substances later than they did previously, trends in alcohol and tobacco initiation continue to be a problem. In teenagers in eighth grade, initiation of both alcohol use and daily tobacco smoking is increased compared to earlier cohorts.

In general, adolescent males use illicit drugs more than females do, with a few exceptions. Males are more likely to use anabolic steroids, but females reportedly use amphetamines, barbiturates, tranquilizers, and over-the-counter diet pills more than their male counterparts. In addition, although annual prevalence rates for overall alcohol use show little gender difference, adolescent males have a higher rate of heavy drinking. Tobacco usage is essentially the same for both sexes.

Non–college-bound adolescents are more likely to use illicit substances than their college-bound counterparts, and these adolescents are also more likely to use drugs more frequently. There is no difference, however, between the two groups in the rates of ever having tried illicit substances. The influence of parental education, socioeconomic status, and race or ethnicity on the use and abuse of illicit substances is difficult to determine.

Risk Factors and Risk Behaviors

The strongest predictor of drug use is having friends who use drugs regularly. In addition, it has been shown that the more risk factors identified, the greater the risk of substance abuse.

Several factors are important precursors (risk factors) to drug use during adolescence. These include association with drug-using peers; attitudinal factors, such as favorable attitudes regarding drug use and low religiosity; school failure, beginning in the late elementary years; young age of initiation of alcohol or drug use; environmental factors, such as the prevalence of drug use in a given community; a family history of alcoholism or drug use; poor parenting practices; high levels of conflict within the family; minimal bonding between parents and children; and early and persistent problem behaviors during childhood.

CLINICAL PRESENTATION

Adolescents who are involved in substance abuse may present to the physician in several different ways. Illicit substance use might be uncovered during the routine interview for an annual physical examination or preparticipation sports physical. Alternatively, the adolescent might have physical complaints including chronic cough, persistent allergies, chest pain, and fatigue.

PATHOPHYSIOLOGY

Although several theories have been proposed to explain why casual substance use develops into abuse and addiction in some adolescents, the most critical factor seems to be the presence of underlying psychopathology. Adolescents who have major depressive disorders, attention deficit disorders and hyperactivity, or schizophrenia, for example, may use mood-altering substances to treat unpleasant feelings of dysphoria and low self-esteem. Although initially temporary, this method of self-medication makes chronic use with some substances likely.

DIFFERENTIAL DIAGNOSIS

The differential diagnosis for symptoms and behaviors associated with substance abuse includes underlying psychiatric disorders. Affective, antisocial, conduct, and attention deficit disorders can be the primary or secondary condition in adolescents who are abusing drugs. Like adults, adolescents may be using illicit drugs to self-medicate. The pharmacology and toxicity of the illicit substances most commonly used by adolescents are summarized in Table 100–1.

EVALUATION

History

The interview should be conducted in a private, quiet area with minimal chance of interruptions. If parents have accompanied adolescents, they should be politely asked to leave the room after issues of confidentiality

TABLE 100–1.   Pharmacology and Toxicity of Substances Commonly Used by Adolescents

Substance	Pharmacology	Toxicity
Nicotine	Potent psychoactive drug, acting on receptors in CNS to produce effects: stimulation, relaxation, focuses attention	Nontolerant individuals: weakness, nausea, vomiting, feeling unwell
Marijuana	Active ingredient (delta-9-tetrahydrocannabinol) is rapidly absorbed into bloodstream from inhaled smoke	Acute: Panic attacks, Psychosis (rare). Chronic: Short-term memory impairment, Amotivational syndrome, Reduced sperm counts
Alcohol	Causes nerve cell membranes to expand and become more "fluid"—interfering with neuronal conduction. Interference of neurotransmitters	
Cocaine	Produces a sense of well-being and heightened awareness, decrease in social inhibition, intense euphoria	Delirium, confusion, paranoia, hypertension, tachycardia, hyperpyrexia, mydriasis
Stimulants Amphetamines Crystal methamphetamine	Heighten awareness. Cause restlessness and agitation. Low doses increase ability to concentrate. Decrease appetite	Hypertension, Seizures, Stroke
Hallucinogens LSD Mescaline Mushrooms	Distortions of reality—"synesthesias" common ("hearing" smells)	Paranoia, Flashbacks, Psychosis, Depression
Phencyclidine (PCP)	Dissociative anesthetic. Dose-dependent euphoria, dysphoria, perceptual distortion	Psychoses, Aggressive, violent behavior, Depression, Seizures
Opiates Opium Heroin Methadone	Sedative analgesics. Euphoria followed by sedation	Respiratory depression, CNS depression, Miosis, Bradycardia, hypotension, Seizures, rhabdomyolysis
Sedatives Benzodiazepines Barbiturates	Sedation. Anxiety reduction	Similar to opioid intoxication
Anabolic steroids	Euphoria. Increased aggressiveness. Induction of mental changes at high doses	Psychosis

are addressed in the presence of both parties. This avoids further awkward moments when parents ask what was disclosed during the interview with their children. After parents have left the room, issues regarding confidentiality and privacy should be reviewed once again with adolescents. Special circumstances, such as disclosures of sexual or physical abuse and possible suicide or homicide, that dictate that confidentiality be broken should also be discussed (see Chapter 4, Talking to Adolescents).

The interview should then proceed in a casual, nonpressured fashion. Initial inquiries should concern nonthreatening general topics such as school, home life, and outside activities, including activities with friends (Table 100–2). The acronym **HEADSSS** allows review of the essential components of the psychosocial history: **h**ome, **e**ducation or employment, **a**ctivities, **d**rugs, **s**exual activity, **s**uicide or depression, and **s**afety (see Chapter 4, Talking to Adolescents).

Some practitioners prefer to use questionnaires to obtain this background information. A questionnaire is given to patients to fill out while they are waiting to be seen, and the responses are reviewed by practitioners during the visit (Table 100–3). Controversy exists regarding the role of such questionnaires, primarily concerning the truthfulness of answers.

More specific questions related to the use of alcohol and tobacco as well as illicit substances should be asked after general subjects have been discussed (Questions Box). If adolescents seem wary of answering these questions, it may be helpful to initially inquire about their friends. Questions should be phrased with the

TABLE 100–2.   Questionnaire Items Relevant to Substance Abuse

		Y	N
1.	Do you smoke cigarettes?	Y____	N____
2.	Do you smoke marijuana?	Y____	N____
3.	Do you often feel "bummed out," down, or depressed?	Y____	N____
4.	Do you ever use drugs or alcohol to feel better?	Y____	N____
5.	Do you ever use drugs or alcohol when you are alone?	Y____	N____
6.	Do your friends get drunk or get high at parties?	Y____	N____
7.	Do you get drunk or get high at parties?	Y____	N____
8.	Do your friends ever get drunk or get high at rock concerts?	Y____	N____
9.	Do you ever get drunk or get high at rock concerts?	Y____	N____
10.	Have your school grades gone down recently?	Y____	N____
11.	Have you flunked any subjects recently?	Y____	N____
12.	Have you had recent problems with your coaches or advisers at school?	Y____	N____
13.	Do you feel that friends or parents just do not seem to understand you?	Y____	N____

Reproduced, with permission, from Schonberg, S.K. (ed.). American Academy of Pediatrics: Substance Abuse: A Guide for Professionals. American Academy of Pediatrics, Elk Grove, Il., 1988.

**TABLE 100–3.   Open-ended Questions Intended
to Provide a Basis for Further Exploration
of Advanced Substance Abuse**

1. What do your friends do at parties? Do you go to the parties? Do you drink? Get drunk? Get high?
2. Do you drive drunk? Stoned? Have you ridden with a driver who was drunk or stoned? Could you call home and ask for help? What would your parents say? Do?
3. Do you go to rock concerts? Do you drink there? Do you get high? Who drives after the concert?
4. After drinking, have you ever forgotten where you had been or what you had done?
5. Have you recently dropped some of your old friends and started going with a new group?
6. Do you feel that lately you are irritable, "bitchy," or moody?
7. Do you find yourself getting into more frequent arguments with your friends? Brothers and sisters? Parents?
8. Do you have a girlfriend/boyfriend? How is that going? Are you having more fights/arguments with him/her lately? Have you recently broken up?
9. Do you find yourself being physically abusive to others? Your brothers/sisters? Your mother/father?
10. Do you think your drinking/drug use is a problem? Why?

Reproduced, with permission, from Schonberg, S.K. (ed.). American Academy of Pediatrics: Substance Abuse: A Guide for Professionals. American Academy of Pediatrics, Elk Grove, Il., 1988.

assumption that the responses will be affirmative (e.g., How many beers do you drink in a week?). It is hoped that this less threatening approach invites more honest answers. An assessment of the risk of suicidal behavior is also indicated. Further questions relevant to substance abuse are given in Table 100–3.

Physical Examination

Positive findings on physical examination are rare, especially in adolescents who use alcohol or other substances only occasionally. In adolescents with a history of chronic substance abuse, however, certain physical findings may be present.

All vital signs should be reviewed. Tachycardia and hypertension occur primarily with acute intoxication with cocaine or stimulants such as amphetamines. The

Questions: Adolescent Substance Abuse

- Do any of the adolescent's friends drink alcohol, smoke marijuana or tobacco, or use any other drugs?
- What drugs, including alcohol and tobacco, are currently being used by the adolescent? For how long and how frequently?
- In what environments does the adolescent use these substances?
- Has the adolescent ever blacked out or been arrested while under the influence of drugs or alcohol?
- Has drug or alcohol use ever interferred with school, work, or other social activities?
- Has drug or alcohol use adversely affected relationships with family, friends, or romantic partners?
- Has the patient ever had sexual encounters while under the influence of drugs or alcohol?
- Does the adolescent ever use drugs or alcohol to feel better or to forget why he or she feels sad?
- Do the adolescent's parents use alcohol, tobacco, or illicit drugs?

current weight also should be recorded and compared to previous values, and any significant loss should be noted. The skin should be examined closely for track marks, skin abscesses, or cellulitis, especially if patients admit to using drugs intravenously. Findings consistent with hepatitis (hepatomegaly and jaundice) may also be present in these individuals. The presence of diffuse adenopathy, thrush, leukoplakia, seborrheic dermatitis, or parotitis should raise the suspicion of human immunodeficiency virus infection. Upper respiratory symptoms such as chronic nasal congestion, long-lasting "colds" and "allergies," and epistaxis can occur with chronic inhalation of cocaine. Signs of nasal congestion, septal perforation, and wheezing may be noted on examination. In addition, smoking crack cocaine can cause chronic cough, hemoptysis, and chest pain. Smoking marijuana over long periods of time can result in similar findings.

The neurologic evaluation is probably the most important part of the examination. Any abnormalities in memory, cognitive functioning, or affect should be noted. Chronic marijuana use is sometimes accompanied by an amotivational syndrome.

Acute intoxication with some drugs such as cocaine may lead to delirium, confusion, paranoia, seizures, hypertension, tachycardia, arrhythmias, mydriasis, and hyperpyrexia. Acute PCP intoxication produces abnormal neurologic signs, tachycardia, and hypertension. Findings such as central nervous system and respiratory depression, miosis, and cardiovascular effects (e.g., pulmonary edema, orthostatic hypotension) are consistent with opiate overdose.

Laboratory Tests

Drug screening in the evaluation of possible substance abuse is usually not indicated. Specific laboratory studies should be performed only in patients who are known substance abusers and are enrolled in a treatment program or in patients with an acute presentation of altered mental status, intoxication, or abnormal neurologic findings. In the office setting, these symptoms are frequently absent, and urine or serum studies to "check" for drug use are not warranted. If these tests are performed, they require the adolescent's consent.

Urine testing is available to detect marijuana and its metabolites, cocaine, amphetamines, PCP, opiates, barbiturates, and benzodiazepines. Blood levels can be obtained for alcohol, marijuana, cocaine, amphetamines, barbiturates, and benzodiazepines. Although salivary or urinary concentrations of cotinine and nicotine concentrations can also be performed, these measurements are primarily used in research studies.

Testing for specific inhalants is not routinely done. The deleterious effects of these substances on the hematologic, liver, and renal systems can be evaluated by performing a complete blood count, liver function tests, prothrombin time and partial thromboplastin time, and blood urea nitrogen and creatinine.

MANAGEMENT

One of several approaches to the problem of substance abuse can be chosen depending on the degree of risk-taking behavior and drug involvement.

Anticipatory Guidance

If adolescents and their peers are not participating in any high-risk behaviors, pediatricians should provide patients with age-appropriate anticipatory guidance. This should include information regarding safety issues, consequences of alcohol and tobacco use, and exposures to illicit drugs. Adolescents should be encouraged to continue their current behavior but should be invited to return to the office if they have any questions or problems. This may be particularly helpful for adolescents whose daily environment exposes them to high-risk situations.

Early Intervention

Primary care practitioners should provide early intervention guidance to adolescents who are engaging in occasional high-risk behavior but whose substance use does not interfere with or disrupt their daily lives. Such use implies only occasional or casual use of illicit substances by patients or peers. Interventional guidance involves discussing potential risks created by adolescents' current behavior. For example, individuals who drink alcohol or smoke marijuana at parties have an increased risk of involvement in a motor vehicle crash afterward. Another common scenario involves alcohol intoxication and poor judgment with regard to sexual behavior.

Specialized Programs

Adolescents who are routinely using drugs but are clearly motivated to stop can often be managed by primary care physicians. Many of these teenagers began using illicit substances at an older age, have a fairly good relationship with their families, have supportive relationships with friends who do not use drugs, and have continued to do well in school and participate in other outside activities. At first, practitioners should identify the problem and establish that adolescents desire to change their behavior. Then they should meet with families, develop an appropriate strategy, and follow adolescents periodically in the office. Periodic reinforcement by physicians is necessary, especially in the beginning. Referral to outpatient programs, such as Alcoholics Anonymous or Narcotics Anonymous, may also be indicated.

Mental Health or Treatment Programs

Referral to a mental health or specialized treatment program is indicated for adolescents who continue to use drugs despite office treatment. In addition, those teenagers who have a suspected psychological or psychiatric condition should be referred immediately for evaluation. Other criteria for specialty treatment include a long history of drug abuse, a serious life-threatening event in conjunction with substance abuse (e.g., attempted suicide), familial strife, or persistent involvement with a drug-dependent crowd.

Primary care practitioners should become familiar with local inpatient programs and residential substance abuse treatment facilities in the community. Although the selection of a program is often dictated by financial resources, it is very important to select an appropriate one. Guidelines exist to aid practitioners in the selection process. These guidelines include total abstinence, appropriate professionals with expertise in drug abuse, familial involvement in the program, family therapy, and appropriate outpatient follow-up.

Prevention Programs

Prevention programs have been developed to assist and influence the decisions young people make about the use of illicit substances. Current programs focus on multiple aspects of the lives of children and adolescents. Programs may involve individual decision making, self-esteem, and basic education regarding drugs. They frequently emphasize communication skills, family values and dynamics, parenting skills, and positive peer associations. Structured curricula have also been created for use in the schools, and community outreach programs have been organized by groups such as local police departments. The actual effectiveness of each type of program is a subject of controversy, but they are all aimed at somehow preventing the initial or continued use of illicit substances.

PROGNOSIS

It is difficult to assess the outcome for adolescents who undergo treatment for substance abuse because definitions of success vary. For some teenagers, success implies periods of sobriety, for others it means complete abstinence, and for still others it is abstinence in addition to recovery from other contributing problems. Specific outcome data that are available, however, reveal that abstinence rates are positively correlated with regular attendance in a support group and parental participation in these groups. In addition, general success rates range from 15% to 45%, depending on short- or long-term assessments. As expected, there is a lifetime potential for relapse among all substance abusers.

Case Resolution

In the case presented above, the adolescent is at high risk for substance abuse given his drug-using friends, tobacco use, possible school failure, and recent change in extracurricular activities (i.e., dropping out of baseball). The findings on physical examination are also consistent with his smoking history. The physician should review these risk factors with the teenager and acknowledge the difficulty in removing one's self from such an environment. The adolescent's motivation to change his behavior should be assessed and referrals to special intervention programs can be discussed. Regardless of the outcome, the physician should continue to see the teenager at an agreed-upon interval to monitor his behavior.

Selected Readings

Alderman, E. S., S. K. Schonberg, and M. I. Cohen. The pediatrician's role in the diagnosis and treatment of substance abuse. Pediatr. Rev. 13:314–318, 1992.

American Academy of Pediatrics. Committee on Adolescence, Committee on Bioethics, and Provisional Committee on Substance Abuse: screening for drugs of abuse in children and adolescents. Pediatrics 84:396–398, 1989.

Brown, R. R., and S. A. Coupe. Illicit drugs of abuse. Adolesc. Med. State of the Art Rev. 4:321–340, 1993.

Comerci, G. D. Office assessment of substance abuse and addiction. Adolesc. Med. State of the Art Rev. 4:277–293, 1993.

Glob, C. B. Substance abuse: what turns casual use into chronic dependence? Contemp. Pediatr. 3:26–41, 1986.

Hawking, J. D., and Fitzgibbon. Risk factors and risk behaviors in prevention of adolescent substance abuse. Adolesc. Med. State of the Art Rev. 4:249–262, 1993.

Hoffman, A. A. Clinical assessment and management of health risk behaviors in adolescents. Adolesc. Med. State of the Art Rev. 1:33–44, 1990.

Morgan, J. P. Amphetamine and methamphetamine during the 1990s. Pediatr. Rev. 13:330–333, 1992.

O'Malley, P. M., L. P. Johnson, and J. G. Bachman. Adolescent substance use and addictions: epidemiology, current trends, and public policy. Adolesc. Med. State of the Art Rev. 4:227–248, 1993.

Schonberg, S. K. (ed.). American Academy of Pediatrics: Substance Abuse: A Guide for Professionals. American Academy of Pediatrics, Elk Grove, IL, 1988.

Schonberg, S. K. Substance use and abuse. In E. R. McAnarney et al. (eds.). *Textbook of Adolescent Medicine.* Philadelphia, W. B. Saunders, 1992, pp. 1063–1077.

Terney, R., and L. G. McLain. The use of anabolic steroids in high school students. A.J.D.C. 144:99–103, 1990.

Werner, M. J. Hallucinogens. Pediatr. Rev. 14:466–472, 1993.

C H A P T E R   1 0 1

EATING DISORDERS

Monica Sifuentes, M.D.

Hx   A 16-year-old adolescent female is brought to the office by her mother because she feels that her daughter is too thin. The mother complains that her daughter does not eat much at dinner and always says she is not hungry. Recently the girl bought diet pills that were advertised in a teen magazine. She claims that the pills are supposed to help her gain weight, so she doesn't understand why her mother is so upset. She says she feels fine and considers herself healthy.

The girl is a tenth grader at a local public school and attends classes regularly, although her friends are occasionally truant. She is involved in the drill team, the swim team, and the student council. She has many friends who have "nicer" figures than she does. Neither she nor her friends smoke tobacco or use drugs, but they occasionally drink beer at parties. The girl is not sexually active and denies a history of abuse. Her menstrual periods are irregular; the last one was approximately six weeks ago.

She currently lives with her mother, father, and two younger siblings. Although things are "okay" at home, she thinks her parents are too strict and don't trust her. They have just begun to allow her to date.

Her physical examination is significant for a thin physique and normal vital signs. On the growth chart, her weight is at the 15th percentile and her height at the 75th percentile, giving her a body mass index (BMI) of 17 (10th percentile). The remainder of her physical examination is unremarkable.

Questions

1. What are the common characteristics of eating disorders in adolescents?
2. What are the important historical points to include when interviewing patients with suspected eating disorders?
3. How is the diagnosis of anorexia nervosa and bulimia nervosa made?
4. What is the treatment plan for adolescents with eating disorders?
5. What are the medical complications of anorexia and bulimia nervosa?
6. What is the prognosis for these conditions? How can primary care practitioners help improve the outcome?

Eating disorders are complex problems that are sometimes difficult to diagnose based on strict DSM-IV criteria (Table 101–1). Adolescents may have partial or atypical forms, a combination of both anorexia and bulimia nervosa, or an underlying affective component

TABLE 101–1. Diagnostic Criteria for Anorexia and Bulimia Nervosa

Anorexia Nervosa

A. Refusal to maintain body weight at or above a minimally normal weight for age and height.

B. Intense fear of gaining weight or becoming fat, even though underweight.

C. Disturbance in the way in which one's body weight or shape is experienced, undue influence of body weight or shape on self-evaluation, or denial of the seriousness of the current low body weight.

D. In post-menarcheal females, amenorrhea, i.e., the absence of at least three consecutive cycles.

Bulimia Nervosa

A. Recurrent episodes of binge eating, characterized by the following:

  (1) eating, in a discrete period of time an amount of food that is definitely larger than most people would consume under similar circumstances and in the same period of time

  (2) a sense of lack of control over eating during the episode

B. Recurrent inappropriate compensatory behavior in order to prevent weight gain (self-induced vomiting, laxative or diuretic use).

C. Criteria A and B both occur on average, at least twice a week for 3 months.

D. Self-evaluation is unduly influenced by body shape and weight.

E. The disturbance does not occur exclusively during episodes of anorexia nervosa.

Adapted and reproduced, with permission, from Diagnostic and Statistical Manual of Mental Disorders (DSM-IV). Washington, D.C., American Psychiatric Association, 1994.

that confuses the issue. In addition, preoccupation with physical appearance and weight is not uncommon or necessarily pathologic in today's society. Both the fashion industry and media promote the idea that thinness and beauty are interrelated. Thus, average adolescents who long to be accepted by peers and who are learning to develop a sense of independence and control are prime targets for the development of eating disorders.

EPIDEMIOLOGY

In general, eating disorders are more common among females and in more affluent communities. Although they occur in other settings, in previous years they were nearly unheard of in lower socioeconomic groups. Today, they can be seen in all ethnic, cultural, and social backgrounds. In addition, males make up an estimated 5 to 10% of all patients with eating disorders.

Although dieting behavior among adolescents and young adults is not uncommon, true anorexia nervosa has a prevalence of approximately 0.5% in these individuals. Estimates have ranged from 1 to 10% in high-risk groups such as upper and middle class white females. Fewer than 5% of these cases are males, with a female:male ratio of 9:1. The age of onset is usually during early or middle adolescence (age 12–16 years). However, anorexia has been reported to have a second peak later in adolescence.

The prevalence of bulimia nervosa is approximately 1 to 4%, although some studies report that as many as 8% of adolescents and college women and 0.4% of men are bulimic. The age of onset tends to be later than for anorexia, with symptoms beginning during late adolescence (age 17–20 years). Females outnumber males by a factor of five.

Several other behavioral and affective disorders have been associated with anorexia and bulimia ner-

vosa. These include major depression in patients as well as first-degree relatives, alcoholism and substance abuse, other addictive behaviors (e.g., laxative abuse), poor impulse control and anxiety disorders, and obsessive-compulsive personality. In addition, suicidal behavior (attempts) is more likely in individuals with bulimia.

PSYCHOBIOLOGY

ANOREXIA NERVOSA

Although several factors predispose individuals to the development of anorexia nervosa, this condition has no single cause. Current theory suggests that a complex relationship among many factors may lead to anorexia.

Biologic Factors

It has been postulated that the normal increase in adipose tissue with the onset of puberty creates a special problem for some females. An eating disorder may develop as an attempt to control or combat this normal pubertal weight gain. Preexisting hypothalamic dysfunction has also been implicated as a contributing factor to anorexia. In addition, changes in neurotransmitter levels have been shown to occur with initial vomiting or dieting. These changes may then lead to specific psychiatric symptoms that may perpetuate eating disorders.

Genetic Factors

A possible genetic predisposition to anorexia has been shown in studies of monozygotic twins. The incidence of the disorder is increased in sisters and other female relatives of patients with anorexia.

Personal Characteristics

In general, patients with anorexia are described as obsessive-compulsive personality types, perfectionists, and overachievers. They also display low self-esteem and high anxiety levels despite their successes. They are the "model daughters" who have never caused any previous problems given their compliant, self-sacrificing, nonassertive nature.

Familial Influences

Researchers have noted that certain family dynamics may serve to initiate and perpetuate anorexia nervosa. Typically, the family is overprotective and rigid, with the mother often enmeshed in her daughter's life. Conflict resolution tends to be poor. An inability to express feelings within the family is often evident.

Social/Environmental Pressures

Both the media and societal standards are believed to play a role in "setting the stage" for an eating disorder. Affluent communities are especially at risk for this. Within these social circles, thinness, food, eating, and exercise can become the prime focus of daily activity.

In addition, young women become caught in what has been labeled a "slender trap" in which thinness is equivalent to attractiveness and success. Food restriction or purging are a means of attaining thinness. An inability to maintain thinness equals failure. Role models in the media, such as fashion models and actresses, also serve as ideals by which young people create their standards.

Other Influences

Involvement in particular extracurricular activities, such as ballet and gymnastics, may contribute to the development of anorexia in females. For male athletes, such influences include participation in sports such as wrestling, in which maintaining a given weight is important and dieting is used to achieve that weight. Chronic medical conditions, such as diabetes mellitus or inflammatory bowel disease (IBD), may also contribute to the development of an eating disorder.

BULIMIA NERVOSA

Several theories have been proposed to explain the etiology of bulimia nervosa. Most likely, multiple factors contribute to the development of this eating disorder.

Familial Influences

Family theory assumes that the eating disorder is a symptom of familial dysfunction and may be associated with physical or sexual abuse. With bulimia, unlike anorexia, conflict is discussed openly but negatively within the family. The relationship between mothers and daughters is distant rather than enmeshed. Parents and relatives have a high rate of depression as well as alcoholism.

Social/Environmental Influences

The sociocultural theory notes the influence of societal pressures to be thin. This thinness is synonymous with success. Thus, the binge-purge cycle is maintained as the adolescent attempts to become successful and avoid failure.

Cognitive-Behavioral Theory

This theory suggests that the eating disorder is a manifestation of irrational thoughts that adolescents have concerning weight, dieting, and self-esteem. Dieting and starvation result from cultural pressures and emotional instability. The binge-purge cycle develops as a coping mechanism for dealing with the disinhibition and guilt associated with these practices.

Psychodynamic Theory

This theory views bulimia as an attempt to control distressful feelings, such as depression, low self-esteem, and ineffectiveness. Adolescents may exhibit impulsive behaviors, including shoplifting and sexual activity. Treatment focuses on identifying these underlying processes.

Addiction Theory

This theory views binging and purging activity as an addictive behavior. Treatment stresses abstinence, support groups, and relapse prevention.

DIFFERENTIAL DIAGNOSIS

It is important to differentiate anorexia nervosa from bulimia nervosa. Differences between these two conditions are listed in Table 101–2. Occasionally, this distinction may be difficult to make, especially if patients display behavior consistent with both conditions. In addition, major affective disorders such as depression, schizophrenia, bipolar disorder, and obsessive-compulsive disorder must be excluded.

Other diagnoses to consider when evaluating patients for anorexia include IBD, diabetes mellitus, malignancies, Addison disease, hyper- or hypothyroidism, hypopituitarism, tumors of the CNS, and substance abuse, particularly with amphetamines and crack cocaine.

EVALUATION

History

A complete medical history should be obtained from all adolescents with suspected eating disorders (Questions box). Inquiries should focus on symptoms associated with complications such as dysphagia secondary to esophagitis from recurrent vomiting, constipation from fluid restriction, or muscle weakness associated with emetine toxicity from chronic ipecac use. A

TABLE 101–2.   Differences Between Anorexia Nervosa and Bulimia Nervosa

Anorexia Nervosa	Bulimia Nervosa
Vomiting or diuretic or laxative abuse uncommon	Vomiting or diuretic or laxative abuse common
Severe weight loss	Less weight loss; avoidance of obesity
Slightly younger	Slightly older
More introverted	More extroverted
Hunger denied	Hunger pronounced
Eating behavior may be considered normal and a source of self-esteem	Eating behavior is ego-dystonic
Sexually inactive	Sexually active
Obsessional fears with paranoid features	Histrionic features
Amenorrhea	Menses irregular or absent
Death from starvation/suicide	Death from hypokalemia/suicide

Reproduced, with permission, from Shenker, I.R. Bulimia nervosa. In E.R. McAnarney et al. (eds.). Textbook of Adolescent Medicine. Philadelphia, WB Saunders, 1992.

thorough psychosocial assessment should be performed. The **HEADSSS** format (**h**ome, **e**mployment and education, **a**ctivities, **d**rugs, **s**exual activity/sexuality, **s**uicide and depression, **s**afety) is useful to direct the psychosocial interview from general topics to more sensitive ones (see Chapter 4, Talking to Adolescents). The use of psychological testing/questionnaires to assess cognition and depression may be beneficial.

A dietary history should be taken as well. Direct questions regarding food intake and weight gain or loss should be asked.

A detailed menstrual history must also be obtained in females, because secondary amenorrhea is frequently present in patients with anorexia. Menses may be irregular or absent with bulimia as well. A family history of eating disorders, substance abuse, or psychiatric disease should also be addressed.

Physical Examination

In both conditions, the patient should undress, wearing only underwear, for the physical examination. This prevents any bulky clothes from hiding the true body habitus. The height and weight should be plotted on a growth chart, and the body mass index (BMI) should be calculated (BMI = weight [kg] ÷ height [m²]). Delayed growth or short stature should also be noted, because it can occur with severe malnutrition as well as other systemic conditions. Vital signs, including blood pressure, should also be recorded. The overall general appearance of patients must be noted. Adolescents with anorexia are often emaciated with an obvious loss of subcutaneous tissue. Patients with bulimia may be mildly obese or of normal weight with a full-appearing facies secondary to parotid and submaxillary swelling. Physical findings in patients with **anorexia nervosa** are consistent with a "state of hibernation." Hypother-

mia, bradycardia, and lanugo (downy hair) on the arms and back are seen. The palms and soles may be yellow, and pigmentation of the chest and abdomen may be increased as a result of malnutrition. Loss of pubic and scalp hair as well as dry skin may also be seen. The breasts should be examined carefully for galactorrhea. The presence of galactorrhea, along with a history of amenorrhea, warrants further investigation for a prolactinoma.

The abdomen should be palpated for tenderness or masses. Bowel sounds are often decreased in patients with anorexia, and stool may be palpated secondary to constipation. A rectal examination should be performed for any evidence of bloody stool, which is a finding consistent with IBD. The extremities should be evaluated for coldness and mottling. Finally, a complete neurologic examination, including a mental status evaluation, should be performed to exclude any signs of a CNS lesion or endocrine disorder.

In patients with **bulimia nervosa,** specific physical findings, if any, are often associated with dehydration and electrolyte imbalances that occur as a result of chronic vomiting or laxative abuse. Vital signs should be reviewed for tachycardia and orthostatic hypotension; their presence indicates hemodynamic instability. The skin should be inspected on the dorsum of the hand over the knuckles for scratches, scars, or calluses from self-induced vomiting. Petechiae and subconjunctival hemorrhages may also be seen as a result of severe retching. The oropharynx should be inspected for dental caries, enamel erosion, or discoloration as well as for parotid hypertrophy. The abdomen should be palpated for epigastric tenderness or midabdominal pain. Positive findings may be due to esophagitis, gastritis, or pancreatitis.

From a musculoskeletal standpoint, any muscle weakness or cramping should be appreciated and may indicate an electrolyte abnormality. Edema of the extremities may be seen in laxative abusers and should be noted.

Laboratory Tests

Table 101–3 lists the laboratory studies necessary in the evaluation of patients with **anorexia nervosa.** A CBC may be helpful because leukopenia, anemia, and rarely, thrombocytopenia can be found with this disorder. Electrolytes (sodium, potassium, chloride, and carbon dioxide) and a BUN are important especially if patients use diuretics, laxatives, or ipecac. The ESR may be low with anorexia and high with IBD or some other inflammatory process. Normal liver function tests aid in excluding other causes of weight loss. Some endocrine tests help differentiate a hormonal problem from anorexia (see Table 101–3). An ECG allows practitioners to diagnose QT_c prolongation, heart block, and arrhythmias.

Laboratory abnormalities in **bulimia nervosa** reflect the type and extent of purging behavior of adolescents. Table 101–3 summarizes the necessary laboratory studies for patients with bulimia.

TABLE 101–3. Laboratory Assessment of an Eating Disorder

Anorexia Nervosa

Complete blood count, erythrocyte sedimentation rate
Serum electrolytes (Na, K, Cl, CO_2)
Blood urea nitrogen/creatinine
Serum glucose
Serum calcium
Serum protein, albumin, cholesterol
Liver function tests
Endocrine labs:
    Follicle-stimulating hormone
    Luteinizing hormone
    Estradiol
    Thyroid function tests: $TSH/T_4/T_3$
    Cortisol
Urine pH and urinalysis
Electrocardiogram

Bulimia Nervosa

Serum electrolytes (Na, K, Cl, CO_2)
Serum glucose
Serum calcium, phosphorous, magnesium
Blood urea nitrogen/creatinine
Serum amylase
Urine pH and urinalysis
Electrocardiogram

MANAGEMENT

It is the role of primary care practitioners to recognize when weight becomes an obsession for adolescents and when abnormal behaviors develop for maintenance of obvious malnutrition. When treating patients with eating disorders, physicians must first establish trust. Patients should be assured that practitioners are not attempting to remove all control. Next, a compromise must be reached between adolescents and pediatricians regarding the minimum acceptable weight given the patient's height. A contract that describes goals of treatment should then be established. Weight gain should be the initial priority, especially in adolescents with anorexia.

Family and individual counseling is also often indicated. Patients must acknowledge the problem and their need for assistance before a referral can be made. This allows them to assert themselves and remain in control. Support groups may also be beneficial.

Numerous studies have shown that eating disorders are best treated by an interdisciplinary professional team experienced in the care of adolescents. This team should consist of the primary care provider, a psychologist or psychiatrist, a nutritionist, and a social worker. Ideally, the team is available to offer both inpatient as well as outpatient services. Criteria for inpatient admission should be established by the team and reviewed with patients and their families. Treatment for depression or any other affective disorder must be provided by a member of the team.

Inpatient treatment is required for weight loss greater than 30% below normal or a BMI less than 16; continued weight loss while on outpatient treatment; or a history of rapid weight loss over three months. Other indications include cardiovascular compromise, such as bradycardia (< 50 beats/min), orthostatic hypotension, or altered mental status; evidence of persistent hypothermia (< 36° C); suicidal or out-of-control behavior; electrolyte disturbances or uncompensated acid-base abnormalities; and significant dehydration. Rarely does confirmation of the diagnosis warrant an inpatient stay.

PROGNOSIS

Overall, the outcome for patients with eating disorders is variable, with the recovery of some patients after minimal intervention and the development of more chronic problems in others. Binge eating, for example, may replace food restriction. The prognosis is more favorable if the patient's condition is identified early and treated aggressively. Predictors of poor outcome include a longer duration of illness, a concomitant personality disorder, a dysfunctional parent-child relationship, and vomiting.

The mortality rate for anorexia nervosa is less than 5%. Exact figures for bulimia have not been determined. The most common cause of death in both disorders is suicide. Medical causes are less common but are often due to cardiac arrhythmias.

Case Resolution

In the case history presented at the beginning of this chapter, the girl does not meet the strict criteria for the diagnosis of anorexia nervosa, but her preoccupation with weight is worrisome. Concerns about her behavior should be discussed with the girl and her family. If she and her family agree, she should be referred to a psychologist and nutritionist for further evaluation, with the continued support and involvement of the primary care physician.

Selected Readings

Comerci, G. D. Eating disorders in adolescents. Pediatr. Rev. 10:1–11, 1988.

Farrow, J. A. The adolescent male with an eating disorder. Pediatr. Ann. 21:769–774, 1992.

Fisher, M. Medical complications of anorexia and bulimia nervosa. Adolesc. Med. State Art Rev. 3:487–502, 1992.

Harper, G. Eating disorders in adolescence. Pediatr. Rev. 15:72–77, 1994.

Joffe, A. Too little, too much: eating disorders in adolescents. Contemp. Pediatr. 7:114–135, 1990.

Kreipe, R. E., and M. Uphoff. Treatment and outcome of adolescents with anorexia nervosa. Adolesc. Med. State Art Rev. 3:519–540, 1992.

Shenker, I. R., and D. W. Bunnell. Bulimia nervosa. In McAnarney, E. R., et al. (eds.). Textbook of Adolescent Medicine. Philadelphia, W. B. Saunders, 1992.

Yates, A. Current perspectives on the eating disorders. I. History, psychological and biological aspects. J. Am. Acad. Child Adolesc. Psychiatry. 28:813–828, 1989.

Yates, A. Current perspectives on the eating disorders. II. Treatment, outcome and research directions. J. Am. Acad. Child Adolesc. Psychiatry 29:1–9, 1990.

DIVORCE

Carol D. Berkowitz, M.D.

Hx A 7-year-old girl who has been your patient for five years is brought in by her mother with abdominal pain that occurs on a daily basis and is not associated with any other symptoms. The pain is periumbilical. In obtaining the history, you learn that the father has moved out of the home and the parents are planning a divorce. The mother believes that her daughter's symptoms may relate to the impending divorce, and she wants to know what else to expect.

Questions

1. What are the problems faced by children whose parents are undergoing divorce?
2. What are the age-related reactions of children in families undergoing divorce?
3. What is the role of pediatricians in counseling families undergoing divorce?
4. What anticipatory guidance can be offered about custody and remarriage?

Divorce represents the "death" of a marriage, and in some ways it may be even worse for children than the death of a parent. When a parent dies, that parent becomes idealized in the mind of children, but when parents divorce, the noncustodial parent is devalued. In fact, each parent is often devalued by the other. For children, parents are no longer the idealized figures that they once were. The challenge for pediatricians is to maintain a neutral position. This may be particularly difficult because much of the contact has been with one parent rather than the other, usually the mother.

Pediatricians play a specific role in managing children going through a parental divorce because other resources are few. Extended families are no longer available to provide help. Religious institutions have often failed to assume a counseling role in this area; some religions view divorce unfavorably. Most families do not seek out mental health services unless the problems are overwhelming. Therefore, it is important for pediatricians to become involved in anticipatory guidance of families undergoing divorce. This guidance focuses on preparing children and families for times ahead. In addition, practitioners serve as child advocates. The parents themselves are so consumed by their emotional turmoil that they are often not available or are not even aware of the stress and trauma their children are experiencing. Physicians should be aware of the effect of the divorce on children and their subsequent psychological development.

EPIDEMIOLOGY

Divorce has become so prevalent that it affects approximately 50% of marriages. An estimated 100,000 couples divorce annually; most often this occurs in the first 14 years of marriage (mean: 7.1 years). Approximately one million children per year are affected by divorce. Children between the ages of 3 and 8 years are the major age group affected. Children involved with parental divorce take 2 1/2 to 3 years to regain their equilibrium and master a sense of control.

Types of custody include single parent custody, joint custody, joint legal custody, and joint physical custody, where parents have physical access to the child with equal frequency. Thirty-two states now allow for joint custody. Issues of remarriage and stepsiblings are also important. Eighty percent of divorced men and 75% of divorced women remarry, and 40% of these remarriages end in divorce. As a result of the high rate of remarriage, one in six children in the United States has a stepparent. Such children often have to readjust to differing roles in differing households and differing relationships between their biologic parents, stepparents, biologic siblings, and stepsiblings.

PSYCHOPHYSIOLOGY

The reaction to divorce that children experience depends, to a large extent, on the age of the child (Table 102–1). In general, children do not have the cognitive ability to understand the meaning of divorce until they are 9 or 10 years of age.

Children between the ages of 2 1/2 to 4 years usually manifest regressive behavior. They become needy and dependent, and their behavior is characterized by irritability, whining, crying, fearfulness, increased separation anxiety, and sleep problems. Both aggression and regression, particularly in the area of toilet training, may develop. One third of children in this age group continue to exhibit regressive behavior one year after divorce.

TABLE 102–1. Children's Reaction to Divorce

Age	Symptoms
2½–4 years	Regressive behavior
3½–5 years	Aggressive behavior
5–6 years	Whiny, immature behavior
6–adolescence	Disequilibrium
	Depression
	Somatic complaints
	Poor school performance

Preschool-age children between the ages of 3 1/2 to 5 years often show more aggressive patterns of behavior with hitting, biting, and temper tantrums. Regressive behavior may also be seen. Young children feel particularly responsible for their parents' divorce (i.e., the parents are divorcing the child). At this point in development, children experience what Piaget has referred to as an egocentric way of thinking. Self-blame, decreased self-esteem, and a high level of fantasy, particularly about parental reunion, are apparent. Approximately one year after divorce, 65% of these children still show decreased levels of functioning.

Children who are 5 to 6 years of age are often depressed and may exhibit immature behavior. Girls in this age group seem to handle a divorce more poorly than boys. Two thirds of girls are less well adjusted one year after the divorce, as opposed to only about one fourth of boys. These children appear moody and daydream. They may also be whiny and have temper tantrums.

School-age children between the age of 6 years and adolescence seem to experience profound disequilibrium with feelings of shame, anger, and loneliness. This anger may be manifested by antisocial behavior. Older children also talk about an overwhelming feeling of sadness and grief. Their somatic complaints include headache, abdominal pain, and an increase in symptoms of preexisting medical conditions such as asthma. Sometimes the somatic complaints of children, particularly those in the school-age group, are attributed by one parent to the poor living conditions at the other parent's household.

It is important for physicians to anticipate that 50% of children involved in parental divorce show a deterioration in their school performance. Therefore, the school should be notified about the divorce and changes in family structure. Decreased school performance is attributed to decreased ability to concentrate, sadness, and depression.

Parental divorce is particularly difficult for adolescents, who describe it as "extraordinarily painful." The experience is worse for younger adolescents. During the first stages of divorce, they experience a personal sense of abandonment and a loss of parental love. Older adolescents are concerned about their future potential as marital partners. They also feel anxious about financial security, especially money for college. Deidealization of both parents is precipitous. Adolescent girls do better than boys early on, but this reverses with time. This pattern is referred to as a "sleeper effect" or "delayed effect," with girls subsequently feeling rejected and unattractive. Divorce during adolescence sometimes leads to "precocious sexual activity" or risk- or thrill-seeking behavior.

DIFFERENTIAL DIAGNOSIS

Children who present with complaints including headache, abdominal pain, enuresis, and poor school performance should always be assessed for environmental factors that may be contributing to their symptomatology. Interestingly, many parents who are under-

going a divorce do not appreciate the impact the divorce is having on their children. They are often caught up in their own personal feelings and are not aware of their children's symptomatology. It is appropriate to consider organic etiologies for any somatic complaint.

EVALUATION

The focus of the evaluation should be on the interviewing process. Determination of the full extent of the impact of the home factors on children's symptomatology may take several visits. It is not appropriate to pursue extensive laboratory tests without first adequately determining what changes are occurring within the household.

History

The medical evaluation of children undergoing a parental divorce should include a review of the medical history and a discussion with the child of factors of change (Questions Box). This may help open up a discussion that reveals that the parents are in the process of divorce or that the father has moved out of the household.

Physical Examination

Any symptom or specific complaint, such as headache or abdominal pain, should also be addressed (see Chapter 83, Abdominal Pain, and Chapter 87, Headache). Depression and the risk for suicide should also be evaluated (see Chapter 104, Depression and Suicide). A complete physical examination is usually warranted because children who are experiencing stress may also develop stress-related medical problems.

Laboratory Tests

Some simple baseline laboratory studies may be warranted, particularly in children who have complaints such as abdominal pain or enuresis. These tests may include a CBC or urinalysis.

MANAGEMENT

Management of children whose family is undergoing divorce is complex. In addition to treating any somatic complaints that may be related to the divorce, physicians play a key role in anticipatory guidance. Physician

---

Questions: Divorce

- Is there anything different about the child's house now?
- Who lives in the house?
- How are things going between the parents?
- Has the child shown any regressive or aggressive behaviors?
- Has the child been eating and sleeping normally?
- How is the child doing in school?

TABLE 102–2.   Talking to Children About Divorce

Who
Who tells?   Both parents
Who is told?   Children, physicians, teachers, neighbors

When
Before either parent leaves
Age-dependent
   Older children: weeks ahead
   Younger children: days ahead

How
Calmly, with emotional control

Where
Privately, in the home

What
Stress that children are not to blame; that the divorce is between parents, not be-
   tween parents and children; it is the parents who cannot get along
Explain expected living arrangements

---

involvement before parents actually separate helps. Initially, physicians should advise parents about how to talk to children and what to expect in terms of their reaction. It is important for parents to tell children that they are separating from one another and not from the children. As stated above, parents undergoing a divorce are in so much turmoil that they themselves may not see their children's problems. In addition, their parenting skills may suffer, and routine procedures such as meals and bedtime may become disrupted, sporadic, and irregular.

Table 102–2 summarizes advice to parents. "When," "how," "who," and "what" to tell should be discussed. Generally, children should be told of impending divorce by both parents with support from the extended family. Unfortunately, studies report that 80% of preschoolers were told by one parent.

The "when" to tell depends on children's age. Younger children should be told a few days before the actual separation. Older children should be told at least several weeks before. Practitioners should advise parents about "how" to tell. Displays of emotion are permissible. Parents should be encouraged to show their emotions, but not to the extent that they appear overwhelmed or uncontrollable.

The "who" to tell includes not only the children but also the neighbors and the school, so that the feeling of shame or secrecy is less. The "what" to tell involves freeing the children of any blame for the divorce and answering their questions.

It is important for physicians not to become involved in custody disputes, but if they are asked to give an opinion, they should try to evaluate the parenting skills of both parents. In the past, custody was given to the mother in 90% of cases, but this is now decreasing. Questions that physicians should ask themselves when advising about custody include: What are the emotional ties between parents and children? Do children indicate a preference for one parent? Children may be overwhelmed by feelings of loyalty and be torn if asked to choose one parent over the other, which makes this a difficult problem. What is the capacity of each parent to provide emotional and physical support for children? It is important to consider a need for continuity, and it is vital to keep conditions as close as possible to the predivorce situation. Children should not have to move. Living arrangements need to be reassessed on a periodic basis.

Physicians should be aware of the factors that support joint custody. Joint custody tends to maintain a parent-child attachment, and children experience less of a sense of loss. They have more cognitive and social stimulation. Joint custody relieves the burden of single parenthood, and parents who have joint custody are less likely to use children as bargaining tools. Parents themselves are freer to enter into different relationships and are less emotionally dependent on their children.

Although physicians should not become involved in monetary issues, concerns related to payment and cost of medical care are appropriate to discuss. Practitioners should consider involving noncustodial parents in children's health care. Such parents could be notified if medical problems occur.

Pediatricians may also be helpful in counseling noncustodial parents about interacting with children. In general, visitation should reflect previous relationships as closely as possible. Noncustodial parents should be advised not to become camp counselors who focus on fun and games but to be influential figures who help the children meet the challenges of normal living such as completing homework and doing chores and tasks. It is also important for noncustodial parents to be consistent. If a meeting is planned, the parents must show up. Although a couple are no longer married, they can still be coparents rather than rivals. Noncustodial parents should be encouraged to participate in school and sports activities.

Custodial parents may attribute children's somatic complaints to poor care while under visitation with noncustodial parents. Allegations related to abuse, most often sexual abuse, may also arise. These allegations should be taken seriously. An appropriate medical and psychological evaluation is necessary (see Chapter 97, Child Sexual Abuse). The most difficult situations involve allegations of sexual abuse of preverbal children, where conclusions may be contingent on the physical findings, which are usually nonconclusive.

Issues related to parental dating and remarriage should be addressed at an early stage. Parents should be advised that pediatricians may be a resource in helping families readjust. Remarriage is often a difficult time for children because they experience feelings of rejection secondary to displacement by stepparents. Grandparents may also be a source of support.

PROGNOSIS

The prognosis for children undergoing a parental divorce depends, in part, on the degree of dysfunction that existed in the family before separation and the ability of the children to communicate their concerns. Supportive intervention by family, friends, and physicians is key to facilitating the necessary adjustment.

Case Resolution

The case history shows that functional somatic complaints are not uncommon, especially in school-age children of divorced parents. The mother and her daughter should be advised about how stressful divorce is for children. A careful medical examination may reassure both the mother and child about the child's physical well-being. Issues related to custody, financial responsibility, and the need for consistency should all be addressed. In addition, the pediatrician should refer the family to outside agencies if necessary.

Selected Readings

Baris, M. A., and C. B. Garrity. Children of Divorce. Dekalb, IL, Psytec, 1988.

Green, M. Reaching out to children of divorce. Contemp. Pediatr. 5:22–42, 1988.

Long, N., and R. Forehand. The effects of parental divorce and parental conflict on children: an overview. J. Dev. Behav. Pediatr. 8:292–296, 1987.

Schmitt, B. D. Helping children cope with divorce. Contemp. Pediatr. 9:81–86, 1992.

Wallerstein, J. S. The long-term effects of divorce on children: a review. J. Am. Acad. Child Adolesc. Psychiatry 30:349, 1991.

Wallerstein, J. S., and J. R. Johnston. Children of divorce: recent findings regarding long-term effects and recent studies of joint and sole custody. Pediatr. Rev. 11:197–203, 1990.

CHAPTER 103

VIOLENCE

Carol D. Berkowitz, M.D.

H$_x$ You are asked to talk to the students of an elementary school where an on-campus shooting of one student by another, older student has occurred. The shooting took place in the school yard at lunchtime and was directly witnessed by over 40 students. Since the episode a week earlier, school absenteeism and disruptive classroom behavior have increased.

Questions

1. In what settings are children exposed to violence?
2. What is the prevalence of violence in these various settings?
3. What is the impact of violence on students' academic performance?
4. What can physicians do to counteract violence in society?
5. What is the impact of gangs in a community?

Children are exposed to violence in various settings. In the home, violence may be between parents, between parents and children, and between siblings. In the schools, violence has escalated in recent years. This is particularly worrisome because the violence has become more lethal with the increase in the number of guns. Corporal punishment may occur at home as well as in school. In the community, violence involves gangs and criminal acts. The large number of innocent bystanders who are shot during gang conflicts makes some neighborhoods especially unsafe.

Concern has also been expressed about exposure to violence through the media, including television and interactive videogames. It is believed that violence in the media has contributed to an acceptance of violence in society, where violence has become an expected phenomenon.

EPIDEMIOLOGY

In 1933, natural causes accounted for more than three times as many deaths as violent incidents or injuries in adolescents. By 1985, natural causes accounted for only 27% of all adolescent deaths. Death from homicide is presently the second leading cause of death in adolescents between the ages of 15 and 24 years. The United States has the highest teenage homicide rate in the industrialized world.

Males and African-Americans are more likely to die by homicide. If current trends continue, five out of every 1000 African-American males who turn 15 this year will die in a homicide before they reach age 25.

A survey of 1035 youngsters in Chicago's South Side found that by age 11, four out of five children had witnessed a beating either at home or in the street. One out of three children had seen a shooting or stabbing, and one out of four had seen a murder committed.

Violence in the school is equally pervasive. In 1989, the National Adolescent School Health Survey reported the following data:

1. Fifty percent of boys and about 33% of girls participated in at least one fight during the year. These once trivial quarrels now frequently escalate to lethal confrontations because of the ready availability of guns.

2. About 14% of boys and 13% of girls were robbed at least once in school, and a similar proportion were robbed on their way to or from school.

3. Seventeen percent of boys and 9% of girls were attacked at least once in school, and 20% of boys and 20% of girls were attacked in the vicinity of school.

4. Weapons frequently accompany youngsters to school. At one school in New York City, 2669 weapons were confiscated from students during the 1988–89 school year. A 1990 report noted that 50% of the boys at one Baltimore high school had brought a gun to school at least once. A Youth Risk Behavior Survey conducted that same year indicated that approximately one out of every five high school students carried a firearm, knife, or club to school during the preceding month. Over 200 million firearms, including 50 million handguns, are privately owned in the United States. Nearly half of all U.S. homes contain firearms and 25 million households have handguns. The average age of acquisition of a gun is 12.5 years, usually as a gift from an older male relative. Access to handguns is simple. When questioned, 41% of boys and 21% of girls said that they could get a handgun if they wanted. It has been said that adolescents find it easier to obtain a handgun than a driver's license.

CLINICAL PRESENTATION

Children who are affected by violence may have various symptoms. Physical evidence of victimization, including bruises or wounds from stabbing or gunshots, may be apparent. Children who are emotionally traumatized often present with somatic complaints such as abdominal pain, headache, or vomiting. These children may also have symptoms consistent with depression such as poor appetite and sleep disturbances.

Children who have witnessed violence in school settings may exhibit school refusal behavior or apparent school phobia because of fears for their safety within the school setting. Poor school performance may also follow a violent episode in the school or be related to an inability to concentrate because of fear in the school setting. Domestic violence and child abuse may lead to symptoms of low self-esteem, poor school performance, and acting-out behavior.

PSYCHOPHYSIOLOGY

Violence that affects children and adolescents has several facets. In violent situations, children fit into one of three categories: aggressors, victims, or bystanders. Aggressors are the initiators of violence, victims are the targets of violence, and bystanders are the observers of violence. Bystanders are often characterized as "inno-

cent," but they can contribute to violent behavior by instigating as well as endorsing it. What are some of the factors that encourage children to participate in antisocial behavior?

Peer group influence is particularly strong, especially in individuals with low self-esteem. The concepts of identity (the "macho" image) and rite of passage—becoming an adult—relate to peer pressure. In addition, teenagers feel invincible, and this contributes to their risk-taking behavior. They wish to assert independence and autonomy from adult authority figures. Learning disabilities, a history of physical abuse, and school or athletic failure, are additional factors contributing to low self-esteem.

Although the majority of teenage homicides are not related to gang activity, the presence of gangs in a community has a deleterious effect on the community and its sense of safety and well-being. Los Angeles, which has 100,000 gang members, is reported to be the gang capital of the United States. Studies suggest that about one-fifth of adolescent males in communities of 10,000 or more belong to gangs. Teenage gangs are of two types. The first type are loosely organized "crews" or "posses" whose members tend to "hang out" together, drink and use drugs together, and engage in vandalism or petty theft. The second type are gangs organized to sell drugs. Gang membership is associated with high morbidity and mortality. In addition, gangs are also responsible for the deaths of uninvolved individuals who are gunned down during drive-by shootings. Such shootings are often adjacent to school grounds and not infrequently occur during school hours.

Substance abuse is another factor associated with violence and violent death. Alcohol and drug use increase risk-taking behavior and impulsiveness. Approximately 50% of all homicide victims have elevated blood alcohol levels. The medical examiner of Washington, D.C., once reported that 80% of homicide victims had cocaine in their bodies.

The role of the media in contributing to violence is more controversial, although research strongly supports the link between viewing violence on television and the subsequent development of violent behavior. These data come from naturalistic field studies, longitudinal studies, and population-based studies. Additional concern relates to the violence against individuals that is portrayed in interactive videogames.

EVALUATION

The evaluation of children to determine the risk of their becoming perpetrators or victims of violence is challenging. Ideally, all children should be assessed at each health maintenance visit. Risk factors for aggressive behavior should be identified. Children at greater risk for antisocial behavior include those who have experienced neurologic injuries and those who have been prenatally exposed to certain drugs such as opiates, cocaine, or alcohol. It is also suggested that lead poisoning may increase the risk for aggressive behavior. In addition, certain psychological attributes, including hyperactivity, impulsivity and cognitive deficit associated with low intelligence, and poor concentration, may also place children at higher risk. Poor bonding between children and parents has been associated with subsequent aggressive behavior patterns.

Children should be questioned about being victimized or witnessing violence either in their school, community, or home environment or viewing violence on television. Statements such as "There seems to be a lot of fighting going on in schools and homes, and I'd like to talk to you about it" facilitate the discussion.

In addition, children should be questioned specifically about their involvement as aggressors in violent acts. They should then be asked about the number of fights they have engaged in. Appropriate questions are: "How many shoving fights have you had in the last month?," "What were they about?," "Did you or anyone else get hurt?," "How did you get out of the fight?," "Have you ever been threatened with a gun?," and "Have you ever carried a gun?"

Parents should also be asked about violent acts within the home. They should routinely be questioned about the presence of guns in the home, whether the guns are kept unloaded and locked up, and whether ammunition is stored in the home, and if so, where. Children who have witnessed violence should be evaluated to determine the effect of such exposure on their day-to-day functioning and school performance. Children should be assessed for their ability to eat and sleep normally and perform daily activities.

Neither physical examination nor laboratory assessment is helpful unless children have sustained specific physical injuries.

MANAGEMENT

Pediatricians can deal with violence in several ways. They can work with aggressors in an effort to reduce violent behavior, treat victims and help them recover from physical as well as emotional injuries, assist schools and communities with violence reduction programs, and advocate for legislation concerning gun control and gun safety and portrayals of violence by the media, including television. Practitioners can work with numerous groups and organizations, such as law enforcement agencies and the American Bar Association, to structure programs and lobby for change.

When dealing one-on-one with aggression-prone children, pediatricians should strive to assist children with their development of nonviolent problem-solving skills such as articulating anger and frustration or enlisting the aid of an adult to resolve conflicts. In addition, families should be instructed to prohibit their access to guns, thereby diminishing the lethality of children's aggressive behavior.

Victims of violence need emotional support. These individuals may develop isolated or multiple somatic complaints. Alternatively, they may manifest symptoms of posttraumatic stress disorder, experiencing depression, anxiety, and sleep and eating disruptions. Children may need referral to mental health counselors to assist them in restoring a sense of control over their lives. Pediatricians as well as mental health specialists may

assist schools where an episode of violence has occurred. Sessions for students allow them to articulate their fears and reactions.

Several interventional strategies may be employed through the schools to reduce violence. Early intervention during grade and middle school is important. Just as drug prevention programs are geared toward younger children, programs to deglorify violence should also be instituted. This is one of the goals of the U.S. Public Health Service for the year 2000. Strategies for achieving this objective include the following actions:

1. Counteracting the cultural acceptance of violence.
2. Decreasing aggressive behavior between parents and their children through child abuse prevention programs.
3. Reducing the exposure of children and adolescents to violence in the media by helping parents select appropriate television programs to watch.
4. Improving the recognition, management, and treatment of adolescent victims and those at high risk for assault.

Schools can use educational interventions that stress nonviolent conflict resolution and teach such skills. One such educational intervention is the Violence Prevention Project of the Health Promotion Program for Urban Youth. This program, which consists of 10 sessions, teaches that anger is normal and uses videotapes and role playing to teach students how to channel anger in a constructive manner.

Schools may also have to use additional means, including metal detectors and campus police, to ensure the safety and well-being of students. School attendance should be enforced, and parents should be called when students are absent. Students who are found to be off campus should be returned to the school and their presence enforced on school grounds.

Concerned parents can use schools to mobilize their efforts. Grass roots organizations similar to Mothers Against Drunk Drivers (MADD) are emerging to address the problem of adolescent violence. Save Our Sons and Daughters (SOSAD), founded over 10 years ago in Detroit, is now a national organization. Other groups include New York City's Mothers Against Violence and Parents of Murdered Children and Atlanta's Mothers of Murdered Sons (MOMS).

Pediatricians can also serve as leaders to encourage the community, through schools, to develop quality youth programs. These programs should provide the following services:

1. Address various needs: remedial services, crisis intervention programs, and enrichment activities.
2. Be open year round with long hours.
3. Serve a wide range of age groups, so youths can interact with people of various ages.
4. Allow for continuity, with no age-based mandatory termination (i.e., participants must leave at the age of 19 or 20).
5. Provide contact with adults who can serve as role models.

6. Provide opportunities for youths to practice leadership.

7. Do outreach and case management.

PROGNOSIS

The prognosis varies with the nature of children's involvement in the violence. Some children sustain significant physical injuries such as neurologic impairment or disfigurement. Other children are emotionally traumatized, and even with psychological counseling, they have difficulty with the normal tasks of childhood such as attending school. Long-term involvement by primary care physicians is needed by children who are the physical or emotional victims of violence.

Case Resolution

In the case history presented at the beginning of this chapter, the physician should discuss the fears and feelings of the students to help facilitate their coping with the violence. Safety should also be discussed to empower the students to avoid violent situations. The use of teaching tapes and role playing helps the students think of solutions to dangerous situations before these conditions develop.

Selected Readings

Christoffel, K. K. Pediatric firearm injuries: time to target a growing population. Pediatr. Ann. 21:430–436, 1992.

Cohall, A. T., et al. Teen violence: the new mortality. Contemp. Pediatr. 8:76–86, 1991.

Hutson, H. R., D. Anglin, and M. J. Pratts. Adolescents and children injured or killed in drive-by shootings in Los Angeles. N. Engl. J. Med. 330:324–327, 1994.

Koop, C. E. Violence in America: a public health emergency. J.A.M.A. 267:3075–3076, 1992.

Prothrow-Stith, D. Can physicians help curb adolescent violence? Hosp. Pract. 27:193–205, 1992.

Ropp, L., et al. Death in the city: an American childhood tragedy. J.A.M.A. 267:2905–2910, 1992.

Senturiam Y., K. K. Christoffel, and M. Donovan. Children's household exposure to guns: a pediatric practice-based survey. Pediatrics 93:469–475, 1994.

CHAPTER 104

ADOLESCENT DEPRESSION AND SUICIDE

Monica Sifuentes, M.D.

Hx A 15-year-old girl is brought to your office by her mother with the chief complaint of easy fatigability. The mother is concerned because her daughter is always tired, although several other physicians have told her that the girl is healthy. The adolescent, who states no complaints or concerns, appears very shy. She is currently in the tenth grade, likes school, receives average grades, and speaks both English and Spanish. She says she has a few friends at school and adamantly denies any drug, alcohol, or tobacco use. She has never been sexually active and reports no history of sexual or physical abuse.

The mother, a single parent, moved to the United States from El Salvador approximately two years ago with her two daughters. They are currently living with relatives in a two-bedroom apartment. The mother is employed as a housekeeper, and the patient and her sister help their mother clean homes on weekends. During the week they make dinner for the rest of the family as a means of contributing to the rent.

The girl's physical examination is entirely normal, although her affect appears flat.

Questions

1. What is the significance of nonspecific symptoms, such as fatigue, during adolescence?
2. What factors contribute to depression in adolescents?
3. What are the classic signs and symptoms of depression in adolescents?
4. What are some important historical points to cover when interviewing adolescents with suspected depression?
5. How is the risk of suicide assessed in adolescent patients?
6. How should suicidal behavior (i.e., suicide attempts) be managed in adolescents?

Depression has been identified as one of the multiple risk factors that predispose adolescents to suicide. However, not all teenagers who try to take their own lives are depressed, and conversely, not all depressed adolescents attempt suicide. This distinction is important to keep in mind when evaluating adolescents for either depression or suicidal behavior.

EPIDEMIOLOGY

Depression

The exact prevalence of depression in adolescents is difficult to determine because depression is both an illness and a symptom. Depressive symptoms have been reported in as many as 47.7% of girls and 41.7% of boys in the 14–15-year-age group. The overall prevalence of depression as an illness is approximately 5%; mild depression is reported in 13 to 28% of teens, moderate depression in 7%, and severe depression in 1.3%. Depression occurs more commonly in adolescents than in prepubertal children and is more frequent in females than males after puberty.

Several risk factors contribute to the development of depressive disorders in adolescents (Table 104–1). Certain psychiatric conditions are also associated with depression, including anxiety disorders, eating disorders, substance abuse, conduct disorders, and borderline personality disorders.

Suicide and Suicidal Behavior

Suicide is the third leading cause of death in the United States in individuals 10 to 24 years of age; only accidents and homicides result in more deaths in young people. In 1960 the annual suicide rate in this age group was 5.2/100,000, and by 1990 it had more than doubled to 13.2/100,000. In particular, the 1990 suicide rate for 15- to 19-year-old adolescents was 11.1/100,000, triple that of 1960. For every suicide that is completed successfully, 50 to 200 suicides are attempted.

According to the 1990 Youth Risk Survey of the Centers for Disease Control and Prevention, 27.3% of all students in grades 9 to 12 had thought of attempting suicide during the previous 12 months. Approximately 16% of these students had made specific suicide plans; about 50% of those students with suicide plans reported attempting to take their lives. Two percent of the individuals who attempted suicide required medical attention.

Several risk factors associated with adolescent suicide have been identified (Table 104–2). Adolescent females are more likely to attempt suicide than males,

TABLE 104–1.   Risk Factors Associated With Depressive Disorders in Adolescents

Family history of psychiatric illness (e. g., parent with an affective condition or another family member with a bipolar or recurrrent unipolar disorder). The age of onset of depression in the affected parent is important; the earlier the age of onset, the greater the likelihood of depression in the children.
History of environmental trauma (e.g., sexual or physical abuse, loss of a loved one)
Chronic illness
Certain medications (e.g., propranolol, phenobarbital)

TABLE 104–2.   Risk Factors Associated With Suicide in Adolescents

History of a previous suicide attempt (most important)
Preexisting psychiatric condition
Alcohol and illicit substance abuse
Family history of psychiatric disorders, especially depression and suicidal behavior
Family disruption, including violence, divorce, or the death of a loved one
Exposure to an unexpected suicide in the school or community
Chronic debilitating illness
History of physical or sexual abuse
Availability of firearms in the home

but males are more likely to succeed. This fact may result from the lethality of the methods, such as firearms or hanging, that males usually choose. Females are more likely to ingest pills. The availability of firearms and alcohol, which varies from state to state, also contributes to the occurrence of suicide. Up to 45% of individuals who have committed suicide show some evidence of intoxication at the time of death. Although most suicide attempts are impulsive, studies have shown that adolescents often have communicated their suicidal intent or ideation to someone before the attempt.

CLINICAL PRESENTATION

Depressed or suicidal adolescents may visit physicians for a variety of reasons. They may present with seemingly nonemergent complaints and a flat affect or with multiple concerns and an anxious appearance. Sometimes adolescents are accompanied by family or friends, and they are often reticent to discuss psychosocial issues. Occasionally, they are referred by school officials for educational problems.

PATHOPHYSIOLOGY

Although depression does not necessarily have one single etiology, three primary theories to explain depression have been proposed. A combination of several factors probably causes depression.

The **psychoanalytic hypothesis** proposes that low self-esteem, which is the result of a critical and punitive childhood, leads to self-destructive anger. This self-destructive thinking and behavior then results in depression.

The **biologic explanation** includes dysregulation of specific neurotransmitters such as norepinephrine, serotonin, and dopamine. Antidepressant compounds induce noradrenergic and serotoninergic responses. The genetic basis of depression is supported by statistics that indicate that 25% of children who take their own lives have a family member or close relative who has committed suicide. Recent studies suggest the incomplete penetrance of a dominant gene as a possible etiology.

The hypothesis known as **"the final common pathway"** states that depression is caused by a number of factors (see Table 104–1) that interact and lead to one common outcome. Specific behaviors triggered by a biochemical alteration, an infectious agent, or an envi-

---

Dx   Adolescent Depression

- Depressed or irritable mood
- Decreased interest in most activities, including school
- Significant weight changes
- Sleeping problems
- Psychomotor agitation or retardation
- Fatigue
- Feelings of worthlessness or guilt
- Diminished ability to concentrate or think
- Preoccupation with death or suicide

Questions: Adolescent Depression

- Does the adolescent occasionally feel sad and not know why?
- Does the adolescent have unexplained crying spells?
- Does the adolescent feel "mad," "bored," or "grouchy"?
- Does the adolescent seem inappropriately jovial?
- Have there been any recent losses in the adolescent's life that may explain his or her feelings?
- Is the adolescent having trouble with concentration or memory?
- Does the adolescent have trouble falling asleep at night or with early morning awakening?
- Has the adolescent lost weight recently or shown any disinterest in food?
- Does the adolescent have feelings of hopelessness and have any desire to hurt himself or herself? Has the adolescent made any previous suicide attempts?
- Do the parents or siblings have a history of drug or alcohol use?
- Is there a family history of affective disorders?
- Is there a history of family violence?

---

ronmental experience may result in depression and self-deprecation.

DIFFERENTIAL DIAGNOSIS

The differential diagnosis of depression includes any condition that may affect the patient's nutritional status and lead to malnourishment (D$_x$ Box). Examples include underlying eating disorders such as anorexia nervosa, cancer, and tuberculosis. In addition, endocrine disorders such as hypothyroidism, hyperthyroidism, and Addison's disease can mimic depression. CNS pathology, although rare, includes postconcussive syndromes and cerebrovascular accidents. Illicit substance abuse and alcoholism should also be investigated. Side effects of both prescribed and over-the-counter medications may also produce depressive symptoms.

EVALUATION

History

The assessment of an adolescent for depression is an important part of any routine encounter, but the diagnosis of depression is difficult to make after just one interview. Initially, a complete **HEADSSS** assessment (**h**ome, **e**mployment and education, **a**ctivities, **d**rugs, **s**exual activity/sexuality, **s**uicide and depression, **s**afety) should be performed on all adolescents (see Chapter 4, Talking to Adolescents). A thorough history should be obtained (Questions Box: Adolescent Depression). Mood changes should be noted; a labile affect can be a symptom of ongoing depression. Physicians should remember that patients who are malnourished for any reason can have a depressed affect.

To identify youths at risk for suicide, practitioners must inquire about specific areas of adolescents' lives. Adolescents who are suspected of being at risk for suicide must be questioned directly about suicide ideation. Initially questions should be nonspecific and become more specific as the interview proceeds, especially if answers to the initial questions are positive (Questions Box: Adolescent Suicide).

Promises to maintain confidentiality with adolescents considered at risk for suicide are discouraged because parental involvement is strongly advised. Precipitating and motivating factors for any previous suicide attempts should be determined prior to the development

of a treatment plan. The lethality of previous attempts should be evaluated.

Physical Examination

A thorough physical examination and a review of systems should be completed to rule out a chronic medical condition or an organic etiology for nonspecific complaints. If patients have a history of sexual abuse or assault or a history of sexual activity, a genital examination should be performed to check for STD. Otherwise, the physical examination is of little help in adolescent patients with a true affective disorder.

Laboratory Tests

No routine laboratory studies are recommended. Psychometric testing may help rule out a learning

---

Questions: Adolescent Suicide

- Is the adolescent experiencing any psychiatric difficulties, social maladjustments, or family or environmental challenges (e.g., recent parental divorce, school expulsion)?
- Does the adolescent have a history of symptoms of depression, conduct problems, or psychosis?
- Does the adolescent have a history of substance abuse?
- How is the adolescent progressing in school?
- Does the adolescent have any legal problems?
- Does the adolescent suffer any social isolation or have interpersonal conflicts with family or friends?
- Has the adolescent suffered any personal losses recently?
- Are there any family problems such as abuse or neglect?
- Is the adolescent at risk for suicide?
  - Has the adolescent ever thought that life was not worth living?
  - Does the adolescent ever feel hopeless?
  - Does the adolescent have a previous history of suicide attempts?
  - Does the adolescent presently have a plan for suicide?
  - Does the adolescent have access to a firearm?
  - Has there recently been a suicide in the school or community?

disability or ADHD. A dexamethasone suppression test or other neuroendocrine evaluation is not necessary to diagnose depression. Before TCAs are prescribed, a baseline ECG should be performed to rule out conduction defects. In addition, liver function tests should be obtained and followed.

MANAGEMENT

Depression

If depressive symptoms are associated with an adjustment disorder and if family, peers, or school factors are involved, **supportive counseling** is indicated. The duration and depth of counseling depends, in part, on how comfortable primary care practitioners feel performing this task. Identification of the problem and development of a reasonable solution with adolescents often helps. **Psychological referral** may be initiated if patients require more prolonged treatment.

If family difficulties are the major problem, family members and physicians or counselors should meet to assess the magnitude of the problem and the motivation required to address it. Physicians should use this opportunity to educate both adolescents and families about depression. The need for individual as well as family therapy should be discussed and the appropriate referrals should be made at the end of the meeting.

Immediate **psychiatric referral** is indicated if adolescents have severe depressive features that interfere with daily functioning or if they are suicidal, homicidal, or psychotic. Such management is also appropriate if supportive counseling has been ineffective. Psychiatric intervention may include pharmacotherapy (e.g., TCAs, serotonin reuptake inhibitors), as well as psychotherapy. TCAs prevent reuptake of catecholamines at the synaptic level and therefore increase serotonin, norepinephrine, or dopamine levels (depending on the particular TCA). Anticholinergic side effects are not uncommon, however, and may limit the usefulness of some medications.

Suicide and Suicidal Behavior

Adolescents who are considered at risk for suicide must be asked directly if they are, in fact, suicidal (Questions: Adolescent Suicide). Response to this inquiry determines whether adolescents should be treated on an inpatient or outpatient basis. Adolescents with no previous suicide attempts, ambivalence regarding suicidal thoughts, no real intent to die, and a good family support system may be managed as **outpatients.** In patients who deny current suicidal ideation, a no-suicide agreement must be made between the physician or psychologist and the adolescent. At this time the precipitants for possible suicidality must be reviewed and alternative methods for coping should be rehearsed. In addition, all potential means of suicide, particularly firearms, must be removed from the home or place of residence. It is not enough to "secure" firearms; they must be removed.

Referral to a therapist is recommended as soon as possible. Preferably, this should be arranged while adolescents are in the office, and they should be given a definite time and date for the appointment. Ideally, the therapist should meet with the family before the first appointment. Detoxification from drugs or alcohol, if necessary, should also be addressed.

All suicidal threats or ideations by adolescents should be taken seriously, and psychiatric referral is required. Adolescents judged to be at serious risk for suicide should be managed as **inpatients.** Patients who have attempted to take their own lives should be admitted to a pediatric or adolescent unit for 24 to 48 hours. The purpose of hospitalization is threefold: (1) to stabilize patients medically, if necessary; (2) to observe and evaluate patient-family dynamics; and (3) to impress on patients and families that the attempt has been recognized and taken seriously. Intervention requires the involvement of mental health professionals in addition to social services. Transfer to an inpatient psychiatric treatment center is indicated for those adolescents who are judged by mental health consultants to have serious suicidal intentions or an underlying psychiatric illness.

PROGNOSIS

The risk of recurrence of major depression in adolescents who have recovered is substantial. A recent study reports that 5% of patients relapse within six months of recovery, 12% within one year, and an estimated 33% within four years.

The risk of repeated suicidal behavior appears to be greatest within the first three months following the initial attempt. Reported reattempt rates are 6 to 15% in the first one to three years following the initial attempt.

Case Resolution

In the case history presented at the beginning of this chapter, the girl's symptoms may be indicative of depression because she seems to have insufficient time for friends and just recently moved to the United States. She appears to be at low risk for suicide, however. The physician should nonetheless inquire about suicidality and then make arrangements to follow the girl's condition closely. If depression is confirmed at future visits or if she becomes suicidal, both she and her family should be referred to a mental health professional for intervention.

Selected Readings

Adler, R. S., and M. S. Jellinek. After teen suicide: issues for pediatricians who are asked to consult to schools. Pediatrics 86:982–987, 1990.

American Academy of Pediatrics, Committee on Adolescence. Suicide and suicide attempts in adolescents and young adults. Pediatrics 2:322–324, 1988.

Berman, A. L., and R. H. Schwartz. Suicide attempts among adolescent drug users. Am. J. Dis. Child. 144:310–314, 1990.

Brent, D. A. Depression and suicide in children and adolescents. Pediatr. Rev. 14:380–388, 1993.

Centers for Disease Control and Prevention. Attempted suicide among high school students–United States, 1990. M.M.W.R. 40:633–635, 1991.

Centers for Disease Control and Prevention. Programs for the prevention of suicide among adolescents and young adults. M.M.W.R. 43(RR-6):3–17, 1994.

Crumley, F. E. Substance abuse and adolescent suicidal behavior. J.A.M.A. 263:3051–3056, 1990.

Grossman, D. C. Risk and prevention of youth suicide. Pediatr. Ann. 21:448–454, 1992.

Hodgman, C. H. Adolescent depression and suicide. Adolesc. Med. State of the Art Rev. 1:81–95, 1990.

Lewisohn, P. M., et al. Major depression in community adolescents: age at onset, episode duration, and time to recurrence. J. Am. Acad. Child Adolesc. Psychiatry 33:809–818, 1994.

Lopez, R. I. Role of the primary care pediatrician in adolescent psychosocial assessment and intervention. Adolesc. Med. State of the Art Rev. 3:147–160, 1992.

Tishler, C. L. Adolescent suicide: assessment of risk, prevention, and treatment. Adolesc. Med. State of the Art Rev. 3:51–59, 1992.

Yaylayan, S., et al. Depressive mood disorders in adolescents. Adolesc. Med. State of the Art Rev. 3:41–50, 1992.

CHRONIC DISEASES OF CHILDHOOD AND ADOLESCENCE

C H A P T E R   1 0 5

CANCER IN CHILDREN

Pamela S. Cohen, M.D.

H$_x$ A ten-year-old boy has a history of intermittent fevers of 102.2° F (39.0° C) for one month. For two days, he has experienced increasing shortness of breath with rapid respirations. His face is dusky and plethoric, and the veins in his neck are prominent. The remainder of the examination is normal.

The blood count is normal, but the ESR is 110. A chest x-ray reveals a large mediastinal mass.

Questions

1. What signs and symptoms are associated with malignant conditions in children?
2. What oncologic emergencies require immediate attention?
3. What factors correlate with the development of cancer in children?

EPIDEMIOLOGY

Cancer accounts for 10.4% of deaths from all causes in children under 15 years of age in the United States, exceeded only by accidents (43.9%). Approximately 8000 new cases of cancer are diagnosed in children in the United States every year. Acute leukemia (30%), brain tumors (19%), lymphomas (13%), neuroblastomas (8%), and other soft-tissue tumors constitute the majority of these cases (Fig. 105–1).

Various epidemiologic factors correlate with the development of cancer in children. Genetics appears to play a large role, although it does not account for disease in every case. Inheritance of mutations in tumor suppressor genes, such as the retinoblastoma gene or the p53 gene, predispose affected children in families with these mutations to particular malignancies at a greater frequency and earlier age than those who do not inherit these mutations. Other syndromes listed in Table 105–1 also predispose children and adolescents to the

development of particular malignancies. All these syndromes can be assumed to result from genetic mutations, some of which have not yet been identified.

Environmental factors associated with carcinogenesis include ionizing and ultraviolet radiation; stilbestrol, androgen, and iron ingestion; and infection with various viruses, such as EBV, papillomavirus type 5, and hepatitis B. These environmental agents can interact with specific genetic traits to give rise to certain malignancies. For example, ionizing radiation given to individuals with mutated retinoblastoma genes may result in osteosarcoma much more often than it might in the general population. Electromagnetic fields are reportedly associated with a higher incidence of acute lymphoblastic leukemia (ALL) in areas in proximity to power sources (e.g., high-energy power lines), but these claims have yet to be conclusively substantiated.

CLINICAL PRESENTATION (Table 105–2)

Children with **leukemia,** whether acute or chronic, commonly complain of diffuse bone pains and can present with symptoms related to anemia, thrombocytopenia, or neutropenia. Mucosal bleeding, particularly from the gums, is commonly seen in children with acute myeloblastic leukemia (AML). Frank DIC is characteristic of AML, especially acute promyelocytic leukemia. Children with leukemia often also have hepatosplenomegaly, lymphadenopathy, or mediastinal masses.

Superior vena cava (SVC) syndrome, seen primarily in ALL, may occur in children with such masses. Children with SVC syndrome have respiratory difficulties and are plethoric and cyanotic due to compression of the mediastinal mass on the trachea and blockage of venous return and lymphatic drainage. Symptoms of SVC syndrome sometimes rapidly progress over a period of hours to pleural or pericardial effusion and respiratory arrest. Involvement of the CNS by leukemia can result in signs of increased ICP (e.g., headache, vomiting, hypertension, seizures, cranial neuropathies). In advanced

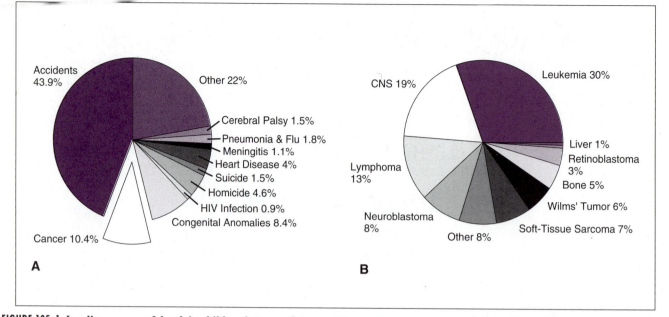

FIGURE 105–1. *Leading causes of death in children between the ages of 1 and 14 years (A).* (Adapted from U.S. Vital Statistics.) ***Distribution of cancers in children less than 15 years of age (B).*** (Reproduced, with permission, from Pizzo, P.C., and D.A. Pollack. Principles and Practice of Pediatric Oncology. Philadelphia, J.B. Lippincott, 1993, p. 4; adapted from Surveillance, Epidemiology and End Results Program.)

situations with tumor cell lysis, the products of dead tumor cells can cause renal sludging and ultimate shutdown. In such situations, patients with leukemia may present in renal failure with hyperkalemia, hyperphosphatemia, hypocalcemia, and hyperuricemia.

Children with **brain tumors** can present with a wide array of signs and symptoms, depending on the anatomic location of the tumor (supratentorial or infratentorial) and on whether the tumor has resulted in ICP. Supratentorial tumors can result in seizures, upper motor neuron signs (e.g., hemiparesis, asymmetric hyperreflexia, clonus), sensory changes, visual dysfunction (e.g., field defect with or without an afferent pupillary defect), and disorders of midbrain function (e.g., paralysis of upward gaze [Parinaud's syndrome]). Infratentorial tumors can lead to cranial neuropathies (often asymmetric), a partial Horner's syndrome (unilateral facial signs [ptosis, miosis, anhidrosis]) or cerebellar signs such as balance deficits (particularly truncal ataxia), appendicular dysmetria, or nystagmus. Signs and symptoms of increased ICP include headaches, especially ones that awaken children from sleep; lethargy; vomiting; weakness; and loss of developmental milestones in infants.

Children with spinal cord involvement may present with back pain, sometimes intense radicular pain (i.e., localized to specific dermatomes), local bony tenderness of the affected spine, bowel and bladder dysfunction, and ultimately, lower motor neuron signs, which are often associated with dermatomal sensory loss.

Lymphomas in children can be divided pathologically into either Hodgkin's or non-Hodgkin's types. Children with **Hodgkin's lymphoma** classically have a protracted history (often at least 2–3 months) of enlarging lymphadenopathy, sometimes in association with constitutional symptoms (i.e., "B" symptoms) that include fever,

night sweats, and weight loss greater than 10% of body weight. **Non-Hodgkin's lymphoma** often can be subdivided into two categories: lymphoblastic and nonlymphoblastic. Children with **lymphoblastic lymphoma** often present with supradiaphragmatic disease and may have cervical or supraclavicular lymphadenopathy, sometimes in association with a mediastinal mass or SVC syndrome. Central nervous system disease in such children is associated with signs of increased ICP. Patients with small, noncleaved, **nonlymphoblastic lymphoma** of the Burkitt's or non-Burkitt's type often present with intra-abdominal disease, intussusception, abdominal obstruction, hepatosplenomegaly, and obstructive jaundice. Children with Burkitt's lymphoma may also present with isolated jaw tumors. In addition, patients with lymphoma can manifest any of a number of paraneoplastic syndromes. These include idiopathic thrombocytopenic purpura, autoimmune hemolytic anemia, nephrotic syndrome, and peripheral neuropathies, which may be mediated by abnormal and lymphoma-driven humoral or cell-mediated processes. In general, patients may either have entirely normal blood counts or a mild anemia, but occasionally their bone marrow may be infiltrated, giving a clinical picture consistent with leukemia with anemia, thrombocytopenia, or neutropenia.

Neuroblastoma, the most common soft tissue tumor aside from brain tumors, is of sympathetic ganglionic cell origin, and as such, can present as intra-adrenal or extra-adrenal (paraspinal) abdominal masses, posterior (paraspinal) mediastinal masses, cervical masses, or in some cases with disseminated disease of the liver, spleen, skin, and bone and bone marrow, sometimes without evidence of a primary tumor (regressed primary). Because of the systemic effects of neuropeptide overexpression, children may have hypertension,

TABLE 105–1.   Selected Single Gene Traits Associated With Childhood and Adolescent Neoplasia

Gene Trait, Neoplasm, or Disorder	Inheritance	Associated Neoplasms
Skeletal		
Paget's disease of bone	AD	Osteosarcoma
Hematolymphopoietic		
X-linked lymphoprolif-erative disorder (Purtilo's syndrome)	XR	Burkitt's and other lymphomas
Kostmann's agranulo-cytosis	AR	AML
Multiple System		
Bloom's syndrome	AR	ALL
Fanconi's anemia	AR	AML
Beckwith-Wiedemann syndrome	AR	Wilms' tumor, hepato-blastoma
Li-Fraumeni syndrome	AD	Sarcomas of bone and soft tissue: young age breast cancer, brain tumors, leuke-mia, lung and laryn-geal cancer, adrenal cortical neoplasia
Inborn Errors of Metabolism		
Tyrosinemia, Wilson's disease	AR	Postcirrhotic hepatoma
Phakomatoses		
von Recklinghausen's disease Neurofibromatosis type I	AD	Sarcoma, schwannoma, optic glioma, pheo-chromocytoma, AML
Nervous System		
Retinoblastoma	AD	Retinoblastoma, os-teosarcoma
Neurofibromatosis type 2	AD	Bilateral acoustic neu-roma, meningioma
Endocrine System		
MEN type I	AD	Adenomas of pancreas, parathyroid, pitu-itary and adrenal glands; malignant schwannoma
MEN type II	AD	Medullary carcinoma of thyroid, neurofi-broma, pheochro-mocytoma
Alimentary Tract		
Peutz-Jeghers syn-drome	AD	Intestinal polyps, colon cancer
Familial polyposis coli	AD	Carcinoma of colon, pancreas, thyroid, and adrenal glands; hepatoblastoma

Adapted, with permission, from Pizzo, P.A., and D.G. Poplack. *Principles and Practice of Pediatric Oncology.* J.B. Lippincott, Philadelphia, 1993, pp. 21–22.

Abbreviations: AD, autosomal dominant; AR, autosomal recessive; XR, X-linked recessive; AML, acute myeloblastic leukemia; ALL, acute lymphoblastic leukemia; MEN, multiple endocrine neoplasia.

TABLE 105–2.   Signs and Symptoms of Childhood Cancer

Disease	Symptoms	Signs
Leukemia	Fatigue	Anemia
	Fever, infection	Neutropenia
	Petechiae, purpura, bleeding	Thrombocytopenia
		Lymphadenopathy
	Disseminated intravas-cular coagulation	Hepatosplenomegaly
		Mediastinal mass
	Superior vena cava (SVC) syndrome	Papilledema
		Cranial neuropathies
	Headache	Renal failure
	Seizures	
	Oliguria/anuria	
Brain tumors	Supratentorial tumors	
	Seizures	Upper motor neuron signs
	Visual dysfunction	Marcus Gunn pupils
	Unilateral motor dys-function	Parinaud's syndrome
		Diabetes insipidus
	Infratentorial tumors	
	Deficits of balance	Appendicular dysmetria
	Difficulty breathing	Sixth nerve palsy
		Cranial neuropathies
		Horner's syndrome
	Increased intracranial pressure	
	Headache	Papilledema
	Vomiting	Systemic hypertension
	Diplopia	Sixth nerve palsy
	Motor weakness	"Setting sun" sign
	Loss of developmen-tal milestones	Large head size
Lymphoma	Supradiaphragmatic (lymphoblastic):	
Non-Hodgkin's lymphoma	Respiratory diffi-culty, cough	Mediastinal mass +/– effusions
	SVC syndrome	Lymphadenopathy
	Enlarged/enlarging lymph nodes	
	Infradiaphragmatic (small, noncleaved):	
	Abdominal obstruction	Abdominal mass
	Intussception	Hepatosplenomegaly
	Abdominal dis-tension	Obstructive jaundice
Hodgkin's lymphoma	Constitutional symp-toms (fever, weight loss, pruritis)	Lymphadenopathy +/– matted nodes
Neuroblastoma	Abdominal mass	Hypertension
	Skin nodules	Hepatosplenomegaly
	Proptosis, "racoon eyes"	Horner's syndrome
	Nystagmus	
	Diarrhea	
	Spinal cord compres-sion symptoms	
Rhabdomyosarcoma	Related to primary site	
Wilms' tumor	Rapid development of abdominal swelling	Abdominal mass
		Hypertension
	Painless hematuria	Associated congenital anomalies:
		Aniridia
		Hemihypertrophy
		Urogenital anomalies
Ewing's sarcoma	Painful swelling of bone	
	Constitutional symp-toms (fever, fatigue)	
Osteosarcoma	Painful swelling of bone	

diarrhea, nystagmus, opsomyoclonus (random dyscon-jugate eye movements), and cerebellar ataxia. Proptosis and hemorrhage due to metastases behind the orbit can result in "raccoon eyes." A mediastinal tumor may be associated with unilateral Horner's syndrome due to compression of cranial nerve VII. Children with widespread disease may have pancytopenia if the bone marrow is diffusely infiltrated.

Rhabdomyosarcoma, another soft tissue sarcoma of childhood, presents primarily with signs and symptoms related to whether the tumor has developed in the head and neck, chest, abdomen/pelvis, or extremities. One classic presentation, sarcoma botyroides, occurs when the tumor is located in the vagina or uterus. Wilms' tumor, which arises in the kidney, usually appears as an abdominal mass that sometimes rapidly enlarges as the result of hemorrhage. Painless hematuria may be present, even in the absence of an abdominal mass. Children may have hypertension and associated congenital anomalies including aniridia, hemihypertrophy, and various urogenital conditions.

The **bone sarcomas** that occur in children include Ewing's sarcoma, osteosarcoma, and other rarer sarcomas. All bone tumors appear as growing, painful swellings of bone; patients with Ewing's sarcoma may also have associated constitutional symptoms such as low-grade fever, fatigue, and weight loss.

PATHOPHYSIOLOGY

Researchers have contributed substantially to the understanding of the pathophysiology of carcinogenesis, but the process of cancer development is still incompletely understood. In general, carcinogenesis is a series of sequential genetic mutations that affect the complex processes that control cell growth, differentiation, and death. Figure 105–2 outlines the pathway of cell proliferation. Growth factors are often responsible for exogenous stimulation of proliferation, and growth factor receptors transduce this signal into the cell via cytoplasmic second messengers such as protein kinase

TABLE 105–3. Types of Genes Altered During Carcinogenesis

Gene Type	Selected Examples
Potential cancer genes	
Dominant oncogenes	c-src, N-ras
Recessive cancer genes	Retinoblastoma gene, p53
Growth regulators	
Growth factors	PDGF, TGF-α, NGF, EGF
Growth factor receptors	EGF receptor, insulin receptor
Cytoplasmic messenger protein	
G proteins	c-ras, G protein subunit of adenylate cyclase
Cyclic-AMP-dependent protein kinases	Protein kinase A
Nuclear regulatory factors	
Transciption factors	c-myc, c-fos

Adapted from Pizzo, P.A., and D.G. Poplack. Principles and Practice of Pediatric Oncology. Philadelphia, J.B. Lippincott, 1993, p. 62.
Abbreviations: PDGF, platelet-derived growth factor; TGF-α, transforming growth factor-alpha; NGF, nerve growth factor; EGF, epidermal growth factor.

C and activated *ras* proteins, which in turn transmit the signal to nuclear regulatory factors. These factors ultimately regulate transcription of new RNA and protein, resulting in the desired cellular response of either stimulation or inhibition of growth. Dysregulation of growth via mutations in genes controlling all of these steps have been identified in tumors (Table 105–3). Similar aberrations in genes regulating differentiation and cell death have also been described.

DIFFERENTIAL DIAGNOSIS

The symptoms of cancer may be varied and mimic common pediatric conditions. Lymphadenopathy, which is associated with leukemia, lymphoma, and metastatic disease, is more frequently due to infection (see Chapter 59, Lymphadenopathy). Not all masses noted on physical examination are tumors; they may represent infection, trauma, or physical anomalies (see Chapter 53, Neck Masses). CNS symptomatology may be related to tumor, infections, hemorrhage, or problems such as seizures or migraine.

EVALUATION

History

The history should focus on the extent of symptoms, associated systemic complaints (e.g., anorexia, fever, night sweats), relevant family history, and unusual environmental exposures (e.g., ionizing radiation) (Questions Box). The impact of the symptoms on daily activities (school attendance, sports) should be determined.

Physical Examination

A full physical examination should be performed, with particular attention paid to symptomatic areas (see Table 105–2). In general, the lymph nodes should be carefully assessed for enlargement, and the abdomen

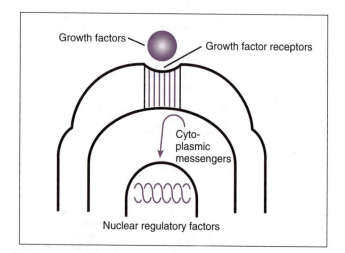

FIGURE 105–2. *Pathway of stimulated cell proliferation.* *Cellular proliferation can be modified by extracellular signals, such as growth factors, that interact with receptors on the surface membrane. These receptors can be transmembrane proteins that transduce the regulatory signal through the membrane, which initiates an intracellular cascade of molecular messages that culminates in the alteration of nuclear proteins. This regulates the expression of genes important for cellular proliferation and tumorigenesis. (Reproduced, with permission, from Pizzo, P.C., and D.A. Pollack. Principles and Practice of Pediatric Oncology. Philadelphia, J.B. Lippincott, 1993, p. 64.)*

for organomegaly. Neurologic symptoms, including headache, vomiting, or focal complaints, warrant a full neurologic examination. Increased ICP may manifest as papilledema, sixth nerve palsy, or systemic hypertension. In infants, increased ICP can manifest with the "setting sun" sign (eyes deviated downward), large head size, or full fontanelles. Both supratentorial and infratentorial tumors can in some situations metastasize to the spinal cord (see Chapter 42, Increased Intracranial Pressure).

Laboratory Tests (Table 105–4)

Children with nonspecific symptoms are usually evaluated with a CBC, ESR, and chemical panels that assess electrolytes and renal and liver function. Certain tumors secrete or synthesize characteristic proteins that are pathognomonic for their diagnosis. For example, elevated levels of the sympathetic neurotransmitter metabolites vanillylmandelic acid and homovanillic acid are found in the urine of individuals with neuroblastoma or pheochromocytoma. The substances α-fetoprotein, β-human chorionic gonadotropin, and carcinoembryonic antigen are sometimes secreted in the blood, urine, or CSF of patients with malignant teratomas. Detection of these proteins in body fluids can also be an indicator of response to therapy and can predict relapse.

Imaging Studies (Table 105–4)

The MRI scan is a valuable tool in the diagnosis and staging of tumors. When performed using contrast with gadolinium, MRI is far more powerful than the CT scan even with contrast, particularly for visualizing lesions in the brainstem area. MRI of the spine with gadolinium contrast are as good as standard myelography without the additional morbidity of the latter. This technique is especially good for visualizing sarcomas (e.g., neuroblastoma, rhabdomyosarcoma, Ewing's sarcoma).

Once the diagnosis of malignancy is made, children should receive the appropriate imaging studies to assess the local and metastatic spread of the disease before the initiation of therapy. Every malignancy has specific areas to which it is more likely to metastasize.

The initial diagnosis of a malignancy or its relapse, regardless of clinical likelihood, *must* be documented pathologically before treatment is initiated. The only exception to this rule is radiologic evidence of a

brainstem tumor, which for all intents and purposes is consistent with the diagnosis of brainstem glioma. Even when a child is in respiratory distress (e.g., with SVC syndrome secondary to a mediastinal mass), coordinated efforts must be made by the pediatrician, oncologist, intensivist, pathologist, and surgeon to obtain

TABLE 105–4. Diagnostic Tests and Imaging Studies Used in the Evaluation of Childhood Cancer

Disease	Diagnostic Tests	Imaging Studies
Leukemia	Bone marrow aspirate and biopsy Cytogenetic analysis of bone marrow CBC with platelet count, differential PT, PTT, fibrinogen Serum electrolytes, Ca, PO_4 BUN, creatinine, uric acid CSF cell count, cytology	None usually indicated
Brain tumors	(None usually indicated except in case of suspected teratoma: serum and CSF α-fetoprotein, β-human chorionic gonadotropin, carcinoembryonic antigen)	CT of head (with/without contrast) or spine MRI of head with gadolinium
Lymphoma	Bone marrow aspirate and biopsy CSF cell count and cytology Serum LDH ESR	Gallium scan CT chest, abdomen, pelvis Lymphangiography (in some centers)
Neuroblastoma	Serum ferritin CBC with platelet count Serum electrolytes, liver and renal panel Serum LDH Bone marrow aspirate and biopsy	CT or MRI of primary tumor site CT of chest, abdomen, pelvis, (+/head) with contrast Bone scan MIBG scan
Rhabdomyosarcoma	CBC with platelet count Liver and renal panel Bone marrow aspirate and biopsy CSF cell count and cytology (head and neck primary tumors only)	CT or MRI of primary tumor site CT of chest, abdomen, pelvis Bone scan
Wilms' tumor		CT of primary tumor site Ultrasound of inferior vena cava CT of chest Bone scan
Ewing's sarcoma	ESR CBC with platelet count Bone marrow aspirate and biopsy Serum LDH	CT or MRI of primary tumor site CT of chest Bone scan
Osteosarcoma		MRI of primary tumor site CT of chest Bone scan

Abbreviations: CBC, complete blood count; PT, prothrombin time; PTT, partial thromboplastin time; BUN, blood urea nitrogen; CSF, cerebrospinal fluid; CT, computed tomography; LDH, lactate dehydrogenase; MRI, magnetic resonance imaging; ESR, erythrocyte sedimentation rate; MIBG, metaiobenzylguanidine.

pathology specimens before the initiation of therapy. In less emergent situations, children with suspected malignancies should, when at all possible, be referred to an experienced pediatric surgeon for evaluation of biopsy versus surgery.

MANAGEMENT

Because the management of malignancies in children is a large topic, this discussion will touch on basic principles of oncologic management in pediatrics.

Four basic therapeutic modalities for the treatment of malignant disease are available; these are **surgery, chemotherapy, radiation therapy,** and **bone marrow transplantation.** Depending on the particular diagnosis, children with malignancies may require treatment with one or more of these modalities, singly or in combination. The reader should refer to a textbook on pediatric oncology to obtain further details concerning "standard of care" treatments for individual tumor types.

The surgeon should utilize the best surgical approach to minimize "tumor spill" and should be familiar with any intraoperative sampling requirements that may be necessary to stage the cancer adequately for further adjuvant therapy postoperatively (e.g., lymph node sampling in neuroblastoma). In addition, in some situations (e.g., a hepatoblastoma that is initially unresectable), an initial biopsy is the appropriate management. Chemotherapy to shrink the tumor to a point at which complete surgical resection is possible should follow.

If the index of suspicion for malignancy is very high, affected children should be transferred to a pediatric cancer center if possible. Optimal outcome depends on several factors: **correct pathologic diagnosis; careful medical management,** including administration of chemotherapy and monitoring of side effects; **precision customization of radiation fields** if radiation therapy is necessary; **optimal surgical resection,** if indicated; and **therapeutic ability and experience** with administration of treatment to small children. Centers that specialize in the treatment of pediatric cancer are experienced in the diagnosis and treatment of rare malignancies and are thus best equipped to treat affected children.

In the interest of cost-containment and convenience as well as children's well-being, it is often more feasible for children to be closer to home between chemotherapy cycles. Primary care physicians should be familiar with the management of various infectious complications to which children undergoing cancer therapy are prone.

Fever in children with neutropenia (absolute neutrophil count $< 500/cm^3$) requires a different therapeutic approach than fever in otherwise normal children. Until proven otherwise, children with fever and neutropenia (usually induced by chemotherapy, sometimes in combination with radiation therapy) must be assumed to have a serious bacterial infection. They should be treated accordingly, with hospitalization, intravenous antibiotics, thorough examination for site of infection and careful hemodynamic monitoring. Initial treatment consists of antibiotic coverage for *Staphylococcus au-*

reus, gram-negative enteric organisms, and *Pseudomonas aeruginosa* (e.g., ceftazidime with or without gentamicin). Additional coverage for anaerobic infection (e.g., mucositis), viral infection (e.g., herpes stomatitis, varicella) and other pathogens (e.g., fungi) depends on clinical findings.

The placement of indwelling venous catheters has revolutionized cancer therapy in pediatrics, making frequent venous access for both diagnostic and therapeutic purposes more easily tolerated by children. Broviac, Hickman, and Port-A-Caths, some of the indwelling catheters used by pediatric oncologists, are all associated with a finite incidence of catheter infections, which can result either from contamination of blood (line infections) or infections around the catheter site itself (tunnel infection). *Staphylococcus epidermidis* and *S. aureus,* the pathogens generally involved in catheter-related infections, can sometimes be cultured from blood drawn from the line; these infections are usually treatable with intravenous vancomycin. Immediate catheter removal with additional antibiotic or antifungal treatment should be performed if a blood culture from

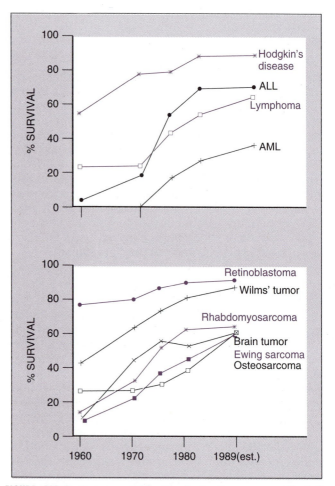

FIGURE 105–3. *Cancer-specific trends in five-year survival for children less than the age of 15 years.* ALL, acute lymphoblastic leukemia; AML, acute myeloblastic leukemia. (Reproduced, with permission, from Pizzo, P.C., and D.A. Pollack. Principles and Practice of Pediatric Oncology. Philadelphia, J.B. Lippincott, 1993, p. 9, Surveillance, Epidemiology and End Results Program, and the National Cancer Institute, NIH Publication No. 91-2789, Bethesda, MD, 1991.)

the line yields *P. aeruginosa* or *Candida* spp., or a tunnel infection is present.

PROGNOSIS

The prognosis for children with all forms of cancer has steadily improved during the last 30 years. Many children can expect to be cured, with minimum long-term side effects in many cases. Figure 105–3 shows the improvement in overall survival of children less than age 15 years with cancer. This increased survival affects the natural history of these diseases; some children develop second malignancies after completion of therapy for the primary disorder. Contributing factors to the development of another malignancy include the carcinogenic effects of treatment, such as chemotherapy and radiation therapy (e.g., the development of AML in patients cured of Hodgkin's disease) and the inheritance of mutant tumor suppressor genes (e.g., Li-Fraumeni's syndrome, familial retinoblastoma) that predispose certain tissues to develop tumors. Continued surveillance of children at known risk should help to optimize a favorable outcome.

Case Resolution

In the case history, the boy undergoes a mediastinoscopic biopsy of the mediastinal mass, which reveals lymphobastic lymphoma. No evidence of disease in the bone marrow or spinal fluid is present, which would indicate a worse prognosis. Treatment involves chemotherapy, and the prognosis is quite good. Symptoms of SVC due to obstruction from the tumor resolve with shrinkage of the tumor secondary to therapy.

Selected Readings

Brodeur, A. E., and G. M. Brodeur. Abdominal masses in children: neuroblastoma, Wilms' tumor, and other considerations. Pediatr. Rev. 12:196–206, 1991.

Donaldson, S. S., and M. P. Link. Hodgkin's disease: treatment of the young child. Pediatr. Clin. North Am. 38:457–474, 1991.

Friedman, H. S., M. E. Horowitz, and W. J. Oakes. Tumors of the central nervous system: improvement in outcome through a multimodality approach. Pediatr. Clin. North Am. 38:381–392, 1991.

Lamkin, B. C., et al. Biologic characteristics and treatment of acute nonlymphocytic leukemia in children. Pediatr. Clin. North Am. 35:743–764, 1988.

Pizzo, P. A. Cancer and the pediatrician: an evolving partnership. Pediatr. Rev. 12:5–6, 1990.

Pizzo, P. A., et al. The child with cancer and infection. I. Empiric therapy for fever and neutropenia, and preventive strategies. J. Pediatr. 119:679–694, 1991.

Poplack, D. G. Acute lymphoblastic leukemia. *In* Pizzo, P. A., and D. G. Poplack (eds.). Principles and Practice of Pediatric Oncology, 2nd ed. Philadelphia, J. B. Lippincott, 1993, pp. 431–483.

C H A P T E R   1 0 6

PEDIATRIC HIV

Carol D. Berkowitz, M.D.

Hx   A 6-month-old girl who was born to a substance-abusing mother is brought in by the maternal grandmother for increasing respiratory distress of two days' duration. The infant has had poor growth, two ear infections, and thrush, which has not responded to treatment with nystatin. On physical examination, the weight is at the tenth percentile, and the length is at the 25th percentile. Thrush is apparent in the mouth, and rales are found in the lungs. The infant is hypoxic, with a pulse oximeter reading of 85%. A chest x-ray reveals diffuse alveolar filling.

Questions

1. What are the risk factors for HIV infection in children?
2. What are the pitfalls associated with diagnosing HIV infection in children?
3. What are the usual manifestations of HIV infection in children?
4. What methods are available for treatment of HIV infection in children?

Human immunodeficiency virus (HIV) may produce a chronic, progressive disease. In the United States, nearly 30,000 children under the age of 13 years are infected. In recent years, early detection of the infection through the use of serologic testing of pregnant women and young infants has resulted in a greater role for involvement of primary care physicians. Subspecialists, such as immunologists and infectious disease experts, are available for consultation, but primary care physi-

TABLE 106–1. Acquisition of Human Immunodeficiency Virus Infection in Children

Infants and Children

Vertical transmission
    Maternal intravenous drug abuse
    Maternal sexual activity
    Maternal transfusion
Transfusion
Breast-feeding
Sexual abuse

Adolescents

Sexual activity
Intravenous drug abuse
Transfusion

cians are responsible for the routine health care of many HIV-infected infants.

Although some children who are HIV-infected may be asymptomatic and their infection may be detected by serologic testing, others may present with an assortment of medical problems related to the HIV infection. HIV infection is protean in its manifestations and may be mistaken for many other illnesses. It is important for physicians to be aware of the prevalence of HIV infection in their geographic location to help assess the patients' potential risk.

EPIDEMIOLOGY

Pediatric HIV, which is defined as infection between birth and 13 years, accounts for 2% of the total number of cases of HIV infection in the United States. Seventy-five percent of pediatric HIV cases involve minority populations, particularly African-American and Hispanic groups. In addition, approximately 75% of the cases come from specific geographic areas, namely New York, New Jersey, Florida, California, and Puerto Rico.

In over 80% of the pediatric cases, transmission has been vertical (Table 106–1). Children have acquired the infection from HIV-infected mothers. The overall rate of vertical transmission is estimated to be about 25 to 30% in the United States. This rate varies geographically. In Scandinavia, it is reported to be 15%, whereas in Africa, it is reported to be as high as 40%.

Intravenous drug abuse, sexual activity with intravenous drug abusers, or any high-risk sexual behavior are risk factors for HIV infection in females. It is estimated that about one-third of infected women have acquired the infection through heterosexual contact with HIV-infected males. In addition, up to one-third of mothers in some areas in the United States have acquired HIV through blood transfusion.

Mother-infant transmission may occur at three different times: (1) in utero, (2) at birth, or (3) during breast-feeding. Transmission at the time of birth involves exposure of infants to maternal genital secretions or blood. Studies to assess the impact of cesarean section have not documented a lower rate of transmission in infants delivered by this method. Zidovudine treatment of mothers during pregnancy and at the time of delivery and of their infants after birth reduces the rate of transmission. Transmission during breast-

feeding occurs because breast milk is rich in lymphocytes, which may contain viral particles.

In approximately 20% of cases, children have been infected with HIV as a result of transfusion, either for hemophilia or for other conditions. Prior to 1985, blood was not screened routinely for the presence of HIV. In countries where routine screening does not occur, children as well as adults may be infected through transfusions.

Children may also acquire HIV if they are the victims of sexual abuse by infected perpetrators. Adolescents acquire HIV infection in a manner similar to adults (i.e., homosexual or heterosexual activity, intravenous drug abuse, transfusion).

CLINICAL PRESENTATION

Following infection with the HIV virus, usually within four to six weeks of exposure, patients experience a flulike illness, with fever and myalgia. These symptoms are often attributed to influenza. Patients regain a sense of well-being within several days, and further symptoms of HIV infection may not appear for many years.

Children who are infected with HIV may present with an assortment of symptoms, depending on their age and method of acquisition of the virus (D$_x$ Box). Children often develop recurrent bacterial infections, including sepsis, meningitis, and recurrent otitis media. These illnesses are similar to those in non–HIV-infected children, but symptoms tend to be more severe, last longer, and recur more frequently. HIV-infected infants not under treatment may also present with FTT, which reportedly affects 50 to 90% of infants infected with HIV. The etiology of the impaired growth is unclear but appears to relate to decreased nutrition and increased caloric needs.

Other symptoms include infection with opportunistic organisms such as *Candida* (recurrent thrush) or *Pneumocystis carinii*. Almost any organ system can be affected in HIV-infected children, and other presenting

D$_x$ Pediatric HIV

- Recurrent bacterial infections
- Opportunistic infections (thrush, *P. carinii*)
- Anemia
- Thrombocytopenia
- Neutropenia
- Failure to thrive
- Diarrhea
- Wasting
- Fever
- Lymphadenopathy
- Parotitis
- Lymphoid interstitial pneumonia
- Hepatosplenomegaly
- Xeroderma
- Neurodevelopmental abnormalities
- Malignancies

problems include anemia, thrombocytopenia, lymphad-enopathy, hepatosplenomegaly, and tumors.

PATHOPHYSIOLOGY

HIV, an RNA retrovirus, synthesizes DNA through reverse transcription after cell invasion. HIV attaches to receptors on CD4 cells and other cells (e.g., mono-cytes, microglia cells). Following attachment, the viral envelope glycoprotein, gp120, interacts with a cell receptor. This then leads to cell invasion and ultimately cell death. By invading CD4 cells, HIV diminishes CD4 cell numbers. CD4 cells are important for cell-mediated immune function, and a reduction in their number makes patients particularly susceptible to infection with a host of organisms. Invasion of the microglia cells in the brain results in impaired neurologic function. Any body organ can be infected. Infection of the heart leads to the development of cardiomyopathy, and infection of the kidneys results in symptoms of ne-phritis.

DIFFERENTIAL DIAGNOSIS

The presence of repeated bacterial infections or certain other infections should suggest the need for an assessment for HIV. HIV-infected children are prone to **bacterial illnesses** caused by common pathogens such as *Streptococcus pneumoniae*. In addition, these children are also susceptible to opportunistic infec-tions. **P. carinii pneumonia (PCP)** is the most common opportunistic infection. Additional organisms causing opportunistic infections include *Candida,* particularly of the esophagus and lower respiratory tract; *Crypto-sporidium,* causing a chronic, watery diarrhea; CMV, although this is not uncommon in non–HIV-infected children under the age of six months; and *Mycobac-terium,* involving both *M. tuberculosis* and *M. avium intracellulare. M. avium intracellulare,* which usually develops late in the course of HIV infection, results in anemia, fever, and diarrhea.

HIV-infected children may also develop **lymphoid interstitial pneumonia (LIP).** This disorder involves the appearance of multiple nodule-like lesions throughout the lungs. Biopsy of these lesions demonstrates the presence of lymphocytes. Although affected children may be relatively asymptomatic, they may experience hypoxia, cough, and occasional wheezing. An associa-tion between LIP and parotitis appears to exist. Parotid enlargement is reported in about 15% of children infected with HIV. X-ray as well as laboratory evalua-tions reveal differences between LIP and PCP. Children with PCP are more symptomatic and often experience acute respiratory distress.

Some presenting complaints are directly related to the HIV infection. Such conditions include hematologic dis-orders, such as anemia, neutropenia, and throm-bocytopenia; skin problems, including dry and itchy skin; and developmental delay, or loss of milestones. Malignancies, particularly lymphoma, may develop. However, malignancies are much less common in chil-dren than in adults.

Questions: Pediatric HIV

- What types of infections has the child had in the past?
- How frequent were these infections?
- How did the child respond to medications? Did the infections resolve rapidly?
- What organs and organ systems were involved in these infections?
- Besides the infections, is the child ill in any other way?
- Has the child's development been normal?
- Did the child acquire the infection from the mother? What are her risk factors?
- Has the child ever had a blood transfusion?
- Is the child now taking any medications?
- Has the child received any immunizations?

HIV-infected children are categorized according to both their clinical and their immunologic status. Immu-nologic categories include no evidence of suppression, evidence of moderate suppression, and evidence of severe suppression, based on levels of CD4 cells. Similarly, clinical categories for signs and symptoms are none, mild, moderate, and severe. Asymptomatic chil-dren under the age of 18 months may have an indeter-minate infection because their antibodies have been passively acquired from their infected mother.

EVALUATION

History

Infants or children who present with signs or symp-toms of HIV infection should be evaluated for risk factors, including maternal factors (see Table 106–1), prior transfusion, or the possibility of sexual abuse. In addition, adolescents should be assessed for high-risk behavior, including unprotected sexual intercourse and intravenous drug abuse. A complete medical history should be obtained in all children and adolescents who may be infected with HIV (Questions Box).

The health status of parents should also be ascer-tained, especially if children have acquired the infection vertically. Parents who are ill may have a difficult time tending to the needs of infected children.

Physical Examination

A complete physical examination should be per-formed. Growth parameters should be plotted on a growth curve, and children's nutritional status should be assessed.

The extent and location of any lymphadenopathy and the presence of organomegaly should be noted. Evi-dence of infection, including thrush and otitis media, should be determined. The lungs should be carefully examined for the presence of abnormal breath sounds such as rales or wheezes.

Laboratory Tests

The laboratory evaluation includes the determination of whether patients have HIV antibodies. Such testing is done using an ELISA assay. If the assay is positive, a Western blot test is routinely done. A positive Western blot is evidence of HIV infection in children over the age of 18 months.

Diagnosis of HIV in infants under 18 months of age has been problematic because antibodies to HIV are transplacentally acquired from the mother. Thus the presence of a positive HIV test in these young children does not necessarily mean they are infected. Other assays have been developed for evaluating HIV in infants. These include determining the presence of IgA anti-HIV antibodies, which usually appear between three to six months of age in infected infants; determining the positivity of PCR testing; looking at immune complex-dissociated p24 antigen, and obtaining cocultures for HIV. These tests are expensive and not readily available, but if positive on two separate occasions, they are indicative of true infection.

To help evaluate the HIV status of patients, the number of CD4 cells should be determined. Table 106–2 lists the normal CD4 cell numbers by age. It is important to note that children maintain higher levels of CD4 cells than adults. In addition, CD8 cell levels should be assessed, and the CD4:CD8 cell ratio should be determined. These values are used as indicators for antiviral therapy and *Pneumocystis* prophylaxis. Periodic reassessment of CD4 and CD8 cells, liver function studies, and complete blood counts is recommended to monitor disease progression.

Another useful laboratory test in HIV-infected children is the quantitative immunoglobulin assay. Circulating gamma globulin is markedly elevated, reflecting abnormal B cell activity. The gamma globulin is often not specific and not functional, and children may fail to develop specific antibodies in response to vaccines or infections, an important consideration when determining a management plan.

If symptoms of infection, such as fever, otorrhea, and dysuria, are present, appropriate specimens (e.g., blood, ear, urine) for culture should be collected. Blood cultures should be obtained if fever without a known source is present. Specimens should also be submitted for opportunistic pathogens such as *P. carinii* if pulmonary symptoms are present.

Evidence of organ impairment may be noted by other laboratory tests. HIV-positive children are often anemic and have mildly decreased platelet levels. They should be evaluated with a CBC and platelet count. Neurodevelopmental testing should be used to determine children's neurologic status as well as their developmental level.

TABLE 106–2. CD4 Cell Numbers (cells/mL) by Age in Children

Age	Normal Level (mean)	Critical Level (Antiretroviral therapy)	Critical Level (PCP prophylaxis)
0–1 yr	3200	< 1750	< 1500
1–2 yr	2500	< 1000	< 750
2–6 yr	1700	< 750	< 500
> 6 yr	1000	< 500	< 200

Abbreviations: PCP, *Pneumocystis carinii* pneumonia.

Imaging Studies

If impairment in the neurodevelopmental level is apparent, children should be evaluated using CT scanning or MRI, which may show cerebral atrophy and calcification of the basal ganglia as well as ventriculomegaly. Chest x-rays should be obtained in children who are experiencing pulmonary symptoms. These x-rays may show evidence of LIP, with a diffuse nodular pattern, or evidence of PCP, as demonstrated by marked alveolar filling.

MANAGEMENT

The management of children who are infected with HIV has several components. Key to appropriate management is delivery of **routine well child care,** particularly immunizations. HIV-infected children can receive their routine immunizations except for oral polio vaccine. Children with HIV should be immunized with an inactive polio vaccine to make certain that they are not infected by the vaccine strain of polio, which can revert in the gastrointestinal tract to a more virulent strain. HIV-infected children should receive influenza vaccine, once they are older than six months of age, and pneumococcal vaccine, once they are over the age of two years.

Antiretroviral therapy may be used. The decision to begin therapy with zidovudine is usually determined by the level of CD4 cells or the presence of significant disease. Zidovudine therapy is presently given at 180 mg/m²/day, divided into four doses. Other therapies include didanosine (DDI), which is approved for use in children, particularly those who cannot tolerate zidovudine or those who have zidovudine-resistant HIV. Zalcitabine (DDC) is presently not approved for use in children. Additional drugs, such as Stavudine (d4T) and Lamivudine (3TC), are currently under investigation.

In addition to antiretroviral therapy, children should also receive **prophylaxis for *Pneumocystis* infection,** which may improve the quality of life and help prolong survival. The decision to institute prophylaxis is determined by the CD4 cell count or the presence of *Pneumocystis*. Trimethoprim-sulfamethoxazole is the mainstay of therapy. Other medications (e.g., pentamidine or dapsone) are used in children who do not tolerate the trimethoprim-sulfamethoxazole.

Intravenous gamma globulin is used in some patients, particularly those who appear to have recurrent bacterial infections or those who fail to mount specific antibody responses to antigens. Infants should be monitored with CD4 cell counts at one month, two months, and six months, and then every three months thereafter. Infections should be managed with the appropriate antibiotic therapy. Children who develop anemia may require transfusion or erythropoietin, and those who develop neutropenia from disease or zidovudine may need granulocyte-stimulating factor.

The nutritional needs of children should be met. This may require the use of supplemental agents (see Chapter 98, Failure to Thrive). In addition, children's emotional and social needs should be addressed. Society still stigmatizes HIV-infected individuals. HIV-infected children are frequently cautioned against disclosing their HIV status to their friends, which may make them feel isolated from their peers. This isolation can be lessened by involving these children in groups or camps with other HIV-infected children. If well enough, HIV-infected children should attend regular school. Federal law prohibits discrimination on the basis of handicapping conditions. Some HIV-infected children are in foster care, which raises other concerns about the emotional strain on the foster parents. Both foster parents and biologic parents who care for HIV-infected children should also be encouraged to join support groups.

PROGNOSIS

The prognosis for children who are infected with HIV is not as bleak as initially indicated, when reports noted that survival was related to symptoms at the time of presentation. With some conditions, such as PCP, postdiagnosis survival was as short as one month. Most infants were symptomatic by two years and died by age six years. Vertically infected children appear to fit into three categories: rapid progressors (onset of disease within a few months of birth), long-term nonprogressors (alive and relatively well eight or more years after birth), and children who lie somewhere between these two groups. Present studies are evaluating nonprogressors to help understand the factors that allow these individuals to stay healthy.

Case Resolution

The infant in the case history has recurrent thrush and has had two episodes of otitis. The past history of maternal

substance abuse is a risk factor for HIV. The acute symptoms suggest an acute respiratory infection, and the x-ray findings of diffuse alveolar filling are consistent with *P. carinii* infection. The infant should be admitted to the hospital. Aggressive antiretroviral and antipneumocystis therapy must be instituted immediately to ensure a good outcome. The hypoxia should also be managed with oxygen administration.

Selected Readings

Centers for Disease Control and Prevention; 1994 revised classification system for human immunodeficiency virus infection in children less than 13 years of age. M.M.W.R. 43:1–11, 1994.

Connor, E. M., et al. Reduction of maternal-infant transmission of human immunodeficiency virus type 1 with zidovudine treatment. N. Engl. J. Med. 331:1173–1180, 1994.

McKinney, R. E., and C. M. Wilfert. Treatment of pediatric HIV infection. HIV Adv. Res. Ther. 4:22–29, 1994.

Mofenson, L. M. A critcal review of studies evaluating the relationship of mode of delivery to perinatal transmission of human immunodeficiency virus. Pediatr. Infect. Dis. J. 14:169–176, 1995.

Oleske, J. M. The many needs of the HIV-infected child. Hosp. Pract. 29:63–69, 1994.

Pizzo, P. A., and C. M. Wilfert (eds.). Pediatric AIDS. Baltimore, Williams & Wilkins, 1991.

Rand, T. H., and A. Meyers. Role of the general pediatrician in the management of human immunodeficiency virus infection in children. Pediatr. Rev. 14:371–379, 1993.

Spector, S. A., et al. A controlled trial of intravenous immune globulin for the prevention of serious bacterial infections in children receiving zidovudine for advanced human immunodeficiency virus infection. N. Engl. J. Med. 331:1181–1187, 1994.

Wiznia, A. A., et al. Virlogic, immunologic, and clinical evaluation of human immunodeficiency virus antibody status of symptom-free children born to infected mothers. J. Pediatr. 125:352–355, 1994.

CHAPTER 107

CHRONIC RENAL FAILURE[1]

Isidro B. Salusky, M.D.

Cheryl P. Sanchez, M.D.

Hx A 6-year-old boy has recently been diagnosed with chronic renal failure. He was healthy until age five, when his pediatrician noted that he was falling off his growth curve. His past history is remarkable for recurrent UTIs, polyuria, and intermittent enuresis. His appetite has remained fair, but his activity level has significantly decreased over the last few months.

Physical examination reveals his height and weight to be less than the fifth percentile for age and his blood pressure more than the 95th percentile for age. His color is pale. He is small and looks younger than his chronological age (six years). When the boy walks, he appears to have "knock knees."

[1]Acknowledgment: This work has been partially supported by U.S. Public Health Service grants DK-35423 and RR-00865 and the Casey Lee Ball Foundation.

Questions

1. What laboratory studies should be obtained during the initial assessment of children with CRF?
2. To pinpoint the etiologic cause of CRF, what additional diagnostic tests are needed?
3. What is the appropriate management for children with CRF?

Chronic renal failure (CRF) is defined as the irreversible reduction in glomerular filtration rate (GFR) to below 25% of normal for more than three months. Because advances in the management of CRF have occurred in the past decade, the early recognition of children with the disease is important. The signs and symptoms of CRF in the pediatric population are nonspecific, and therefore it is important that the primary medical caretaker, usually the pediatrician or family practitioner, recognize the earliest signs and symptoms and institute proper medical care. Prompt referral to a pediatric nephrologist must be made, and concomitant, close follow-up by both physicians should be performed for the optimal management of children with CRF.

EPIDEMIOLOGY

It is difficult to determine the true incidence of CRF in children because estimates are based on the number of children accepted for dialysis and renal transplantation. Some children do not require dialysis or renal transplantation until adulthood, so this underestimates the true incidence. Based on these figures, the incidence of CRF is about 0–2 per million total population in infants and about 1–5 per million total population in children and adolescents.

The incidence various considerably in children of different age groups in different geographic locations. In younger children (0–5 years), the incidence of congenital urinary tract malformations predominantly affects boys. Chronic glomerulonephritis and pyelonephritis are primarily seen in older children. Some geographic locations exhibit a preponderance of certain renal diseases (e.g., congenital nephrotic syndrome in Finland, hemolytic-uremic syndrome in Argentina).

CLINICAL PRESENTATION

Children with CRF are often asymptomatic, and the abnormality is detected during routine examination or screening. A small percentage of these children are "accidentally" discovered when they present with another illness. Patients may be referred to the physician because of growth retardation, hypertension, or anemia (D_x Box). It is also not uncommon to uncover the presence of ureteral reflux or recurrent UTIs. Children may complain of vague symptoms, including malaise, anorexia, and vomiting, which may be associated with advanced renal failure. At present, children do not usually develop advanced kidney disease without previous medical contact.

Growth Failure

About half of children with CRF are below the fifth percentile in height for age, particularly if renal insufficiency began during the first two years of life. FTT is by far one of the most frequent clinical presentations of children afflicted with CRF. Maximum growth occurs during the early years in life, and children with congenital renal problems are most affected (see Chapter 98, Failure to Thrive). In addition, affected children frequently present with anorexia, feeding difficulties, and vomiting. Sexual development is often delayed in children with CRF.

Anemia

The anemia of CRF is normochromic and normocytic. Anemia is frequently accompanied by decreased serum iron levels, increased total iron binding capacity, and low reticulocyte counts. Insufficient production of erythropoietin has been demonstrated to occur when the GFR is below 30 mL/min/1.73 m^2. Bleeding becomes a major problem in uremic patients because of platelet dysfunction (see Chapter 58, Bleeding Disorders).

Electrolyte and Metabolic Abnormalities

Children with advanced renal failure usually have impaired sodium excretion leading to water retention, edema, and hypertension. In patients with congenital renal problems such as obstructive uropathy and dysplasia/hypoplasia, salt-wasting may be a prominent feature.

Water balance may be a problem for children with CRF. Hyperkalemia is not an unusual component of CRF, and it becomes evident when the GFR is below 10 mL/min/1.73 m^2. Hypokalemia is a less common problem and could be secondary to excessive use of diuretics or strict dietary restriction.

As renal function deteriorates below 50%, metabolic acidosis ensues. The acidosis of CRF, irrespective of etiology, is mainly due to the overall decrease of ammonia excretion. Bicarbonate wasting may be a prominent feature in patients with renal tubular acidosis, particularly Fanconi's syndrome.

Glucose intolerance may also be a prominent feature of CRF even though insulin levels are elevated.

Both cholesterol and triglyceride levels may be elevated in children with CRF. The characteristic plasma lipid abnormality is a moderate hypertriglyceridemia. More than 50% of children develop hyperlipidemia by the time they have end-stage renal disease.

D$_x$ Chronic Renal Failure

- Growth retardation/growth failure
- Anemia
- Bone disease
- Metabolic acidosis

Renal Osteodystrophy

The development of bone disease is present in all patients with progressive renal insufficiency. The primary clinical indicators are growth retardation and skeletal deformities, including genu valgum, ulnar deviation of the hands, pes varus, and less commonly, limping secondary to slippage of the capital femoral epiphysis.

Hypertension

The incidence of hypertension in pediatric patients with CRF varies from 38 to 78%. An acute rise in blood pressure usually results in seizures in children. Other clinical manifestations may include headache, congestive heart failure (CHF), palsies, and not uncommonly, intracerebral hemorrhage.

Cardiac Dysfunction

CHF may be a prominent finding in children with fluid overload, uncontrollable hypertension, or uremic cardiomyopathy.

Neurologic Dysfunction

Children with CRF may have impaired neurodevelopment. Memory deficits, lack of concentration, depression, and weakness may occur. In smaller children, microcephaly, hypotonia, and lack of maturation on EEG may be apparent. Research has shown that the degree of neurologic delay is related to the severity of renal impairment and the age of the child. Younger children (< 6 years) are more affected because significant brain growth and maturation occur during the early years in life. Children who are severely uremic may suffer from global developmental retardation and seizures. Unless neurodevelopmental delays are recognized promptly and intervention is begun early, problems are most often progressive.

PATHOPHYSIOLOGY

The steady decline in the capacity of the kidney to perform its excretory and endocrine functions is caused by the progressive loss of nephrons. The body is unable to excrete water and electrolytes; it retains "uremic toxins," leading to clinical symptoms of uremia; and it is incapable of producing erythropoietin and 1,25-dihydroxyvitamin D.

Inadequate nutrition, metabolic acidosis, renal osteodystrophy, and (currently) insensitivity to growth hormone may lead to growth retardation in children with CRF. Although the serum levels of growth hormone are normal, several studies have documented decreased production of insulin-like growth factor 1 (IGF-1) and accumulation of its binding protein, resulting in reduced levels of unbound IGF-1.

Metabolic abnormalities, including metabolic acidosis, develop once the kidney is unable to excrete nitrogenous wastes. In addition, fluid and electrolyte imbalance, most notably hyperkalemia, may accompany this problem. Excessive fluid and salt accumulation and increased production of renin secondary to a poorly functioning kidney usually lead to severe hypertension that requires immediate intervention. Prolonged hypertension and chronic fluid overload contribute to the development of cardiac dysfunction.

Various uremic toxins have been identified (e.g., parathyroid hormone [PTH]) that may be responsible for the clinical manifestations of uremia. No specific cause has been found for impaired neurodevelopment; previously, this was attributed to aluminum toxicity because of the widespread use of aluminum as phosphate binders. Aluminum has been replaced by calcium in the past decade, but the developmental delay continues.

Delays in sexual development are also encountered in adolescents. This problem has been ascribed to several factors, including primary gonadal dysfunction, insufficient production of gonadal steroids associated with pituitary dysfunction, and elevated gonadotropin concentration. In addition, pulsatile hormone secretion is frequently impaired in these children.

Several closely interrelated factors, including phosphorus retention, decreased production of 1,25-dihydroxyvitamin D (calcitriol), abnormal parathyroid gland function, and hypocalcemia, result in renal osteodystrophy. Phosphorus retention coupled with inadequate diet restriction lead to elevated phosphorus levels, hypocalcemia, and increased serum PTH levels. Furthermore, the diseased kidney is incapable of producing 1,25-dihydroxyvitamin D, which is the active component of vitamin D necessary for bone regulation. More recently, skeletal resistance to PTH has been described. These factors all contribute to the development of a condition called secondary hyperparathyroidism. With the advent of the radioimmunoassay to measure the intact PTH and the availability of calcitriol, the diagnosis and management of patients with secondary hyperparathyroidism have changed in the past 10 years.

In addition to the problems with 1,25-dihydroxyvitamin D production, decreased erythropoietin production leads to the development of anemia.

DIFFERENTIAL DIAGNOSIS

First-time CRF must be differentiated from acute renal failure. Children with CRF usually present with growth retardation and radiologic and clinical evidence of renal osteodystrophy. Renal ultrasound usually reveals small, shrunken kidneys, which reflect the chronicity of the kidney problem. Anemia, hypertension, and fluid and electrolyte abnormalities are seen in children who present with acute renal failure.

A variety of kidney problems, whether congenital, hereditary, acquired, or metabolic, may result in CRF. In infants and young children, congenital and anatomic malformations account for the largest percentage of patients who progress to CRF; more than half of these patients require kidney transplantation. These conditions include hypoplastic/dysplastic kidneys, obstructive uropathy, and reflux nephropathy. The hereditary diseases most commonly encountered are hereditary nephritis (Alport's syndrome) and juvenile nephronophthisis. Acquired diseases such as chronic glomerulonephritis, membranoproliferative glomerulonephritis, and focal and segmental glomerulosclerosis affect a large percentage of older children who progress to CRF.

Even though specific cures for some of these renal conditions (e.g., renal dysplasia) may not be available, it is essential to perform a complete diagnostic workup to determine the exact etiology of the renal problem. Such information may identify the presence of an inherited problem that may require genetic counseling or suggest future kidney transplantation. Some renal diseases may recur in the renal allograft; parents and children must be informed early about this possibility in preparation for renal transplantation.

EVALUATION

It is of the utmost importance to differentiate between acute and chronic renal failure because management strategies for the two conditions may be different.

History

A thorough history must be obtained (Questions Box). A detailed family history is an essential part of the clinical evaluation, and it may provide an important clue to diagnosis.

Physical Examination

A complete physical examination is important. Blood pressure, using appropriate cuff size, must be taken by the primary physician. Any heart murmur and other abnormal heart sounds that may indicate pericardial involvement should be noted. Gross eye examination should be performed, including fundal evaluation, to assess for evidence of chronic hypertension. In addi-

tion, macular abnormalities and hearing problems may provide clues to an inheritable disease (e.g., Alport's syndrome). Any ear abnormalities (e.g., preauricular pits, ear tags) require special attention, because they are associated with some forms of renal disease (e.g., brachio-otorenal syndrome). Undescended testes may be evident in some children with urologic problems.

Laboratory Tests

Laboratory studies, including CBC, electrolytes, BUN, creatinine, and urinalysis, are important in the initial diagnostic workup (Fig. 107–1). Glomerulonephritides usually present with abnormal urinalyses; RBCs and WBCs are present along with a variety of urinary casts or enhanced urinary protein excretion. If nephrotic range proteinuria is suspected (protein excretion > 40 mg/kg/hour), a 24-hour urine protein collection may be indicated. In infants and very small children, however, a random urine protein-creatinine ratio greater than 0.2 is a good predictor of the magnitude of proteinuria: both methods are highly correlated. Immunologic studies, such as C3, C4, antinuclear antibody, and antidouble-stranded DNA, should be obtained if the renal disease suggests the presence of an immune complex–mediated nephritis (e.g., membranoproliferative disease, SLE, postinfectious glomerulonephritis).

Imaging Studies

Ultrasound is by far one of the best radiologic tools in the assessment of patients with CRF. Renal ultrasound yields important information (i.e., kidney size, echogenicity, presence of hydronephrosis) that may help establish the diagnosis of the renal problem. The presence of small kidneys compared to age controls usually indicates chronicity that may date back to fetal development. Increased echogenicity but normal size is associated with the presence of medical renal disease in more than 90% of cases (48%, tubulointerstitial disease; 30%, glomerular disease; 16%, end-stage renal disease; 6%, no detectable kidney disease).

Renal ultrasound does not yield much information in patients with recurrent UTIs unless the UTI has caused major parenchymal kidney disease. In patients with recurrent UTIs, a voiding cystoureterogram is indicated to diagnose vesicoureteral reflux and evaluate bladder anatomy and obstruction in the lower urinary tract. An IVP is seldom used, especially in very small infants, unless the upper urinary tract needs to be evaluated.

Renal nuclear studies have played a major role in the workup of patients with CRF. In general, however, they are not routinely done unless specifically indicated. Measurement of the GFR may be helpful but does not have a significant impact on the long-term management of children with CRF. GFR measurements can be performed using technetium-99m-DTPA, which yields an estimate of the GFR within 5% of the true value. In some centers, the newer Tc-99m-MAG3 is being used to evaluate effective renal plasma flow. More recently,

---

Questions: Chronic Renal Failure

- Does the child have a history of prolonged illness, pallor, weakness, vomiting, or loss of appetite?
- Does the child have any family members (immediate and distant) who have had kidney diseases (including hematuria, proteinuria, cysts in the kidney, recurrent UTIs, or urologic surgery)?
  - Have any family members ever been on dialysis or undergone kidney transplantation?
  - Do any family members have any ear/hearing or eye abnormalities?
  - Did the mother have any problems during the pregnancy (e.g., oligohydramnios, polyhydramnios)?
- What is the child's micturition history?
- Does the child have daytime or nighttime enuresis?
- Does the child have polyuria or polydipsia?
- What is the child's growth and developmental history (In relation to other siblings, friends, etc.)?
- What is the child's dietary history?
- Does the child have any headaches, visual problems, or hearing problems?

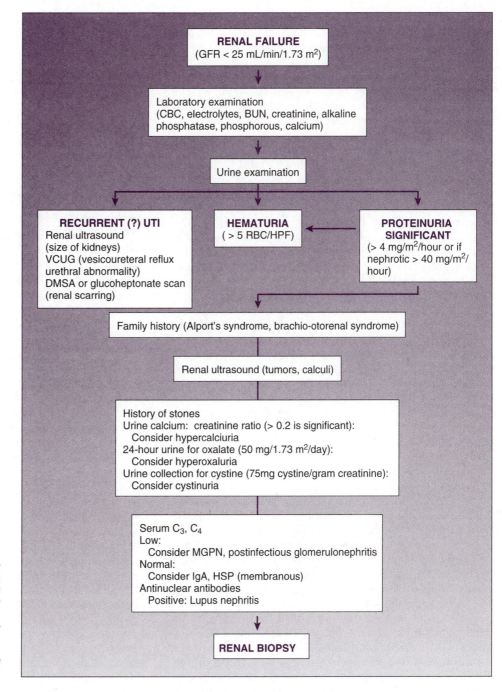

FIGURE 107–1. *Initial diagnostic workup of a pediatric patient with chronic renal failure. BUN, blood urea nitrogen; CBC, complete blood count; DMSA, dimercaptosuccinic acid; GFR, glomerular filtration rate; HSP, Henoch-Schönlein purpura; MPGN, membrano-proliferative glomerulonephritis; UTI, urinary tract infection; VCUG, voiding cystourethrogram.*

physicians have been using Tc-99m-DMSA to help in the assessment of renal parenchymal problems. Because this study provides an excellent image of the renal parenchyma, it has been used in the detection of renal scars in patients with a history of recurrent UTIs. Renal scars portend the development of hypertension later in life in the affected child.

MANAGEMENT

The management of children with CRF has improved over the last decade. Newer modes of therapy and early intervention have made tremendous improvement in the life-styles and psychological well-being of affected children.

Dietary management remains an important and challenging part of the overall treatment of patients with CRF. Frequently, anorectic patients require supplementation with fat, carbohydrate, or sometimes tube feedings. Children with CRF should receive the recommended daily allowance for protein and calories according to age and sex. Several ongoing investigations are studying the effects of protein restriction on the preservation of kidney function and its effect on growth in small children. Currently, restriction of dietary protein is not routinely implemented unless the patient has persistently elevated and rising BUN. Dietary controls should also be used to manage hypertension. A low-sodium diet must be imposed to avoid excessive water retention.

The use of **recombinant human growth hormone** (rhGH) in the last few years has revolutionized the management of stunted growth in patients with CRF. Growth velocity increases in patients undergoing treatment with rhGH.

In the 1990s, the use of **recombinant human erythropoietin** in children with CRF has become standard. The correction of anemia with this new mode of treatment results in improved appetite, physical activity, and sense of well-being, and more importantly, avoids the risks of blood transfusion. Prior to the availability of recombinant human erythropoietin, patients with severe anemia were given frequent RBC transfusions, thereby increasing the risk of infection, transfusion reaction, and development of antibodies.

Potassium excretion declines rapidly once the GFR starts to deteriorate. Initially, dietary intervention may be sufficient, but this becomes a problem in infants and small children because their diet is usually limited to formula and few solid foods. In these cases, patients may require **pharmacologic treatment** (i.e., diuretics, polystyrene sulfone) to help in the management of hyperkalemia. In instances of an acute rise in serum potassium level, emergency measures must be instituted (Table 107–1). Recently, it has been shown that intravenous and inhaled β_2-agonists (e.g., salbutamol) acutely decrease serum potassium by facilitating intracellular potassium uptake. If hyperkalemia becomes uncontrollable with medical management, dialysis must be performed immediately (Table 107–2).

The use of diuretics in children with CRF should be individualized. Indications include fluid overload and hyperkalemia (potassium-sparing diuretics should not be used). Diuretics should be avoided in patients with disturbed concentrating and diluting mechanisms because some of these children may have polyuria and would develop dehydration.

Medication should be started if hypertension is unresponsive to conservative management in patients with end-organ damage and those who are symptomatic. Drugs currently available include diuretics, angiotensin-converting enzyme (ACE) inhibitors, adrenergic blockers, adrenergic agonists, peripheral vasodilators, and calcium channel blockers. Treatment with ACE inhibitors has been shown to be beneficial in slowing kidney damage in patients with renal failure.

TABLE 107–1. Treatment of Hyperkalemia

Calcium gluconate, 0.5 mL/kg of 10% solution, or calcium chloride, 0.2 mL/kg of 10% solution (intravenous)

Sodium bicarbonate, 2 mEq/kg/dose (intravenous)

Glucose-insulin solution, 0.5 g/kg glucose with 0.25 units of insulin per gram of glucose (intravenous, monitor serum glucose closely)

Diuretics (do not use potassium-sparing diuretics): furosemide, 1 mg/kg/dose (intravenous)

Polystyrene sulfonate (Kayexalate), 1 g/kg/dose orally (if awake) or rectally

If unable to control using the above measures, start dialysis

---

TABLE 107–2. Indications for Initiation of Dialysis

Fluid overload
   Congestive heart failure
   Uncontrollable hypertension
Uremic neuropathy
   Paresthesia
Uncontrollable electrolyte abnormalities
   Intractable metabolic acidosis
   Hyperkalemia
Pericarditis
Severe renal osteodystrophy
   Metastatic calcification
   Severe skeletal deformities
Progressive malnutrition and severe growth retardation, especially in the first year of life
Severe anemia or bleeding diathesis

Caution must be observed in patients receiving ACE inhibitors who have solitary kidney and renal vascular stenosis because of the agent's propensity to decrease kidney function acutely. ACE inhibitors can also aggravate hyperkalemia. Diuretics are the drug of choice in patients with salt and water retention. In cases in which blood pressure is extremely elevated, calcium channel blockers (e.g., nifedipine) can be administered orally or sublingually because of their rapid onset of action. Clonidine is currently available in the form of transdermal patches, which are appropriate in patients with poor compliance with daily medications. Patients must be warned, however, of rebound hypertension and CNS side effects if the patch is removed abruptly.

Patients with long-standing hypertension must have regular echocardiograms to evaluate for left ventricular hypertrophy and serial ophthalmologic examination to follow eye-ground changes.

In the presence of these complications, aggressive fluid removal with diuretics and control of hypertension must be instituted. Pericarditis, on the other hand, is usually a manifestation of severe uremia that may require pericardiocentesis. In some instances, the lack of response to medical management may be used as additional criterion for the initiation of dialysis treatment.

Several studies are currently being performed to assess the effect of pharmacologic treatment on lipid and cholesterol abnormalities in patients with CRF.

Treatment with phosphate-binding agents and vitamin D sterols (e.g., calcitriol) are primarily used in the management of renal osteodystrophy. Dietary phosphorus restriction (i.e., 800 mg/day) should be reinforced but generally is not followed well in children because of unpalatability of food. Phosphate-binding medications, are therefore, an integral part in the management of hyperphosphatemia in children with renal failure. Aluminum-containing phosphate-binding agents are seldom used today because of the danger of aluminum toxicity. Precautions must also be taken in children who are concomitantly being treated with citrate-containing medications, because citrate enhances the absorption of aluminum, thus increasing the risk of aluminum intoxication.

Recent developments in the understanding of the interaction between vitamin D and PTH have led to new treatment modalities. Vitamin D in the form of calcitriol has been used more frequently over the last few years. Many investigators have demonstrated that intravenous and oral preparations given as intermittent or "pulse" therapy (2–3 times a week) markedly lower serum PTH levels and decrease the size of the parathyroid gland. The determination of the serum biochemical markers calcium, phosphorus, alkaline phosphatase, and serum PTH is required at regular intervals to monitor progression of disease or response to treatment.

PROGNOSIS

The prognosis of children with CRF has changed dramatically in the last decade. Options for dialysis (hemodialysis or peritoneal dialysis) and kidney transplantation (cadaveric or live-related) must be discussed prior to occurrence of end-stage renal disease. The current technical advances in dialysis have allowed the pediatric nephrologist to offer dialysis options to children of any age. These advances have made long-term survival possible while children await renal transplantation.

Kidney transplantation is the ultimate treatment for children with CRF. With the improvement in immunosuppression, survival of grafts in children has improved significantly. Full rehabilitation can be achieved after children have a successful renal transplant. Further studies utilizing new immunosuppressive regimens must be done to prevent the occurrence of acute and chronic rejection.

Case Resolution

In the case history presented at the beginning of this chapter, the initial evaluation of the young boy reveals anemia (hematocrit [25%]) low serum bicarbonate (17 mEq/L), slightly elevated creatinine (1.0 mg/dL), high serum phosphorus (> 7.0 mg/dL), and normal serum calcium. Diagnostic workup shows bilateral ureteral reflux, which is worse on the right side, and the presence of a small rim of kidney parenchyma on the right side.

Long-term management involves dietary intervention and treatment of the metabolic acidosis, anemia, hyperphosphatemia, and hypertension. Because the boy is young and severely growth retarded, growth hormone therapy must also be considered. In addition, he should also be on a prophylactic antibiotic for the ureteral reflux to prevent further UTIs and should be referred to a pediatric urologist.

Selected Readings

Drukker, A. Hypertension in children and adolescents with chronic renal failure and end-stage renal disease. Child. Nephrol. Urol. 11:152–158, 1991.

Fine, R. N. Recent advances in the management of the infant, child and adolescent with chronic renal failure. Pediatr. Rev. 11:277–282, 1990.

Fine, R. N., et al. Growth after rhGH treatment in children with chronic renal failure: report of a multicenter randomized double-blind placebo-controlled study. J. Pediatr. 11:146–151, 1994.

Foreman, J. W., and J. C. M. Chan. Chronic renal failure in infants and children. J. Pediatr. 113:793–800, 1988.

Geary, D. F., and K. Haka-Ikse. Neurodevelopmental progress of young children with chronic renal disease. Pediatrics 84:68–72, 1989.

Gusmano, R., and F. Perfumo. Worldwide demographic aspects of chronic renal failure in children. Kidney Int. 41:S31–S35, 1993.

Kist-van Holthe, J. E., et al. Protein restriction in chronic renal failure. Arch. Dis. Child. 68:371–375, 1993.

Liou, H. H., et al. Hypokalemic effects of intravenous infusion or nebulization of salbutamol in patients with chronic renal failure: Comparative study. Am. J. Kidney Dis. 23:266–271, 1994.

Salusky, I. B., J. A. Ramirez, and W. G. Goodman. Recent advances in the management of renal osteodystrophy in children. Curr. Opin. Nephrol. Hypertension 2:580–587, 1993.

Schaefer, F., O. Mehls, and E. Ritz. New insights into endocrine disturbances of chronic renal failure. Miner. Electrolyte Metab. 18:169–173, 1992.

CHAPTER 108

DIABETES MELLITUS

Helen DuPlessis, M.D., M.P.H.

H$_x$ A seven-year-old girl presents with a three-week history of nocturnal polyuria. Her mother reports that her daughter seems to have lost weight in the past two months although she has had a good appetite. Laboratory tests reveal that the girl's serum sodium level is 130 mEq/L; potassium, 3.2 mEq/L; glucose, 324 mg/dL; and 1+ ketones. Urinalysis reveals specific gravity of 1.025 and moderate glucose and ketones. Her physical examination is unremarkable.

Questions

1. What are the objectives of therapeutic interventions in children with IDDM?

2. What diagnostic evaluations constitute the ongoing assessment of children with IDDM?
3. What are the acute and chronic complications associated with IDDM?
4. Does "tight control" of glycemia influence these complications?

Insulin-dependent diabetes mellitus is the second most common chronic illness among children. The diagnosis rarely poses a serious challenge to health care providers, but adequate management of the medical, nutritional, emotional, and behavioral aspects of the disease, which are critical to improving patients' quality of life and preventing long-term complications, is a serious undertaking. In recent years, much progress has been made in understanding the pathogenesis, treatment, and outcomes associated with diabetes.

EPIDEMIOLOGY

Over 97% of cases of childhood diabetes are of the IDDM type. According to the World Health Organization Multinational Project for Diabetes, the incidence of IDDM among children under 15 years of age shows tremendous variation; the lowest rates are in Korea (0.6/100,000), and the highest are in Finland (35/100,000). The incidence in the United States is approximately 15/100,000, with the highest rate among Caucasian youths. The peak onset of IDDM is between 7 and 13 years of age. The disease affects boys and girls equally.

CLINICAL PRESENTATION

Children may initially present with a range of symptom severity. The classic triad of polydipsia, polyuria, and polyphagia may be elicited through careful assessment of patient history (D_x Box). Increased urinary frequency, manifested as nighttime polyuria or secondary enuresis, is the most consistent presenting complaint. Alterations in appetite and thirst are most commonly recognized when disease onset occurs in the preschool years (probably because parents are most able to monitor eating and drinking behaviors during the first few years of life). Weight loss is a variable finding. Ketoacidosis occurs in 10 to 40% of children

---

D_x Insulin-Dependent Diabetes Mellitus

- Polyuria, polydipsia, and polyphagia (with weight loss) together with a random plasma glucose of over 200 mg/dL
- Asymptomatic individuals must have an abnormal oral glucose tolerance test:
  - fasting plasma glucose of over 130 mg/dL *and*
  - peak plasma glucose of over 200 mg/dL (at some other time during the sample)

TABLE 108–1. Predictive Tests for Individuals Susceptible to IDDM*

Immunologic Marker(s)	Risk of Developing IDDM *(within 5 to 8 years)*
Islet cell antibodies (ICA)	25–70%
Insulin autoantibodies (IAA)	Variable (may not be specific to islet cell tissue)
Reduced first-phase insulin release (FPIR)	100%
ICA + IAA	90%
Human leukocyte antigen with index case	25–30%

*Individuals with first-degree relative with IDDM.

---

with IDDM and presents with vomiting, polyuria, dehydration, and Kussmaul respirations.

PATHOPHYSIOLOGY

The pancreatic beta cell destruction, which is the hallmark of IDDM, occurs as a function of genetic and environmental factors that are as yet not entirely understood. Over 90% of affected individuals carry either human leukocyte antigen DR3 or DR4. This information, along with studies of twins and other familial cases, indicates a clear genetic etiology, although the exact pattern of inheritance is unclear (Table 108–1).

Disordered immune function, in which some antigenic components of pancreatic islets cells are not recognized as self, appears to be the pathogenetic mechanism for the development of IDDM. It is generally believed that at least 90% of beta cell mass must be destroyed before problems with glycemic regulation are manifest. Endogenous insulin deficiency, occurring as a natural consequence of islet cell destruction, results in the inappropriate utilization of carbohydrate. Cellular uptake of glucose by liver, muscle, and adipose tissue is blocked. Synthesis of glycogen, protein, and fat is reduced, and a catabolic state marked by lipolysis, proteolysis, and ketone body formation ensues. Increased serum glucose and ketones presents an overwhelming osmotic load to the kidneys, resulting in urinary losses of volume and cations (Na^+, K^+, NH_4).

The autoimmune phenomena described above are not evident in cases of NIDDM, also known as type II diabetes. This disease, which is characterized by resistance to insulin, may assume one or two chemical presentations in childhood. The more traditional form of NIDDM occurs in association with obesity and has no familial pattern. More recently authors have described a heritable form in nonobese individuals that presents at puberty that is known as maturity-onset diabetes of youth (MODY). Individuals with either presentation may have a short-term insulin requirement or need for glycemic control that can be treated with dietary manipulation or oral hypoglycemics (e.g., tolbutamide, glipizide); long-term insulin replacement is not required.

DIFFERENTIAL DIAGNOSIS

The diagnosis is usually straightforward given the symptomatology, except in children who present at a very young age. Although the onset of IDDM is rare before one year of age, the disease does occur but symptoms are nonspecific (e.g., irritability, vomiting, tachypnea, and poor weight gain). Chemotherapeutic agents (e.g., L-asparaginase) and a variety of medications (e.g., corticosteroids, diuretics, oral contraceptives, diphenylhydantoin, epinephrine, etc.) may induce glucose intolerance. Glycosuria without evidence of ketosis or elevated blood glucose occurs in certain renal conditions (e.g., Fanconi's syndrome, carbohydrate malabsorption syndromes, heavy metal intoxication). Transient hyperglycemia, with or without glycosuria, may occur in response to physiologic stress (e.g., burns, trauma, hyperosmolar dehydration, etc.). In most of these cases, glucose regulation returns to normal within several days.

EVALUATION

History

The history should focus on classic symptomatology and rule out exogenous causes of diabetes (Questions Box).

Physical Examination

Growth parameters should be measured and plotted on standard growth curves. Such parameters are among the most important aspects of the physical examination. Any weight loss should be documented. Otherwise, the physical examination may be unrevealing in cases of uncomplicated IDDM. An intercurrent infection may trigger the symptomatology and should always be sought in cases of ketoacidosis. Children who present with ketoacidosis may have evidence of vomiting, dehydration, Kussmaul respirations, and, in severe cases, altered mental status.

Laboratory Tests

Delays in making the correct diagnosis may occur if serum and urine are not evaluated for the presence of glucose and ketones. Oral glucose tolerance tests are rarely necessary to confirm the diagnosis of IDDM.

Questions: Insulin-Dependent Diabetes Mellitus

- Is the child having increased urination (e.g., nighttime urination, unusual bed-wetting)?
- Is the child drinking or eating more than usual?
- Has the child experienced any weight loss?
- Has the child been taking or had access to any kind of medications (e.g., corticosteroids, L-asparaginase, diuretics ["water pills"], birth control pills)?

Two-hour postprandial values in excess of 180 mg/dL or a fasting serum glucose level of greater than 120 mg/dL are evidence of IDDM. The introduction of the intravenous glucose tolerance test with measurement of first phase insulin release has allowed early diagnosis of individuals at risk for the disease prior to development of diabetic ketoacidosis.

MANAGEMENT

Early diagnosis together with a comprehensive program of education and aggressive management are essential to prevent acute and long-term complications. In general, children with newly diagnosed IDDM are admitted to the hospital to correct any electrolyte and acid-base disturbances, determine the insulin requirement, and educate the family and child about the disease and management plans. Long-term objectives of therapeutic intervention in children with IDDM are (1) to facilitate normal physical growth and psychological and sexual maturation, (2) to promote normoglycemia through regulation of glucose metabolism, (3) to prevent acute complications (i.e., hypoglycemia, ketoacidosis), (4) to prevent or delay long-term sequelae, and (5) to accommodate physiologic changes that alter therapeutic needs (e.g., exercise, adolescence, intercurrent illness).

Effective management necessitates a multidisciplinary team of professionals skilled in handling the myriad issues that arise for families and children with IDDM. Most clinics specializing in the care of children with diabetes include a nurse educator, dietician, social worker, psychologist or therapist, and a pediatric diabetologist. In settings where such special care centers are available, the primary care physician serves as a key adjunct, underscoring the importance of ongoing patient-family involvement in disease management and ensuring optimal growth, development, and nutrition. In the absence of special care centers, the primary care physician assumes responsibility for all aspects of management, including the treatment of acute complications, monitoring compliance and control, and surveillance for long-term complications.

Effective therapeutic intervention is based on individual needs for energy, insulin, and exercise. A number of factors, including physical growth, insulin requirement, glycemic control, and activity level, influence those needs and must be assessed on a regular basis. Growth parameters using standard growth curves should be measured at regular intervals. At the time of diagnosis, these parameters often indicate a state of negative energy balance that must be made up with additional caloric intake (more than basal requirements). Subsequent evaluation of physical growth using growth curves should occur at intervals of three to six months, depending on the child's age.

Insulin

The purpose of insulin therapy is to enable children to approach normoglycemia in response to adequate

TABLE 108–2. Commonly Used Insulin Preparations*

Type	Onset of Action	Duration of Effect
Short-acting Regular	0.5 hour	5–12 hours

Intermediate-acting
    (zinc or protamine)
    Lente
    NPH
	1.5–2.5 hours	18–24 hours

Long-acting Ultralente	2–4 hours	20–28 hours

*Twice daily injections: One half of the total daily dose before breakfast and dinner. Each dose should be made up of intermediate- and short-acting insulin in 2 : 1 ratio.
Basal bolus: Intermediate/long-acting insulin at bedtime with regular insulin before each meal.

amounts of food, insulin, and exercise. Average children with diabetes require 0.6–0.8 units of insulin per kilogram of body weight in a 24-hour period. Within three to four months of diagnosis, most individuals experience a partial remission, or "honeymoon" phase, during which time their insulin requirements decline dramatically. Conversely, illness, anxiety, and adolescence (i.e., pubertal changes) may cause the insulin requirement to increase. Even under conditions of increased need, reported daily insulin dosages in excess of two units per kilogram of body weight should stimulate investigations into patient compliance.

A number of insulin regimens are currently in use that take advantage of the variable onset of action of the different insulin preparations (Table 108–2). The regimen used by individual patients must be tailored to their needs for glycemic regulation and fit their lifestyles, yet allow for rapid adjustments when necessary. Children with newly diagnosed diabetes should use semisynthetic or recombinant human insulin preparations to minimize the possibility of allergic reactions. Any change in insulin preparation should be undertaken cautiously and only under medical supervision, because brands vary in strength, purity, and glycemic response.

Morning hyperglycemia may result from one of two phenomena, which must be distinguished, because the appropriate therapeutic responses are opposite. The "dawn phenomenon" probably involves a nocturnal surge of growth hormone, resulting in hyperglycemia that is present during the night (2:00 to 4:00 AM) and is sustained until morning. The treatment involves increasing the evening dose of intermediate-acting insulin. In the Somogyi phenomenon morning glucose is high as a physiologic response to nighttime hypoglycemia. Treatment of this condition requires decreasing the evening intermediate-acting insulin or increasing the carbohydrate content of a bedtime snack.

Adolescents require special consideration. The sexual maturation process occurs in the setting of relative insulin resistance, other hormonal alterations, and a burden of developmental tasks, which make glycemic control problematic at best. Daily insulin requirements may increase to 1.5–2 units/kg during adolescence, but return to prepubertal levels at the end of the teenage years. Particular efforts must be made to ensure physical and psychological growth in the context of these special tasks. Dietary manipulation and consideration of alternative (usually more intensive) insulin and monitoring regimens is critical for successful glycemic control during this challenging period.

External infusion pumps are not widely used in young children because of the danger of mechanical malfunction (leading to hypo- or hyperglycemia). Their use may be considered, however, in children with unstable diabetes or severe, chronic, intercurrent illness.

Glucose Monitoring

Self-monitoring of glycemic response through the in-home assessment of blood glucose levels is critical to effective therapy. The introduction of reflectance meters (glucometers) has obviated the need for inaccurate, visually read strips of glucose-sensitive paper. Some protocols for home blood monitoring involve a single morning test, whereas others measure glucose three to four times daily. Most diabetologists advocate testing before each meal and at bedtime during the first year after diagnosis. An acceptable range for glycemic control is 80–150 mg/dL. Patients also need to monitor their urine for ketones whenever their blood glucose readings exceed 240 mg/dL.

Glycosylated hemoglobin (HbA_{1C}) measurements reflect glucose control over the preceding two to three months. The normal value is 4 to 6% of total hemoglobin. HbA_{1C} values of 9 to 13% indicate very good to good control, and values in excess of 15% indicate poor control. HbA_{1C} measurements should be obtained every three to six months and more often during adolescence and other stressful periods. Whenever children's routines undergo dramatic change, stepped-up home monitoring and medical consultation are advisable. Caution should be used in interpreting HbA_{1C} values in infants and others in whom fetal hemoglobin is present, because this may falsely elevate the value of glycosylated hemoglobin. Although compliance with intensive regimens is an indisputable challenge (particularly as responsibility for management shifts from parent to child), increasing evidence underscores the importance of "tight control" (defined by HbA_{1c} value).

Nutrition

The timing, amount, and types of foods eaten for meals and snacks should be relatively consistent from one day to the next to match the relative constancy of the exogenous insulin. Daily caloric requirements should be distributed in the following way: carbohydrate, 50 to 60% (< 10% in the form of sucrose); protein, 12 to 20%; fat, less than 30% (6–8% polyunsaturated, < 10% saturated). Snacks are an important part of the nutrition regimen for children with diabetes. Most nutritionists recommend three snacks for young children (between meals and at bedtime) and two for older children. Dietary discipline is a tremendous challenge for many children. Introducing one change at a time may make such dietary manipulations more acceptable over the long run.

Exercise

Exercise contributes to glucose control by facilitating the utilization of glucose without the assistance of insulin. If not carefully undertaken on a regular basis, exercise can precipitate acute hypoglycemia. Physical activity enhances the body's sensitivity to insulin and can even decrease the daily insulin requirement. Thoughtful planning of exercise involves compensatory changes in food intake and insulin doses. For example, extra energy intake at bedtime may offset the nighttime hypoglycemia that accompanies late afternoon exercise. Seasonal physical activities may necessitate an adjustment in the insulin regimen at certain times of the year.

Education

The role of education is pivotal to the successful management of diabetes in childhood and throughout life. During childhood, educational efforts must be focused on the entire family unit. Affected children must be involved as early as possible and in ways that are developmentally appropriate. The process should involve the early introduction of basic survival information, such as insulin therapy and management of complications. This can be followed by more detailed information, including strategies to reduce long-term sequelae.

PROGNOSIS

Although the mortality rate from IDDM has decreased with improvements in management, life expectancy is still reduced, primarily because of the devastating effects of long-term complications. **Hypoglycemia** and **ketoacidosis** are acute complications of IDDM. Clinical signs of hypoglycemia in older children include shakiness, blurred vision, and dysarthria. Concerns about the neurodevelopmental impact of hypoglycemia in young children have led to the recommendation of more liberal glycemic control in early onset disease. Diabetic ketoacidosis, precipitated by an intercurrent infection or poor compliance, is a metabolic derangement that always requires urgent medical attention and often necessitates hospitalization. Replacement of fluids, attention to electrolyte abnormalities, and insulin therapy are the mainstays of treatment in the face of this complication.

Long-term complications include **proliferative retinopathy, nephropathy, peripheral and autonomic neurologic impairment,** and **early onset of cardiovascular disease**. Ophthalmologic evaluation, overnight urine protein measurement, and a detailed neurologic examination should occur once or twice each year depending on the duration of disease. Intensive therapeutic intervention results in significant reduction in retinopathy, nephropathy, and cardiac and peripheral vascular disease. Preliminary evidence warrants consideration of such therapy with the expectation of benefit in long-term outcomes.

Case Resolution

The girl in the opening case history is admitted to the hospital to help determine appropriate insulin dosing. She and her family require ongoing education. Careful management is necessary to optimize normal growth and development as well as delay or prevent long-term sequelae.

Selected Readings

Allen, D. B., and M. J. MacDonald. Pancreas and islet cell transplantation for type I diabetes mellitus: does it have a role for children? Adv. Pediatr., 37:391–412, 1990.

Bertrand, J., R. Rappaport, and P. Sizonenko (eds.). Pediatric Endocrinology, 2nd ed. Baltimore, Williams & Wilkins, 1993.

Connell, J. E., and D. Thomas-Doberson. Nutritional management of children and adolescents with insulin-dependent diabetes mellitus: a review by the diabetes care and education dietetic practice group. J. Am. Diet. Assoc. 91:1556–1564, 1991.

Diabetes Control and Complications Trial Research Group. The effect of intensive treatment of diabetes on the development and progression of long-term complications in insulin-dependent diabetes mellitus. N. Engl. J. Med. 329:977–986, 1993.

Drash, A. L., and S. A. Arslanian. Can insulin-dependent diabetes mellitus be cured or prevented? Pediatr. Clin. North Am. 37:1467–1487, 1990.

Dunger, D. B. Diabetes in puberty. Arch. Dis. Child. 67:569–570, 1992.

Gianani, R., et al. Prognostically significant heterogeneity of cytoplasmic islet cell antibodies in relatives of patients with type I diabetes. Diabetes 41:347–353, 1992.

Karvonen, M., et al. A review of the recent epidemiologic data on the incidence of type I diabetes mellitus. Diabetologia 36:883–892, 1993.

CHAPTER 109

CHRONIC LUNG DISEASE

Helen DuPlessis, M.D., M.P.H.

H_x A 3-month-old male infant is seen for routine health maintenance after discharge from the neonatal intensive care unit. He was born by emergent cesarean section after a precipitous labor at 30 weeks' gestation. Symptoms of respiratory distress were present in the delivery room and the newborn was treated with surfactant, endotracheal intubation, and mechanical ventilation for the first 15 days of life. The course was complicated by the discovery of a grade I intraventricular hemorrhage on day three of life, apnea of prematurity, and slow feeding until approximately one week ago. The infant received a six-day course of corticosteroids prior to extubation and is currently maintained on 0.5 L of oxygen, theophylline, spironolactone, iron, and vitamins.

On physical examination, the infant is small but well-nourished and has nasal cannula in place. Auscultation of the lungs reveals occasional expiratory wheezes in both lung fields.

Questions

1. What monitoring is appropriate in the outpatient care of infants who required intubation in the newborn period?
2. What considerations should be made for the routine health care needs of children with chronic lung disease?
3. What are the long-term sequelae associated with bronchopulmonary dysplasia? Cystic fibrosis?
4. What medical advances have affected the natural history of bronchopulmonary dysplasia? Cystic fibrosis?

Chronic lung diseases in the pediatric population are associated with significant morbidity and mortality. Missed school days, developmental and emotional difficulties, and superimposed acute respiratory illnesses and premature death are among the many serious sequelae experienced by children with these diseases. Asthma, bronchopulmonary dysplasia (BPD), and cystic fibrosis (CF) can be characterized as chronic lung diseases. For a complete discussion of asthma in children, see Chapter 55, Wheezing and Asthma. This chapter includes a separate discussion of the evaluation and management considerations unique to BPD and CF, followed by discussion of the common preventive and health maintenance measures with which the primary care physician should be familiar.

EPIDEMIOLOGY

Bronchopulmonary Dysplasia

Approximately 15% of neonates admitted to neonatal intensive care units (tertiary level nurseries) in the United States develop BPD. As care of very premature infants has improved over the past three decades, the distribution of BPD by birth weight has changed (i.e., increased incidence among infants weighing < 1500 g) while the overall incidence of BPD has remained the same.

Cystic Fibrosis

The incidence of CF is 1:2500 among Caucasians, with a carrier rate of 5%, but drops to 1:17,000 in African Americans. The condition is inherited in an autosomal recessive manner, and girls and boys are equally affected.

CLINICAL PRESENTATION

Bronchopulmonary Dysplasia

BPD is a disorder seen in infants who have the following three criteria at or beyond 28 days of age: (1) supplemental oxygen required to maintain the PaO_2 above 50 mm Hg, (2) radiographic findings characteristic of BPD, and (3) clinical symptoms of respiratory disease (e.g., tachypnea, retractions, increased work of breathing) (D_x: Bronchopulmonary Dysplasia).

Cystic Fibrosis

Most children with CF present during the first year of life with symptoms related to pancreatic insufficiency or pulmonary disease. FTT, steatorrhea, and obstructive liver disease are common indications of the malabsorption that affect 80% of patients (D_x: Cystic Fibrosis). Children may present with wheezing, airway hyperreactivity, and frequent lower respiratory tract infections, often with unusual organisms such as *Pseudomonas*, *Klebsiella,* and *Staphylococcus*.

D_x **Bronchopulmonary Dysplasia**

- Supplemental oxygen requirement to maintain PaO_2 above 50 mm Hg
- Radiographic findings consistent with BPD (e.g., hyperinflation, fibrotic changes)
- Clinical symptoms of respiratory distress (e.g., tachypnea, retractions, increased work of breathing)

Dx   Cystic Fibrosis

- Evidence of exocrine glandular dysfunction (e.g., pancreatic insufficiency, chronic pulmonary disease, intestinal malabsorption) *plus*
- Sweat chloride content greater than 60 mEq/L *or*
- Definitive genetic screening

PATHOPHYSIOLOGY

Bronchopulmonary Dysplasia

Although the pathophysiology of BPD is not clearly understood, it appears that prematurity, oxygen exposure, positive pressure ventilation, and idiopathic respiratory distress syndrome predispose infants to the disease. Additional research indicates that lung repair mechanisms also interact to perpetuate the chronic changes characteristic of BPD.

Cystic Fibrosis

CF is a disorder of exocrine glandular dysfunction characterized by severe pulmonary disease, pancreatic insufficiency, and intestinal malabsorption. The basic defect in CF involves malfunction of chloride transport through the chloride channel. Sodium accompanies the chloride. The recessive mutation responsible for 70% of cases is a chromosomal deletion on chromosome 7 that codes for a transmembrane protein involved in the regulation of chloride transport.

DIFFERENTIAL DIAGNOSIS

Bronchopulmonary Dysplasia

Pulmonary infections, congenital heart disease, and congenital lung malformation (e.g., bronchogenic cysts, adenomatoid malformations) may all result in symptoms of respiratory distress. The history and classic radiographic findings usually distinguish BPD from other diseases.

Cystic Fibrosis

In the absence of family history or neonatal screening programs, children with CF may go undiagnosed for years until the severity and multiplicity of exocrine dysfunction is recognized. Children who present with acholic or "fatty" stools (i.e., steatorrhea) may undergo diagnostic evaluation for the myriad causes of intestinal malabsorption. Wheezing and recurrent pulmonary infections may prompt diagnostic considerations of asthma (or reactive airway disease), congenital lung malformation, α_1-antitrypsin deficiency, or an immunodeficiency. Children who present with FTT may be suspected of having endocrinologic, genetic, or environmental disorders (see Chapter 98, Failure to Thrive).

EVALUATION

BRONCHOPULMONARY DYSPLASIA

History

The history should focus on respiratory events in the neonatal period as well as the severity of pulmonary disease since discharge from the nursery (Questions: Bronchopulmonary Dysplasia). In addition, a review of the patient's most recent radiographs is essential to facilitate accurate interpretation of any future x-rays, because chronic scarring may be present.

Physical Examination

The physical examination should focus on growth, development, nutritional, and respiratory status. Growth parameters and anthropometric measurements should be obtained regularly. A careful lung examination should be part of every assessment.

Laboratory Tests

In infants with BPD, pulse oximetry should be performed and the usefulness of supplemental oxygen should be evaluated. Oxygen saturation should be measured at times when oxygenation is expected to fall (e.g., while feeding and sleeping). Regular chemistries such as serum electrolytes are indicated for infants with BPD before they are given diuretics and other medications that may cause electrolyte and acid-base disturbances. Steroid therapy is associated with biventricular hypertrophy and systemic hypertension, necessitating regular blood pressure measurements.

Imaging Studies

Pulmonary function should be assessed frequently. These children are at risk for excessive and unnecessary radiation exposure. Radiographs are probably not indicated for minor infections; much more can be gained from microbiologic evaluations of sputum and blood and from objective evaluations of pulmonary function (e.g., spirometry, oximetry, blood gas).

Questions: Bronchopulmonary Dysplasia

- Was the infant delivered prematurely? If so, how may weeks before term?
- Did the mother take any medications?
- How much did the infant weigh at birth?
- Did the infant ever require mechanical ventilation or oxygen in the newborn period? If so, for how long?
- Has the child had frequent respiratory infections or problems? How many times has he or she been to the emergency department or spent a night in the hospital as a result of respiratory illness?
- Does the child currently require oxygen during feeding?

CYSTIC FIBROSIS

History

The history should focus on nutritional symptoms and intestinal and respiratory function in children with CF (Questions: Cystic Fibrosis).

Laboratory Tests

The clinical test accepted as the "gold standard" for the diagnosis of CF is the quantitative pilocarpine iontophoretic sweat test. Sweat glands in the skin of the forearm are stimulated using topical pilocarpine gel and a measured electrical current. Premeasured filter paper is utilized for the collection of sweat, which is then analyzed for chloride concentration.

The sweat test is sometimes problematic in children under three months of age. Stool trypsinogen has been of some use in small infants. A definitive genetic screen exists for another 4% of affected individuals. However, at this time these screens are not widely accessible. Although prenatal genetic screening is available for at-risk pregnancies, population-based testing has not been recommended because screening does not diagnose approximately 25 to 30% of cases.

Imaging Studies

Radiographs should be used as they are for children with BPD (see Bronchopulmonary Dysplasia: Imaging Studies). In addition, children with CF may require CT of the sinuses to aid in the diagnosis and management of recurrent sinus infections.

MANAGEMENT

BRONCHOPULMONARY DYSPLASIA

Respiratory support and pharmacologic therapy are the mainstays of treatment of BPD.

Inpatient Therapy

Supplemental oxygen is required by most premature infants, regardless of the presence of infantile respiratory distress syndrome. The route of delivery and concentration varies among institutions. Some neona-tologists promote the early use of continuous positive airway pressure via nasal cannulae as an effective method of preventing alveolar collapse while minimizing potential barotrauma to premature lungs. This method has been effective in some institutions, but it has not been successful in others. Most neonatologists strive to minimize the duration of mechanical ventilation in an effort to reduce barotrauma, although intubation of the smallest premature infants is routine in many nurseries. The application of high-frequency ventilatory techniques may potentially decrease the amount of barotrauma to which infants are exposed. The use of these techniques is too new to allow evaluation of the possible impact on the incidence of chronic lung damage.

A variety of **pharmacologic agents,** most notably bronchodilators, diuretics, and corticosteroids, have been used in the treatment of BPD. The rationale for using **bronchodilators** was questioned for many years until researchers demonstrated that even very premature infants have sufficient bronchial smooth muscle to respond to a variety of agents. Indeed, smooth muscle may undergo hyperplasia during the development of BPD. Although multiple effects are attributed to methylxanthines (e.g., diuretic action, facilitation of cyclic AMP metabolism, respiratory stimulant), the relatively weak impact of these drugs on bronchial smooth muscle and potential for erratic metabolism results in their infrequent use as a primary therapy for BPD. However, methylxanthines are still used in the treatment of apnea of prematurity, which often complicates the course of infants who go on to develop BPD. Beta-adrenergic agents such as albuterol and metaproterenol can be quite effective in treating the acute episodes of bronchospasm, which makes them ideal for intermittent therapy. Reports do not support their use in long-term therapy of BPD. The results of studies of cromolyn sodium have been mixed.

Diuretics are frequently used in the management of BPD in premature infants both for treatment and prevention. Although well-controlled clinical trials are limited, many researchers believe that fluid restriction and diuresis decrease the likelihood of chronic lung damage through some mitigating effect on the development of pulmonary edema. The use of loop and thiazide diuretics improves short-term oxygen exchange and lung function. The mechanism of action is uncertain. The use of several other diuretics, including antioxidants and pulmonary vasodilators, is still experimental.

Corticosteroids have been used both for prevention and treatment of BPD. Although prenatal administration of corticosteroids before delivery has been effective in minimizing acute lung disease in premature infants, such use has not yet gained widespread acceptance. Results of numerous clinical trials designed to evaluate the effectiveness of corticosteroids in the treatment of BPD seem to indicate that long-term (> 6 weeks) therapy with corticosteroids is more effective in minimizing bad outcomes from BPD than short-term treatment. Protocols for corticosteroid administration vary greatly among institutions. Short-term therapy may hasten the time to extubation and decrease the need for ventilator support. The potential for serious side effects with prolonged use is a deterrent.

Surfactant therapy is now widely used in most tertiary facilities because of its ability to improve survival and decrease the duration of time that surfactant-deficient infants require supplemental oxygen. Although it may be too early to determine the impact of surfactant therapy on the incidence of BPD, it appears that the surfactant primarily decreases the risk of chronic lung disease in infants with birth weights in excess of 1 kg.

Discharge Planning

Discharge planning for neonates with pulmonary problems requires the mobilization of a multidisciplinary team including social service workers, representatives of developmental/rehabilitation centers, health educators, and primary providers, all of whom participate in health care on discharge. Caregivers often need time to become accustomed to the special needs of chronically ill infants and their impact on other members of the household. Ongoing support for both psychosocial and physical stressors should be available.

Providing in-home care for infants with chronic lung disease should be encouraged, not only as an appropriate and cost effective use of scarce health care resources, but as the ultimate fulfillment of the attachment process between caregivers and children. Judicious determination of when infants are ready for discharge goes a long way toward ensuring the success of in-home care. Needs of infants for pulmonary support and physiotherapy should be minimal. Infants should have a well-established and consistent growth trajectory after attaining a reasonable postconceptual age and weight. Caregivers must be trained in basic life support and feel confident about the use of any special equipment such as apnea monitors, suction devices, and oxygen tanks.

Outpatient Management

Management of infants with BPD following discharge focuses on **health maintenance** as well as on any residual problems related to prematurity (see Chapter 19, Well Child Care for Preterm Infants).

Chronic lung disease and the alterations in respiratory dynamics affect nonrespiratory systems. The increased work of breathing raises metabolic demands. Children with BPD often require more than 180 to 200 kcal/kg of body weight/day to maintain acceptable growth. Intercurrent illnesses, posttussive emesis, and bronchospastic episode challenge even those metabolic requirements. **Nutritional supplements** such as energy-dense formulas (i.e., 24 kcal/ounce) and fat-soluble vitamins may be necessary to sustain adequate growth and nutrition. The cardiovascular system may be challenged by the respiratory requirements or by medications. Chronic hypoxemia leads to hypertrophy of smooth muscle in the pulmonary vasculature, which can progress to pulmonary hypertension and cor pulmonale.

Infants with BPD have increased airway reactivity, decreased lung compliance, and increased number of upper respiratory tract infections. These altered lung dynamics and decreased pulmonary reserve underscore the need for early medical attention in the face of respiratory infections. **Pulmonary toilet** and early, judicious use of **antibiotic and antiviral therapies** can prevent further lung damage and allow the reparative process to proceed.

CYSTIC FIBROSIS

The management of CF focuses on the maintenance of adequate growth and development and the minimization of progressive lung disease (Table 109–1). **Adequate nutrition** is critical. Although children with CF often have substantial appetites, recurrent pulmonary infections, increased energy requirements, and malabsorption may result in a negative energy balance. Pancreatic insufficiency can be documented through quantitative fecal fat analysis and enzyme replacement started early in life. Dietary intake and an assessment of basal caloric requirements should occur annually along with evaluation of serum protein, electrolytes, and fat-soluble vitamins (especially A and E). Anthropometric measurements (e.g., height, weight, head circumference, and triceps skinfold thickness) should be recorded quarterly so that growth failure can be recognized early and appropriate intervention undertaken. Ongoing **education of children and families** is an important process that facilitates compliance and improves the quality of patients' lives.

Respiratory hyperreactivity, pulmonary obstruction, and frequent infections inevitably lead to fibrotic lung disease and cor pulmonale. The early and judicious use of **antibiotics, antiviral agents** (e.g., ribavirin), **mucolytics** (e.g., acetylcysteine), and **bronchodilators** may halt this progression but cannot prevent it. The development of effective **antipseudomonal treatments** has improved the outlook for adolescents with CF, but the potential musculoskeletal morbidity associated with these drugs makes their use in younger patients

---

TABLE 109–1. Management of Cystic Fibrosis

Clinical Complication	Diagnostic Evaluation	Therapy
Growth and nutrition	Frequent assessment of basal caloric requirements	Caloric supplements and dietary adjustments
Pancreatic insufficiency	Fecal fat analysis	Pancreatic enzyme replacement
		Fat-soluble vitamins (A, D, E, K) replacement
Pulmonary disease	Pulmonary function tests (every 3 months)	Routine percussion and postural drainage (P and PD)
		Appropriate antibiotic or antiviral therapy

controversial. **Lung transplants** are used with increasing frequency in this population, with good pulmonary outcomes and two-year survival rates in excess of 60%. At present transplants are by no means optimal therapies because of the morbidity and mortality associated with lifelong immunosuppression.

Health Maintenance and Prevention

Although specific therapies for BPD and CF and their complications may differ, some basic health practices are common to both diseases. These children deserve the protection of active immunization at least as much as well children, and full doses should be administered at ages recommended for nonaffected children. In addition, children over six months of age should receive an annual influenza vaccination. Children with BPD or CF have no inherent increased susceptibility to pneumococcal or meningococcal infection, and vaccines against these infections are probably not necessary. Conversely, children with either lung disease should receive early consideration for antiviral therapy in the face of infections with respiratory syncytial virus or varicella.

PROGNOSIS

The long-term outcome of children with BPD still leaves much to be desired. Although repair of chronic lung injury occurs, the mortality from BPD is 10 to 25%. Fifty-four percent of premature infants have CNS se-

quelae. Hospitalizations are significantly increased in infants with BPD.

Advancements in therapeutic modalities and lung transplantation have improved survival of individuals with CF, but the morbidity associated with the disease and these therapies results in a shortened lifespan. Once the biochemical basis of CF is better understood, biomolecular intervention may be effective in the treatment of this disease.

Case Resolution

The infant in the case scenario will benefit most from a well-informed, methodical, well-coordinated approach to preventive and primary health care. His growth and neurodevelopment should be monitored, and his serum electrolytes should be assessed periodically. He should receive appropriate immunizations for age.

Selected Readings

Northway, W. H., Jr. Introduction to bronchopulmonary dysplasia. Clin. Perinatol. 19:489–495, 1992.

Lemen, R. J., et al. Pediatric lung disease. Chest (supplement) 102:232S–242S, 1992.

Ramsey, B. W., P. M. Farrell, P. Pencharz, and the Consensus Committee. Nutritional assessment and management in cystic fibrosis: a consensus report. Am. J. Clin. Nutr. 5:108–116, 1992.

Stern, R. The primary care physician and the patient with cystic fibrosis. J. Pediatr. 114:31–36, 1989.

CHAPTER 110

OSTEOMYELITIS

Helen DuPlessis, M.D., M.P.H.

Hx A 2-year-old boy is evaluated for refusing to walk. He has been in good health and his immunization status is appropriate for age. He has been walking normally since 12 months of age. Three days before presentation, the boy began to favor his left leg when he walked and played, and this morning he refused to put any weight on the leg. He had a tactile temperature last evening. The boy fell from a park slide two weeks before his current symptoms began.

His physical examination is remarkable for a temperature of 100.4° F (38.0° C) and tenderness in the left lower leg that is poorly localized.

Questions

1. What pathogens are most commonly responsible for bone infections?
2. What is the appropriate evaluation for children with suspected osteomyelitis?
3. What therapeutic regimens are appropriate for the treatment of osteomyelitis?
4. When is surgical intervention indicated in children with osteomyelitis?
5. When is outpatient management appropriate for children with osteomyelitis?

Osteomyelitis is an infection of bone, most commonly of bacterial origin. The diagnosis and management of osteomyelitis may be problematic because of the nature of the clinical presentation and the lack of well-controlled, prospective studies of diagnosis and treatment. Despite the paucity of extensive scientific data, progress has been made in the radiographic diagnosis, antimicrobial treatment, and outpatient management. As with most serious health problems, a high index of suspicion leading to early diagnosis and prompt initiation of therapy can prevent the serious morbidity that may befall children with this condition.

EPIDEMIOLOGY

Osteomyelitis affects individuals of all ages. Acute osteomyelitis generally affects children; the duration of symptoms is short (2–7 days), and bone destruction at the time of presentation is minimal or nonexistent. Good epidemiologic data are not available, but many large centers report 5–10/10,000 cases of acute osteomyelitis each year. Chronic osteomyelitis refers to bone infections presenting after a long duration of symptoms (> 3 months) or after failure of previous antimicrobial therapy. Although acute osteomyelitis may become chronic in some children, the majority of chronic cases occur in adults.

CLINICAL PRESENTATION

Pain and, in toddlers, refusal to bear weight are the most common presenting symptoms of osteomyelitis, often giving rise to a limp or other manifestation of limited function. Fever is sometimes present, but may be absent in as many as 50% of cases (D_x Box). Careful examination may reveal tenderness to palpation. Late signs include erythema, warmth (calor), and induration overlying the infected part.

PATHOPHYSIOLOGY

Osteomyelitis results from infection of the bone and may be attributed to certain predisposing factors in addition to various bacteria. The microorganisms responsible for most cases of osteomyelitis are those implicated in other serious childhood infections. However, the success of the *Haemophilus influenzae* type B vaccine program has all but eliminated this organism as a significant pathogen in invasive diseases such as osteomyelitis.

D_x. **Osteomyelitis (two or more of the listed findings)**

- Tenderness to palpation over bone
- Erythema, swelling, or warmth over affected extremity (late)
- Fever, leukocytosis, or elevated sedimentation rate
- Positive culture (blood, bone, or subperiosteal aspiration)
- Scintigraphic or radiologic changes

Staphylococcus aureus is the most common organism to infect bone from birth through adulthood. Causative organisms vary significantly depending on the age of the host, however. Streptococci and other gram-positive bacteria, followed by gram-negative organisms, are second in frequency to *S. aureus.* Some studies indicate that specific gram-negative bacteria, particularly *Pseudomonas aeruginosa,* have accounted for an increased percentage of cases of osteomyelitis in the last 25 years. *Salmonella* is frequently the causative pathogen in osteomyelitis in patients with sickle cell anemia.

Seeding of skeletal tissue with microorganisms can occur by a variety of different mechanisms. Blood-borne dissemination is by far the most common route of bone infection in children, giving rise to the term acute hematogenous osteomyelitis. In adults with skeletal infections, direct inoculation of bone with bacteria frequently occurs as a consequence of trauma (e.g., penetrating injuries, compound fractures), invasive orthopedic procedures, or contiguous spread of infections in joint spaces or soft tissues. In bacteremic animals, bone infections have readily been established following blunt trauma involving the skeleton, which has led to speculation about the role of nonpenetrating trauma in osteomyelitis in humans.

The predilection for infection of long bones to occur through the hematogenous route can be explained by developmental changes in the skeleton and the associated vasculature. The vasculature at the ends of long bones is composed of tiny capillaries through which blood flow is sluggish. It is postulated that blood-borne bacteria coursing slowly through these capillaries may exit the vessels and inoculate surrounding bone, particularly if the vessels have been traumatized. In newborns, tiny vessels traverse the metaphysis, cross the growth plate, and penetrate the epiphysis. This anatomy may explain the relatively high incidence of contiguous joint and soft tissue infection in neonates (as high as 70%). These vessels involute toward the end of the first year of life, after which time metaphyseal capillaries end in blind loops and the growth plates serve as a barrier to the egress of infected material. In toddlers and older children, infection is often confined to the metaphysis. Furthermore, if the infection has been present for more than a few days, decompression of the purulent material may progress underneath the periosteum or, in rare instances, lead to the formation of a sequestrum, a piece of necrotic bony material that has been separated from surrounding healthy bone and vascular supply.

DIFFERENTIAL DIAGNOSIS

Osteomyelitis must be differentiated from trauma, inflammation of the joint (e.g., infectious or rheumatologic disease), malignancies affecting bone, leukemic bone involvement, myositis, diskitis, and age-related orthopedic abnormalities such as Legg-Calvé-Perthes disease and slipped capital femoral epiphyses (see Chapter 76, Evaluation of Limp).

The organisms responsible for osteomyelitis may be affected by a number of factors related to host defenses and the particular circumstances of infection. The age and the immune status of the host and the mechanism of infection may all be associated with peculiar microbiology.

Osteomyelitis is an uncommon infection in the neonatal period, and morbidity and mortality are high when diagnosis and treatment is delayed. The clinical features, causative organisms, and long-term outcome vary dramatically when compared to bone infections at other periods of childhood.

In the majority of affected neonates, osteomyelitis has a benign course characterized by absent or low-grade fever. Swelling or decreased mobility near the affected site is difficult to detect without a high index of suspicion and a focused examination. Consequently, most infections with this indolent presentation are diagnosed after a delay of 5–10 days. In 15 to 25% of neonates with bone infections, the illness is acute. Septic emboli seed the bone during an episode of serious bacteremia. The presence of transphyseal vessels results in a much larger incidence of contiguous spread to joints and soft tissues in infants. In addition, multiple bony foci may be present in up to 50% of cases.

Staphylococcus aureus is the most common etiologic agent in all age groups. Group B streptococcus (GBS) and enteric gram-negative rods (GNRs) are also significant causal microorganisms in neonates. Long-term morbidity is relatively uncommon with GBS infections, although infection with other organisms, including *S. aureus* and GNRs, may result in residual deformities as a consequence of growth plate disruption.

Bone infections with mycobacteria and fungi are uncommon in all age groups and almost impossible to diagnose without a high index of suspicion. Skeletal infection with tubercle bacilli is primarily a disease of older children and adults who were never or inadequately treated for their primary infection. Vertebral body involvement (Pott's disease), the most common form of mycobacterial osteomyelitis, is characterized by spinal rigidity secondary to paraspinous muscle spasm. Nighttime pain is a common complaint occurring when the protective spasms relax. Ultimately, destruction of the vertebral body results in a wedge-shaped collapse called a gibbus deformity. The current epidemic of tuberculosis along with the increasing number of individuals with HIV or otherwise compromised immune systems may make chronic infections from mycobacteria and fungi more prevalent.

Much has been written about the association of *Pseudomonas* osteomyelitis with puncture wounds through tennis shoes. Although no well-controlled studies of puncture wound infections have been conducted, provocative evidence exists to warrant consideration of infection by *P. aeruginosa* in certain situations. Apparently the bacteria reside in the foam of tennis shoes, and puncture wounds through this colonized material into the forefoot may result in deep infection because of the propensity of *Pseudomonas* to infect cartilaginous structures. Comprehensive management of puncture wound infections should include tetanus prophylaxis, wound cleansing, diagnostic radiography, and an aggressive search for a retained foreign body when appropriate.

No evidence indicates that prophylactic antipseudomonal therapy is warranted for these puncture wounds. However, afebrile, apparently healthy children who present with localized pain, swelling, and decreased ability to bear weight one to three weeks after a puncture wound should stimulate an aggressive search for bone infection. If the workup indicates an underlying bone infection, surgical debridement should be considered in addition to postoperative antibiotic regimens to cover both *Staphylococcus* and *Pseudomonas* (ceftazidime, gentamicin).

Bone pain in children with sickle cell disease requires the physician to distinguish between infarctions due to vaso-occlusive phenomena and true osteomyelitis. The initial clinical presentation may differ only in the degree of fever or the unusual severity of pain. More commonly, however, osteomyelitis should be seriously suspected when pain symptoms fail to respond to conventional treatment for sickle crises such as rest, analgesia, and hydration.

Salmonella is clearly an important infective agent, although which microorganisms most often infect skeletal tissue is the subject of some debate. It is speculated that the integrity of the intestinal mucosa is regularly compromised by microinfarcts in individuals with sickle cell anemia. *Salmonella* use this route to invade the blood stream, where they ultimately reach metaphyseal vessels in which blood flow is possibly even more sluggish than in hematologically normal persons. Faulty splenic clearance mechanisms also may contribute to the risk of infection. *Salmonella* osteomyelitis is often multifocal and sometimes symmetrical. Unlike neonatal osteomyelitis, it tends to respond to treatment rapidly and without long-term sequelae.

Radiographic diagnosis is also plagued by similarities in the pathophysiologic changes of bone infarcts and bone infection. Hyperemia and osteoclastic activity are characteristic of both infarcts and infection, rendering most nuclear medicine imaging techniques ineffective in distinguishing between these two conditions. Technetium sulfur colloid imaging of the marrow and MRI have been utilized with some success, but as yet there has been little scientific evaluation of the merits of these techniques.

EVALUATION

History

Most cases of osteomyelitis come to medical attention during the first week of illness. A thorough history should be taken (Questions Box).

Questions: Osteomyelitis

- Has the child suffered any recent trauma?
- Has the child ever had any of the following symptoms: fever, weight loss, rashes, joint swelling?
- How long have the symptoms been present?

Physical Examination

Localized findings may be missed on physical examination even in the most systematic evaluation. Refusal to move an extremity may be found. Tenderness to palpation is often elicited in older children in the early stages of infection. Fever and localized swelling or erythema are late findings.

Laboratory Tests

Routine laboratory evaluation should include CBC, ESR, and cultures of blood or bone. Leukocytosis is present in 50 to 67% of cases, and ESR is elevated over 90% of the time. ESR is a nonspecific test, but it can be extremely useful for monitoring response to therapy.

Imaging Studies

Radiographic findings on plain films are not usually evident before 10 to 14 days, and as a result, they are useful only for eliminating other entities that may be considered in the early stages of disease. Radionucleotide imaging techniques can be extremely helpful in the early diagnosis of osteomyelitis. Technetium-99m, which localizes in areas of increased vascularity or osteoblastic activity, is very sensitive in diagnosing osteomyelitis outside of the newborn period. Gallium- or leukocyte-labeled indium scans are useful adjuncts if the results of Tc-99m scans are equivocal or when infection is superimposed on conditions characterized by increased turnover of bone (e.g., trauma).

The use of CT and MRI is still being studied. These techniques give much better anatomic detail, which often helps determine the extent of abscesses that require surgical intervention. They may also be useful in the diagnosis and management of chronic osteomyelitis and bone infections in individuals with sickle cell anemia.

MANAGEMENT

Management involves **antibiotic therapy,** which must be tailored to age and situation-specific pathogens; when symptoms persist or pus or devitalized bone is present, **surgical intervention** may be necessary. The initial choice of antibiotics must be sufficiently broad to cover the predominant pathogens under specific prevailing conditions. In all cases of suspected osteomyelitis, coverage for *Staphylococcus* and other gram-positive organisms is necessary (neonates: nafcillin and a third-generation cephalosporin or aminoglycoside; infants and children: cefuroxime or nafcillin and chloramphenicol) (Table 110–1).

The route, duration, and location of antibiotic therapy are constantly reconsidered as new antimicrobial agents become available and the pressures for cost-effective treatment increases. At this time, therapy for acute osteomyelitis should be initiated with parenteral antibiotics in an inpatient setting. Once acute signs and symptoms have resolved, and children are able to bear weight, consideration should be given to outpatient management. Depending on the causal organism and the

TABLE 110–1. Antibiotic Treatment for Children With Osteomyelitis

Likely Organisms	Recommended Antibiotics
Neonates	
Group B streptococcus	Nafcillin and third-generation
Staphylococcus aureus	cephalosporin or amino-
Coliform bacteria	glycoside
Other gram-negative bacteria	
Infants and Children	
S. aureus	Cefuroxime or nafcillin and
Haemophilus influenzae type B	chloramphenicol
Group A streptococcus	
Streptococcus pneumoniae	
Pseudomonas	

availability of effective oral antibiotics, this may be undertaken with either parenteral or oral medication. Intramuscular ceftriaxone, administered once daily, has also been used, but its effectiveness must be documented in cases of staphylococcal infections.

Regardless of the route, serum bactericidal concentrations (peak > 1:8; trough > 1:4) and ESR should be followed to document treatment effectiveness. Therapy for less than 35 days has been associated with treatment failures in infections with staphylococci or GNRs. Shorter treatment courses may be undertaken in the face of uncomplicated infections with *H. influenzae* type B or streptococcus. Some investigators suggest the continuation of therapy for one week beyond the point at which the ESR returns to normal.

Although antibiotic therapy is curative in most cases of acute osteomyelitis, surgical intervention may be critical when the diagnosis occurs late in the course of the disease. In these instances, abscesses and sequestra form, which antibiotics are incapable of penetrating. Bacteremia and constitutional symptoms (e.g., fever and pain) that persist 72 hours after the initiation of antimicrobial therapy may be an indication for either diagnostic or therapeutic surgical intervention. Because neonatal osteomyelitis may result in growth plate disruption, some institutions advocate aggressive surgical drainage and debridement. Surgery is also indicated in the face of sinus tract formation and other signs of chronic osteomyelitis.

PROGNOSIS

Although mortality from osteomyelitis is rare, delays in diagnosis or inadequate treatment of skeletal infections can result in significant morbidity because of the proximity of the infection to growth plates of long bones. Abscess formation, recurrent infections, and contiguous joint involvement are much more common when adequate treatment is begun more than four days after the onset of clinical symptoms. Leg-length discrepancies, resulting from delayed or inadequate therapy, may occur years after the initial infection. Children who have had osteomyelitis need long-term follow-up.

Chronic osteomyelitis may exist as a complicated or recurrent infection of the original organism, or as an infection with unusual pathogens—mycobacteria or fungi—that resists surgical and antimicrobial therapy. Unifocal recurrences uncomplicated by additional organisms frequently respond to appropriate combinations of surgery and antimicrobial agents.

Multifocal and culture-negative cases of chronic osteomyelitis may wax and wane for months following aggressive antimicrobial and surgical treatment, however. Girls are more often affected by chronic multifocal disease than boys and often present with weeks to months of malaise, pain, loss of function, and swelling of adjacent joints. Therapy beyond adequate surgical drainage and a six-week regimen of antibiotics rarely affect the course of these cases; they usually resolve spontaneously.

Case Resolution

In the case history, a high index of suspicion leads to early diagnosis via blood cultures, which are positive for

S. aureus, and bone scans. After a short course of parenteral antibiotic therapy, the boy completed a six-week course of antibiotics in the hospital as an outpatient and had no orthopedic disabilities.

Selected Readings

Asmar, B. I. Osteomyelitis in the neonate. Infect. Dis. Clin. North Am. 6:117–132, 1992.

Dagan, R. Management of acute hematogenous osteomyelitis and septic arthritis in the pediatric patient. Pediatr. Infect. Dis. J. 12:88–93, 1993.

Knudsen, C. J. M. Neonatal osteomyelitis. J. Bone Joint Surg. Br. 72B:846–851, 1990.

Nelson, J. D. Skeletal infections in children. Adv. Pediatr. Infect. Dis. 6:59–78, 1991.

Schauwecke, D. S., E. M. Braunstein, and L. J. Wheat. Diagnostic imaging of osteomyelitis. Infect. Dis. Clin. North Am. 1:463–490, 1990.

Scott, R. J., et al. Acute osteomyelitis in children: a review of 116 cases. J. Pediatr. Orthop. 10:649–652, 1990.

CHAPTER 111

JUVENILE RHEUMATOID ARTHRITIS

Helen DuPlessis, M.D., M.P.H.

H$_x$ A 4-year-old girl is evaluated for pain in the legs and arms of six to eight months' duration. Symptoms began with pain and swelling in the left elbow that lasted for approximately two and one-half months. After an initial evaluation, including radiographs, the girl was diagnosed with a "bad sprain" and was treated with a two-week course of an NSAID. The elbow improved, but it still caused discomfort occasionally. About five months ago, the child was evaluated for painful knees and diagnosed with "growing pains." She has had no trauma, fevers, or rashes, but her activity level has decreased since the symptoms began. The mother has noted swelling in all three of the joints at one time or another but reports no erythema. On physical examination the vital signs are normal. Both knees are swollen but not erythematous. Range of motion in the knees and left elbow is decreased.

Questions

1. What findings are indicative of juvenile rheumatoid arthritis (JRA)?

2. What is the role of diagnostic imaging in the diagnosis and treatment of JRA?
3. Are any prognostic factors associated with JRA?
4. What are the indications for orthopedic intervention in children with JRA?
5. What medical therapies are currently used in the management of JRA?

Juvenile rheumatoid arthritis (JRA) is a diagnostic term applied to a specific collection of disorders characterized by a chronic inflammatory process of joints. JRA initially affects children under the age of 16 years. The diagnosis is particularly difficult to make because of the tremendous variability in clinical presentation, unpredictable disease course, and limited laboratory findings. A number of terms other than JRA have been proposed to describe the broad spectrum of arthropathies affecting children. These include juvenile arthritis, juvenile chronic arthritis, and juvenile chronic

---

Dx Juvenile Rheumatoid Arthritis

- Joint swelling
- Joint pain
- Limitation of motion of joints
- Fever
- Iridocyclitis
- Limitation of ability to open mouth (temporomandibular joint involvement)

---

polyarthritis. Conditions other than JRA included in these diagnostic categories are mentioned briefly in Differential Diagnosis.

EPIDEMIOLOGY

Any discussion of the epidemiology of JRA is imprecise at best for the reasons stated above. The reported incidence of the disease is 9.5–25/100,000 in children 16 years of age or less. African-American and Asian populations are much less likely to suffer from JRA, whereas Native Americans are more frequently affected. The age at presentation has a bimodal distribution, with an initial peak in the preschool age range (1–4 years) and a second peak before puberty (8–12). Overall, girls are affected two to three times more often than boys, but this varies with disease subtype and age of onset. In prepubertal children the sex distribution is relatively equal.

CLINICAL PRESENTATION

Swelling and inflammation (i.e., warmth) of joints is present in all cases of JRA, although the timing, location, and number of joints involved may vary with the stage of disease and specific type of JRA (D$_x$ Box). Young children may have decreased activity, inability or refusal to bear weight, or exhibit behaviors that appear to be developmentally regressive before joint effusion and inflammation is appreciated.

Fever (temperature: >100.4° F [38.0° C]) may be present in either the systemic or polyarticular subtype, but additional symptoms are more common in systemic JRA. In systemic JRA, fever spikes occur once or twice each day, and are usually accompanied by a characteristic ephemeral rash that occurs in discrete, small (< 1 cm) macules on the trunk or extremities. The rash may be missed because it usually occurs in the evening hours and is quite transient.

PATHOPHYSIOLOGY

A precise etiology for JRA has not been fully elucidated. Disturbances in traditional immunoregulatory mechanisms play a significant role in the development of the disease. Genetic factors are also evident. Studies of twins and family clusters demonstrate increased incidence and strong concordance of onset subtype and course. In addition, the recent advances in immunogenetics have uncovered striking associations between certain human leukocyte antigen (HLA) genes and particular subtypes of JRA, providing evidence for a genetic component to JRA.

DIFFERENTIAL DIAGNOSIS

The diagnosis of JRA is primarily based on clinical features, which may evolve over a period of weeks to months. During the early stages of JRA, associated clinical symptoms may be similar to those in infective arthritis, Lyme disease, and a variety of orthopedic conditions such as Legg-Calvé-Perthes disease, slipped capital femoral epiphyses, and Osgood-Schlatter disease. The distinction between JRA and other forms of childhood arthritis such as SLE, juvenile ankylosing spondylitis (JAS), and arthritis associated with immune deficiencies, in particular, is the most difficult to make. SLE is a multisystem disease, and as organ systems other than the musculoskeletal system become involved, the diagnosis becomes more apparent. JAS may be distinguished from JRA by the presence of characteristic sacroiliac joint involvement and the frequent presence of the HLA B27 antigen. Children with immunologic deficiencies may present with joint symptoms, like children with JRA, but an evaluation of immunoglobulins and complement usually indicates the deficiency.

Children under 16 years of age with persistent arthritis (≥ 6 weeks) who do not meet the criteria for other types of arthritides may be considered for the diagnosis of JRA (Table 111-1). The particular clinical manifestations evident within three to six months of initial presentation often allow the disease to be classified into one of three subtypes.

Pauciarticular JRA, which accounts for more than 40% of all cases of JRA, is characterized by involvement of fewer than five joints during the early stages. Girls are most frequently affected, and those with positive antinuclear antibody (ANA) are at significant risk of developing chronic uveitis. Immunogenetic studies indicate an association with HLA alleles DR8, DR5, and to a lesser extent, DR6. Systemic symptoms of pauciarticular disease are rare, but after the first 6 to 12 months the disease pattern may become polyarticular.

TABLE 111-1. Criteria for the Classification of Juvenile Rheumatoid Arthritis

Age of onset less than 16 years
Arthritis in one or more joints defined as swelling or effusion or presence of two
  or more of the following signs:
    Limitation of range of motion
    Tenderness or pain on motion
    Increased heat
Duration of disease for six weeks or more
Type of disease during the first six months classified as:
    Polyarthritis (≥ 5 joints)
    Pauciarticular disease (oligoarthritis) (≤ 4 joints)
    Systemic disease (Still's disease): arthritis with intermittent fever
Exclusion of other forms of juvenile arthritis

Reproduced, with permission, from Cassidy JT, and R.E. Petty. Juvenile rheumatoid arthritis. In *Textbook of Pediatric Rheumatology*, 2nd ed. New York, Churchill Livingstone, 1990, pp. 113–219 and Cassidy JT, Levinson JE, Bass JC, et al: A study of classification criteria for a diagnosis of JRA. Arthritis Rheum. 29:274, 1986.

Polyarticular JRA involves more than four joints during the first six months of illness. This subtype can be divided into two categories based on laboratory findings and clinical course. Children with positive rheumatoid factor (RF) who account for 10 to 15% of all cases of JRA make up the first group. They are primarily adolescent females whose clinical course more nearly resembles adult rheumatoid arthritis, with severe erosion and degeneration of joints. Furthermore, there is a strong association between RF-positive JRA and the DR4 antigen, which is the predominant HLA association in adult rheumatoid arthritis. Children with negative RF, the second group, have variable clinical manifestations. Although seronegative, they may have an increased prevalence of the DR4 antigen and develop severe erosive disease. Alternatively, they may manifest a pauciarticular pattern with uveitis and an association with the pauciarticualr HLA antigens.

Systemic onset arthritis, often referred to as Still's disease, accounts for 10% of all cases of JRA. The hallmark of this subtype is the presence of systemic features such as fever, which can be quite elevated (temperature: 102.2° F [39.0° C]), hepatosplenomegaly, and rash. Joint involvement may be variable, as in RF-negative polyarthritis. HLA associations seem to fall into the two patterns indicated above; children with severe disease are more likely to have the DR4 antigen, and others may have DR5 or DR8.

EVALUATION

History

The history should focus on joint symptoms (arthritis rather than arthralgias), specific extra-articular manifestations such as uveitis, and systemic signs such as fever and skin rashes (Questions Box).

Physical Examination

A thorough physical examination should be performed, with special attention paid to the assessment of all joints and extremities. The examiner should also look for evidence of skin rashes, lymphadenopathy, or organomegaly. Although joint involvement in JRA may be variable, swelling and inflammation, rather than simple arthralgias, are present in all cases. Larger joints (e.g., wrists, ankles, knees, shoulders, elbows) are usually involved. The pattern of arthritis is often symmetric, except in pauciarticular JRA. In the poly-articular subtype, smaller joints including the phalanges and temporomandibular joints may also be affected.

Because of their ephemeral nature, skin rashes may not be evident during an office visit. Nevertheless, a careful inspection of the skin of a completely unclothed child in a well-lighted room should still be performed.

In children with Still's disease, a careful abdominal examination may reveal organomegaly, which involves the spleen more often than the liver.

Laboratory Tests

Although laboratory studies are sometimes confirmatory, they may be negative, and the absence of a positive test does not rule out JRA. RF serology may be performed, but fewer than 10% of children with confirmed JRA are seropositive, making this a very poor screening test. ANA may be positive in pauciarticular JRA. The pattern of ANA immunofluorescence and the presence of multisystem disease distinguishes SLE from JRA.

Analysis of joint fluid aspirates may distinguish infectious arthritis from JRA. At present, serologic titers against *Borrelia burgdorferi* (the infectious agent in Lyme disease) are frequently uninterpretable. The physician should rely on the clinical pattern of disease progression to rule out this entity. An ESR is a nonspecific finding that may be helpful in encouraging repeat clinical assessments of children whose diagnosis is not yet certain.

Imaging Studies

Plain radiography is a useful adjunct in making the diagnosis of JRA because the resulting synovial proliferation may destroy articular surfaces, leading to erosion and ankylosis of bone. However, such studies may actually underestimate the extent of joint damage. The earliest radiographic findings in JRA are soft tissue swelling and periarticular osteopenia. As increasing amounts of cartilage are destroyed, joint space narrowing occurs. The most severe cases progress to bony erosion and other evidence of joint destruction.

MRI has proven to be much more useful in identifying early cartilage loss, changes due to avascular necrosis, and other intra-articular pathology. The increased sensitivity of MRI may prove useful in guiding medical and orthopedic interventions.

MANAGEMENT

The management of children with JRA necessitates a multidisciplinary approach designed to address not only the progression of inflammatory joint symptoms but also children's functional, nutritional, and emotional well-being. If possible, children should receive care where such support is readily available. The primary care physician can best serve the patient by overseeing the coordination of health care activities, providing routine preventive care, and treating minor illness or flare-

---

Questions: Juvenile Rheumatoid Arthritis

- Has the child ever had any swelling, warmth, or redness of joints?
- Does the child have any difficulty walking or running? If so, does this occur at any particular time of the day?
- Have the parents ever noticed any type of skin rash? If so, are the rashes temporally related to the joint swellings?
- Has the child ever had any serious eye problems?
- Has the child had any other health problems (e.g., kidney, lung, or brain diseases)?
- Has the child traveled recently or been bitten by a tick?

TABLE 111–2. Medical Therapy for Juvenile Rheumatoid Arthritis

Drug	Dosage	Toxicities	Comments
NSAIDs			
Aspirin	60–100 mg/kg	GI effects, Reye's syndrome	Salicylate level (20–25 mg/dL)
Various NSAIDs	Dosage varies with product	GI, renal effects; platelets, anemia	Urinalysis, CBC; indomethacin, naprosyn, ibuprofen available in liquid formulations
Steroids			
Oral	Dosage varies with drug	GI effects, infection, growth retardation, glaucoma, osteoporosis, endocrine derangements	Ongoing ophthalmologic care; infection surveillance
Ophthalmic	1–2 drops 4–6 times daily		
Intraarticular	10–30 mg (prednisolone)		

ups in close communication with the rheumatologist. In settings where access to subspecialists is limited, the primary care physician must accept a much more active role in the ongoing assessment and management of children with JRA. Affected children and their families must be kept informed of the child's condition and appropriate therapies. In addition, they must be counseled about the unpredictable nature of JRA, advances and controversies in therapies, and the importance of their participation in treatment decisions.

Physical and Occupational Therapy

Children are most likely to maintain their normal routine when adaptations and interventions that address their limitations, maximize their functional status, and minimize their deformities are used. Carefully selected **physical activities,** such as swimming and bicycling, interspersed with periods of rest, decrease the incidence of bone demineralization, muscle atrophy, contractures, and advanced joint damage. For children who are unable to bear weight, **range-of-motion exercises** are necessary substitutes. **Splints** and other orthotics are useful to prevent contractures and maximize the functional status of joints.

Medical Treatment

The traditional protocol for medical therapy begins with **NSAIDs** (Table 111–2). Many NSAIDs are frequently used in the treatment of childhood arthritides, but only a few are approved for this purpose. **Corticosteroids** are often the next line of therapy and have been used for the treatment of joint inflammation, uveitis, and systemic manifestations. **Slow-acting antirheumatic drugs** and **immunomodulators** are currently considered for refractory cases of JRA, but as more scientific evidence accumulates, these drugs may be relied on much earlier in the disease process.

The approach to medical therapy for JRA may change significantly in the future as the merits of the traditional approach are questioned. Some rheumatologists argue that reliance on the least toxic pharmaceuticals as the mainstay of therapy may result in missed opportunities to modify or curtail disease progression. Data from longitudinal studies of JRA combined with the increased sensitivity of diagnostic imaging techniques appear to indicate that (1) joint damage occurs more readily than

previously thought and (2) children once believed to be in remission have ongoing inflammation and joint destruction as they enter into adulthood. To date, no convincing studies prove the existence of so-called disease-modifying antirheumatic drugs, but this an active area of research.

Orthopedic Intervention

Orthopedic procedures play a critical role in the management of JRA. Although **soft tissue releases, tendon lengthening,** and **synovectomies** do not alter the course of the disease, they do much to improve function and relieve pain. **Reconstructive surgery** is sometimes necessary for joints that have been destroyed by severe erosive disease. Collaboration between the surgeon, the medical team, and physical or occupational therapists lead to optimal functional outcomes for children with JRA.

PROGNOSIS

Mortality is not increased in children with JRA, but morbidity affecting growth, emotional well-being, and functional capacity may be high. Progressive joint destruction and pharmacologic therapy, especially steroids, may adversely affect the linear growth rate and final adult height. Disease progression may severely limit children's ability to perform self-care activities and participate in age-appropriate physical activities. These and other factors related to chronic disease may also threaten their sense of emotional well-being.

Certain attributes such as the presence of RFs or ANAs in the serum have universally well-delineated prognostic implications. Progression from a pauciarticular or systemic presentation to polyarticular involvement indicates a worse prognosis. Severe joint destruction is more likely to occur in children with the systemic subtype of JRA who have persistent fevers and thrombocytosis.

Case Resolution

The girl in the case scenario has both signs and symptoms of pauciarticular JRA. Three joints (both knees and left elbow) are involved. Initial laboratory evaluation should include a CBC, ESR, RF, and ANA. The absence of fever eliminates an infectious etiology for the symptoms. X-rays of the affected joints are also appropriate, as is consultation with a pediatric rheumatologist.

Selected Readings

Athreya, B. H., and J. T. Cassidy. Current status of the medical treatment of children with juvenile rheumatoid arthritis. Rheum. Dis. Clin. North Am. 17:871–889, 1991.

Cassidy, J. T., and R. E. Petty. Juvenile Rheumatoid Arthritis. *In* Textbook of Pediatric Rheumatology, 2nd ed. New York, Churchill Livingstone, 1990, pp. 113–219.

Fink, C. W. Medical treatment of juvenile arthritis. Clin. Orthop. 259:60–69, 1990.

Nepom, B. The immunogenetics of juvenile rheumatoid arthritis. Rheum. Dis. Clin. North Am. 17:825–842, 1991.

Singsen, B. H. Rheumatic diseases of childhood. Rheum. Dis. Clin. North Am. 16:581–599, 1990.

Wallace, C. A., and J. E. Levinson. Juvenile rheumatoid arthritis: outcome and treatment for the 1990s. Rheum. Dis. Clin. North Am. 17:891–905, 1991.

CHAPTER 112

NEPHROTIC SYNDROME

Elaine Kamil, M.D.

H$_x$ A two-year-old boy is brought to the office because of abdominal distention. He has just recovered from a runny nose that lasted a week, with no fever or change in activity. His mother complains that his eyelids were very swollen that morning, and she says that his thighs look "fat." She has noticed that he has fewer wet diapers. He has always been a healthy child, and his immunizations are up-to-date. The family has a history of asthma and allergic rhinitis.

Physical examination shows an active two-year-old boy. Head and neck examination is clear, except for a few shotty anterior cervical lymph nodes and some minimal periorbital edema. Chest examination reveals some decreased breath sounds at the bases. The abdomen is moderately distended; bowel sounds are active and a fluid wave is detectable. There is 2+ pitting edema of the lower legs, extending up to the knees. The urine has a specific gravity of 1.030; pH 6; 4+ protein; and trace, nonhemolyzed blood. Microscopic examination shows four to six RBCs per high-power field and 10 to 20 hyaline and fine granular casts per low-power field.

Questions

1. What is the differential diagnosis of edema and ascites in previously healthy young children?
2. What criteria are used to determine if children require hospitalization or can be managed as outpatients?
3. What laboratory evaluation and therapy are instituted initially?
4. What are the important issues to address in parent education?
5. What is the prognosis of young children with nephrotic syndrome?

Although nephrotic syndrome is not a common childhood disease, every pediatrician can expect to care for at least one nephrotic child at some time. Nephrotic syndrome may have serious or even fatal complications, and the disease tends to follow a chronic, relapsing course. Thus it is important for the pediatrician to become familiar with the signs and symptoms of the disease, and with the most current treatment modalities aimed at keeping affected children healthy and active.

Nephrotic syndrome occurs when an individual excretes a sufficient quantity of plasma proteins, primarily albumin, in the urine to cause hypoalbuminemia. Substantial urinary protein losses, hypercholesterolemia, and hypoalbuminemia characterize nephrotic syndrome. The condition is usually accompanied by obvious edema, but occasionally this is not clinically detectable (D$_x$ Box).

In children, proteinuria of more than 40 mg/m^2/hr (> 50 mg/kg in 24 hours) is considered nephrotic range proteinuria. (In adult-sized patients, proteinuria of more than 3.5 grams in 24 hours is associated with nephrotic syndrome.) Collection of a 24-hour urine sample is cum-

---

D$_x$ **Nephrotic Syndrome**

- Heavy proteinuria (> 40 mg/m^2/hr or 50 mg/kg/24 hr in children)
- Hypoalbuminemia
- Hypercholesterolemia
- Edema

bersome in children, and the urinary total protein/ creatinine ratio (U TP/CR) done on a random urine sample is a useful alternative. Whereas a ratio greater than 3.5 is considered nephrotic range proteinuria in adults with normal renal function, a ratio greater than 1.0 is considered diagnostic in children (see Chapter 66, Proteinuria). Twenty-four hour urine protein losses (g/ m^2/day) in children can be estimated by multiplying the U TP/CR by 0.63.

EPIDEMIOLOGY

Minimal change disease (MCD) is the most common form of nephrotic syndrome in childhood. The annual prevalence of new cases of nephrotic syndrome is 2–3/100,000 children in the population less than 16 years of age. The cumulative prevalence of this chronic disease is 16/100,000. Ninety percent of childhood cases are not associated with any systemic disease, and two-thirds of cases of childhood nephrotic syndrome present before age five years. The ratio of boys to girls with nephrotic syndrome is 2:1. By late adolescence, both sexes are equally affected.

CLINICAL PRESENTATION

Typical children with nephrotic syndrome are preschool-age boys who usually present because they appear swollen to the parents. Some children are active and relatively asymptomatic despite the edema, whereas others may be very uncomfortable, with markedly swollen eyelids, abdominal discomfort, scrotal or labial edema, and even respiratory compromise. Usually children have a history of preceding infection, most typically a URI. Occasionally children may develop diarrhea secondary to edema of the bowel wall.

Occasionally children with nephrosis are critically ill due to peritonitis, bacteremia, or (rarely) a major thrombotic episode. Because their immune state is compromised, rapid evaluation and treatment of children with these complications of nephrotic syndrome are essential for survival. The primary peritonitis associated with nephrotic syndrome may be confused with an acute abdomen, such as may be seen with appendicitis. Some children who are experiencing a severe relapse have hypotensive symptoms secondary to intravascular volume reduction.

PATHOPHYSIOLOGY

The exact cause of MCD and focal segmental glomerulosclerosis (FSGS) is not known. Although controversial, many nephrologists consider FSGS to result from severe, treatment-resistant MCD. The best current theory postulates that some stimulus (usually infectious) causes a clone of lymphocytes or monocytes to proliferate and produce a cytokine or several cytokines that are toxic to the glomerular epithelial cells or the glomerular basement membrane. This cytokine induces a reduction in the net negative charge across the glomerular basement membrane. The constituents of this membrane and of the chemicals coating the glomerular epithelial and endothelial cells normally bear a net negative charge. The presence of these negatively charged chemicals creates a charge-selective barrier to filtration. This barrier plays a significant role in the ultrafiltration of macromolecules present in the plasma, enhancing the filtration of molecules bearing a positive electrical charge and retarding the filtration of molecules bearing a negative electrical charge. During episodes of relapse, patients with MCD show a breakdown in the normal charge-selective barrier to filtration, often resulting in massive proteinuria. Kidney biopsies from patients with nephrotic syndrome have demonstrated a net reduction in anionic sites during periods of relapse.

Evidence indicating that the proteinuria may be due to some soluble factor is threefold. One, some patients who develop end-stage renal disease from idiopathic nephrotic syndrome (particularly FSGS) have experienced a relapse of the nephrotic condition with massive proteinuria immediately after transplantation of a normal kidney. Two, infusion of peripheral blood mononuclear cell products from nephrotic children induces albuminuria in rats. Three, removal of serum proteins by adsorption to a protein A Sepharose column has led to remission of proteinuria in some patients who have experienced a recurrence of nephrotic syndrome after transplantation. The remission of the proteinuria after treatment with immunosuppressive medication provides further evidence that the nephrotic syndrome is mediated in some way by the immune system.

Normal adults are able to synthesize 12 grams of albumin per day in the liver, and adults with nephrotic syndrome may synthesize 14 grams of albumin per day. Therefore the **hypoproteinemia** characteristic of nephrotic syndrome cannot be explained completely by measured amounts of urinary protein losses (about 3.5 g/day). The difference between the hepatic synthetic capacity for albumin and the measured urinary losses can be explained by protein catabolism in the kidney. Renal tubular epithelial cells reabsorb filtered plasma proteins and catabolize them to amino acids, which then reenter the amino acid pool of the body. Thus the magnitude of losses of plasma proteins at the glomerular level is far greater than the amount measured in a 24-hour urine sample.

The **hypoalbuminemia** seen in nephrotic syndrome is a result of the massive proteinuria, and the **hypercholesterolemia** occurs as a consequence of the hypoalbuminemia. The hyperlipidemia is partially the result of a generalized increase in hepatic protein synthesis that also involves the overproduction of lipoproteins. In addition, less lipid is transported into the adipose tissue, because the activity of lipoprotein lipase is reduced in adipose tissue during active nephrotic syndrome. Hyperlipidemia is most pronounced in children with MCD. Serum albumin and serum cholesterol are generally inversely correlated.

DIFFERENTIAL DIAGNOSIS

Nephrotic syndrome is considered either primary or secondary. Primary nephrotic syndrome is not associated with a systemic disease. Secondary nephrotic syndrome is a feature of a systemic disease such as anaphylactoid purpura or SLE. The vast majority of children with nephrotic syndrome have the primary form of the disease.

Children with primary nephrotic syndrome are also classified according to their response to steroid therapy. Affected individuals may be categorized as steroid-sensitive, steroid-dependent, or steroid-resistant. Typically, children who are steroid-sensitive and remain so have MCD, although strictly speaking, a renal biopsy must be performed before the diagnosis of MCD is made. Sensitivity to or dependence on corticosteroids is a critical factor in determining children's prognosis.

Nephrotic syndrome is also classified by the appearance of the glomeruli on renal biopsy. A summary of the histologic lesions causing nephrotic syndrome appears in Table 112–1. About 95% of children with nephrotic syndrome have MCD. In these children, light microscopy shows normal-appearing glomeruli. Immunofluorescent microscopy is generally negative but may show some mesangial IgM deposits, and electron microscopy simply shows foot process effacement of the visceral epithelial cells. In individuals with FSGS, light microscopy may show enlarged glomeruli and glomeruli with segments of sclerosis. Immunofluorescence may reveal some IgM and complement in the sclerotic segments, and electron microscopy shows areas of foot process effacement of glomerular epithelial cells. Biopsies performed later in the disease course show some totally sclerotic glomeruli, areas of interstitial fibrosis, and atrophy.

Other primary renal diseases that can cause nephrotic syndrome in children include membranous nephropathy, membranoproliferative glomerulonephritis, IgA nephropathy and other forms of chronic glomerulonephritis, congenital nephrotic syndrome, and diffuse mesangial proliferative glomerulonephritis. Chronic hepatitis B infection may cause membranous nephropathy or membranoproliferative glomerulonephritis. Rarely, poststreptococcal acute glomerulonephritis and other forms of postinfectious acute glomerulonephritis may also cause nephrotic syndrome. With the exception of congenital nephrotic syndrome, all of these diseases show (1) the presence of immune deposits in the glomerular mesangial regions or along the glomerular basement membrane and (2) some element of cellular proliferation, which may be severe.

TABLE 112–1.   Distribution of Histologic Type by Age of Onset in Children With Nephrotic Syndrome

Age (years)	MCD*	FSGS	MN	MPGN	Other GN
1–4	95%	3%	2%	—	—
4–8	75%	15%	1%	7%	2%
8–16	52%	15%	2%	25%	6%

*MCD remains the dominant histologic type through midadolescence but becomes relatively less important in later childhood and adolescence.

Abbreviations: MCD, minimal change disease; FSGS, focal segmental glomerulosclerosis; MN, membranous nephropathy; MPGN, membranoproliferative glomerulonephritis; other GN, other forms of glomerulonephritis.

> ### Questions: Nephrotic Syndrome
>
> - Has the child recently had any infections, such as pharyngitis or a URI?
> - Are the child's eyelids swollen? Do they look more or less puffy at other times during the day, especially on awakening or after crying?
> - Does the child have a history of rashes characteristic of diseases that are associated with nephrotic syndrome?
> - Is there a history of fever, oliguria, or abdominal pain?
> - Is the child playful and active, or is the edema so significant that movement is uncomfortable?
> - Are the ascites and pleural effusions so severe that some respiratory compromise is evident?

In these disease states, the presence of nephrotic syndrome is indicative of marked injury to the glomerular capillary wall. Infants with congenital nephrotic syndrome have been found to have diminished numbers of anionic sites along the glomerular basement membrane, suggesting that the biochemical composition of the membrane is abnormal.

Because of the varying distribution of edema fluid, nephrotic syndrome may be confused with sinusitis or an allergic reaction (periorbital edema), obesity (ascites), or an abdominal mass (ascites). Other causes of generalized edema such as congestive heart failure or liver disease can be easily excluded.

EVALUATION

History

The clinical evaluation should include a careful history (Questions Box).

Physical Examination

A complete physical examination is necessary. Blood pressure should be monitored, because hypertension or hypotension may occur. The extent of the peripheral and central edema, including swelling of the eyelids, should be assessed. The physician should obtain a reliable, overall impression of the child's level of comfort and activity. The examination should also include a careful search for infection, particularly life-threatening infections such as pneumonia or peritonitis. Examination of the head and neck should focus on signs of recent infection such as otitis media. The presence of dullness to percussion at the bases of the thorax is consistent with large pleural effusions. Ascites may be minimal or massive. With severe ascites, scrotal or labial edema may occur. If the child has a history of abdominal pain, a careful check for signs of peritoneal irritation should be made. The skin should be inspected for infection and rashes.

Laboratory Tests

The laboratory evaluation of children with nephrotic syndrome begins with a urinalysis. The dipstick shows 3+ or 4+ protein, although a dilute urine may be only 2+.

Hematuria may be evident; up to 25% of children with MCD have microscopic hematuria. The presence of associated glycosuria in a nephrotic child who is not on steroid therapy raises a concern for FSGS. Careful microscopic examination is necessary. Casts are seen frequently because urinary proteins precipitate in the tubules. The casts are hyaline, fine, and coarse granular. WBC casts are sometimes seen because some children with nephrotic syndrome also have increased amounts of leukocytes in their urine. Large amounts of RBCs and RBC casts are not seen in uncomplicated MCD, and if present, indicate another cause for the nephrotic syndrome. If RBC casts are seen together with substantial hematuria, an antistreptolysin-O titer should be added to the preliminary evaluation. A random U TP/CR should be sent to determine whether children have nephrotic range proteinuria.

If the urine shows only proteinuria, with perhaps some microscopic hematuria, blood tests should include a CBC, serum creatinine and BUN, serum albumin, cholesterol, C3, and antinuclear antibody (ANA). The CBC may show a high hematocrit from hemoconcentration, because many children experience volume contraction as a complication of hypoproteinemia. Children may also have very high platelet counts (sometimes > 1,000,000/μL). The BUN and creatinine help assess renal function. The serum albumin and cholesterol are required to differentiate nephrotic syndrome from other edematous states. A low level of C3 is associated with other renal diseases such as membranoproliferative glomerulonephritis, acute postinfectious glomerulonephritis, and SLE. The ANA is useful in screening for SLE and other collagen vascular diseases. Hepatitis B serology is helpful in children who come from a population at risk for hepatitis B infection, such as recent immigrants from southeast Asia or children of intravenous drug abusers. Although not part of the routine laboratory evaluation, measurement of quantitative immunoglobulins often shows low IgG levels and elevated IgM levels.

Imaging Studies

Chest x-rays help assess the severity of pleural effusions in children with marked ascites and respiratory compromise.

MANAGEMENT

Hospitalization

The decision to admit a child with nephrotic syndrome to the hospital is determined by the child's functional status. All children with severe edema compromising ambulation or respiration should be admitted. Other indications for admission include unstable vital signs, fever, marked oliguria, and severe hemoconcentration (hematocrit > 48–50%).

Most children with nephrotic syndrome are hospitalized for control of edema or treatment of a complication such as infection. The management of children in relapse is aimed at minimizing edema and preventing complications until the disease can be controlled with immunosuppressive therapy. Intake, output, and weight need to be closely monitored. Blood pressure should be followed, although hypertension is uncommon.

If children have a fever (temperature: > 100.7° F [38.2° C]), blood and urine cultures should be obtained and antibiotics started pending culture results. If signs of peritoneal inflammation are evident, paracentesis should also be performed to obtain samples of the ascites fluid for Gram stain, cell count, and culture. Broad-spectrum antibiotics should be given to cover respiratory pathogens, especially pneumococcus, and enteric pathogens. All children who are newly diagnosed with nephrotic syndrome should have a purified protein derivative (PPD) test, because immunosuppression associated with steroid therapy may facilitate reactivation of tuberculosis infection.

Intravenous albumin (25%) should be used selectively, because albumin infusions are very expensive, and much albumin is excreted very rapidly in the urine. Infusions are indicated in children with marked ascites, scrotal or labial edema, or significant pleural effusions. They are also helpful in maintaining blood pressure and renal perfusion in septic children with nephrotic syndrome. The usual dose is 1 g/kg, up to 25 g, infused over 60 minutes, with close monitoring of blood pressure. Furosemide (1 mg/kg intravenously) is usually administered postinfusion. The albumin infusions may be repeated every 6 to 12 hours as necessary. If children with oliguria fail to increase their urine output after the first or second albumin infusion, they need to be evaluated immediately for the presence of acute renal failure (see Chapter 43, Acute Renal Failure). Mobilization of edema fluid in children with acute tubular necrosis precipitates pulmonary edema.

Supportive Therapy

Diet

Because sodium plays a key role in edema formation, children with nephrotic syndrome should be placed on a no-added salt diet that limits dietary sodium to three grams per day. Technically, sodium restriction is indicated only during times of relapse, but a constant no-added salt diet helps entire families maintain a consistent regimen. In general, fluid restriction is not necessary except in unusual circumstances (e.g., a steroid-resistant patient with severe fluid retention problems). Although earlier teachings recommended the use of high-protein diets, newer research has shown that these diets increase urinary protein losses.

Activity

In the past, children with nephrotic syndrome were treated with bed rest, because the supine position reduces urinary protein losses somewhat. No evidence shows that bed rest has a significant impact on children's clinical state, however. Therefore most pedi-

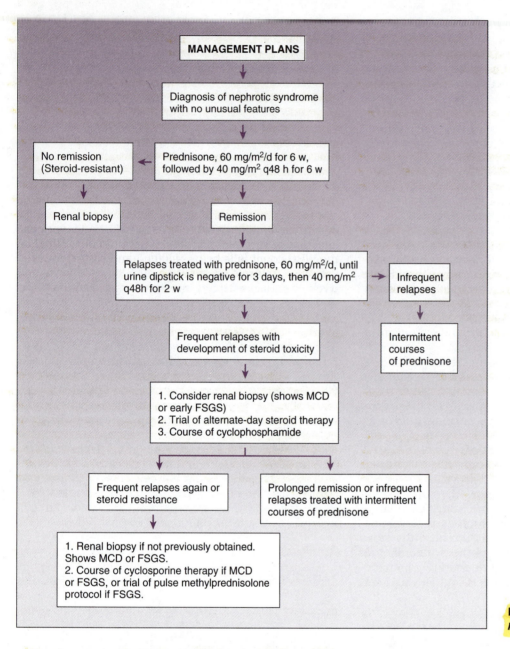

FIGURE 112–1. *Management of nephrotic syndrome in children.*

atric nephrologists recommend that children be allowed full activity. Boys with marked scrotal edema may be more comfortable resting in bed while diuresis is being initiated. Children with nephrotic syndrome should not be isolated from other children, and they should be allowed to attend school.

Diuretics

Diuretics are often helpful in children in relapse, particularly in children with steroid-resistant disease. Serum potassium levels, as well as clinical signs of intravascular volume, should be monitored. If children have moderate intravascular volume contraction, the injudicious use of diuretics could precipitate hypotension and increase the risk of thrombosis and acute tubular necrosis. The most commonly used diuretic is furosemide (1–2 mg/kg per dose given orally or intra-

venously). Spironolactone is sometimes added to the diuretic regimen for its potassium-sparing effect.

Long-term Management

The goal of long-term management is induction and maintenance of remission from active nephrotic syndrome. At the same time, the side effects of medications should be minimized. Spontaneous remission eventually occurs in children with MCD, but the 70% historical mortality rate makes waiting for a spontaneous remission unacceptable. Remissions are induced and maintained with the use of immunosuppressive medications. Figure 112–1 summarizes an approach to the overall management of nephrotic syndrome with these agents. A list of commonly used medications and dosages appears in Table 112–2.

TABLE 112–2. Treatment Options in Childhood Nephrotic Syndrome

Medication	Dose	Length of Therapy
Prednisone	60 mg/m²/day	Varies
Cyclophosphamide	2–3 mg/kg/day (cumulative dose < 200 mg/kg)	12 weeks
Chlorambucil	0.15–0.2 mg/kg/day (cumulative dose ≤ 8.2 mg/kg)	8 weeks
Cyclosporine	3 mg/kg/q12h	Varies
Levamisole	2.5 mg/kg qod	Varies

Corticosteroids and Alkylating Agents

Over 90% of children with primary nephrotic syndrome respond to corticosteroid therapy. Steroids are therefore both diagnostic and therapeutic, because failure to respond to steroids can be a marker for disease other than MCD. Even so, some children with MCD are steroid-resistant at some time in their disease. Steroids can be started in children who are newly diagnosed with nephrotic syndrome if they have no signs of systemic disease, no more than microscopic hematuria, a normal C3 (or results pending), and normal renal function. Acute infection should be managed with specific antimicrobial therapy to avoid infection-related steroid resistance.

Prednisone is usually started at 60 mg/m²/day. It can either be given once a day, in the morning, or divided into two or three daily doses. Proteinuria resolves within two weeks in many children with MCD and by four weeks in more than 90%. Serum albumin normalizes soon after proteinuria clears, but hypercholesterolemia may take many weeks to return to normal.

The pediatrician can easily manage steroid-sensitive children, but children with more difficult nephrotic syndrome should be managed in conjunction with the pediatric nephrologist. Children with relapses are treated with daily prednisone (60 mg/m²) until the urine is protein-free for three days. This regimen is followed by two weeks of 40 mg/m² every other morning. An increased incidence of side effects (e.g., cushingoid appearance, hypertension, obesity, glucose intolerance, cataracts, osteopenia, decreased growth rate) occurs when children require frequent courses of prednisone therapy. In frequently relapsing children, a chronic course of alternate-day steroid therapy may eliminate relapses and reduce steroid toxicity. Usually 60 mg/m² of prednisone is given every other morning initially. The dose is then gradually tapered over several months to the lowest dose that keeps the child in remission.

If alternative-day steroid therapy fails to maintain remission, cyclophosphamide or chlorambucil is administered. Both of these alkylating agents induce long-lasting remission in children with steroid-dependent or frequently relapsing nephrotic syndrome. Either of these agents is started while children are on steroid therapy, and the steroids are gradually tapered during the course of treatment with the alkylating agent. In the past a diagnostic renal biopsy was routine prior to starting an alkylating agent. Many pediatric nephrolo-

gists now consider such therapy in steroid-sensitive or steroid-dependent children without a biopsy, however, providing renal function is normal. Initially a daily dose of 2 mg/kg of cyclophosphamide was recommended for eight weeks. Recent studies, however, have shown that a 12-week course is more likely to induce prolonged remission and still be safe.

Potential toxicities of cyclophosphamide include bone marrow suppression with increased risk of infection, alopecia, hemorrhagic cystitis, gonadal toxicity, and a small but indeterminately increased risk of developing a malignancy at some time. CBCs should be monitored weekly, and parents should be cautioned about the increased risk of overwhelming varicella infections in children who have not yet had a varicella infection or vaccination. The dose should be withheld if the WBC count falls below 4000/μL and restarted when the WBC returns or exceeds 4000/μL. Alopecia and hemorrhagic cystitis are rare when the recommended dose is used. A 12-week course of cyclophosphamide (2 mg/kg/day) does not appear to increase the risk of infertility, but longer courses are associated with oligospermia, aspermia, and ovarian dysfunction. Postpubertal individuals may be at greater risk for gonadal toxicity than prepubertal children.

When steroid-sensitive or steroid-dependent children have failed to achieve prolonged remission after cyclophosphamide therapy, a diagnostic renal biopsy should be performed. Renal biopsy is indicated early in the course of illness for steroid-resistant children. If FSGS is identified on biopsy, treatment involves a prolonged course of intravenous methylprednisolone therapy or cyclosporin. Therapeutic options for children with MCD who continue to be steroid-dependent after a course of cyclophosphamide include treatment with cyclosporin or levamisole. Although cyclosporin is more likely to induce prolonged remission, it only maintains remission while being administered. Children trade steroid dependence for cyclosporin dependence. Nevertheless, for children with steroid toxicity, a 6–12-month course of cyclosporin allows resolution of the adverse effects of steroids and is generally well tolerated when administered by the experienced physician. Side effects such as hirsutism and gingival hyperplasia are frequent at the onset of therapy. These effects regress as the dose is decreased or the drug is discontinued, however. Hypertension is not uncommon. The most common metabolic abnormality seen with cyclosporin use is hypomagnesemia. Long-term therapy may lead to significant nephrotoxicity, and rarely patients experience liver toxicity.

Because of potential toxicity, cyclosporin A should only be prescribed by a physician familiar with the drug. Cyclosporin requirements may change with remission and relapse, and the family and physician should be aware of several drug interactions. Any medication interfering with the P450 enzyme system in the liver, such as erythromycin, greatly increases cyclosporin A levels and should be used only under extraordinary circumstances. Children who require prolonged treatment with cyclosporin A should have follow-up kidney biopsies performed after a year of therapy to assess for any nephrotoxicity.

Immunization Issues

Because of the unusual susceptibility to pneumococcal infections, children with nephrotic syndrome over the age of two years should receive the pneumococcal vaccine. The vaccine is best administered while the children are in remission, but it produces protective titers even in children who are on alternate-day steroid therapy at the time of immunization. Influenza vaccine should be administered each fall to children with nephrotic syndrome using the age-appropriate schedule and dosage.

Some of the routine childhood immunizations (diphtheria-tetanus-pertussis, *Haemophilus influenzae* type B, hepatitis B) should be administered by the usual schedule but while children are in remission (see Chapter 17, Immunizations). Some controversy exists concerning the use of live virus vaccines in children who require long-term immunosuppressive therapy. No vaccines should be administered if children are currently being treated with an alkylating agent. The parenteral polio vaccine (IPV) may be substituted for the oral vaccine, and IPV may be used for "boosters." The measles-mumps-rubella (MMR) vaccine could potentially cause a relapse.

Parent Education

Because nephrotic syndrome follows a chronic, relapsing course, parent education is essential for effective long-term management. Parents need to be instructed about using urinary dipsticks (Albustix) to monitor protein excretion. Generally urine dipsticks should be used daily during periods of active relapse and when medication is being tapered. Otherwise, the dipstick should be checked whenever children have infections, including URIs, or whenever they look "puffy."

Weight should also be monitored, especially during relapse. Children should be weighed each morning when they awaken. Urine output should be measured in more difficult cases. As parents become more familiar with the nephrotic syndrome, they may contact the physician about medication changes. Parents should also contact the physician about "danger signs" such as fever (temperature: > 100.7° F [38.2° C]), significant abdominal pain, or exposure to varicella. If children do not have protective antibodies against varicella and if they are taking any immunosuppressive medication (including prednisone), the varicella-zoster immune globulin should be administered within 72 hours of exposure to varicella. If varicella infection develops, acyclovir should be instituted.

PROGNOSIS

In the preantibiotic era, nephrotic syndrome was frequently fatal, usually because of overwhelming infec-tion. After the introduction of antibiotics, the mortality rate fell. The use of corticosteroids has led to a further reduction in mortality. Currently, the mortality rate is about 5%, almost exclusively due to infections from encapsulated organisms or from thrombosis. The greatest risk of death in children with nephrotic syndrome is among the children with resistance to corticosteroid therapy.

The long-term outlook for the majority of children with nephrotic syndrome is favorable, particularly for steroid-sensitive patients. Relapses often disappear by the completion of puberty. Occasionally children continue to have relapses into adulthood. Approximately 20% of children with steroid-sensitive MCD still experience relapses 15 years after the onset of their disease. Disease recurrence is highly unlikely if eight years pass without a relapse. Less than 10% of initially steroid-sensitive children with nephrotic syndrome develop end-stage renal disease. This occurs almost exclusively in children with FSGS. FSGS may recur after kidney transplants, particularly in young children with aggressive FSGS.

Case Resolution

In the opening scenario, the child most likely has MCD. He appears stable enough to be managed as an outpatient and should be placed on a salt-restricted diet and prednisone. The overall prognosis depends on a close interaction among the parents, pediatrician, and consulting pediatric nephrologist.

Selected Readings

Arbeitsgemeinschaft Für Pädiatrische Nephrologie. Short versus standard prednisone therapy for initial treatment of idiopathic nephrotic syndrome in children. Lancet I:380–383, 1988.

Bernard, D. B. Extrarenal complications of the nephrotic syndrome. Kidney Int. 33:1184–1202, 1988.

Brodehl, J. Conventional therapy for idiopathic nephrotic syndrome in children. Clin. Nephrol. 35:S8–15, 1991.

International Study of Kidney Disease in Children. Minimal change nephrotic syndrome in children: deaths during the first 5 to 15 years' observation. Pediatrics 73:497–501, 1984.

Kher, K. K., M. Sweet, and S. P. Makker. Nephrotic syndrome in children. Curr. Prob. Pediatr. 18:203–251, 1988.

Lewis, M. A., et al. Nephrotic syndrome: from toddlers to twenties. Lancet I:255–259, 1989.

Mendoza, S. A., et al. Treatment of steroid-resistant focal segmental glomerulosclerosis with pulse methylprednisolone and alkylating agents. Pediatr. Nephrol. 4:303–307, 1990.

Niaudet, P., et al. Treatment of severe childhood nephrosis. Adv. Nephrol. 17:151–172, 1988.

Thabet, M. A. E. H., J. R. Salcedo, and J. C. M. Chan. Hyperlipidemia in childhood nephrotic syndrome. Pediatr. Nephrol. 7:559–566, 1993.

CHAPTER 113

SEIZURES AND EPILEPSY

Kenneth R. Huff, M.D.

Hx A 6-year-old boy is evaluated for unusual episodic behaviors. The previous week his mother was awakened by the boy's brother and found her son lying in bed unresponsive and drooling, with his head and eyes averted to the right, his right arm slightly raised, and his body stiff. His face was jerking intermittently. When the paramedics arrived, the boy's posturing and movements had stopped. After the event he could speak but was somewhat incoherent. He was taken to the local emergency department, where his examination and mental status were normal. Screening blood and urine tests were normal, and he was discharged. His family was instructed to see his pediatrician for further recommendations.

His father remembers two or three other episodes of a somewhat different nature in the past month. These occurred as the boy was being put to bed. They involved some body stiffening and facial grimacing, with the mouth slightly open and the tongue twisted and deviated to one side. The child could not speak but appeared to be trying to talk. The episodes lasted 20 to 30 seconds. Afterwards the boy was his usual self and could tell his father what had been said to him.

The child has had no intercurrent illnesses or abnormal behavior apart from these "spells," and he has lost no abilities. A paternal cousin and grandfather had seizures during childhood but "grew out of them." The examination is completely normal.

Questions

1. Is it likely that the episodic behavior was a seizure?
2. What historical data about an event support the diagnosis of a seizure disorder?
3. How does the EEG help in classifying the type of seizure disorder?
4. What rationale should be used to formulate short-term and long-term treatment plans?

Seizures are a common medical problem in children. Diagnosing a seizure that is not a generalized tonic-clonic convulsion is sometimes problematic. Seizures are defined as episodic, stereotypic behavior syndromes of abrupt onset that result in loss of responsiveness and that generally are not provoked by external factors. Correlation with scalp-derived, brain electrical discharges on EEG is likely but not absolute.

A detailed history of the nature of the episodic behavior from an eyewitness is paramount both in making the diagnosis of a seizure disorder and in elucidating the type of seizure problem. The EEG is an adjunct. It is abnormal in many individuals who do not have clinical seizures, and it may be normal interictally

in many patients with clinical seizures, because of its sampling limitations. Special techniques can sometimes help alleviate these limitations.

The type of seizure problem directs the treatment plan. Seizures can simply be classified as primary generalized seizures or partial seizures. Some partial seizures can secondarily generalize, thereby clinically mimicking primary generalized seizures. This development illustrates the importance of eyewitness information. Many treatment options are available, and the therapeutic plan must often be individualized to optimize seizure control and minimize side effects. With appropriate treatment, the majority of children with seizure disorders are handicapped neither scholastically nor socially and can enjoy normal lives.

EPIDEMIOLOGY

About 0.5 to 1.0% of all children experience at least one afebrile seizure. Febrile seizures are as much as 10 times more common, however (see Chapter 35, Febrile Seizures). Some types of seizures have a familial predisposition. Seizure disorders are more common following hypoxic/ischemic attacks, severe head trauma, and encephalitis or meningitis.

CLINICAL PRESENTATION

Children present with a history of an episode of abrupt onset characterized by a loss of ability to respond to external stimuli. They may experience preliminary symptoms before losing consciousness and may feel sleepy following the period of lost responsiveness. During the seizure, observers may note only an akinetic or staring spell or dramatic, rhythmic spasms of the face, extremities, or torso, depending on the type of seizure (Dx Box). With major motor seizures, autonomic system changes, including those related to skin vasculature, sweating, saliva production, and sphincter control, frequently occur. Most seizure disorders are not af-

Dx Seizures

- Abrupt loss of responsiveness
- Rhythmic clonic movements
- Sustained changes in posture or tone
- Simple automatic movements
- Staring without change in tone
- Changes in cerebral electrical activity

fected by environmental factors. Between episodes, the examination may be entirely normal.

PATHOPHYSIOLOGY

A seizure represents a sudden, synchronous change in the electrical organization of a large group of neurons that can be propagated by those neurons. Partial seizure disorders may result from a focal cortical lesion, such as a glial scar caused by a prior insult (e.g., an infarct), that disrupts the electrical organization and allows for periodic, propagated abnormal transmission of impulses.

Exactly what produces the synchronous depolarization of the neurons and the propagation is not well understood. Several physiologic mechanisms, including neuronal circuitry, membrane ion channels, and glial transmitter precursor metabolism or uptake, are probably involved. An understanding of the mechanism involved in familial epilepsy syndromes awaits the definition of the various gene products.

Seizure Types

Seizures can be simply classified as either **primary generalized seizures,** which include grand mal, generalized tonic-clonic convulsions, and petit mal (absence) seizures, or **partial seizures,** which include focal motor, psychomotor, and other partial disorders (Table 113–1). In addition, a number of age-related seizure syndromes exist that may be related to maturational events in brain circuitry. The examples presented here should not be considered an exhaustive list of such syndromes but some of the more common types of problems encountered in practice.

The majority of all seizures in older children result from partial seizure disorders. **Psychomotor seizures** are partial seizures that have a wide range of ictal (seizure) behaviors, including focal clonic jerking, aversive or asymmetric hypertonic posturing, and more complex stereotypic fumbling or fingering behaviors. These seizures are usually preceded by sensory auras or emotional manifestations and may be followed by postictal drowsiness. In some instances, children may have partial sensory awareness during seizures. In other cases, however, they are completely unconscious, and

TABLE 113–2. Partial Complex Versus Absence Seizures

	Partial Complex	Absence
Aura	Frequent	None
Loss of consciousness	Sometimes partial	Complete
Motor movements	Sometimes complex	Blinking
Postictal state	Frequent	None
Duration	> 30 seconds	< 15 seconds
Frequency	Few per day	Many per hour or day
Hyperventilation provoked	No	Yes
EEG	Variable or normal	3/sec spike-wave
Prognosis past adolescence	Frequently persists	Rarely occurs

the initial partial motor manifestations can rapidly generalize. Partial seizures are more highly associated than generalized seizures with demonstrable focal brain pathologic processes, including traumatic lesions, infarcts, malformations, infections (e.g., viral encephalitides, cerebral cysticercosis), and mesial temporal or hippocampal sclerosis (seen on MRI).

Sylvian or rolandic seizures are a relatively common familial partial seizure syndrome with a good prognosis. These episodes commonly occur when children are drowsy or awakening. Sensory auras precede the seizures, and motor manifestations involve the tongue, mouth, or face but can partially or completely generalize. The clinical syndrome is accompanied by a characteristic focal EEG discharge over the central temporal region of the scalp.

Absence seizures may sometimes be difficult to distinguish from partial seizures (Table 113–2). They are brief (2–15 seconds) losses of consciousness without loss of tone. Staring and minor lip, tongue, or semipurposeful-appearing finger movements are often the only observed behaviors. There is no postictal period. Because absence seizures occur several times a day and children are often unaware of them, parents may dismiss the subtle behavior change and inattention as daydreaming. These seizures may adversely affect learning. Hyperventilation, a diagnostic test that can be performed in the office, may provoke absence seizures. The EEG is confirmatory and distinguishes classic petit mal seizure syndromes from variant types. The classic petit mal is more often familial with dominant transmission, age-specific manifestation (4–16 years), and sensitivity to ethosuximide.

DIFFERENTIAL DIAGNOSIS

Seizures are distinguished from nonepileptic paroxysmal disorders on the basis of history. **Syncope** is often accompanied by premonitory symptoms of lightheadedness, nausea, tinnitus, and eventually a gradual darkening of vision, sometimes without loss of auditory perception. The syncopal episode is also frequently situational, unlike a seizure. It occurs when children are in hot, stuffy environments; when they have been standing in one place for a long time; or when they see or experience a painful or traumatic event such as an

TABLE 113–1. Classification of Epileptic Seizures

Partial seizures (seizures beginning locally)
    Elementary symptoms: focal seizures
    Complex symptoms: psychomotor seizures
    Partial seizures evolving secondarily to generalized seizures
Generalized seizures (bilaterally symmetric; onset not local)
    Absence seizures (petit mal): typical and atypical
    Tonic-clonic seizures
    Tonic seizures
    Clonic seizures
    Myoclonic seizures (minor motor)
    Atonic seizures (drop attacks)
    Infantile spasms
Unclassified seizures (includes neonatal "subtle" seizures)

injection or phlebotomy. In boys syncope may occur during early morning micturition.

Breath-holding spells are characterized by apnea and loss of responsiveness with change in color to a cyanotic or pallid shade. Children may throw themselves backward and stiffen, and they may even have a few clonic jerks. Breath-holding spells are also "situational." Infants or children are often upset and very frequently cry just before such spells. They may be frightened by a seemingly minor injury or angry after a toy is taken away or a disciplinary action is administered.

Selective attention is frequently mistaken for minor motor or absence seizures. This behavior often occurs when children are involved in passive activities (e.g., watching television, playing a video game, daydreaming) and do not respond to verbal stimuli such as their own name. Generally, attention lapses do not occur when children are involved in activities in which they are actively engaged (e.g., talking, eating). Electrically generated brain discharges occur even during these activities.

Seizures must also be differentiated from **pseudoseizures,** which actually occur most often in patients who have true seizures. Such episodes may resemble true seizures, and the psychodynamics of secondary gain or other motivation for the behavior may not be apparent. Pseudoseizures should be suspected in children who have witnessed seizures in relatives or close friends, who have seizures that recur in common situations, who do not experience a change in seizure frequency with therapeutic levels of anticonvulsants, and who appear suggestable. Diagnosis can often be made in suggestable children, with the caregiver's consent, in the following manner. Patients are connected to an EEG machine, told that an injection will produce a seizure, and then given an intravenous injection of a placebo. It is hoped that the placebo will produce a pseudoseizure that the EEG monitoring will confirm. Children with pseudoseizures have an unusual need (perceived or real) for attention. All major causes of psychological trauma (e.g., sexual abuse) should be further investigated.

EVALUATION (Table 113–3)

History

The history should determine the exact events surrounding the seizure episode. A detailed history of the

---

TABLE 113–3.   Initial Evaluation of Seizure Patients

Eyewitness account of the episode

Description of children's own experiences before, during, and after the episode if they are articulate

Past history from caregiver concerning remote injuries to the nervous system, progressive neurologic symptoms, or intercurrent illness

Careful neurologic examination looking for signs of cerebral hemisphere lateralization

Brain imaging study when a partial seizure is observed, a crescendo history of neurologic symptoms is obtained, or focal neurologic signs are found on interictal examination

Waking and sleep electroencephalogram with hyperventilation

Questions: Seizures

- Where was the child and what was he or she doing when the episode began?
- Did the child experience a loss of responsiveness?
- Did the child show any warning behavior or aura (e.g., a cry, a facial expression of fear, fearful behavior, irritability)?
- Did any part of the child's body become stiff? Was any shaking or jerking apparent?
- What did the child's eyes do and was saliva produced at the mouth?
- Did the child's skin change color?
- Did the child experience a loss of sphincter control?
- How long did the episode last?
- Has the child been well recently?
- Did the child have a complicated birth, head trauma, meningitis, or other previous brain damage?
- Have episodes of a similar nature occurred previously? If so, when did they begin and how frequently do they occur?
- Has the child's development and school experience progressed normally?
- Does the child have any relatives who have had seizures?

---

nature of the behavior from an eyewitness is essential (Questions Box). The physician should find out whether children experienced any loss of responsiveness. Most often this change in mental status is abrupt, although a warning behavior or aura that lasts for a few seconds may precede complete loss of responsiveness. The warning behavior may be a cry, an expression of fear, or irritability. If children are articulate, they may be able to describe a sensory phenomenon or relate an indescribable sensation.

A change in muscle tone and activity is frequently associated with the abrupt change in mental status unless the spell is an absence seizure. Most often, the tone is increased as manifested by general extensor posturing, more focal hypertonicity, or more complex posturing such as torsion or aversive upper extremity posturing. The patient may fall if not supported. Rhythmic jerking or clonic movements (focal or general), including the trunk, limbs, face, and eyes, may occur concomitantly. Respirations may involve rhythmic grunting or nearly imperceptible movements. Swallowing may not occur, so that saliva pools or forms at the lips. Autonomic changes including skin color change (circumoral cyanosis), increased pulse, and loss of sphincter control frequently occur with major motor spells. The ictal period generally lasts 30 seconds to two minutes, although observers frequently overestimate this time. Postictal periods of sleepiness or lethargy may be seen. Their length is often correlated with the length or intensity of the seizure.

Physicians should note that children and individuals around them are often unaware of the occurrence of minor motor or absence seizures. Often an observant teacher brings a child's problem to a physician's attention. During a spell, a child may have only subtle facial or hand movements, the duration of the episode is short, and there are no preictal or postictal behaviors.

Historical information can help determine potential etiologies of the seizure disorder. A distant brain insult or hereditary disposition may be the cause.

Physical Examination

Children should be examined carefully for focal neurologic signs, particularly asymmetries. This examination should include a developmental assessment and a mental status examination. The physician should look for signs of potential genetic problems, such as dysmorphic features, indicating potential cerebral dysgenesis; abnormal skin pigmentation, suggesting a neuroectodermal disorder; and bony deformities, indicating a possible storage disorder. Children who are old enough to cooperate should be asked to hyperventilate to provoke an absence spell if the history is suggestive of this type of seizure.

Laboratory Tests

An EEG should be requested to help with the diagnosis of the type of seizure disorder. Children with typical or atypical petit mal disorders rarely have normal EEGs. In children with partial seizure disorders, the interictal discharge is helpful in localizing the site of genesis of abnormal electrical activity. Sleep is often essential to observing abnormalities. If a normal EEG is obtained without sleep and seizures continue to recur, it is sometimes useful to ensure sleep during the test. Caregivers can be instructed to deprive children of sleep before the EEG. Special techniques (e.g., prolonged monitoring with telemetry or special anatomic electrode placements) can sometimes help overcome EEG limitations of sampling time and lack of contiguity between the scalp and some areas of the cortex.

Electrolytes are rarely abnormal in older children who have been well prior to the seizure. The Dextrostix should be checked in acute cases, however. Neonates and infants with recurrent, unexplained seizures should have metabolic screening including organic acid and amino acid levels. Urine screens, specific assays, and tissue histologic biopsy may be indicated for diagnosis when physical signs suggest a neurologic storage disease.

Imaging Studies

An MRI scan should be requested, especially in the following situations: if a progression in neurologic symptoms or signs has occurred, if an asymmetry of strength or tone is noted on examination, if there is a history of prior neurologic insult, or if signs of dysgenesis are present in other parts of the body. In the absence of these factors, partial or focal seizure disorders have a higher yield of abnormal imaging results. Intravenous contrast should generally be given because loss of focal blood-brain barrier with inflammatory or neoplastic lesions can lead to seizures. Recurrent, resistant seizures are sometimes further elucidated with functional imaging studies such as positron emission

tomography (PET), single photon emission computerized tomography (SPECT), and functional MRI.

MANAGEMENT

Anticonvulsants are the mainstay of management of seizure disorders. These drugs are prescribed if the risk of recurrence of seizures is significant. A structural lesion seen on imaging studies or the clinical situation and the EEG may suggest a high risk of recurrence. The choice of anticonvulsant agent depends on age, neurologic diagnosis, other conditions or medications, and social factors. Many anticonvulsants are available (Table 113–4). Short- and long-range treatment plans depend on the type of seizure disorder, the seizure history, and the individual patient's situation.

Carbamazepine is often recommended for partial seizures. Toxicity is generally mild; adverse effects include GI upset, dizziness, and headaches. Diphenylhydantoin is also effective for these types of seizures. This can be given intravenously for status epilepticus. Phenobarbital is effective in neonatal seizures but may have deleterious effects on behavior and learning in older children. Ethosuximide is used for classical petit mal seizures. Valproic acid is used for atypical petit mal and other seizure disorders that are resistant to other anticonvulsants. Newer anticonvulsants, including gabapentin, lamotrigine, and vigabatrin, have not yet been used as extensively in children but may prove helpful, especially in an adjunctive way.

Periodic monitoring of efficacy and side effects is essential in children who take anticonvulsants daily on a long-term basis. A log of seizures helps assess medication efficacy. Drug levels are useful in monitoring dosages, compliance, and the likelihood that symptoms are the result of drug side effects. Organ toxicity (bone

TABLE 113–4. Drugs Useful for Treating Seizures

Seizure Type	Dose (mg/kg)	Toxic Symptoms
Partial seizures		
Carbamazepine	approx. 30	Gastrointestinal distress, headache
Diphenylhydantoin	4–8	Ataxia, nystagmus
Primidone	12–25	Drowsiness, ataxia
Newer medications		
Lamotrigine	4–7	Dizziness, sedation
Gabapentin	4–8	Somnolence, ataxia
Vigabatrin	15–50	Drowsiness, behavioral disturbances
Neonatal seizures		
Phenobarbital	5	Lethargy, irritability
Generalized seizures		
Valproic acid	30–60	Tremors, sedation
Myoclonic seizures		
Clonazepam	0.15	Drowsiness, ataxia
Absence seizures		
Ethosuximide	30	Nausea, hiccups
Valproic acid	30–60	Tremors, sedation
Infantile spasms		
Adrenocorticotropic hormone	40 units/m^2	Increased appetite, acne
Valproic acid	30–60	Tremors, sedation

marrow and liver) must be considered and monitored with many medications.

The individualized decision to discontinue medication is often complex. The prognosis for recurrence of seizures, the parents' and children's reactions to the seizures and to the prospect of their recurrence, and social factors such as school participation may all contribute to the decision. Children and parents must be aware that none of the prognostic factors, whether considered individually or in combination, are absolute predictors of seizure recurrence.

PROGNOSIS

In general, the majority of children who have experienced a seizure have a good prognosis for prevention of recurrence and little or no problem with side effects of medication. They can lead normal lives without handicap. The etiologic diagnosis is the most important prognostic factor. The type of epilepsy, the EEG findings, the child's age, the difficulty of initial seizure control, and the time since the last seizure are also important.

Some seizure types have intrinsically poor prognoses. For example, infantile spasms are prognostically ominous because even in the absence of a metabolic or morphologic diagnosis, children frequently suffer head growth and developmental arrest, unless the seizures are controlled with medication. Partial complex seizure disorders and the atypical variant of petit mal syndrome sometimes have a poorer prognosis for early resolution and may be more resistant to treatment with anticonvulsants. However, some of the familial disorders such as Sylvian seizures and typical petit mal seizures have a relatively good prognosis for both control by medication and ultimate complete resolution.

Case Resolution

The boy described in the case history at the beginning of the chapter had a generalized seizure when he was taken to the emergency room. The previous episodes recalled by the father had characteristics of partial seizures. The tonic-clonic seizure was probably a secondary generalized rather than a primary generalized seizure. The possibility of sylvian seizures are suggested by the circumstances of the prior episodes, which occurred when the boy was drowsy; their "facial" symptomatology; and the family history. This diagnosis was confirmed by EEG. Carbamazepine was prescribed. The boy experienced no side effects or seizure recurrences and was successfully able to discontinue the medication three years later.

Selected Readings

Holmes, G. L. Diagnosis and Management of Seizures in Children. Major Problems in Pediatrics, vol. 30. Philadelphia, W. B. Saunders, 1987.

Pellock, J. M. (ed.). Seizure disorders. Pediatr. Clin. North Am. 36:265–461, 1989.

Scheuer, M. L., and T. A. Pedley. Current concepts: the evaluation and treatment of seizures. N. Engl. J. Med. 323:1468–1474, 1990.

Wyllie, E. The Treatment of Epilepsy: Principles and Practice. Philadelphia, Lea & Febiger, 1993.

INDEX

Note: Page numbers in *italics* refer to illustrations;
page numbers followed by t indicate tables.

Head, circumference of, in normal growth, 35, 36, 36t
  examination of, in newborn, 26, 27t
  trauma to, 153–157, *154, 155,* 156t
    and increased intracranial pressure, 153–155, 157, 158
    in automobile-pedestrian crashes, 146, *146*
Headache, 373–376, 374t, 376t
  migraine, vs. increased intracranial pressure, 160
Health maintenance organizations, 3
Hearing, assessment of, in preterm infant, 79
  disorders of, 55–58, 56t, 57t, 181–185, *182,* 183t, 184t
    in Down syndrome, 71–72, 74t
    with cleft lip and palate, 170, 171
    with microtia, 170, 171, 183
Hearing aids, 58, 184
Heart, congenital diseases of, and cyanosis, in newborn, 247–252, 248t, *250*
  congestive failure of, 244–246, 252t, 252–255, *253,* 254t, 255t
  disorders of, in anaphylaxis, 217–220
    in athletes, 24
    in Down syndrome, 69, 70
    in renal failure, chronic, 457, 460
    in sudden infant death syndrome, 142t–144t, 142–145
  examination of, in newborn, 27, 27t
  murmurs of, 244–247, *245,* 245t
Heart rate, variations of, with age, 136, 136t
Heartburn, gastroesophageal reflux and, 336
Height, in normal growth, 35, 36, 36t
Helicobacter pylori infection, and peptic ulcers, 355–357
Hemangiomas, in neck, *210,* 212–213, 215
Hematemesis, 340–341
  gastroesophageal reflux and, 336–337
Hematochezia, 340–343
Hematoma, cephalic, examination for, in newborn, 26
  head injury and, 154, *155*
  of gum, with tooth eruption, 47
  of scalp, 386
Hematuria, 265t–267t, 265–270, *268*
Hemiballismus, vs. tics, 378
Hemoccult test, 342
Hemoglobin, disorders of, screening for, in newborn, 16, 17t, 18
  in anemia, 230–234, 231t–233t
  oxygen dissociation from, in cyanosis, in newborn, 250, *250*
Hemolytic anemia, autoimmune, and lymphadenopathy, 241t
Hemolytic-uremic syndrome, 237
  and hematuria, 269–270
  and renal failure, acute, 163
Hemophilia, 235–238, *236,* 239t
Hemorrhage. See *Bleeding.*
Hemorrhagic telangiectasia, hereditary, and epistaxis, 193
Hemotest, 342
Henoch-Schönlein purpura, 239t
  and abdominal pain, 355
Hepatitis, 364–368, *365, 366*
  and abdominal pain, 355
  and jaundice, 359, 361, *361, 362,* 363
  drug abuse and, 427
  immunization against, 63t–66t, 64–66
Hepatosplenomegaly, with lymphadenopathy, 240, 241t
Hermaphroditism, 261, 263t
Hernia, hiatal, and gastroesophageal reflux, 336
Herniation, of brain, after head trauma, 157
  with increased intracranial pressure, 159, *160*

Heroin abuse, 426t, 427
  maternal, and disorders in infants, 420–423, 421t, 423t
Herpangina, 175, 176
Herpes gladiatorum, 403
Herpes infection, and gingivostomatitis, 173–175
  and hearing loss, 56
  and jaundice, 359–360, 362
  and roseola, 397, 398
  and sore throat, 187
  and vesicular rash, *401,* 401–403
  and whitlow, *401,* 402, 403
  genital, epidemiology of, 284
    sexual abuse and, 414, 414t
  in atopic dermatitis, 395
  in uncircumcised males, 33
  of eye, 202, 203, 205
  of scalp, 386, 388
Heterophoria, 196, 198, *199*
Heterotropia, 196, 198
Hiatal hernia, and gastroesophageal reflux, 336
Hip, disorders of, and limp, 320–324
  dysplasia of, developmental, 296–299, *298, 299*
    with torticollis, 325, 327
  examination of, in newborn, 27
  rotational deformities of, 300–305, 302t, *303, 304*
Hirschsprung's disease, bleeding in, 340, 343
  constipation in, 350–352
  diarrhea in, 346
  encopresis in, 125
Histiocytosis, and diaper dermatitis, 391
  and lymphadenopathy, 241t
Histoplasmosis, and lymphadenopathy, 241t, 242
History, in examination, before athletics, 21–22, 22t
  in screening, of adolescents, 19t, 20
    of children, 20
  prenatal, 26
  taking of, by telephone, 14
HIV infection, 451–455, 452t, 454t
  and lymphadenopathy, 241t, 242, 243
  epidemiology of, 284
Hodgkin's lymphoma, 211, 241t, 241–243, 446, 447t, *450,* 451
Homicide, 437, 438
Homocystinuria, screening for, 17t
Homovanillic acid, in Tourette's syndrome, 377–378
Hordeolum, 202, 204, 205
Horner's syndrome, 446–448
Human immunodeficiency virus infection, 451–455, 452t, 454t
  and lymphadenopathy, 241t, 242, 243
  epidemiology of, 284
Human leukocyte antigens, in diabetes, 462
  in juvenile rheumatoid arthritis, 475, 476
Human papillomavirus infection, genital, 283–284, 286t, 288–289
Humidifiers, for nosebleeds, 194
Hydrocephalus, increased intracranial pressure with, 159
Hydrocortisone, for papulosquamous eruptions, 395
21-Hydroxylase deficiency, in adrenogenital syndrome, 262, 264
Hydroxyzine, for allergy, 220
Hygroma, cystic, *210,* 212, *213,* 215
Hymen, examination of, after sexual abuse, 413–414, *414*
Hyperactivity, with attention deficit, 404–407, 405t, 407t
  and temper tantrums, 109
Hyperammonemia, in hepatic encephalopathy, 367

Hyperbilirubinemia, 357–363, *358, 360–362*
  in anemia, 230, 231, 232t, 233, 234
  in hepatitis, 365
Hypercalciuria, and hematuria, 267, 267t
Hypercholesterolemia, in nephrotic syndrome, 478, 479, 481
Hyperdontia, 172, 174
Hyperexplexia, vs. tics, 378
Hyperglycemia, in diabetes, 464
Hyperkalemia, in renal failure, acute, 165
  chronic, 456, 460, 460t
Hyperlipidemia, in nephrotic syndrome, 478, 479, 481
Hypertension, 256–260, 257t–259t
  in chronic renal failure, 457, 458
Hyperthyroidism, vs. attention deficit/hyperactivity disorder, 405
Hyperventilation, in management of head trauma, 157
Hypnagogic hallucinations, 44
Hypodontia, 172, 174
Hypoglycemia, in diabetes, 464, 465
Hypokalemia, in chronic renal failure, 456
Hypopharynx, in croup, 140, *140*
Hypotension, gastrointestinal bleeding and, 340, 341, 343
Hypothyroidism, and constipation, 350, 352
  in Down syndrome, 69–72, 74t, 75
  screening for, in newborn, 16, 17, 17t
Hypotonia, 369–373, *370,* 370t–372t
Hypovolemic shock, after trauma, 146–147, *147,* 147t
  to abdomen, *151,* 151–152, 152t
  gastrointestinal bleeding and, 340, 341
Hypoxia, in cyanosis, in newborn, 250, *250*

I

Ibuprofen, for dysmenorrhea, 294, 294t
  for headache, 376t
  for orthopedic injury, 319
Icterus (jaundice), 357–363, *358, 360–362*
  in anemia, 230, 231, 233
  in hepatitis, 365
Ignoring, in discipline, 107
Ileus, meconium, in cystic fibrosis, 347
  and jaundice, 360
Imipramine, for enuresis, 122
Immune globulin, for bleeding disorders, 238
  for Kawasaki disease, 399
  in hepatitis prevention, 367–368
Immune system, development of, breast-feeding in, 37
  disorders of, and hemolytic anemia, with lymphadenopathy, 241t
    in diabetes, 462
    in allergy, 216–221, 218t, *219*
    in asthma, 222–223, *223*
Immunization, 62–67, 63t–67t
  active, vs. passive, 63
  against hepatitis, 367–368
  against rubella, and synovitis, with limp, 322
  against varicella, 402
  contraindications to, 65, 65t
  history of, in adolescents, 21
    in older children, 21
  in nephrotic syndrome, 484
  in public health programs, 66–67, 67t
  of preterm infant, 78
  schedule for, 63t, 63–65, 64t
  side effects of, 65
Immunodeficiency, acquired, 451–455, 452t, 454t
  and lymphadenopathy, 241t, 242, 243
  epidemiology of, 284